Fragrance and Wellbeing

by the same author

Essential Oils
A Handbook for Aromatherapy Practice
ISBN 978 1 84819 089 4
eISBN 978 0 85701 072 8

A Sensory Journey
Meditations on Scent for Wellbeing
ISBN 978 1 84819 153 2 (card set)

Fragrance and Wellbeing

Plant Aromatics and Their Influence on the Psyche

JENNIFER PEACE RHIND

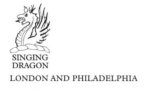

SINGING
DRAGON

LONDON AND PHILADELPHIA

First published in 2014
by Singing Dragon
an imprint of Jessica Kingsley Publishers
73 Collier Street
London N1 9BE, UK
and
400 Market Street, Suite 400
Philadelphia, PA 19106, USA

www.singingdragon.com

Library of Congress Cataloging in Publication Data
Rhind, Jennifer.
  Fragrance and wellbeing : an exploration of plant aromatics and their influences on the psyche / Jennifer Peace Rhind.
     pages cm
  Includes bibliographical references.
  ISBN 978-1-84819-090-0 (alk. paper)
  1. Odors--Psychological aspects. 2. Perfumes--Psychological aspects. 3. Aromatherapy. I. Title. II. Title:
Fragrance and well being.
  RM666.A68R52 2014
  615.3'219--dc23
                              2013011089

British Library Cataloguing in Publication Data
A CIP catalogue record for this book is available from the British Library

ISBN 978 1 84819 090 0
eISBN 978 0 85701 073 5

Printed and bound by Bell & Bain Ltd, Glasgow

For my husband Derek,
our lovely 'little person' Leeloo,
my mother Elizabeth,
and in memory of my father James Mackie

Contents

Preface

It is no secret that I have a love of all things fragrant; perhaps we all do. I know mine started in early childhood. Like many little girls I made rose 'perfume' from flowers in the garden, but that wasn't enough! I also tried out carnation, marigold, flowering currant and southernwood, but with little success. My earliest ambitions were 'to be a lady who worked in a flower shop and/or who made perfume' – none of the nurse or ballerina aspirations, then! My mother's and grandmother's perfumes reflected the times of my childhood – Coty's *Muguet de Bois* and *L'Aimant*, *Chanel No.5*, Bourjois' *Soir de Paris* in its vibrant blue bottle, one (it was particularly pungent) called *Californian Poppy*, and another called *Jasmine* (a favourite), my father's *Old Spice* – and I wore them all! I remember 'eating' soap, biting into a solid block of pipe tobacco, and, when I was older, attempting to inhale the smoke from joss sticks. The memory of the fragrances I wore in adolescence remains vivid; even their names are hugely evocative for me – Yardley's *Sea Jade*, Goya's *Aqua Manda*, and Lentheric's *Tramp*. When I was a student I wore Carven's *Ma Griffe* (a bottle fell out of my bag in a corridor in the old Royal College Building of Strathclyde University; it shattered, and scented the area for quite some time, provoking some interesting reactions), and then Dior's *Diorella*, and Guerlain's *Shalimar*. They all remind me of my sense of 'self' in those days. In fact, I still wear the last two, although the three of us have changed, just a bit, since the 1970s. My internal olfactory landscape is populated by the scents in the natural world that have made their indelible mark on my psyche. Even thinking about them – roses, peonies, sweet peas, carnations, honeysuckle and flowering currant in our various, much-loved family gardens; the exotic blossoms of lemon and frangipani at the Andromeda Gardens in Barbados; the fragrance of sweet clover on the grass behind the sand dunes of Westport beach on the Kintyre peninsula; the seaweed tang on shores of Loch Fyne, and the deep, earthy, resiny scent in ancient pine forests that surround Loch Maree; aromatic wild thyme on the hillsides of the Greek islands; even the scent of cut timber, wood shavings and diesel in my father's garage – brings back breathtaking and fond memories of happy times. I relish the aromas of food and drink too – for me it is unthinkable to cook without savouring the smells of herbs and spices, and exploring how they interact to give ever-changing aroma and taste sensations; I enjoy discerning the different notes in wines and malt whisky, and sensing how different botanicals influence the aroma and flavour of gins. I usually light a joss stick when I sit down to write – not just for its fragrance but also as an acknowledgement to 'the Muses' – I like the ritualistic aspects of fragrance too.

But perhaps best of all is the gentle scent of loved ones, human and canine. I even dream about scent, and have always been aware of its subtle significance in my life.

Since 1987 my professional life has revolved around aroma too, or perhaps I should say it has surrounded me! Initially working with food flavours, and then studying aromatherapy, led me along the essential oil trail and to studies in perfumery. I have worked in aromatherapy and essential oil education since 1993, latterly on the degree programme at Edinburgh Napier University. My focus now is on scent education in the broader sense, because I believe that the benefits of cultivating the sense of smell can be considerable; the process itself is therapeutic, and it leads on to a greater appreciation and enjoyment of scent, whether in the natural world or in the form of aromatic plant extracts or fragrances. Scent makes our experience of the world so very much better... Fragrance allows us to exist 'in the moment', and to be totally free and absorbed in that moment.

There are many excellent books about the sense of smell, aromatherapy, incense, essential oils, perfumery and the fragrance industry, and there is a considerable body of research too, on many aspects of odours, both fair and foul. Here, I have made every attempt to draw together the many disparate strands and compose a work on fragrance that I hope will be of interest to a wide range of readers. If even a few find this inspirational, I know I will have succeeded. It has been challenging to bring together subjects such as biology, neuroscience, behavioural science, psychology, social science, theology, anthropology, ethnobotany, natural product chemistry, psychotherapy, aromatherapy, ancient Greek philosophy, mythology, history, folk traditions, healing practices, essential oils, hallucinogens, fine perfumery, meditation, spirituality and wellbeing. However, in order to do fragrance justice, this was necessary, because fragrance reaches and permeates all of these realms. The biggest challenge has been to write about this in a way that is accessible and understandable to a potentially wide audience. If I have oversimplified or overcomplicated anything, I hope that the reader will understand why – it is simply because of the wide range and nature of the underpinning disciplines, and my educational background is in biology, microbiology, mycology and latterly essential oils. I make no pretence to be an 'expert' in all of these disciplines, and do hope that I have represented the subject-matter fairly.

I have written a book that I would like to read, and this is because fragrance itself has been my guide and messenger. It has been a fascinating journey, and although I did not fully realise this when I started, I would revisit much that has inspired me over the years, such as my fascination with the myths and legends of ancient Greece and Rome (thank you Miss Fisher, my classics teacher), and curiosity about life in ancient times.

There are many people to whom I would like to express my thanks. It is difficult to know where to start, so I will begin by thanking Kareen Hogg and the students at Edinburgh Napier University – the very last cohort – who worked with me on scent meditation and gave me such wonderful feedback. I know that there were times when we perhaps inhaled rather than sniffed, but what a valuable and fun lesson that was! Thanks are also due to my friends, colleagues and managers at Edinburgh Napier, especially Dr Christine Donnelly, and also Derek Baird and Wendy Cairney; thank you for your time, friendship, encouragement and support. The Edinburgh Napier library facilities gave me a wonderful opportunity to conduct a thorough cross-disciplinary literature search. There are also individuals who, in different ways, have had a profound influence on how I have come to think about wellbeing. These are Dr Peter Strigner and Heather Strigner – thank you for your time, care and insight; Linda Downey, my friend and spiritual companion, who, amongst very many other things, reminded me to pause and be mindful when my world was moving too quickly. Thanks to my sister Dr Janice Whittick and Dr Ian Anderson, Gregor and Alison Law, Richard and Karen Marshall – for friendship, fun, for being such good 'sounding boards' and for convivial company, hospitality and excellent food! Thank you, Courtney and Susan Wilding, for your friendship, sage advice, sharing your insights and for such good times in France; and thank you, Arthur and Liz Johnstone, for stimulating conversations, generosity and introducing my palate to some excellent French wines and foods. There is another individual who had a profound influence on the way that I now think and feel about fragrance, and that is the late Alec Lawless. I attended his last course on Artisan Perfumery, exactly a year ago as I write these words, and this showed me how the process of composing and creating a fragrance can be, in itself, therapeutic. He was a truly inspiring individual, with an infectious enthusiasm for his subject and indeed life – and yes, the course was hugely informative and fun too. I would like to thank Alec's colleague, the journalist Lila Das Gupta, for her constructive review of my first attempts at composing natural fragrances, her encouragement, and her friendship through the sad time that followed. Thanks also to Carlotta Zorzi of Scent Sciences, for her boundless energy and enthusiasm, and for promoting my work via the Scent Sciences blog.

Special thanks are due to Jeannie Fatimeh Graham, practitioner of Unani Tibb medicine at the Pomegranate Garden, Edinburgh, who contributed Chapter 12 on attars. This specialist area absolutely epitomises 'fragrance and wellbeing', and I am delighted to be able to include it here.

As always, thanks are due to Jessica Kingsley, Jane Evans, Victoria Peters and Alex Fleming at Singing Dragon, for their ongoing support of my work, and for their patience as this book emerged from a scented haze and then just kept on evolving, and to Anne Oppenheimer the copyeditor, whose input is, as always, greatly valued.

Finally, thanks to my husband, Derek, for absolutely everything: love, companionship, support, encouragement, sense of humour and patience throughout; and to our furry companion – Leeloo the Tibetan terrier – who, with her beautiful, gentle spirit, quirkiness and sense of fun (and gorgeous scent), makes our family complete.

Introduction

When exploring fragrance and wellbeing, the only place to start is with the sense of smell; understanding this is crucial if we are to follow the scent trail. Chapter 1 gives an overview of our olfactory sense: how we detect odours, and their biological significance. Some important concepts are presented in this chapter, and their full significance will become apparent in the concluding chapters. Chapter 2 leads us into a discussion about the many ways in which odours influence us, and how this can happen. Here, we will use some examples from research in neuroscience, psychology and the behavioural and social sciences to illustrate the effects of odours on cognition, moods and behaviours. The concept of wellbeing is also introduced in this chapter, and thus the two themes of this book, fragrance and wellbeing, are established.

It has been said that fragrance is a shadow or mirror of societies, and that our history can be told from its perspective. Chapter 3 is an exploration of scented smokes, while Chapter 4 looks at the evolution of perfumery. David Williams, the late and much respected perfumery educator, did say that 'a historical survey can always be bettered' (Williams 1995a, p.16), and so to tackle a survey, one has to start with what others have already written. Therefore, a variety of sources have informed these chapters. The works of Morris (1984), Corbin (1996), Classen, Howes and Synnott (1994), Goody (1993), Lawless (1994), Manniche (1999) and Stamelman (2006) are excellent resources, and have been consulted on a regular basis. More recent texts such as those by DuBois (2009), Jay (2010), Kaiser (2006) and Pennacchio, Jefferson and Havens (2010) have been invaluable, and are also destined to become 'classics'. Some insightful papers, such as those of Craffert (2011), Moeran (2007, 2009), Dannaway (2010) and Tonutti and Liddle (2010), have also been invaluable and are cited, especially where the historical account is not simply about fragrance but also about how it has influenced and reflected human culture.

The use of fragrance is a global human phenomenon. In Chapter 5 we explore the different philosophies that can explain why we use scent, and how our preferences are formed. We return to some of the ideas presented in Chapters 1 and 2, and progress these towards a fuller understanding of our relationship with fragrance.

Chapter 6 is an introduction to the 'language' of scent, and so here, along with the guide to fragrance classification in Appendix 1, the reader who is unfamiliar with the words used to describe odours can quickly learn to negotiate this aspect of the fragrance world.

In Chapters 7 to 11 we explore many of the aromatic plants and their scents that have been enjoyed and exploited since early times. These chapters are led by fragrance; the discussions follow the different scent types, from the deep, woody base notes, resins and lighter coniferous notes in Chapter 7, to the pungent spicy notes in Chapter 8, the herbaceous, green, cineolic smells and the world of agrestic fragrances, the scents that recall the natural world, in Chapter 9, the outstandingly beautiful floral odours that dominate perfumery in Chapter 10, and the sparkling citrus, lemony and fruity aromas in Chapter 11. Fragrance can be quite 'elusive'; it is tangible but temporary, and a simple profile-by-profile account of the aromatic plants and their products is simply not fitting – they cannot be pinned down or tackled in a formulaic manner. So this discussion is guided by their messages and stories, which reflect their unique natures, and thus gives us a real sense of what they mean to us. For this reason, Chapters 7 to 11 are more of a narrative than a reference section or guide, and many different sources have been consulted to let the fragrances 'talk' to us and tell their own tales.

Where appropriate, myth has been used as a metaphor to illustrate the characteristics and 'personality' or 'signature' of some aromatic plants and their fragrances. In Jung's *The Structure and Dynamics of the Psyche*, it was suggested that mythology could be a type of projection of the 'collective unconscious',[1] and the characters in myth are archetypes which represent human behaviour. Hunt (2012) revisited Jung's concepts of archetypes and the collective unconscious in terms of contemporary psychology, finding that they are indeed close 'in spirit to a socio-cultural collective unconscious based on metaphoric imagination' (p.76), and thus validating his key observations. For this reason, mythology can give us a glimpse of the way the world was perceived by our ancestors, and so if we view aromatic plants through their lens, we gain a different perspective, and perhaps a deeper understanding of the early uses of some species. Apart from symbolic significance, these fragrances have been used to enhance health and beauty, and as medicines. Many scents are deeply integrated within our sensorial and sensual experiences, and thus give some fascinating insights into traditional practices across the globe. Some of them have played unseen but important roles in societies, from differentiating gender and culture, to policy making and communicating with the divine. Fragrances span therapeutic, personal, social, cultural and spiritual realms. In recent times many have also been investigated in terms of their chemistry and biological actions. Therefore, in order to give the broadest perspective, and to present hitherto scattered insights in one place, a wide range of sources inform these chapters.

---

1   The collective unconscious is part of the unconscious mind, which is expressed in humanity and all life forms; a part of the psyche that autonomously organises experience, and consists of pre-existent forms (archetypes) that represent all knowledge and experience.

Grieve's *A Modern Herbal* (1992 [1931])[2] and Gordon's *A Country Herbal* (1980) have been useful sources regarding traditional beliefs and uses, and Graves' *The Greek Myths* (1992) has been used to elaborate when required. Weiss' *Essential Oil Crops* (1997) has been used to inform most aspects in relation to the botanical and geographical origins of aromatic plants, and the extraction of their volatile oils, and Kaiser's *Meaningful Scents around the World* (2006) gives valuable insight into some of the most important cultural fragrances and some rare ones, but when experienced *au naturel*. The literature search also revealed a rich seam of information, from chemical analysis of some rare and exotic fragrances and studies on the biological actions of some well-known essential oils, to some ground-breaking anthropological analyses. It was never the intention to present a critique of these studies; the methodology has not been described in many instances, and the research design has been neither applauded nor criticised. The research presented herein is all considered to be of high quality and worthy of inclusion.

Naturally, the aromatic plants also command our attention within the art of perfumery. For this, four sources in particular have been invaluable. First, the enormous contributions of David Williams (1995a–d; 1996; 2000); second, Calkin and Jellinek's *Perfumery: Practice and Principles* (1994); third, the *Haarmann and Reimer Fragrance Guide* (Glöss 1995), which lists the primary and secondary fragrance 'notes'[3] in commercial and mainstream perfumes; and last, but not least, Turin and Sanchez's *Perfumes: The A–Z Guide* (2009). This last source is not 'academic', but is written by two very knowledgeable individuals who are also willing and able to critique mainstream and niche perfumes. So although this could be described as an opinionated and subjective work, it is also accessible and considered to be reliable, and appropriate in the context of these chapters. Readers are free, of course, to form their own opinions!

Chapter 12 has been contributed by Jeannie Fatimeh Graham, and places attars within an historical context. It outlines their earliest uses in the Middle East and their subsequent role in Unani Tibb medicine, used either alone or alongside herbal and other therapeutic treatments. This chapter includes a brief review of how Unani Tibb works in rebalancing the individual, with respect to *mizaj* (temperaments), *akhlat* (humours) and their relations to *arkan* (temperaments). We then look more deeply into the effects attars have on the physical, mental, emotional and spiritual aspects of the individual, and the specific ways in which they are used in these realms, including the spiritual realm of the sufis.

---

2   In 1931 *A Modern Herbal* was published, the first encyclopaedia of herbs since Culpeper in 1649. It has been revised and republished, but still retains the writings of the older herbalists such as Dioscorides, Gerard, Parkinson and Culpeper, and traditional plant lore. *A Modern Herbal* is considered to be indispensable for those interested in the history of herbs.

3   A perfume 'note' refers to the structure of a perfume in terms of the relative volatility of the component materials, so we have top, middle and base notes that emerge as the perfume evaporates. However, the term has also come to mean a distinctive odour within a fragrance which can be recognised and identified.

Finally, in Chapter 13, by exploring the cultivation of the sense of smell, the development of an olfactory memory, reflective awareness, meditative trance and noetic insight, we emerge with a deeper awareness of our scented world. Two outstanding papers deserve mention here, those of Glicksohn and Berkovich Ohana (2011) and Hewitt (2011), which, although not directly concerned with the sense of smell or scent, have provided us with new insights regarding the possible effects of fragrance. In Chapter 13 we also consider how we can cultivate our sense of smell, and reap the considerable benefits of doing so. A guide to this process is provided in Appendix D.

A comprehensive glossary is included at the end of the book, with terminology pertaining to a wide range of disciplines, to help the reader when perhaps less familiar territory is encountered.

PART I

Scent

A Pan-Dimensional Perspective

CHAPTER 1

The Fallen Angel

Ackerman (1990) wrote that:

> Smells spur memories, but they also rouse our dozy senses, pamper and indulge us, help define our self image, stir the cauldron of our seductiveness, warn us of danger, lead us into temptation, fan our religious fervour, accompany us to heaven, wed us to fashion, steep us in luxury. Yet, over time, smell has become the least necessary of our senses, 'the fallen angel' as Helen Keller dramatically calls it. (p.x)

Despite this viewpoint on the diminishing importance of our olfactory sense, it is well recognised that, historically, the use of aromatic substances to elicit particular responses via the sense of smell was integral to many cultures and life practices. These uses include sacred and ritualistic practices, such as anointing with fragrant oils and offering rites to gods; embalming and medicinal practices; as cosmetics, fumigants and mood-altering substances; as spiritual and philosophical healing systems; and for ritual stimulation of dreams and visions (Classen *et al.* 1994; Lawless 1994).

In order to even begin to understand how odours can affect us, first we need to take a very brief look at what is understood about our sense of smell. The olfactory system is our 'receptor' system, and is thus the direct interface for our connection with the world of smells.

The sense of smell

For any substance to have an odour, it must be able to exist in the form of a vapour – where its molecules are light enough to evaporate into the atmosphere, where they can reach the nose or mouth. The part that detects the smell is known as the *olfactory organ*, and consists of very thin, twin membranes which are located on each side of the bony part of the nasal septum. It is thought that the olfactory organ contains in the region of 800 million nerve endings, known as *olfactory hairs*. These are connected with the secondary neurons of the adjacent structure, called the *olfactory bulb*, which extends to form the *olfactory nerve* (Williams 2000). Via the olfactory nerve tract, an olfactory signal is transmitted to the brain. Neurons from the olfactory tract project to several parts of the brain that constitute the *limbic system* (*limbus* means 'border'). The limbic system is situated in the temporal lobes of the brain; it is a diffuse region associated with emotional response, memories, motivation and pleasure – and where there is no conscious control. It comprises a loop of structures surrounding parts of the brain known as the *corpus callosum* and the *thalamus*. It was, in the past, known as the *rhinencephalon* – the primitive 'smell brain', or olfactory centre. Therefore, the limbic system is the central control over the expression of emotions, instinctive behaviours, drives, motivations and feelings, and it is frequently guided, at least in part, by the sense of smell. In addition, the neurons from the olfactory tract also project to the thalamus, where sensory integration occurs, and to the *frontal cortex*, where recognition of the odour occurs.

There are many connections between these two systems; and so there are two interrelated responses to olfactory signals – the cognitive, interpretative aspects at the frontal cortex, and the emotional response at the limbic system. A smell can trigger emotional and physical reactions, even without our conscious awareness of it. Olfactory signals, unlike other sensory inputs, do not always have to pass through the thalamus to reach the cerebral cortex.

The process of olfaction – theories and mysteries

Although much about the anatomy of olfaction is clear, there are many aspects of the actual process of olfaction that remain unknown. We do not yet know how an odour molecule binds to the olfactory receptor cells, or how olfactory signals are generated. We do not know how odour is interpreted by the brain, and we cannot yet fully explain olfactory sensitivity. There are several hypotheses that attempt to elucidate such aspects of olfaction. The prevalent theories have revolved around what has become known as the 'Steoric Theory of Odour' first proposed by Moncrieff in 1949, and elaborated upon by Amoore in 1963 (see Leffingwell 1999). This is more commonly described as the 'lock and key' theory: the surface of each olfactory nerve ending has receptor sites, which are specific to odour molecules of a particular size and configuration. When an odour molecule is trapped by and then penetrates the layer of mucus, it can fit into the receptor site; this stimulates the nerve, which then forms an olfactory signal. The signal gives rise to the sensation and interpretation of a specific odour.

The steoric theory goes some way towards explaining why we can detect an infinite number of different odours at even very low concentrations, because of the very large number of chemical odorants (humans can detect more than 10,000 smell molecules) and the huge number of receptor sites. The steoric theory may partly explain why molecular isomers (molecules that have the same chemical formula but differences in the way their component atoms are arranged) will have different odours. In 1999 Buck and Malnic of Harvard Medical School with Hirono and Sato of the Life Electronics Centre, Amagasaki, Japan, demonstrated that single receptors can recognise multiple odorants, that a single odorant is typically recognised by multiple receptors, and that different odorants are recognised by different combinations of receptors (Malnic *et al.* 1999). They proposed that the olfactory system used a combinatorial coding scheme to encode the identities of odours. This explains why a thousand receptors can describe many thousands of odours (Leffingwell 1999).

So, instead of the traditional steoric theory that one type of odour receptor is dedicated to a specific odour, the combinatorial diversity theory proposes that the olfactory system uses *combinations* of receptors, analogous to musical chords or computer processing, to reduce greatly the number of actual receptor types that are required to detect a vast number of odorants.

> Each receptor is used over and over again to define an odour, just like letters are used over and over again to define different words. (Buck, cited in Howard Hughes Medical Institute 2004)

Malnic *et al.* (1999) demonstrated that even slight changes in chemical structure activate different combinations of receptors, and that a large concentration of an odorant binds to a wider variety of receptors than smaller amounts of the same odorant (Leffingwell 1999). In 2004 Axel and Buck were awarded the Nobel Prize in Physiology and Medicine for their discovery of 'odorant receptors and the organisation of the olfactory system' (Miller 2004).

However, in 1996, Luca Turin, then a biophysicist at University College, London, had proposed his Vibrational Induced Electron Tunnelling Spectroscope Theory. Turin claimed that central to the process of olfaction was the frequency at which the bonds of an odorant molecule vibrate. He proposed that olfactory receptors are tuned to the vibrational frequency of odorants. When an odorant binds to the receptor protein, electron 'tunnelling' occurs across the binding site if the vibrational mode is equal to the energy gap between filled and empty electron tunnels (Turin 1996). Turin (2006) maintains that we still do not really understand these 'lock and key' mechanisms, and points out that 'something has to turn the key' (p.193).

Olfactory significance – the biological perspective

So, what is the biological significance of our sense of smell – a chemical sense that, unlike our other senses, is 'hardwired' to both the conscious and unconscious parts of our brain? It is recognised that in other species, in the wild, the sense of smell is used to find food, to sense threat from predators, to find and attract mates and to communicate within and between species. However, in humans, the sense of smell is not used consciously for such fundamental activities. We do use our sense of smell when we are curious, or checking if food is fresh and edible, or sensing danger, such as smoke, burning or noxious fumes (Williams 1995a). Stevenson (2010) suggested that there are three classes of olfactory function in humans, namely ingestive behaviour, avoidance of environmental hazards and social communication.

Throughout the following chapters, we will explore the other facets of our olfactory sense, such as the pleasure it brings, its therapeutic potential and its relationship to memory and altered states of consciousness. However, first we will focus on the biological aspects of olfaction, as identified by Stevenson (2010).

Ingestive behaviour

The sense of smell can assist in locating food and assessing whether or not it is suitable for consumption (which can be dependent on prior experience); the volatile flavour compounds released when food is placed in the mouth and chewed will also give a sense of whether it is safe to consume. Smell and flavour combined can both stimulate and repress appetite.

Avoidance of environmental hazards

Stevenson (2010) observed that there are two fundamental types of hazards characterised by volatiles – microbial and non-microbial – which evoke the emotions of disgust and fear. For example, faeces, vomit, urine, decay of organic matter and cadavers are sources of pathogens and are thus microbial hazards (Curtis and Biran 2001). These odours invariably provoke a sense of disgust and avoidance behaviour, although this is more obvious in adults than in children aged two to three years, reflecting an element of learned behaviour (Stevenson *et al.* 2010). In many other animal species we do not see expressions of disgust, but avoidance behaviour can be observed, such as in sheep avoiding contaminated grazing pasture; many animals such as domestic dogs and cats will not defecate or urinate in their sleeping places, and omnivorous and carnivorous species will not eat their dead conspecifics (companions) (Stevenson 2010).

Non-microbial hazards, however, generally provoke sensations of fear rather than disgust. These hazards are not usually related to food, but rather to some environmental volatiles. For example, chlorine, mustard and phosgene gases were used in the World Wars I and II. These gases have odours that can become associated with (i.e. learned behaviour) impending danger in war zones – chlorine is distinctive and very recognisable, phosgene is hay-like, and mustard gas has an odour that is reminiscent of geranium (Stevenson 2010). The smell of burning, smoke and domestic gas will also provoke fear and avoidance behaviour.

Subtle communication

It is very possible that humans communicate by means of biological odours, although Stoddart (1988) suggested that man may have repressed this ability for a variety of ecological and behavioural reasons. However, human olfactory communication can be witnessed from the moment we are born – babies bond with their mothers through the sense of smell, which is fully functional at birth. This capacity for neonates to learn their mother's odour 'signature' has been demonstrated on several occasions (Cernoch and Porter 1985; Schleidt and Genzel 1990; Schaal, Marlier and Soussignan 1998, cited in Stevenson 2010). As we grow and gain life experiences, we will also start to identify the 'odour signatures' of individuals (Porter et al. 1986; Weisfeld et al. 2003; Olsson, Barnard and Turri 2006, cited in Stevenson 2009a), which in turn carry different sets of associations. Therefore, from birth and throughout life, we recognise olfactory cues and establish odour associations, and thus odour and emotional memory become inextricably linked (Engen 1988).

Chen and Haviland-Jones (2000) investigated the potential for human communication of emotional states via body odour, by asking participants to identify whether the underarm odours collected on gauze pads and then presented in bottles were from 'happy' donors (who had watched an excerpt from a funny movie) or 'afraid' donors (who had watched a frightening movie). This study revealed that women chose the correct bottles significantly more often than by chance, and that there are gender differences too. Men seem to be more sensitive to 'happy' female odours than the male counterparts, and both women and men are able to detect fear in male odour more readily than in female odour. They concluded that there is indeed olfactory information in human body odour that is indicative of emotional states, and that this adds further complexity to the way humans interact. This study also highlighted that there were differences in the way males and females responded. This was witnessed again in research conducted by Wysocki et al. (2008) who suggested that responses to stress-related odours were gender-specific.

It was, and still is, believed by some that olfaction plays a role in sexual attraction, partly because of the presence of chemicals known as *pheromones*. These biological chemicals are a means of communication between insects and animals of the same species, which elicit predictable social, behavioural and neuroendocrine responses. For some time it was thought that they might stimulate an accessory part of our olfactory apparatus known as the *vomeronasal organ*, or VNO – originally called Jacobson's organ (Jacob 1999). This is located at the base of the septum, or the roof of the mouth, in mammals and also amphibians and reptiles. However, there is controversy over whether adult humans actually have a VNO, although endoscopic and microscopic evidence would suggest that most of us have an organ on at least one side of the nasal septum – a blind-ending diverticulum in the septal mucosa, opening around two centimetres from the nostril (Meredith 2001). It was suggested that in mammals the VNO functioned to detect pheromones, and therefore was involved in reproductive and social behaviours, such as identifying and attracting a mate. In 1994 one group of researchers had described the vomeronasal system as the 'long-neglected sixth sense' (Jennings-White, Dolberg and Berliner 1994). At that time, researchers suspected that it was responsible for spontaneous feelings between people such as 'love at first sight' or 'getting bad vibes'. Messages from the VNO were believed to bypass consciousness, so resulting in an inexplicable impression, rather than a distinct perception of an odour.

Human pheromones do have a scent, although they are not particularly volatile (that is, they do not evaporate quickly, and it takes some time before they enter the vapour state necessary for detection by the nose). We all produce them, all of the time, and they are found on the skin – especially in the proximity of the exocrine glands in the axillae and groin. Our pheromones were thought to elicit physiological and behavioural effects mediated by the VNO, even at subliminal levels. However, recent studies indicate that perhaps this is not the function of the VNO after all. In 2001 Meredith published a critical review of the VNO, commenting that at best the VNO had a minor role in human olfactory communication, and at worst it was not functional at all. However, early evidence produced using the electrovomeronasogram (EVG) had supported the notion that there was a sensitive and selective response to human-derived scents in the region of the VNO (Monti-Bloch and Grosser 1991, cited in Meredith 2001), so it may well have some degree of chemosensitivity. Meredith therefore concluded that although it was likely that the main olfactory system was responsible for human olfactory communication, the positive evidence from the EVG merited further investigation before the notion was discarded.

Prehn-Kristensen *et al.* (2009) investigated how the smell of sweat caused by anxiety could induce feelings of empathy. The chemosensory stimuli used in the study were judged to be of low intensity, and in fact only around half of the participants even recognised the presence of an odour. However, it was found that the anxiety-sweat samples activated the same brain areas that are involved in the processing of social anxiety signals, and this also happens during odour perception. The anxiety-sweat also activated brain areas that are implicated in feelings of empathy for others. It was concluded that conscious mediation is not involved in our responses to such chemosensory signals, and that 'smelling the feelings of others could be termed as an incorporation of the chemical expressions and thus the feelings of others' (Prehn-Kristensen *et al.* 2009, p.8).

The idea of the VNO and pheromones has also been discarded in a recent series of experiments by Frasnelli *et al.* (2011). They explored the possibility that the VNO was responsible for processing social chemosensory signals, as there had been much speculation, but little evidence, to support this hypothesis. None of their experiments supported the role of the VNO; it was suggested that chemosensory signals in humans are processed via the main olfactory system.

Immune system connections

As early as 1995, Kirk-Smith suggested that, in the light of evidence that olfactory 'conditioning' (along the lines of classical 'Pavlovian' conditioning, where odours act as cues that evoke associated learning) can stimulate the immune system, there may be a link between our olfactory and immune systems, and that this could be important for species survival. Hosoi and Tsuchiya (2000) subsequently demonstrated that olfactory stimuli could regulate cutaneous allergic reactions. Then, exploring the hypothesis that odours which provoked disgust could help prepare the immune system for microbial attack (Stevenson 2010), Reither *et al.* (2008) showed that olfactory conditioning could, via the central nervous system, either stimulate or supress peripheral immune responses such as allergic reactions. If such effects, which are all mediated by associative learning, are considered in tandem with the apparent olfactory cues that perhaps prevent inbreeding in animal species, and indicate attraction between prospective mates (Stevenson 2010), we can begin to see the profound implications of the intricate connections between olfaction, immunity and reproduction.

It is well established that inbreeding can cause serious birth defects and compromised immune function in offspring, and, in humans, incest is a taboo. Outbreeding is naturally preferable – and optimal outbreeding involves the selection of a mate that is genetically different, but not too different (Bateson 1983, cited in Stevenson 2010). The *major histocompatibility complex* (MHC) is a set of genes that is important in immune function; it is indicative of genetic relatedness but also influences the available selection of antigens, and hence potential protection against infection. In mice and rats, MHC genotypes can be detected by volatile compounds in the urine; so mice and rats may learn to recognise not only their own olfactory signatures but also those of close relatives, and olfaction might have a role in the prevention of inbreeding. Humans also have their own distinct odour signatures, including the smell of volatile organic acids in the sweat and urine (Zavazava, Westphal and Muller-Ruchholtz 1990), which will be partially conferred by their MHC, notably the *human leucocyte antigens* (HLA). Stevenson (2010) cites studies that have shown that if there is a high degree of similarity in partners' HLA, there is a higher risk of miscarriage or low birth weight. Additionally, McClintock *et al.* (2005) had noted that matching MHC alleles in human odours affected emotional, as opposed to cognitive, processing, and increased the perceived pleasantness of the odour.

For centuries it has been recognised that there is a link between scent and sex. Several studies have shown that smell is the overriding most significant factor for females regarding male sexual attractiveness (Franzoi and Herzog 1987; Herz and Cahill 1997; Herz and Inzlicht 2002, cited in Stevenson 2010). In 2001, Milinski and Wedekind explored the link between perfume preferences and the MHC. It had already been demonstrated that mice and humans prefer the body odour of partners who have a dissimilar MHC genotype; in an earlier study women preferred the smell of T-shirts worn by men whose MHC genes were dissimilar to their own (Wedekind *et al.* 1995). Again, this could potentially produce heterozygous offspring and contribute to genetic diversity. Their study supported the hypothesis that perfumes that are self-selected for personal use might in some way amplify body odours that resonate with the individual's immunogenetics. We will return to this idea in Chapter 5.

Sensitivity to odour

The degree of sensitivity to odours varies among individuals. The neurobiologist Andreas Keller maintains that 'everybody's olfactory world is a unique private world' because of the immense variation in the ways that individuals report their responses to smells (Spinney 2011). Keller suggests that we perceive smells differently because of the variability of our odorant receptor genes – we all have different and unique sets of receptors. However, he also acknowledges the part that culture and environment play in this. It is also possible that, over time, the genes that encoded our olfactory receptors began to mutate as our sense of smell became less important than that of sight, and eventually became *pseudogenes* – ones which no longer encode a functioning receptor. Therefore, if we all have different combinations of these pseudogenes, we have what the geneticist Doron Lancet likened to a 'barcode' situation (Spinney 2011).

It has also been noted that we all have olfactory 'blind spots'; that is, there is at least one smell to which we are insensitive (Spinney 2011). In perfumery, this is described as *partial* or *specific anosmia* – the inability to perceive a particular odour. This is often associated with synthetic musks in perfumery, and sandalwood constituents; also with some perfumery materials such as ambergris and methyl ionone (Williams 1995b). The artisan perfumer Alec Lawless commented that if we all have these blind spots, then we should also have particular sensitivities. For example, he has observed that many people can detect even tiny amounts of cumin in a fragrance, very often provoking an adverse reaction. Cumin can impart a note that is, for some, reminiscent of an unwashed body odour, therefore perceived as an unpleasant 'dirty' note. Others, however, do not find this note objectionable. Lawless also disputes the idea that we all have a unique olfactory palate. Drawing on his experience as a sommelier, he commented that the aroma of wine made with grapes infected by *Botrytis cinerea* (a fungus that concentrates sugar in the grapes) has a strong Seville orange note; some people cannot detect this, but they do pick up on notes of wet wool, or lanolin, while others can detect both notes. So, he reasons, this is not a unique private sensation, but one experienced by two or three groups (Lawless 2011).

Olfactory abnormalities

Individuals can also have pronounced olfactory abnormalities, which can cause a very different perception and experience of the world. The loss of the sense of smell is known as *anosmia*. Most of us will have experienced a temporary or partial form of this (*hyposmia*) caused by, for example, an upper respiratory tract infection, and it is probable that it is more noticeable in terms of the loss of the sense of taste rather than smell. Hummel and Nordin (2011) noted that it is estimated that complete loss of the sense of smell is found in at least 1 per cent of the US population, and that up to 24 per cent of adults aged 53–97 have impaired olfactory function.

Stevenson (2010) cites the American Medical Association's (AMA 1993) assertion that anosmia constitutes a small 3 per cent impairment of the 'whole person', compared with 35 per cent for hearing loss and 85 per cent for loss of sight. However, it is well known that permanent anosmia can have a much greater impact than these figures would suggest. Sacks (1986) described the distress of a man whose olfactory tract was damaged because of a head injury:

> 'Sense of smell?' he says, 'I never gave it a thought. You don't normally give it a thought. But when I lost it – it was like being struck blind. Life lost a good deal of its savour – one doesn't realise how much "savour" is smell. You smell people, you smell books, you smell the city, you smell the spring – maybe not consciously, but as a rich unconscious background to everything else. My whole world was suddenly radically poorer...' (p.152)

Rachel Hertz is a psychologist who has observed a type of emotional shutdown that follows the loss of the sense of smell. She notes that initially there is a sense that the loss will have little impact, but over time it is devastating – sensual experiences are hugely diminished, and there is a 'general, progressive blunting of their emotional lives' (Hertz 2000, p.38). The journalist Gabrielle Glaser has an acute sense of smell; she has experienced periods of hyperosmia (see below), but experienced a spell of temporary but complete anosmia following surgery on her sinuses. She claimed that words could not describe this loss, even although she had interviewed other anosmics and clearly empathised with their experiences. Glaser relates that anosmia affected her emotional responses to most daily activities, but perhaps the most dramatic moment was her inability to smell leaking gas – 'Finally I went outdoors. I couldn't smell my kids, I couldn't smell myself, I couldn't even detect danger. I just stood and sobbed in the snow' (Glaser 2002, p.245).

Over the years there have been a few studies that attempted to actually quantify the effects of the loss of this sense, such as Van Toller's 1999 survey/review, investigations by Santos *et al.* (2004) and Bonfils *et al.* (2008) of potential dangers associated with smell impairment, such as failure to detect gas leaks and smoke, and the Aschenbrenner *et al.* (2007) study of the influence of anosmia on eating habits (cited in Stevenson 2010). Less obvious and indirect effects of anosmia, such as the deleterious effects on mood, the increased propensity for depression and even the effects on immune and reproductive functions, have not been quantified.

Congenital anosmia is not common; however, if the sense has been missing since birth, it is much less likely to cause stress and depression than anosmia resulting from injury. *Parosmia* is more common, and often occurs in anosmics. This term relates to the illusion or hallucination of a smell – usually a bad odour such as drains or faeces (Douek 1988). We can also all experience *olfactory fatigue*, the temporary loss of the ability to perceive a particular odour after a short period of overexposure. For example, we may use a liberal amount of perfume which is noticeable on application, but imperceptible after a short while, and we are only reminded of the scent when someone else makes a comment! At the other extreme, *hyperosmia* is enhanced olfactory capability. Again, Sacks (1986) describes a hallucinogenic drug-induced case of hyperosmia that persisted for three weeks, where the sense of smell was so heightened that the male subject reported, '…and now I awoke to an infinitely redolent world – a world in which all other sensations, enhanced as they were, paled before smell' (p.149). When he returned to his previous level of olfactory sensitivity, he reported feeling a sense of loss.

Odour versus fragrance

So far, we have looked at our sense of smell, encompassing all types of odours, from those regarded as foul and disgusting to the interesting and the pleasing. However, beauty is in the nose of the beholder. We must always be cognisant of the fact that very personal judgements and preferences exist; however, we will be considering the pleasing end of this spectrum, at least according to the general consensus, and we will use the term 'fragrant' to denote this. The next chapter will look at the many ways in which odours impact on us.

CHAPTER 2

Smell and the Psyche

In this chapter we will look at concepts of the psyche and wellbeing, and examine the ways in which odour can influence our perceptions and experiences. This will include an exploration of the impact of natural, plant-derived fragrances and aromatic mood stabilisers, enhancers and modifiers. To do this we will draw on research from various disciplines, including the biological and social sciences, and on observations from aromatherapy practice.

Concepts of the psyche

The Greek word *psyche* means the 'soul', the 'spirit' and the 'self'. Aristotle, the Greek philosopher, proposed that there were three psyches – the vegetal soul, the animal soul and the rational soul. His works were developed by Galen (see footnote 1 on p.46), who then proposed that there were three spirits or *pneumae*. Much later Freud and Jung, the pioneers of analytical and depth psychology, also focused on the concept that there are forces which influence ways of being, thinking and behaving, and that these forces shape the personality. Freud suggested that there were indeed three parts that comprised the psyche, namely the *id*, the *ego* and the *superego*. The id described the unconscious drives and instincts, the ego the conscious part of the individual that deals with reality, and the superego the conscience, the part that 'civilises' us, our sense of morality, ethics, right and wrong, and so influences our ways of behaving. However, Jung maintained that the psyche was a comprehensive, overarching term that related to all aspects of being. He also suggested that the soul, in terms of psychology, was a part of the personality, rather than the spiritual aspect of being. Jung also introduced two further terms – *anima* and *animus*, pertaining to the female and male aspects of the personality respectively.

Eastern philosophies also embrace the idea of the energy and the psyche in their healing traditions. For example, in Chinese 'five element theory' there are five phases/cycles of *Yin* and *Yang* energy (*Qi*) that are representative of the natural forces within us and our environment – and these are named Water, Wood, Fire, Earth and Metal. There are also five aspects of the psyche. These are *Shen* (the Mind, associated with Fire), *Yi* (the Intellect, associated with Earth), *P'o* (the Bodily Soul, associated with Metal), *Zhi* (the Will, associated with Water) and the *Hun* (the Ethereal Soul, associated with Wood) (Hicks, Hicks and Mole 2011). Along similar lines, the ancient Sanskrit texts, the Vedas, tell us that humans are spiritual beings in physical form – we are fields of energy manifesting as matter. Ayurvedic medicine is derived from the Vedas, and is based on the perspective that humans can live healthily in body, spirit and mind through an understanding of their own nature and their interactions with the world. The spirit or soul is on a journey of enlightenment to reunite with pure consciousness. In that journey, the human spirit manifests as matter on the planet, to learn the great spiritual lessons that it has forgotten, such as love and compassion, in order to bring about the uniting or yoking (*yoga*) with the unknown (Svoboda 2003).

So, when we come to explore the effects of fragrance on our emotions, moods, thought processes, ways of behaving, social patterns, interactions with nature and the environment, and spirit, it is perhaps more useful to think in terms of the psyche, rather than 'the mind' or 'the emotions' or 'the spirits', as it could be said that odours can influence every level of being.

Odour and the psyche

It has long been noted that, via the sense of smell and the limbic system, odours can act directly on the psyche, and that different odours can enhance, modify or stabilise cognitive and emotional states. Aromatherapy is the only contemporary therapeutic modality that has developed around this observation, and in practice the different odour characteristics of plant essential oils and absolutes are used to impart positive mood benefits. This aspect of aromatherapy is often termed 'psycho-aromatherapy', to differentiate between this and the wider health-enhancing effects of essential oils.

Psycho-aromatherapy and aroma-chology

In 1923, well before aromatherapy had become established as a discipline that used essential oils in a specifically therapeutic manner, Giovanni Gatti and Renato Cajola published a comprehensive review of the effects of essential oils on the nervous system, and their influences on moods and emotions (cited in Tisserand 1988). They had investigated the states of anxiety and depression, and identified specific oils for use as sedatives, which counteract anxiety, and stimulants, which counteract depression. They also documented, for the first time, the phenomenon that initial, light exposure to an aroma, which resulted in stimulation, sometimes led to a state of sedation if exposure was prolonged or repeated. Later, in 1973, Professor Paolo Rovesti of the University of Milan identified that specific essential oils could be used to alleviate depression and anxiety, but he also noted that essential oil combinations were often deemed more pleasant than single oil odours (cited in Tisserand 1988). This has underpinned the aromatherapy practice of prescribing individual 'synergistic' essential oil combinations, which aims to address an individual's particular circumstances and needs, developed by Marguerite Maury, one of the early proponents of the discipline.

However, the emergence of aroma-chology is more recent. In 1982, Annette Green of the Fragrance Foundation introduced aroma-chology as a science that is:

> ...dedicated to the study of the interrelationship between psychology and fragrance technology to elicit a variety of specific feelings and emotions – relaxation, exhilaration, sensuality, happiness and well-being through odours via stimulation of olfactory pathways in the brain, especially the limbic system. (Fragrance Research Fund 1992, cited in Jellinek 1997a, p.25)

Despite some similarities with aromatherapy, aroma-chology is only concerned with the *temporary* effects of natural and synthetic fragrances, not their therapeutic potential (Jellinek 1997a). There have since been numerous studies which investigated the effects of essential oils on human and animal behaviour, mood and cognition, many of which support the belief that essential oils can be used as olfactory therapeutic agents. Some of these studies have been concerned with the effects of the odours, while a few explore the ways in which these odours might be producing their effects. In his influential paper 'Psychodynamic odor effects and their mechanisms' (Jellinek 1997a), the perfumer Stephan Jellinek suggested that there are four ways in which smells can exert their effects on our states of mind. He named these the *quasi-pharmacological, semantic, hedonic valence* and *placebo* mechanisms. By exploring the considerable body of research into the myriad effects of odour, we can find examples of these mechanisms at work.

The quasi-pharmacological mechanism

When some aromatic molecules, such as those typically found in plant essential oils, are inhaled, they are able to enter the bloodstream via the mucus membranes that line the nasal cavity and the lungs mucosa. This is because they are small enough and possess an optimal degree of fat and water solubility – in other words, their chemical and physical characteristics confer this ability. Once in the blood, they can reach nervous tissues and thereby elicit effects on the nervous system. Early studies using mice (Buchbauer *et al.* 1993) showed that inhalation of lavender essential oil consistently decreased motor activity. The main chemical constituents of lavender are linalool and linalyl acetate, and these too decreased motor activities. However, thymol (found in thyme oil), nerol (neroli oil) and geraniol (geranium oil) all increased motor activity. This demonstrated that fragrance compounds can have direct pharmacological effects. More recently Linck *et al.* (2010) conducted animal studies to investigate the anxiolytic (anxiety-relieving) potential of inhaled linalool in mice. The study also focused on its effects on social interaction and aggressive behaviour, and a memory task. Their results confirmed the anxiolytic action of inhaled linalool – at a 3 per cent concentration, but not at 1 per cent, which was comparable with diazepam. It was also shown that memory was impaired, and again the effect was comparable with diazepam administration. In relation to social interactions, 1 per cent increased social interaction time compared with controls, and reduced aggressive behaviour. It was postulated that the lack of effect with 3 per cent in this instance was because it might have antagonistic actions on NMDA (N-methyl-D-aspartate) receptors, thus reducing social interactions. Practical recommendations emerged too; it was suggested that 0.74 per cent and 2.55 per cent inhaled linalool, administered for one hour, produced the optimal anxiolytic effect, and that this could be used in the development of olfactory treatments for anxiety in humans.

In humans, the effects of odours can be examined and measured using the electroencephalogram (EEG), which reveals brain wave activity; aspects of this, such as contingent negative variation (CNV), are sensitive to changes in activity and also reflect anticipation (Torii 1997). Early investigations, such as those conducted by Torii and Fukada (1985) and Torii et al. (1988), used CNV measurements, and demonstrated that some odours, such as lavender, had a sedative effect, and others, such as jasmine, had a stimulating effect. Other studies have used different measurements, such as systolic blood pressure, heart rate, peripheral vasoconstriction, electrodermal activity, pupil dilation and constriction, and the 'startle probe reflex', to investigate the physiological effects of odours.

The quasi-pharmacological mechanism naturally infers that specific odours will elicit the same responses in everyone. Perhaps one of the most obvious examples to illustrate this is that of the familiar aromas of lavender and rosemary. It is a notable feature of aromatherapy literature that lavender essential oil is always described as having a sedative effect, while rosemary essential oil is invariably said to stimulate. So, it is not surprising that these two aromas have been the focus of some investigation, and two studies in particular have confirmed not only that this is the case but that the quasi-pharmacological mechanism is probably responsible.

In 1998, Diego et al. reviewed aromatherapy research which had already demonstrated that essential oils could modify alertness, reduce, sustain or enhance attention, enhance performance on visual tasks, modify behaviour and mood, and decrease anxiety and tension. Their placebo-controlled study investigated the effects, on healthy adults, of lavender and rosemary on mood, EEG patterns (which can be used as a measure of alertness) and mathematical computations. They were able to demonstrate that the scent of lavender promoted feelings of relaxation and drowsiness/sleep, in contrast to that of rosemary, which promoted a temporary increase in alertness. Interesting is the finding that both lavender and rosemary brought about an improvement in speed and accuracy with maths computations, but lavender was most effective – possibly because of the added relaxation factor. Therefore, this study supports the quasi-pharmacological theory – although it is possible that any recognition of the aromas and consequent preconceptions about their well-publicised effects might have influenced the study.

Moss et al. (2003) also investigated the olfactory impact on mood, working memory and secondary memory, speed of attention and cognitive performance with the same aromas, lavender and rosemary essential oils. However, their placebo-controlled study was designed to prevent any preconceptions – the participants were deceived in relation to the true aim of the research. By removing this variable, the study indicated that the inhalation of ambient essential oils could significantly affect aspects of cognitive performance, irrespective of the subjects' expectations. As before, the study found lavender to be relaxing and rosemary arousing, and that the quasi-pharmacological mechanism proposed by Jellinek (1997a) was the most likely mechanism involved in producing these effects. Other interesting factors that emerged from this study were that lavender impaired the quality of memory in comparison with rosemary, and that rosemary produced effects on alertness that were comparable with that of oxygen or ginseng administration. However, in both cases the actual speed of memory was impaired, although accuracy was improved. Speed of attention was also affected – it was significantly reduced in the case of lavender, but also slightly reduced with rosemary, compared with the controls. It was postulated that the reason for this unexpected result with rosemary may be that its scent raises arousal to an extent where attentional tasks are impaired, but memory consolidation and retrieval tasks are enhanced.

This aligns with an earlier study conducted by Degel and Köster (1999) where it was found that the odour of lavender reduced errors in maths and letter counting tasks, in comparison with no odour, or the odour of jasmine. They suggested that this result can be explained by the Yerkes-Dodson law, which states that when the arousal level passes a maximum, the performance will decrease. In this case, the lavender would relax the test subjects, leading to a better task performance, but the jasmine would cause further stimulation and arousal, so that performance was not enhanced. They commented that, because of this type of result, it is inadvisable to predict the effects of odours on physiological measures such as CNV variations alone. Moss, Hewitt and Moss (2008), in a further study on the effects of aroma on cognition, supported the quasi-pharmacological mechanism, suggesting the concept of substance-specificity, where each odour would deliver a unique pattern of influence. This particular study focused on the effects of ylang ylang and peppermint, two oils that are commonly used in aromatherapy, and supported the use of ylang ylang as a relaxing scent, and peppermint as a scent that does not slow down reaction times and can perhaps increase task motivation.

This research is very supportive of the aromatherapy concept that specific aromas could be prescribed to elicit specific and reproducible effects; however, other mechanisms are at work too, which make everything less predictable but even more interesting.

The semantic mechanism

Most of the time, we experience smells in the context of life situations. As Engen (1988) noted, smells, memory and associations quickly and irreversibly become linked. This means that each odour will carry an emotional memory, the impact of which can also lead to physiological changes such as an increase in heart rate or blood adrenalin. Odours rapidly become infused with emotional meanings, which can be personal and unique to the individual (King 1988). There may also be some common responses to similar or shared experiences. Most individuals will have their own story to tell in relation to the evocative power of a smell.

Perhaps the best-known example of the semantic mechanism is the Proustian phenomenon. Here we can see a profound link between odour and emotion, where an odour can elicit emotional memories of an episode in the past, or a feeling of being transported back in time. (In Marcel Proust's novel *Swan's Way*, the odour of a madeleine, a type of sweet cake, when dipped in linden-blossom tisane, produces emotionally charged memories of a childhood event that had been forgotten for many years.) Herz, an experimental psychologist, comments that smell is a 'mental tag', or a trigger, which can provoke old, vivid and emotionally laden memories, but cautions against claims that odours are the best memory cues (Herz 2000). Her research has indicated that memories evoked by sight, sound and touch can be just as accurate. Köster, Degel and Piper (2002) agree that odour memories are long-lived because of their uniqueness and emotional charge, but challenge Herz's assertion that this type of memory can be imprecise, and her hypothesis that older olfactory memories are less likely to be weakened by new experiences than memories related to verbal or visual cues. However, it is perhaps this emotionally charged, intense 'feeling' quality that typifies memories triggered by smells, along with a sense that the memory is accurate, and of being brought back to the original event, that defines the Proustian phenomenon – because of the interconnections between olfaction, emotion and memory in the brain. Another distinguishing feature is that the particular odour cue may be experienced just once when it is linked to the event. If an odour is smelled on a frequent basis, it is much less likely to trigger a Proustian memory (Hertz 2000). It has also been suggested that the olfactory part of an autobiographical memory can outlast the other elements of the experience (Chu and Downes 2000), and that the link between smell, emotional arousal and the reactions that arise is mediated by the amygdala (Cahill *et al.* 1996, cited in Chu and Downes 2000). Proustian memories are usually characterised by nostalgia, which facilitates the continuity of our identity, because nostalgia gives us a benchmark – an earlier version of our self in comparison to our current self (Davis 1979, cited in Waskul, Vannini and Wilson 2009). This clearly underpins the practice of Reminiscence Therapy for those with dementia. Waskul *et al.* (2009) found that smelling could play a vital part in the active reminiscing process to establish a somatic sense of self in the past and the present.

The semantic mechanism can also be witnessed in the field of olfactory conditioning – an adaptation of Pavlovian or classical conditioning, where a sensory trigger becomes associated with a specific response. King (1983) demonstrated that, using unconscious conditioning (where the participant is not aware of the process), a smell could be paired with a positive emotional state, and future exposure to the odour could reproduce the same feeling. Researchers at Warwick University showed that it was also possible to pair an odour with a negative emotional state, in this case a stress response, and that the same emotions could be evoked at a later stage in response to that odour (Kirk-Smith, Van Toller and Dodd 1983). More recently, in 2008, Chu showed that olfactory conditioning could not only positively influence behaviour but also enhance performance in the classroom.

Away from the concept of olfactory conditioning in controlled environments, we can still find robust research that shows how our behaviour is influenced by the smells that surround us. The following two examples demonstrate how the quasi-pharmacological and semantic mechanisms may work in parallel. Holland, Hendriks and Aarts (2005) showed that the aroma of a citrus-scented household cleaning agent increased the cleaning activities of students, although the majority reported that they had been unaware of a smell. Citrus is an activating aroma, which can increase perceived energy levels and has become associated with cleaning products such as 'multi-surface' detergents and disinfectants, so here we may be witnessing a combination of nervous system arousal (activity) and the evocative effect (hygiene), resulting in a particular behaviour (cleaning). Schifferstein, Talke and Oudshoorn (2011) investigated the influence of the activating aromas of peppermint, citrus (orange) and 'seawater' on behaviour in a nightclub – and observed that the attendees danced and partied for longer, and rated the music better, than those in the control experiment. Again, this could be due to the arousing effects on the nervous system (feeling energised), coupled with the fresh, invigorating, 'feel-good' associations of the ambient aromas (the music was better). Of course, the social interactions may have been positively influenced too, thus making the whole experience preferable to the control. So, it may be reasoned that if ambient or subtle environmental odours become associated with significant emotions, they can also influence conscious behaviour in our daily and social activities.

The hedonic valence mechanism

This is the name given to the situation where the effects of an odour depend on the subject's state of pleasure or displeasure with that odour, such that if an individual finds an odour pleasing, the perceived effect on the psyche will be positive, and vice versa. This is a very personal mechanism, which can work alongside the semantic mechanism; however, within the hedonic valence mechanism there may well be an element of 'field dependency' – where individuals are influenced by cultural, contextual and environmental factors. Our perception of, and reaction to, odours is affected by 'hedonics' – we respond in a way that is influenced by our personal and cultural experiences (Engen 1988; Jellinek 1997a). Hedonic discrimination is learned behaviour. For example, babies do not discriminate between pleasant and unpleasant odours; and young children do not express disgust with the smell of, for example, faeces, in the same way as adults (Stevenson *et al.* 2010).

In 1997, in her review of the behavioural effects of ambient odours, Susan Knasko highlighted the importance of odour hedonics in relation to 'approach' and 'avoidance' behaviours. Approach behaviour is where an individual is attracted to an area, where they will linger and interact with the surroundings and other individuals; avoidance behaviour is exactly the opposite. Clearly, many other factors will be involved in this – the other senses will be implicated, as we are also influenced by what we see, hear and feel. However, Knasko cited several studies which demonstrated that hedonically pleasant odours encourage people to stay longer in stores than in unscented stores (Knasko 1989; Teerling, Nixdorf and Koster 1992), and that ambient malodours can decrease the time spent in an environment and produce negative responses to strangers and objects in these areas (Rotton *et al.* 1978; Rotton 1983).

Interestingly, but perhaps not surprisingly, studies relating to the effects of ambient human body odours (such as underarm odour) yielded more complex results (Cowley, Johnson and Brooksbank 1977; Kirk-Smith and Booth 1992); we will return to this in Chapter 5. However, Knasko (1989) commented that, along with hedonics, odour congruency plays an important role in approach/avoidance behaviour. Therefore, a hedonically pleasant odour can influence approach behaviour differently, according to its appropriateness within the surroundings or environment. A later study confirmed this observation, where it was found that congruent pleasant ambient odours encouraged consumers to spend longer making purchasing decisions; they would take a more holistic approach, would look beyond the information given, seek variety, and spread their choices more evenly across the range, than when in the presence of an incongruent odour (Mitchell, Khan and Knasko 1995).

In 1997 Baron conducted studies in a shopping mall, to investigate the effect of pleasant ambient fragrances on social behaviour. The shopping mall environment offered a range of pleasant ambient odours, as well as plentiful opportunities for spontaneous acts of 'helping' behaviour. The preliminary study revealed that passers-by were much more likely to offer help in the form of retrieving a dropped object or offering change for a dollar to a same-sex individual (this was designed as an attempt to avoid a 'soliciting' scenario within the study) in the presence of the scent of baking bread or cookies, or roasting coffee beans. In the second study the passers-by were also asked to rate their mood. Here it was found that helping behaviour correlated with a positive mood; and this could mediate the effects of the fragrance on helping behaviour.

Gilbert (2008) highlights the importance of ambient odour in marketing, merchandising and shopping behaviours, giving numerous examples of how hedonically pleasing scents are currently being applied to enhance approach behaviour and selling. He, too, stresses the importance of congruency. He gives the example of potential sales of satin sleepwear, where female students responded more favourably if exposed to the scent of 'lily of the valley' than to 'sea mist', which was equally pleasant. 'Lily of the valley' was perceived as being more feminine, and evoked a bedroom ambience, whereas 'sea mist' did not. Gilbert also relates how researchers demonstrated that an ambient scent of 'feminine vanilla' in a clothing store increased sales of womenswear, while menswear sales decreased, but if the ambient scent was replaced with 'masculine rose maroc', the reverse effect was observed.

These studies have verified the belief that supraliminal odours (that is, those above our detection threshold) and even weak ambient odours can affect mood and behaviour. However, it is also likely that subliminal odours (those below our detection threshold) can also impact on our social behaviour. Li *et al.* (2007) conducted one of the first studies designed to investigate this, testing the full range of odour valence and not just reliant on the participants' self-reporting. They set out to test the hypothesis that the hedonic content of undetectable odours alters social likeability judgements of human faces. The results demonstrated that subliminal odours could influence social preferences, and that it was odours below conscious detection that evoked greater effects. They suggested that subliminal smells influence likeability judgements and autonomic responses because they prevent 'top-down regulation', and thus cognitive input in our behaviour, and that conscious odour detection may in fact disrupt these effects.

In contrast to these behavioural studies, Alaoui-Ismaïli *et al.* (1997) investigated the effects of a range of odours on autonomic nervous system activity, using a range of physiological parameters. It was demonstrated that unpleasant odorants produced higher autonomic arousal than pleasant odorants. Acetic butyric acids were perceived as hedonically unpleasant, and produced a longer duration of electrodermal responses, high skin blood flow and increased heart rate. Lavender and ethyl acetoacetate odorants, rated as pleasant, produced the opposite effects. Camphor was perceived as being pleasant, but the responses produced were between those of the unpleasant and pleasant odorants, probably because the odour can stimulate the trigeminal nerve. The researchers discussed the observation that, when analysing the effects of odours, a 'strong and clear hedonic factor always emerges' (p.246).

When we come to look at associative learning and odour preferences, we can see the overlap between the semantic and hedonic valence mechanisms. Associative learning is a crucial part of cognition and behaviour, and there is strong evidence to show that it is integral to our development of odour preferences. In other words, if an emotion is paired with an odour, it gives the odour a personal meaning, so the odour becomes either liked or disliked. Exposure to the odour can then elicit emotion, and thus influence behaviour (Herz 2005).

The placebo mechanism

Here, we need to consider how expectation can influence the outcome: if an individual is told that a certain odour will have a specific effect, and this becomes a belief, then the chances are that the odour will indeed elicit the expected effect. The only other influences could be the environment or field dependency. Robbins and Broughan (2007) conducted a study that demonstrated the placebo effect in relation to odour. It had been suggested previously that the scent of the essential oil of Spanish sage could improve memory. The participants were randomly assigned to three groups and given a word memory test. Then a similar test was repeated in the presence of the odour of Spanish sage. Prior to the second test one group had been told that the odour would impair their memory, while another group was informed that it would improve their memory. The third group was the control, and was given no information about Spanish sage. Perhaps unsurprisingly, the negative expectancy group performed less well in the second test, and the positive expectancy group had an improved performance, while the control group performed as in the first test. This study demonstrates that the manipulation of expectations can have a very strong influence, and consequently research design should take the placebo effect into account. Even the very suggestion that an odour is present can influence motivation and behaviour (Knasko, Gilbert and Sabini 1990, cited in Ilmberger *et al.* 2001).

So, it is very likely that all four mechanisms are active in humans, and it is very difficult to separate them and look at their discrete effects in experimental situations. In 2001 Ilmberger *et al.* observed that because there are individual differences in the perception of odours (like/dislike, previous exposure, expectation), there will be differential effects on, for example, reaction times. They had also highlighted that, within subject groups, the initial levels of (for example) alertness and motivation will be varied, and this can lead to even more variability in responses. For example, an individual who is already feeling alert will benefit less from an activating scent, such as peppermint, than someone who is feeling inattentive.

The studies explored above have given us a glimpse of the many ways in which odour affects us at physiological and psychological levels, but the mechanisms of this are intricate and interrelated, and quite inextricable. The studies have also shown the many ways in which hedonically pleasing odours can contribute to wellbeing.

Emotional responses to odours

Our responses to odours are linked with their hedonic 'tone'. Chrea *et al.* (2009) commented that, despite the many studies, very few have explored the nature of the affective states that can be elicited by odours. In most of the studies participants have been asked to complete a forced-choice, self-report questionnaire, and this means that the respondents are unable to describe their responses. Alternatively, studies use the 'bi-dimensional' theory, which reduces emotions to positions within a space, using scales defined by arousal and pleasantness. Chrea *et al.* argue that the small number of primary emotions included in such questionnaires is ill-equipped to convey the rich and varied responses to odours, and that the bi-dimensional studies do not give explicit qualitative information. So their research attempted to identify a taxonomy that could verbally measure the subjective experience, and to find out whether emotions could be elicited that were not dependent on the hedonic valence of odours. Their well-designed study, which used a rich array of discriminating terms for both the intrinsic qualities of the odours tested and the affective states, produced some interesting results. A relationship between the intrinsic quality of the odours and the participants' subjective experiences was identified; the emotional experience was finely differentiated across the odour types, and this was influenced by the perceived qualities of the odours, such as delicacy, heaviness, healthiness and sweetness. The research also revealed that the taxonomy used to measure frequently experienced emotions, in terms such as guilt, shame, anger and sadness, is not particularly relevant to the emotional experience of odours. The only word here that was relevant was 'disgust'. The vocabulary for pleasant odour-induced feelings was much richer. Chrea *et al.* suggest that it is possible that odour-induced negative feelings require an appropriate context if they are to be explored in relation to the feelings elicited. This could be, for example, a social context. In studies, odours are not usually presented in a context that facilitates negative feelings, and so impact of context on the semantic affective space needs to be explored. This research culminated in the development of the 'Geneva Emotion and Odor Scale' (GEOS).

The following year, Porcherot *et al.* (2010) published the results of a study which adapted the GEOS to meet commercial and development needs, specifically in the realm of flavours (strawberry was investigated), perfumery oils and fine fragrances. They commented that reliability of the GEOS is well established and relevant not only for the measurement of feelings induced by odours but also for product development and screening. Some of their findings regarding the effects of the oils and fine fragrances will be mentioned in Chapter 5.

Odour, mood and wellbeing

One study in particular is worth mentioning at this point, because it is the only one that has considered the impact of natural odours in an experimental fragrant garden rather than the laboratory. Weber and Heuberger (2008) conducted this research in the *Duftgarten* (fragrant garden) at the University of Natural Resources and Applied Life Sciences in Vienna. This is an experimental garden which is designed with fragrant plant species to give a harmonious blend of scents throughout the days and evenings, and over the growing season. They set out to determine how the scent of fragrant plants in a natural outdoor setting affected mood, alertness and calmness. The first experiment showed that the pleasant scents of the blooming plants in the garden increased calmness and alertness, and improved mood; however, it was acknowledged that the visual impact of the garden may have contributed to this, and neutral and less pleasing scents were not evaluated. Further experiments were designed, and it was found that the beneficial effects of the natural, complex scents were long-lasting, that unpleasant or neutral odours did not compensate, and that unpleasant odours had only a transient negative effect. The garden was also used at night, so that the visual impact was removed. This, incidentally, is the time when the scent of some plants increases in intensity to attract night-pollinating insect species. It was found that, again, the natural odours improved affective states independent of visual input. This particular study is of relevance when we come to look not only at how aromatic plants have been enjoyed and exploited over the millennia but also at the role of the natural world in human wellbeing.

Concepts of wellbeing

Human needs

Maslow produced a model to assist our understanding of human behaviour and what we need in order to reach our fullest potential. Using the visual analogy of a pyramid, he suggested that the most fundamental human needs of water, food and shelter were found at the base of the pyramid. The next level up was safety and freedom from stress, followed by social needs, such as friendship and love. The higher levels were self-esteem and confidence, and at the very top was self-actualisation, or reaching full potential (cited in Benson and Dundis 2003). Each level needs to be achieved, or the higher levels cannot be reached. So it is obvious that we need safety and security in our material, physical and social realms before we can even begin to approach a sense of wellbeing.

However, we live in times where many on the planet live in poverty or in broken communities where even the most fundamental and social needs are not met. Many others live in more affluent circumstances, but perhaps in circles where consumerism is rife or where the only perceived value is monetary. Obsession with the self can take precedence over concern for others and our environment, and this too may eventually contribute to a growing sense of isolation and dis-ease.

The search for meaning is also important – another human 'need'. In many western societies we can observe the misuse of alcohol, sedatives and narcotics. This could be viewed as a reflection of the individual's attempts to escape from, or repress, the negative feelings of despair, or lack of purpose in life, and perhaps to seek heightened sensations as a substitute for meaning (Deikman 1982).

Clearly there is a need for many to reconnect with what is important for physical, mental, emotional and spiritual health; to seek and find a sense of wellbeing. There are many therapies and practices that claim to help us achieve this potentially elusive state, but we still need to explore what we really mean by wellbeing. To do this, first we need to address the concept of the 'ordinary mind'.

The ordinary mind

Like the little stream
making its way
through the mossy crevices I, too, quietly
turn clear and transparent.

Ryokan (1758–1831, cited in Lawless 2010a)

Lawless (2010a) used these lines by the Japanese poet Ryokan to illustrate the nature of the 'ordinary mind' – a simple, uncluttered, healthy state of mind. He also gives the example of the old Zen master Rinzai who, hoping to provoke the arising of 'ordinary mind' in his monks and nuns, asked the question 'Going in and out of the gates of your face is a person of no ranks or title, who is it?'

In his blog 'The Ordinary Mind, Perfume and Natural Health' (2010a), Lawless connected how scents and the natural world can be an integral part of wellbeing. He observed how the sense of wonder that arises when making time to appreciate nature – the stars, the wilderness, or beautifully tended gardens – can lead to a sense of gratitude and contentment. Then, because self-centredness is diminished, the past and the future become irrelevant, and we experience only the present moment and the health of the ordinary mind. A love of the natural world, which provokes these feelings of awe and being 'at one' with nature, is known as *biophilia*, and Wilson (1984) reasoned that this is the source of the human 'religious instinct' (Bloom 2011).

Landscape and wellbeing

The word 'paradise' is derived from *pairi-daeza*, an old Persian word meaning an enclosed park or orchard. Sumerian, biblical and Koranic scriptures refer to such paradise gardens. There are many examples, perhaps the most spectacular being the fragrant Hanging Gardens at the Palace of Nabuchodonosor in Babylon, the *gulistans* (Persian rose gardens) and the garden of Shalimar in Kashmir, variously described as an 'abode of love', a 'bestower of joy' and 'paradise on earth'. In India, China and Japan, gardens surrounded temples and shrines – and these are often filled with sacred and aromatic plants. Natural landscapes – cedar-clad mountains, mountain springs, rivers and tree sanctuaries – also feature in ancient texts. In many cultures there are sacred groves. Celtic spirituality places particular significance on trees, and Druids consider the oak, ash and thorn to be especially important. In India, sacred groves are located in the Parinche valley in Maharashtra. As well as having ecological significance, sacred groves play important roles in village life. They are dedicated to deities and have significance to the local community. In these groves, ceremonies are conducted, festivals are held, medicinal herbs are collected – they are small, natural sanctuaries, with a wide variety of plant life (Waghchaure *et al.* 2006). What all of these landscapes have in common is that they support every aspect of human wellbeing, from fundamental physical needs to spiritual practices (Morris 1984; Thompson 2011).

Similarly, Homer's *Aeneid* describes the paradisiacal Elysian Fields, and here we find references to natural scents – such as fragrant groves of bay laurel – further enhancing the experience of the landscape. In Greco-Roman times sanctuaries were often places protected within the hills, with spring waters and groves of trees. Pliny the Younger wrote about his second home in rural Tuscany, where it was beautiful, green, peaceful and with clean air, to which he would retreat to maintain his physical and mental wellbeing.

The concept of multisensory gardens and landscapes for both the healthy and the sick continued: for example, the cloisters of mediaeval Europe, herb gardens, monastery gardens, fields, meadows, woods and forests. Later, in the eighteenth and nineteenth centuries, the English landscape garden movement echoed the classical Greek and Roman gardens, and reinitiated discussions about landscape, aesthetics, emotions and behaviour. Since then, many studies have demonstrated the importance of the landscape in health and wellbeing, corroborating these long-held beliefs (Thompson 2011).

This may also lead us to question how gardening affects gardeners. Christopher Tilley, an anthropologist, conducted an ethnographic study to explore the sensory dimensions of gardening. He found that 'The sensory feeling for the garden is deeper and much more profound than most gardeners can, will (for fear of sounding silly), or do acknowledge. Such synesthetic experience was frequently implicitly expressed by the use of the term "harmony"' (p.329). He showed that no one sense is more important than another, but it is interesting that smell/scent was highlighted as the second most significant sense, after sight/visual appearance. Tilley suggests that it is the multisensorial aspects of gardening that reconnect us with the natural world (Tilley 2006).

Scents of sanctity

Although humans have lived for millennia in a multisensory world dominated by vision, many otherwise diverse cultures do not make a distinction between the visible, tangible material world and the unseen spirit world. For example, the Greek philosopher Aristotle suggested that nature had powers, and Malawi cultural beliefs are characterised by vitalism and pantheism, where the natural world, plants and animals have inherent powers (Morris 1998). Like the unseen world, scent is invisible, but it is tangible.

Scent has always played an important role in spiritual practices – particularly in marking transition and in connecting with the divine, transcending death and sharing immortality. In ancient Greece, the gods were characterised by their smells, and it was believed that they responded positively to fragrant offerings at altars. Ambrosia (from the Greek word *ambrotos*, meaning immortal) was a sweet, fragrant liquid that both sustained and perfumed the gods. In Islam, scent could evoke paradise; the Sufis meditated in fragrant rose gardens (Morris 1984). In Christianity, specific aromas are associated with martyrs and saints (Evans 2002). St Lyddwyne de Schiedam is said to have had the scent of cinnamon, cut flowers, ginger and clove, lilies, roses and violets, while St Teresa of Avila had the scent of lily and orris root, and after her death this transformed into violet and jasmine, the sweet, fresh smell persisting even after twelve years. The odour of a saint's body, or 'the odour of sanctity' is always said to be 'sweet' – a word with multisensory connotations: sweet taste, sweet melodious sound, agreeable to the senses and the mind. When a saint's soul was released from the physical body at death, a sweet, fragrant odour accompanied the immortal soul, symbolic of heaven and salvation. In the case of St Lambert, the sweet scent was noticed at the funeral ceremony and even around the tomb after burial, accompanied by the sound of his voice amid sweet celestial singing. In early Christianity, incenses were considered to be idolatrous, but sweet scents eventually became representative of divinity and immortality (Saucier 2010).

The theologian St Ephrem the Syrian (circa 306–373 CE), wrote about the 'Fragrance of Life'. Since smells were integral to religious rituals, he connected scents with the divine and salvation – exploring knowledge that does not belong to the cognitive domain but is nonetheless revelatory. We will return to St Ephrem in Chapter 13; at this point it is worth noting that he maintained that extraordinarily beautiful scents revealed divine presence (Harvey 1998). Similarly, Evans (2002) writes that the fragrance of sanctity is frequently said to be an 'incomparably beautiful perfume', and gives examples such as the scents of flowers (often roses, lilies and violets), various spices, and foods (usually apples and bread). He comments that scent is a form of communication that can spread the faith, unhindered by the barriers of human communications such as literacy and linguistics, and the passage of time.

Defining wellbeing

So far, we can see that some important elements of wellbeing may be the 'ordinary mind' and a connection with the natural world, or experiencing spirituality via the natural world and its fragrances. Could we define wellbeing as a state of being where we are calm but alert, perhaps feeling a sense of wonder, or being engaged in a creative activity, or observing and immersing the self in beauty and connecting with the natural world, centred in awareness rather than mental activity and, most important of all, being completely and utterly in the moment?

In the Upanishads of Vedic literature, this condition is described as undifferentiated unity, where the division between the self and the material world ceases to exist – a state of bliss. (In the West, we might begin to equate this with the expression of being 'at one with nature'.) There are two phases to this: the first is known as *dhyana* – which is the point where the focus of attention becomes an unbroken flow of concentration. Then *samadhi* can follow; this is where the boundaries between self and the object of concentration disappear, and this leads to state of dispassion (or non-identification), where identification with the thoughts and contents of the mind are diminished. However, achieving this state has become very difficult for many of us. This is because we are, according to eastern traditions, trapped in *maya* – the transient world of the mind – where we are identified and caught up by, and then fixated in, our feelings, thoughts and emotions (Wolinski

1991). These inner worlds, which feel like realities to the individual, can be defined as states of *maya*, and can also be described as *trance states*.

Wolinski (1991) likened these trance states to tunnels that we walk through so that we can navigate the world around us – they are rather like a coping mechanism. We may experience many trance states every day – perhaps when driving a familiar route and suddenly not remembering passing through a particular village, or a walk along a shoreline which allows us to become caught up in memories of happy childhood days on a beach, or when meeting a litter of puppies or kittens; time passes without our attention as we allow ourselves to be charmed by the little creatures. There are many, many examples of such trance states, sometimes likened to daydreaming, where we are totally self-absorbed, and the mind wanders. Some of these states serve us well; they can help us achieve our goals, and can bring much pleasure. However, trance states which are formed around difficult, unpleasant or traumatic associations can be destructive or even pathological. Such negative trance states can create and sustain symptoms of mental ill-health. Clearly, it is not healthy when an individual's consciousness has a restricted and narrow focus on just a few of these inner 'realities', and the person becomes trapped within a total identification with their inner world.

Within the Eriksonian framework,[1] where trance is viewed as a 'special but natural state of consciousness that is optimally suited for mediating therapeutic work' (Wolinski 1991), we can begin to see that the concept of the trance state is very useful when exploring the ordinary mind, and the potential of fragrance in the search for self-actualisation or wellbeing. In fact, we are looking at the transcendence of these limiting states of mind – where we are free of the trance state, or have entered a *therapeutic* trance.

Fragrance and wellbeing

Our sense of smell can keep us safe, enable subtle communication, affect our social behaviour, and even influence our immune system and our choice of mate. Odours can also help us on the path to wellbeing – through their effects on alertness, their ability to reduce, sustain or enhance attention and task performance. They can stabilise, enhance and modify our moods, decrease anxiety and tension, evoke autobiographical memories and give us a benchmark of our somatic selves, and aid us on a spiritual journey. However, it is their complex relationship with our emotional world, their relationship with trance states, and their ability to bring about altered states of consciousness that is perhaps the real key to their role in enhancing wellbeing. It is also probable that the very process of educating the

---

1   Eriksonian psychology is derived from the work of Milton Erickson, an American medical doctor and psychiatrist, who is known as the 'father of hypnotherapy'. He is noted for his use of therapeutic metaphor and the creative and solution-generating aspects of the unconscious mind, which can be harnessed via trance states to facilitate change and personal growth. His work has also influenced the development of Neurolinguistic Programming (NLP).

olfactory palate is, in itself, therapeutic; we shall return to these ideas in Chapters 5 and 12.

In the next chapter we will explore our long history and relationship with the world of plant aromatics; specifically, via combustion.

CHAPTER 3

Per Fumum

It is often explained that the word 'perfume' is derived from the Latin *per fumum* ('through smoke'). In this chapter we will explore the world of plant-derived smoke, its medicinal and ritual uses; and incenses, which were, and indeed are, integral to spiritual practices across many cultures. It is not intended to give a full account of the history of incense or perfume here, as these topics have been covered admirably elsewhere (Morris 1984; Lawless 1994, 2009). Indeed, Morris's text clearly has served as an invaluable resource for many subsequent histories of aromatics, including this version. However, the following words attributed to Goethe should be heeded:

> Not all that is presented to us as history has really happened; and what really happened did not actually happen the way it is presented to us; moreover, what really happened is only a small part of all that happened. Everything in history remains uncertain, the largest events as well as the smallest occurrence. (Antoninetti 2011, p.383)

It is hoped that the historical highlights presented here and in Chapter 4 will serve to contextualise the perspectives set out in this book.

Plant-derived smoke as a medicine and preventative strategy

Many of the fragrant and therapeutic constituents of aromatic plant materials can be liberated by combustion and accessed via the smoke that is produced. We do not know when this practice began, but it is likely that plant-derived smoke has been used by humans since the discovery of fire, so it possibly dates back 1.6 million years, or more. Pennacchio *et al.* (2010) estimate that currently there are at least 1460 plant taxa, with 2383 ethnobotanical uses in 125 countries. They also comment that the main uses are medicinal – via inhalation of the smoke and by fumigation – followed by their ceremonial and ritual applications.

Aromatic smoke inhalation allows the therapeutic constituents rapid access to the body, and has been used to treat a myriad of disorders in many cultures, including digestive problems and respiratory disorders, including asthma, as well as rheumatism, inflammation and fever. Plant-derived smoke can also be an effective analgesic, and its main application is for headache. Perhaps the best known plant analgesic, apart from opium, is *Cannabis sativa*, whose medicinal uses date back 5000 years in China. Today, it is better known as a recreational drug. In areas of South America, the leaves of *Brugmansia* species were smoked, along with tobacco, by the women and slaves who were to be buried alive along with their dead husbands and masters; the smoke would dull their senses (Pennacchio *et al.* 2010).

However, even without passive inhalation, or actively smoking, fumigation has medicinal and preventative applications. For example, the indigenous Australians treated wounds and facilitated childbirth with aromatic fumigations, as was traditional practice also in parts of India, North and South America and Africa. Fumigation with plant aromatics has been used to purify the surroundings since ancient Egyptian times; it is said that Hippocrates (460–377 BCE) saved Athens from a plague epidemic in 430 BCE by burning aromatic fires, and it would seem that juniper berries were included in the bonfires. *Juniperus communis* is widely distributed in the northern hemisphere, and has been accessed by many cultures, so it has since acquired an impressive array of applications in addition to its disinfectant actions – including repelling insects and driving away evil spirits (Pennacchio *et al.* 2010). Juniper berries and wood, along with rosemary, were used as fumigants in Europe until the mid-eighteenth century, to disinfect the air. At that time the doctors referred to the practices of Hippocrates and Galen[1] – at one point there were plans to protect the city of London from the plague by means of aromatic smoke; it was believed that smoke from burning rue had protected one district during the Great Plague of 1666 (Corbin 1996). During the seventeenth-century plague epidemics, the professional perfumers became 'plague doctors' – who, dressed in bizarre protective garments, would seal infected houses and fumigate them with scented smoke, but apparently with little success (Stamelman 2006).

So the practical uses of aromatic smoke and incense were considerable. Their scent would disguise unpleasant odours, such as burning flesh, putrefaction, decay due to heat and humidity, and poor sanitation, while repelling insect pests, and this would certainly help to reduce chances of the spread of disease. Therefore, it was also seen as a way of purifying places and activities, such as the ancient Assyrian practice of offering incense after sexual intercourse (Moeran 2009), although here we may also see a connection between scent, intimacy and eroticism.

Incense, ritual and ceremony

Scented smoke also acquired ceremonial, religious and ritual uses. This probably originated in the belief that the smoke of some plants could afford protection from

---

1 'Galen of Pergamum' was Aelius or Claudius Galenus (130–201 CE), a Greek born in Pergamum (modern day Turkey). He was a physician, philosopher and writer, and an early medical investigator, who became physician to Marcus Aurelius of Rome, and his successors. His theories persisted for 15 centuries after his death.

evil, which was thought to be the source of illness, and that scented smoke not only pleased the gods but also afforded a way of connecting with the unseen world. At some point it would have been noticed that exposure to the smoke of some plants, entheogens – psychoactive substances that literally 'generate the divine within' – could produce altered states of consciousness or hallucinations, thus enabling communication with the spirit world or the divine. For this reason the practice of using plant-derived smoke in divination, shamanism, ritual and ceremony evolved (Dannaway 2010).

The word 'incense' means 'to set on fire', and refers to any material that is burned or heated to release fragrant smoke or fumes. In western Asia this was done quite simply by placing resins and woods over hot coals. In eastern Asia the process was more sophisticated. Here, resins, wood chips, dried leaves and spices were ground to a powder and sifted; sometimes inorganic saltpetre would be added to help with the burning process. Water or wine was then added to make a paste that could either be formed into cones, or extruded to form spirals, coils or straight sticks (the forerunner of joss sticks). The paste could also be moulded to form 'incense seals' that would burn for extended periods if placed on a bed of ashes, and even incense 'clocks' were made from the sticks, as the time intervals could be marked and measured by the progress of the burning stick (Morris 1984).

Psychoactivity

For some time there has been speculation about the psychoactivity of some incense ingredients, including frankincense (the resin from *Boswellia* species), one of the earliest known incenses, whose use has become widespread (Dannaway 2010). It is said that the ancient Greek philosopher Pythagoras used frankincense to enable him to prophesy. The cross-cultural observations of the effects of incense on the psyche – such as heightened senses and awareness – have been partially explained in terms of neurophysiology.

Iijima *et al.* (2009) demonstrated that the scent of incense could enhance cortical activity. In a controlled study, brain activity was measured by EEG (electroencephalograms) and ERP (event-related potentials, including contingent negative variation (CNV); see page 31). Incense (dominated by agarwood) was compared with the scent of rose; both scents were liked, but 90 per cent of the subjects preferred that of incense, which may also have elicited emotional responses and memories (it was described by some participants as fresh, calm, sweet and 'hometown'), so this may have influenced the results. It was found that alpha 2 activity in the brain increased significantly during exposure to the incense. Generally, alpha activity is reduced under emotional stress. In this study the EEGs showed that an increase in alpha 2 occurred without an increase in theta, slow alpha or beta activity (which are associated with relaxation and sedation), and the authors suggested that this might be because the incense not only caused relaxation but also increased vigilance. The ERP element of the study showed motor responses to the scents. The locations for these responses are in the orbitofrontal and anterior cingulate cortices of the brain – which are connected with the olfactory and limbic systems and the behaviour and inhibitory control processes respectively. The results suggested that the incense enhanced the function of the inhibitory control processes. The authors did not investigate the possible pharmacological effects of incense; however, they did comment that some of the sesquiterpenoids found in incense, including agarwood-based products such as the one used in this study, have sedative and pain-relieving effects (Okugawa *et al.* 2000, cited in Iijima *et al.* 2009).

Magical smokes

The ancients would certainly have made detailed observations of the effects of the smoke from burning plants, noting their aromatic characteristics, any toxic effects and magical (that is, psychoactive) properties. From this, incense cults were formed, and secret recipes for incenses used in divination, or when seeking wisdom in an altered state of consciousness, were closely guarded (Dannaway 2010). The ancient Greek medical papyri refer to 'magical smokes'. Then, there was no distinction between magic and medicine, and there were several routes to achieving altered states of consciousness. The cults that have become known collectively as the 'Greek mystery traditions' all used incense and entheogens, and have elements of the shamanic complex. Examples include the cult of Dionysus, the cult of Orpheus, the brotherhood of Pythagoras and the cult of Mithras.

The cult of Dionysus was a secret society with elaborate initiation rites and 'Bacchic revels' which emerged between 1000 and 3000 BCE. Dionysus, son of Zeus and Demeter or one of the 'corn' goddesses, became associated with intoxication, wine (or, more accurately, the spread of the vine cult, which had been introduced by the Cretans), and also wild animals. Dionysus was a 'horned child' and often took on animal form. He travelled widely with his tutor Silenus and a troop of wild Satyrs and Maenads (Graves 1992). The cult rituals were inspired by his expeditions, travels, exploits and violent murder(s), from which he emerged transformed. For example, at birth he was torn apart by the Titans, his body parts were boiled in a cauldron, and then he was rescued and recreated by his grandmother Rhea. She raised him as a girl until puberty, and later initiated him into her mysteries. According to myth, Dionysus sometimes took on the form of a panther, and transformation into big cats can be seen in other shamanic cultures too. The ancient Greeks maintained that panthers emitted a beautiful, seductive scent. Theophrastus wrote, 'The panther emits an odour agreeable to all other animals, and thus it can hunt by remaining in hiding and attracting animals to it by its smell' (Le Guérer 1993, p.19). Dionysus's associations with intoxicants, animal transformation, 'dying' and subsequent recreation, and gender ambiguity have strong parallels with shamanism (DuBois 2009).

Later on, circa 500 BCE, the cult of Orpheus emerged. Orpheus was a poet and musician who undertook a spiritual journey; he travelled to the underworld to retrieve the soul of Euridice, his dead wife, and returned. Although he found her, she did not survive the journey home. This symbolic journey, with its elements of travelling to the underworld, soul retrieval, and transformation, inspired the development of a major cult following. It is known that the Orphics would inhale incense smoke and experience frenzy and ecstasy. The Orphic incense contained aromatic and psychoactive ingredients in a synergistic combination, and included frankincense, myrrh, styrax resin, saffron, various types of seed, and other aromatics that were sacred to the god being invoked (Dannaway 2010).

The Brotherhood of Pythagoras, the philosopher and mathematician, is another example of a mystery tradition, originating in the sixth century BCE. The cult followers were strict vegetarians, who believed that killing an animal was murder, because animals shared the right of life and possessed souls. At the time, bird and animal sacrifice to the gods, accompanied by incense, was common, but the Pythagoreans offered incense alone as a bloodless sacrifice (Classen *et al.* 1994).

In Rome between the late first and early fourth centuries CE, the cult of Mithras was prominent; this had Persian or Zoroastrian origins, but the Roman version focused on Mithras, who was born out of a rock and was usually depicted slaying a bull. Again, the rituals involved the inhalation of incense smoke. Dannaway (2010) suggests that the cult of Mithras was one of the main cults that has retained and preserved its mysteries for later generations of mystics. The western mystery tradition underwent a revival in the twentieth century. We can find, for example, in the writings of Dion Fortune,[2] reference to rites performed in the Orphic and Dionysian traditions, and also to the burning of sacred woods and incense to release smoke that evoked visions. Although the protocols for daily living, rituals and initiations varied within these mystery traditions, what they had in common was a focus on the wheel of rebirth, transmutation of the soul, transmigration of the soul, advantages in the afterlife, and, of course, the use of incense and entheogens.

Dannaway (2010) explores the cultural exchange between Egypt, Greece, the Holy Land and India in terms of the oldest trade route, the 'Incense Road'. Here, in relation to 'fire rites' and incenses, obvious themes emerge, especially in relation to the *soma* – the sacred elixir of the Brahmins. *Soma* might be *Cannabis sativa*, or *Peganum harmala*, or *Ephedra distachya*, which was burned in fire rites, or it might have been the psychoactive mushroom *Amanita muscaria* (as suggested by Wasson 1963, cited in DuBois 2009). Could it be the same as the Persian *haoma* in ancient Zoroastrianism, or the Vedic *homa*, or the *goma* of Tantric Buddhism in Japan? The same plants were burned by the Shia of Iran and the early Shia Imams. Another term seems to highlight the cultural connections: *bhanga*, referring to cannabis and henbane. The ancient Iranian word *banga* means 'a psychotropic plant', and the later Arabic word *banj* refers to henbane or *Datura stramonium*; in Ethiopia and Somalia, the variation *banji* remains in use (Margetts 1967). The Arabs were heavily influenced

---

2   'Dion Fortune' or Violet Mary Firth (1946–1981) was an influential occultist who championed the western mystery tradition. She founded the 'Society of the Inner Light' in the 1920s, which was grounded in her Christian ethic and morality.

by the Chinese, especially in relation to alchemy, but their incense customs were their own. Hallucinogenic doses of *Datura* seeds are used in Morocco, where they are also used for exorcism. The Sufis refer to *harmal* (*Rhazya stricta*), which is a Dhofari Arabic name. The prophet Muhammad prescribed incense for worship that contained *harmal* and frankincense; however, *harmal* is better known for its use in exorcism and for its apotropaic[3] uses. Paradoxically, *djinns* are also said to like *harmal* smoke, and there are numerous tales of djinns appearing when powders are thrown on fires, or when magical powders are ignited.

If ancient philosophers, seekers of the truth, mystics and religious leaders used incense and entheogens, how did the practice eventually become linked with the occult and witchcraft, leading to persecution? This is a very complex question, because of the many other cultural and social influences of the ages. However, strictly from the incense perspective, 'foreign' influences, that is, the worship of false gods, had been noted in the Israelite incense cult, and by the second century CE fire rites and incense burning were already becoming associated with magic and witchcraft. The early Christian church leaders equated magic with heresy; later on the Church created an institution, the Inquisition, which hunted and persecuted witches (DuBois 2009), who used entheogens in their flying ointments and cauldrons. Dannaway (2010) suggests that:

> From the foreign wives of kings and prophets to the persecuted 'women of the hedge', spinsters and witches, the misogyny of the priest-class can be seen to arise from a fear of the botanical knowledge of women that challenged their monopoly. (p.494)

Psychotropics, aromatics and the senses – an integral part of human culture?

Some plants and fungi produce *secondary metabolites*. These are substances which are not essential for growth and development, and they often have complex biological roles. The scents of the volatile oils and resins in aromatic plants are due to secondary metabolites, such as the terpenes and their derivatives, and the phenylpropanoids. Many medicinal and psychotropic drugs are also plant secondary metabolites. For example, the nitrogen-containing alkaloids include quinine (found in recipes for tonic water), caffeine (coffee, tea, guarana) and theobromine (cocoa). The alkaloids also include hallucinogens found in several species of the Solanaceae family, which have played a major role in human drug culture. These are *Atropa belladonna* (deadly nightshade, containing atropine, a compound that typically dilated the pupils

---

3   The use of incense-based objects for apotropaic use is widespread. In Java *djimats* are small pieces of inscribed paper wrapped around an incense stick, and kept on the person. At certain times, they can be exposed to the smoke of the incense, which provides protection from harm. In ancient Egypt perfumes were worn to protect from the hexes that emanated from the stars and the moon, or unlucky places.

of the eyes), *A. mandragora* (mandrake, containing atropine and other alkaloids), *Datura stramonium* (datura or Jimson weed, containing hyoscyamine), *Brugmansia* species (tree-daturas, containing hyoscine), *Hyoscyamus niger* (henbane, containing hyoscyamine), *Nicotiana rusticum* and *N. tabacum* (wild and cultivated tobaccos, containing nicotine – not a known hallucinogen, but hallucinogenic β-carbolines are also present), *Peganum harmala* (Syrian rue, containing harmine and harmaline alkaloids) and *Solanum nigrum* (black nightshade, containing steroidal alkaloids). Other notable psychotropic alkaloids are mescaline (found in the cactus *Lophophora williamsii*), ephedrine (*Ephedra* species), cocaine (*Coca* species), papaverine and morphine (*Papaver somniferum*, opium poppy). *Ololiuqui* was the name given by the Aztecs to the hallucinogenic seeds of a climbing plant, *Rivea corymbosa*, which is closely related in its constituents and actions to the 'morning glory', *Ipomoea tricolor*. Both contain lysergic acid, from which lysergic acid diethylamide (LSD)[4] is derived. With the exception of cannabis, which contains tetrahydrocannabinols (THCs), the principal hallucinogenic plants contain alkaloids that are related to the human neurotransmitters noradrenalin and serotonin.

The main hallucinogenic fungi are also poisonous. *Amanita muscaria* is the fly agaric used in Siberia; it contains the isoxazone alkaloids, ibotenic acid and muscimol. Hallucinogenic Mexican mushrooms include *Psilocybe mexicana*, *Conocybe cyanopus* and *Stropharia* species; these were known to the Aztecs as *teonanácatl*, 'flesh of the gods'. Their active constituents are the tryptamine derivatives psilocybin and psilocin, both related to serotonin. Puffballs (*Lycoperda* species) are used by the Mixtecs of southern Oaxaca in Mexico to produce auditory hallucinations and a state of half-sleep.

Jay (2010) considers that 'drugs, and our response to them, are the product of an elaborate evolutionary dance between the plant and animal kingdoms that has been underway for at least 300 million years' (p.10). It is acknowledged that many animals seek out intoxicating and hallucinogenic plants. Jay gives numerous examples. The domestic cat becomes ecstatic with catnip, Siberian bears and reindeer clearly enjoy the fly agaric mushroom, and baboons chew tobacco. He suggests that sometimes it was the observation of animal behaviours that led humans to use particular drugs. For example, goats become frisky when they consume coffee beans; perhaps the Ethiopian farmers noted this and were prompted to experiment. Perhaps the peoples of the South Pacific made the ceremonial and ritual stimulant drink *kava*, because they observed rats eating the tubers of *Piper methysticum* and becoming intoxicated. Even in very early times, drug taking acquired a sense of ritual and required paraphernalia. Pipes, dated prior to 2000 BCE, containing the residue of *Anadenanthera* seeds were found in the Andes of northwest Argentina. In the ceremonial centre of Chevin, in the Peruvian Andes, there is visual evidence of the effects of mind-altering drugs in carved stone heads, which exhibit the transformation from human to jaguar. It

---

4   LSD was 'discovered' in 1943, by the chemist Albert Hoffman, who was investigating the vasoconstrictive actions of derivatives of the ergot fungus. He took a small experimental dose and experienced massive changes in his perception of the world.

is thought that this shape-shifting phenomenon was again due to *Anadenanthera*, which contains dimethyltryptamine (DMT), a powerful hallucinogen. Some drugs have important cultural roles, especially in relation to social interactions – witnessed in the kava culture in the South Pacific, tobacco in the Native American peace pipe, betel chewing in Indonesia, and the peyote cult in Mexico (Jay 2010).

Jay (2010) also gives an insight into the botanist and taxonomist Linnaeus, who called himself 'God's registrar' and has much to tell us about early European attitudes to, and uses of, the psychotropic drugs that were arriving from the Old World and the New World. In 1749 Linnaeus published his *Materia Medica*, which included all known medicinal plants, and in 1753 he completed his *Species Plantarum* that described over 8000 plants in great detail. However, he was also interested in mind-altering drugs, and published an inventory called *Inebrianta*. By inebriants, he meant the psychoactive drugs, and he included drugs from Europe, such as poppies and the nightshades, Turkish *hashish* and Persian *bhang*, the seeds of *Pegamum harmala*, and the New World drugs such as tobacco, coffee, cacao and tea. Despite his global perspective, his classification of these drugs was interesting. He maintained that there were three types – natural, artificial (which included alcohol and distilled spirits) and mythical, which referred to the drugs of classical antiquity and those of mythology. Linnaeus was horrified by the deleterious effects of distilled spirits, which he had witnessed in his travels, and even some of his own students had indulged in excessive drinking. In *Inebrianta* he used mythology to illustrate the dangers of drugs. For example, he suggested that Circe's potion which transformed Odysseus's men into pigs was a warning that an uncontrolled appetite for intoxication could lead to 'mental and physical degradation'. He was very suspicious of coffee which 'drained vigour and induced early senility' (p.69), but he did smoke tobacco, which he maintained would prevent infection.

In the West, the hippie movement of the 1960s returned to the use of entheogens and incense in order, at least initially, to stress the importance of the inner experience, of fantasy as an 'inner landscape' and transcendence (Durgnat 1969). In the middle decades of the twentieth century we can also see ethnographers becoming psychonauts. For example, Aldous Huxley described his experience with mescaline in *The Doors of Perception* (1954). Perhaps the most notable example is Carlos Castaneda (circa 1925–1995), who ingested entheogens such as the mescaline-containing peyote, *Datura innoxia*, and *Psilocybe* mushrooms under the guidance of a Yaqui Indian, Don Juan Matus. Castaneda, through his experiences and writing, clarified many aspects of shamanism, thus inspiring neoshamanism, which has influenced New Age ideologies (DuBois 2009). The psychedelic drug tradition can also be seen in many of the popular song lyrics of the era, such as 'Lucy in the Sky with Diamonds' (The Beatles) and 'White Rabbit' (Jefferson Airplane). Saniotis (2010) analysed the use of psychotropics from both evolutionary and anthropological perspectives. This investigation led him to conclude that since prehistoric times psychotropic agents have served several purposes, including promoting altered states of consciousness for religious and recreational purposes, cognitive enhancement, strengthening group identity, reproductive success, and as food. Because of this close association, and the importance of these human drives, 'psychotropic and mood-altering substances will continue to have a considerable impact on future human societies' (p.482).

Heffern's paper 'The catechism of our senses: earth and spirit' (2010) eloquently reflects the return to a healthy perspective on scent and the senses within a spiritual context. He says that 'in the catechism of our senses we can taste and see that God is good', and: 'My own religious upbringing was scented with candle wax, wine and incense. Good healthy religions have always held sacred the senses, both in sacrament and ritual.' This echoes the view held by Howes (1998), who stresses the importance of the senses in healing. He commented that biomedicine 'does little to engage the senses' and that the cosmological integration and multisensory character that are prevalent in diverse ethnomedical traditions have much to teach us about our practice of separating the senses and letting the visual dominate. He comments that many studies have shown the use of ritual with chants, music, percussion, movement, dance, touch and scent to be vital to the healing process. Many of these cultures are 'polyphasic' – that is, cultures where knowledge emerges from altered states of consciousness (ASC) rather than ordinary states of consciousness. Such cultures have used incense, smoke and entheogens in a very specific context – shamanism.

Smoke and the shamanic state of consciousness

Craffert (2011) broadly defines shamanism or the shamanic complex as:

> ...a family of traditions which, as a regularly occurring pattern in many cultural systems, consists of a configuration of controlled ASC experiences and certain social functions that flow from these experiences and that benefit a community. (p.152)

A shaman is essentially a practitioner who enters an ASC to commune with the spirit world in order to act as a diviner, healer or teacher. Sometimes this trance state is called a shamanic state of consciousness (SSC). Early evidence for shamanic practice is found in rock art in South Africa, dated 27,000 BCE (DuBois 2009; Witzel 2011), and many elements of shamanism can be seen in ancient Hindu, Zoroastrian and Greek practices. The first recognition of the shamanic complex was in the Siberian hunting tribes, and the word 'shaman' comes from their word šaman, used by the Tungus people to mean 'one who is excited, moved, raised', or the Tungus–Mongol word meaning 'to know'.

Most versions of shamanism involve concepts such as the shamanic or soul journey, where the consciousness is freed from the physical body and travels to the realms of the specific cosmology of the culture – usually an upper, middle or lower world. The SSC may also involve visions, possession by spirits or transformation into animal form, again dependant on the cultural beliefs. The shaman will usually undertake this to serve the community. Healing will often involve soul retrieval, exorcism, in cultures where spirit possession appears, or removal of malevolent influences from demonic or human sources. Shamans may also act as psychopomps, guiding souls to the afterlife. They can act as mediators with the spirit world to ensure protection and the wellbeing of the community, especially when affected by natural elements such as weather, fire or flooding. Hunting is assisted too, as the shaman will release the soul of the animals so that they are not angered or hurt. Shamans are also the sages, teachers and prophets of their societies, creating and preserving myths, tribal knowledge and traditions (Menezes Júnior and Moreira-Almeida 2009; Craffert 2011).

There are several routes to entering an ASC, which is essentially a biopsychosocial phenomenon. In religious contexts we see sleep deprivation during vigils and prayer, and fasting will also bring about visions. Ritual practices can involve chanting, drumming and dancing to induce an ASC brought on by a sensory overload. Craffert (2011) lists several of the hundreds of identifiable states of consciousness: dreams, daydreams, nightmares, sleeping, drowsiness before sleep, semi-consciousness preceding waking, hallucinations, illusions, visions, a loss of the sense of self or of reality, sexual ecstasy, mystical ecstasy, hysteria, trance, stupor, coma and expanded consciousness. He goes on to discuss the many ways in which ASCs are reached: deliberate (meditation, breath control), accidental (highway hypnosis), artificial (natural or synthetic drugs), natural setting (drumming, dancing); how the states can vary from light to deep, and how they can be religious or pathological.

Menezes Júnior and Moreira-Almeida (2009) conducted a literature review to identify some of the criteria that would differentiate between spiritual experiences and mental disorders of religious content. Freud considered that religion was an 'obsessive neurosis', and in psychiatry the mystical experience is often regarded as a psychotic episode or borderline psychosis. In order to bring about a balanced perspective on the SSC, we do need to consider what constitutes pathological and non-pathological mystical experiences. The main distinguishing criteria of the *non*-pathological mystical experience are absence of suffering, absence of lasting functional impairment, short duration, a critical attitude regarding the objective reality of the experience, compatibility with the individual's cultural background, absence of comorbidities, control over the experience, and that the experience promotes personal growth over time and is directed towards others. Although these criteria have not been tested in controlled studies, we could reasonably assume that the SSC is indeed a spiritual experience, and not a pathological disorder.

In polyphasic cultures it is believed that the world is also inhabited by spirits who affect all living beings and societies. These spirits may be good or bad, and it is the shaman who can communicate with them. Sixty-five thousand years ago humans moved out of Africa, from west to east. Shamanic 'heat' is a feature of non-Siberian, 'southern shamanism' – a very ancient form of practice. The *Khoi-San* bushmen of central Tanzania have a communal dance accompanied by singing, which ends with a trance collapse, and produces 'heat' from which energy may be drawn. *San* shamans master the art of drawing the heat up from the base of the spine, and use the energy for healing. Here there are obvious similarities with kundalini yoga. Andamanese shamans off the Burmese coast are known as *Oko-Jumu*, meaning 'dreamers'. Rather than dancing, they dream, meet with the spirits in the jungle, 'die' and return to life. Here the heat is called *kimil*, meaning 'hot'. The Australian Aboriginal shamans are known as *karadji* and *maban*, 'clever men'. Their initiation involves a symbolic death and recreation, complete with internal rainbow snakes, crystals and totem animals – all symbolic of the transformation. Their shamanic journey is accomplished by riding on the Rainbow Snake. Again, learning to control the heat that rises from the base of the spine is a feature of their practice (Witzel 2011).

In the Siberian tradition the adept usually has a crisis, sometimes in dreams, which leads them to believe that they have been chosen to be recreated and educated by the spirits; this involves an initiation followed by a long apprenticeship. The shamanic initiatory crisis appears very similar to psychosis, with involuntary shaking, and is coupled with physical illness or a near-death experience. The initiation involves travel to the spirit world, being taken apart and reassembled; tokens and crystals may be implanted – again, all features of transformation. Eventually the shaman embodies their spirit guardian, and when the SSC is reached through ritual, the shaman can travel to the other worlds and communicate with the spirits. Animal guides can be evoked to aid on the vision quest. Often the journey is symbolised by a tree or pathway – the *axis mundi*. Shamanic knowledge includes an understanding of local plants and rocks, especially quartz, as it can animate spirits. There are risks; some of the plants used are toxic, some spirits are dangerous, there may be enemy shamans – and if a shaman does not return from the journey, they will die. The Siberian variety of shamanism is found in northern cultures, such as in Scandinavia, Europe, South and Southeast Asia, Korea, Japan, Nepal, Borneo, and many tribes in the Americas.

Entheogens and hallucinogens in shamanic practice

DuBois (2009) explores some of the entheogens used in shamanic practice, noting the powerful link with music, which, like the psychotropic agents, often defines and frames the ritual. Not all of the entheogens he discusses are noted aromatics, or burned in incense, but they are well-known hallucinogens. *Amanita muscaria*, the fly agaric mushroom, is used in Siberia; plants belonging to the genus *Datura* are used in North America and in Europe, and *Atropa belladonna* (deadly nightshade) was used in North America and Europe for magical purposes – it was known as 'sorcerer's cherry' or 'witch's berry'. He also highlights peyote, from the cacti *Lophophora williamsii* and *L. diffusa*, which are widespread in the desert areas of northern Mexico and southern Texas. Peyote is considered to be a central element in the spiritual lives of the Huichol Indians and it is used widely by Native American communities. Peyote is usually shared and dispensed by the shaman, so that he may guide the community on a collective journey under his protection. Collins (1968) described the peyote ceremony of the Taos Indians of Central Mexico in detail. Incense is part of the material paraphernalia, along with the shaman's staff, drum and rattle, altar and fireplace complex, ritual foods and water, and, of course, peyote. The ceremony itself involves prayer, songs, drumming and preaching, underpinned by references to the gods, the supernatural and supporting myths.

Native peoples of the Americas also used tobacco, *Nicotiana rustica* and *N. tobacum*, for blessing and purification. Shamans would use it to drive away evil influences and remove disease. Smoking tobacco also allowed the sharing of spiritual experiences. Alderete *et al.* (2010) analysed ceremonial tobacco use in the Andes, with special reference to the *Pachamama* ceremony. This ceremony reflects the Andean world view that the land, the people and the cosmos are interrelated. In Andean societies, spiritual significance is implicated in the activities of daily life; *Pacha*, or 'Mother Earth', is honoured and respected, and in return provides life, healing and sustenance. The *Pachamama* ceremony is a ritual in which tobacco honours and allows communication with Mother Earth; as its magic is released in smoke, it diffuses upwards with messages to and from the world of the spirits. The spirits' responses are read in the ashes, by the elders, who have the knowledge to interpret and decipher the signs.

The Huichol Indians of Mexico use wild tobacco, *Nicotiana rustica*, known as *yé*, in ceremonies such as those held for deer hunting and peyote hunts and feasts. Wild tobacco itself is said to induce visions; the Warao Indians of Venezuela smoke tobacco and fast, producing an ecstatic dream state or trance, while the *shreipiari*, the Campa shamans of Peru, use massive doses to see and communicate with the spirit world. The Huichols sometimes use a system of violent inhalation and swallowing the smoke to induce stupor and intoxication. In several New World societies tobacco is often mixed with other substances in shamanic practice. For example, the Warao Indians mix tobacco with the aromatic resin of *Protium heptaphyllum*, and in Mexico tobacco is mixed with the leaves of *Ephedra nevadensis*. *Chimó*, a mixture used in Venezuela, contains many aromatics such as tonka bean (for a sweet, vanilla-like flavour), anise (to sweeten and reduce harshness), cloves, *Agave cocui* liquor, nutmeg (a hallucinogen), vanilla, crude sugar, opium and the leaves of *Palicourea chimó*. The medicine pipe of the Shoshone Indians of North America contained not only tobacco but also desert trumpet (*Erigonium* species), and the Paiutes added *kinni-kinnick* (quinine bush, bear berry, prince's pine and sandwort) to their tobacco. A mixture of tobacco and sumac (*Rhus glabra*) leaves is also widespread – not only for recreational use, but also as a purifying smoke. The Huichols are noted for their use of *tumutsáli* or *yahutli* – *Tagetes lucida* (a type of marigold) – either on its own or mixed with tobacco. This was an important plant, with a pungent and fragrant scent, and narcotic and mildly toxic properties. It was used to alleviate fear, and one of its uses was to dull the senses of those about to be sacrificed to *Heuheuotl*. The Huichols enjoy the scent of this plant, removing the flowering tops, and holding them to the face for hours, simply as an aromatic inhalation, or offering bunches in temples and shrines. When smoked with *yé*, it was thought to help with inhalation and also facilitate intoxication and visions; however, in ceremonies led by the *mara'akame* this is often accompanied by ingestion of peyote and fermented beverages producing vivid hallucinations (Siegel, Collings and Diaz 1977). So, until the components of the *yé/tumutsáli* smoking mixture are identified, we will not know for sure if it is a psychotropic. Siegel *et al.* (1977) quote a salient observation from Brooks (1952), who identified why tobacco had become so important in ritual and shamanic practice:

> Tobacco fully met the conditions which primitive people required of a plant set aside at first for magic or ritualism. It contained an element which could induce a form of trance, it was readily consumed by the cleansing power of fire, its perfumed smoke arose subtly to the abode of the gods and it had other virtues of magic. From the immaterial, visible substances of smoke, dreams could be materialised. (p.21)

This is all in stark contrast with the western, materialistic world view, and the secular use of tobacco and psychotropic drugs. However, Pennacchio *et al.* (2010) comment that nowadays, across the globe, most people smoke tobacco for pleasure, or indeed to help ease social interactions or deal with the pressures of modern living, and that its active constituent, nicotine, is 'one of the most physiologically demanding and addictive substances on Earth.' (p.17). In the East the opium poppy, *Papavera somnifera*, was smoked in Middle Eastern and Asian shamanism. Jay (2010) explores the text of Thomas De Quincey's *Confessions of an English Opium Eater* (1822), which claimed that opium 'brought a profound sense of order to the conscious mind, allowing it to explore its own hidden byways and secret passages' (p.81); perhaps this is an insight into the experiences of the eastern shamans?

In the Amazon region a variety of plants, including *Banisteriopsis caapi* (Saniotis 2010), are brewed to form a thick liquid known as *ayahuasca*, the recipe being tailored for specific hallucinogenic effects. Usually, the ceremony consists of a small group sitting in semi-darkness, while a shaman sings songs with rapid rhythms, known as *icaros*, to maintain the experiential flow. Ayahuasca contains dimethyltryptamine (DMT), which is associated with transformation into animal form – usually that of powerful predators such as big cats (especially jaguars), pythons or snakes. This is apparently a very traumatic, agonising and terrifying ordeal; so this practice is certainly not for pleasure, but for immersion in the spirit world, perhaps in other than human form (Jay 2010).

Aromatic smoke in shamanic practice

There are numerous examples of the use of aromatic smoke in shamanic practice. Dannaway (2010) writes: 'The shaman, standing between the two worlds, was the master of the fire, inhaling the smoke for ecstatic trances and bathing in the smoke for healing and the power to heal' (p.485). The idea of bathing in smoke is seen in Native American Indian sweat lodges and the smudging ceremony: smudging is the burning of specific herbs, and the smoke is taken in the hands and directed, or 'brushed' over the body or a place, accompanied by prayer; sometimes a feather may be used. The purpose is purification and to drive out negative influences. In the ceremonial context this is carried out by an elder or shaman so that the ceremony is entered in the right spirit. The most significant aromatics in smudging are various species of *Salvia* (sage) and *Artemisia*, 'cedar' (usually species of *Juniperus* and *Thuja*, and *Calocedrus decurrens*) and sweetgrass (*Hierochloe odorata*). The main use of sage is to drive away bad influences and keep them away during the ceremony. The floors of sweat lodges are often strewn with sage, and the leaves are used to wrap ceremonial pipes. The common sage, *Salvia vulgaris*, is used, as are sagebrush (*Artemisia californica*) and mugwort (*A. vulgaris*). Cedar is burned during prayers, so that the rising smoke carries the prayer to the Creator. It may also accompany sage on the sweat lodge floor – like sage, it drives away negativity, but brings in good influences too. Desert white cedar (*Juniperus monosperina*), eastern red cedar or Virginian cedar (*Juniperus virginiana*), western red cedar (*Thuja occidentalis*) and California incense cedar (*Calocedrus decurrens*) have all been used in smudging ceremonies. Sweetgrass is also known as 'vanilla grass' and 'holy grass'; its botanical name is *Hierochloe odorata*. The grass is usually formed into braids, and burned after sage and cedar to bring in good spirits and to accompany prayers to the Creator.

Bathing in smoke which is generated in sauna-like chambers can also be seen in Ethiopia. Women would cleanse and scent their bodies with the smoke of *Hildebrandtia* and *Acacia* species in this traditional cleansing method. These species were also burned as incense. For a selection of smokes used in shamanism and smudging, and other traditional practices, please refer to Table 3.1.

Table 3.1 A selection of plants used for purposes including incense, smoke and shamanism

Compiled and adapted from Pennacchio *et al.* (2010).

Botanical species	Location	Incense or shamanic use
Abies balsamea (balsam fir)	Iceland, North America.	Incense in Iceland. Used by Native Americans as incense in sweat baths to relieve coughs and colds.
Abies lasiocarpa (Rocky Mountain fir)	Montana, Wyoming, Oklahoma, Oregon.	The Crow used the twigs as incense and in ceremony. The Blackfoot used it in smudges. The Cheyenne used it to drive out bad influences, and the Nez Perce burned the boughs in sweat lodges.
Abies spectabilis (Himalayan fir)	Nepal.	Incense.
Abies species (firs)	Germany, Switzerland. Unspecified location.	The resins and needles of fir trees are used to make incense candles at Christmas. The resin and needles are used in shamanic incense along with black henbane, juniper, common mugwort, yew and wild thyme.
Acacia senegal (gum Arabic)	Ethiopia, Kenya.	The wood was used as incense.
Acer negundo (box elder)	North America.	Native Indians used this as incense.
Achillea millefolium (yarrow)	North America.	The Potawatomi used yarrow in a smudge to repel evil from comatose patients. Many other tribes smoked the dried flowering heads for ceremonial purposes.
Acorus calamus (sweet flag)	India.	A sacred herb; used in incense and as a fumigant.
Alyxia species	South Vietnam, Thailand, Java, North America.	The root, bark or the entire plant is used in incenses.

Botanical species	Location	Incense or shamanic use
Amyris balsamifera and *A. elemifera* (balsam torchwood and torchwood)	Latin America, Caribbean.	Balsam torchwood – resin is a popular incense in Cuba, Jamaica, and Puerto Rico. Torchwood resin is used as incense and for voodoo ceremonies in Montserrat.
Aquilaria species (agarwood)	Indo-Malaysia.	Widely used as incense.
Artemisia indica and *A. japonica* (mugwort and Japanese wormwood)	Nepal.	Incense.
Artemisia ludoviciana (white sagebrush)	North America.	The Sioux and the Meskwaki prepared smoke smudges and purification incenses from the white sagebrush.
Artemisia vulgaris (common mugwort)	Nepal.	Used as incense in the Manang District.
Aster species (aster)	North America.	Used by several Native American communities in smudges and sweat baths for reviving unconscious patients, and for warding off evil influences.
Atropa mandragora (mandrake)	Ancient Greece (Delphic Oracle).	Used by the Pythia to induce visions.
Boswellia carteri (frankincense)	The Middle East, Mediterranean.	This oleo-gum resin has widespread use as incense.
Boswellia serrata (Indian frankincense)	India.	Sacred throughout India; the resin is used as an incense in magico-religious ceremonies to drive away evil and hasten the recovery of the sick.
Brugmansia species	South America.	The leaves were added to tobacco and smoked. This material was given to women and slaves who were to be buried alive, to deaden the senses.
Bryonia dioica (white bryony)	Egypt.	Used by the ancient Egyptians as an incense to drive demons away.

Bursera bipinnata (copal)	Mesoamerica.	The resin was used by the Huichol as incense.
Bursera gummifera (mastic tree)	Mesoamerica.	The Maya used this as incense.
Bursera species	Mesoamerica.	The smoke of the resin was associated with hunting and purification of the prey – notably by the Chorti Maya of Guatemala and the Sierra Popoluca of Tehuantepec.
Calea zacatechichi (Mexican dreamherb)	Mesoamerica.	The Chontal of Mexico used this to communicate with spirits.
Calophyllum inophyllum (Alexandrian laurel)	East Africa.	In the former Tanzanian area the leaves were pounded and macerated in oil; this mixture was cooked on a fire and the fumes would be inhaled by people said to be possessed by the devil.
Cananga odorata (ylang ylang)	Indonesia.	Incense.
Canarium luzonicum (pili nut; elemi tree)	Philippines.	Elemi resin is used as incense.
Cannabis sativa (hemp)	Global.	Kathmandu, India – smoked in preparation for meditation. Gaddi Tribe, Pradesh – smoked the resin of female plants to produce hallucinations. Buganda, Africa and Gilgit District, Pakistan – smoked the leaves and flowers to produce euphoria. Ancient Assyrians – a fumigation to dispel sorrow or grief. Ancient Greece – the smoke was used to inspire visions at the Delphic Oracle, perhaps along with bay laurel. The Tenethara of Brazil – smoked the flowers and leaves for their psychoactive properties. Also used by many cultures for its medicinal properties and as an insect repellent.

Botanical species	Location	Incense or shamanic use
Cedrus libani (cedar of Lebanon)	Iran.	The pulverised wood was mixed with herbs and resins to make incense.
Chamaemelum nobile (Roman chamomile)	England.	The dried flower heads were used to flavour tobacco.
Cinnamomum burmanii (Indonesian cassia)	Indonesia.	Used in Java as incense.
Cinnamomum camphora (camphor tree)	India, China.	Used as incense in Hindu temples. Venerated by the Chinese.
Cinnamomum verum (scent of paradise)	Ancient Egypt and others.	Burned with herbs and resins for incense purposes.
Commiphora abyssinica (Abyssinian myrrh)	Ethiopia.	Known as *kerbe*, incense.
Commiphora erythraea (opopanax)	Ancient and classical world.	This was a major aromatic in ancient times; it was the main species of myrrh; the resin was used as incense.
Commiphora myrrha (Harobol myrrh)	Arabia, Somaliland, Ethiopia.	The resin is burned as incense.
Commiphora wightii (Indian bdellium tree)	India.	Rajasthan – the smoke from the burning resin was used to drive away evil spirits and please the gods. Sacred throughout India, burned on holy occasions. Known to the Bengali as *guggul*.
Cornus species (dogwood)	North America.	Smoked, sometimes mixed with tobacco, for pleasure and in ceremony.
Cryptomeria japonica (tsugi pine)	Nepal.	Incense.

Cupressus lusticana (cedar of Goa)	Uganda (Bulamogi County).	Smoke kept spirits at bay.
Cupressus torulosa (Himalayan cypress)	Nepal.	Incense.
Cymbopogon densiflorus (lemongrass)	Tanzania.	The shamans of Tanzania smoked the flowers (sometimes with tobacco) to induce prophetic dreams.
Cyprus bulbosus (galangal)	Maldives.	The fragrant roots and tubers are used as incense.
Cyprus species (flatsedges)	East Africa.	Called *muudiudi*, preparation of incense sticks.
Cytisus canariensis (genista)	Mexico.	Dried flowers were smoked by the Yaqui shamans for psychotropic effects.
Datura innoxia (prickly burr)	India, Pakistan.	Sacred in the north. Seeds and leaves smoked in southern Pakistan; small doses are euphoric but large doses cause 'madness'.
Datura stramonium[5] (jimsonweed and other) *Datura* species (thorn apple)	Global use.	The common name is derived from Jamestown in Virginia, USA, where British troops consumed the leaves in a salad; its effects (they 'went crazy' for 11 days) meant that they failed to quell a slave rebellion. India – sacred plant, used for narcotic purposes.

5   *Datura stramonium* is a herbaceous annual with large (8–10cm long) white or purple blossoms. These are closed during the day and open at night, when they emit a pungent odour which attracts their pollinators, the night butterflies. The plant is known as 'devil's grass' or 'witchgrass' and it has been widely used by spiritual shamans in Native American Indian culture, and earlier by European Druids. Its extracts can be used therapeutically, but for hallucinogenic effects the seeds are chewed or the dried leaves are smoked. It has been banned because of its toxicity; between 5 and 8 per cent of those who have experimented out of curiosity have died as a result. This is because there is a very narrow range between the active and lethal dose, and even if the dose is not lethal, serious poisoning can result. Despite this, it is thought that the use of *D. stramonium* is more widespread than reported – for example occurring in the USA, France and Italy – and the plant is widely available (Stella *et al.* 2010).

Botanical species	Location	Incense or shamanic use
Datura stramonium (jimsonweed and other) *Datura* species (thorn apple)	Global use.	North India – known as *dhatura*. Used by the shamans (*dumbus*) of the Shuhi, a Tibeto-Burman ethnic group in southwest China. Native American Indians (including the Cherokee, and in the Appalachians) – smoked as a hallucinogen. Ancient Greece – used at the Delphic Oracle. *Datura* is highly toxic; there is a worldwide ban on smoking jimsonweed and related species.
Erigeron canadensis (horseweed)	North America.	Native Americans smoked the flowers for pleasure; they were also smoked as hunting charms and used in sweat lodges.
Erythrophleum suaveolens (coca)	South America.	Originally chewed by the aboriginal peoples of the Andes to promote endurance; now snorted or smoked to induce euphoria. In southern Bolivia the plant is used in smoke offerings to the gods.
Geijera parviflora (Australian willow)	Australia.	The baked and powdered leaves were smoked with other narcotics to induce drowsiness in ceremonies.
Gonstylus species (including aloe wood)	Java, Indonesia, Malaysia.	The wood and its oil are used in incense.
Guaiacum species (lignum vitae)	Mexico.	The Aztecs burned the resin for medicinal and aphrodisiacal purposes.
Hanghomia marseillei (hanghomia)	Laos.	The roots were burned as incense in the pagodas.
Hedychium spicatum (perfume ginger)	Ethiopia.	Incense; known as *afer kocher*, it is sold and burned in the markets at Jima.

Helichrysum italicum (curry plant)	Italy.	In Tuscany, on Christmas Eve, the smoke from burning branches is used to ward off the evil eye.
Helichrysum species (everlasting)	South Africa.	Many species are used by peoples such as the Zulu, as an incense to ward off evil and invoke the goodwill of the ancestors, and smoked by the shamans to induce trance for healing and for hallucinogenic effects.
Heracleum lanatum (hogweed)	North America.	The Native Americans would burn this because the smoke drove away the spirit Sokênau who could steal hunting luck. The Gitskan mixed it with red elder bark and juniper berries for a smudge to repel witchcraft.
Hierochloe odorata (sweetgrass)	North America.	The Kiowa of New Mexico – incense purposes. The Cheyenne – ceremonial purification incense; and as a smudge in homes to repel evil. The Blackfoot and Sioux – burned to purify sundancers. The Blackfoot – smoked leaves mixed with tobacco, for pleasure. The Montana tribes – burned for protection and purification. Other Native Americans – burned leaves to summon the tribe's guardian spirits for protection against thunder and lightning.
Hoslundia opposite (orange bird lantern)	Tanzania.	As part of a smoke that was inhaled to drive away the devil.
Hymeaea courbaril (stinking toe, known locally as copal)	Caribbean.	Rosin (a 'fossil' resin that collects in the soil around the roots) is made into incense cakes for use in churches.
Hymenaea species (locust, palo jiote tree)	Amazon, Caribbean, Guatemala.	The resins were used as incense.

Botanical species	Location	Incense or shamanic use
Hyoscyamus species *H. albus* (white henbane)	Europe.	Used in the Delphic Oracle of ancient Greece, for prophesy. It was also a common ingredient in witches' brews.
H. boveanus (Egyptian henbane)	Egypt.	The flowers were mixed with tobacco and smoked as a psychotropic by the Bischarin and Khushmaan Bedouins; the Arabic name is *saykaran*, 'to become intoxicated'.
H. muticus (henbane)	Egypt.	The smoke could induce a state of narcosis; used by Bedouin thieves on their victims.
H. niger (black henbane)	Europe.	This is the most toxic of the henbanes, but it has a long tradition of use. In Europe the seeds were burned on St John the Baptist's birthday (23 June) since the fourth century CE – to protect farm animals and children from evil, witches, illness and misfortune. Nowadays the fires are made with brushwood. It was also used by witches for its hallucinogenic effects, either in brews or smoked.
	India.	In India and Europe the smoke also had medicinal uses.
	Kashmir.	In Kashmir it was smoked as a hallucinogen.
Ipomoea crassipes (morning glory) *I. pellita* (ground morning glory) *I. purpurea* (common morning glory)	South Africa.	The Zulu used the smoke from the roots as a charm for fertility and protection of the fields.

Iris missouriensis (Rocky Mountain iris)	North America.	In an example of unscrupulous practice, the shamans of the Klamath would mix the dried roots with tobacco and poisonous *Camassia* species for their patients to smoke. This would make them ill, so they would then pay the shaman for more help.
Iris versicolor (harlequin blueflag)	North America.	Native Indians treated their clothing with the smoke; it afforded protection from bites during snake dances.
Juniperus communis (juniper)	Europe, North America. Italy. Alaska.	Widespread use as a disinfecting fumigant. In Tuscany and other parts of Italy branches are burned on Christmas Eve to ward off the evil eye. The Dena'ina of Alaska use the needles as incense.
Juniperus excelsa (Greek juniper)	Iran.	The needles are burned as incense.
Juniperus horizontalis (creeping juniper)	North America.	The Cheyenne burn the needles and twigs in ceremonies to drive away thunder. The Crow use it in incantations.
Juniperus macropoda (pencil cedar)	Pakistan. India.	The Hanzahut of Pakistan shamans (*bitans*) inhale the smoke of the pencil cedar, dance and drink fresh blood from goats' heads to aid communion with the spirit world, where they receive advice on healing the sick. It is used as incense (*dhup*) in the Ladakh region. In the Lahoul valley the Lamas of the Yurnat tribe use its smoke, along with chanting, to drive away evil spirits who have possessed their patients.
Juniperus scopularium (Rocky Mountain juniper)	North America.	The Cheyenne use smoke from the leaves and twigs as incense, and to afford protection from thunder and lightning.

Botanical species	Location	Incense or shamanic use
Juniperus virginiana (Virginian cedar, eastern red cedar)	North America.	The smoke was used by Native Americans as incense, to eliminate nervousness and bad dreams, for purification in ceremonies and rituals. The Kiowa burned the needles as incense during prayers at peyote meetings.
Juniperus species (juniper)	North America. Scotland. Nepal.	Widely used by the Comanche, Dakota, Omaha, Pawnee and others as a fumigant, for purification, to stop bad dreams, as incense during prayer. On Colonsay (an island in the Inner Hebrides) juniper smoke was used to cleanse houses and stables not only of pests and diseases, but also of evil spirits. Burned during the *puja* ceremony before attempts at climbing Mount Everest.
Lantana viburnoides (lantana)	Tanzania.	The dried and powdered leaves were burned to drive away the devil.
Laurus nobilis (bay laurel)	Delphi, Greece.	Smoke from the leaves (possibly along with cannabis) was used by the Pythia to induce a trance.
Liquidambar orientalis (oriental sweetgum)	Asia, Asia Minor.	The semi-solid gum – Levant storax – was used as a fumigant.
Liquidambar styraciflua (sweetgum)	Cyprus. Central and North America.	Bark and wood were burned as incense in the orthodox liturgy. It is known as *xylon tau Aphenti* (wood of the Lord). The resin was burned; known as American storax. The Aztec used it with tobacco, and as incense.
Lobelia tupa (devil's tobacco)	Chile.	The Mapuche smoke the leaves for their psychoactive effects.

Matricaria chamomilla (chamomile)	Libya.	The flowers were added to smoking tobacco to enhance the flavour.
Melilotus officinalis (yellow sweet clover)	Siberia, Ukraine.	The top leaves and flowers were used to enhance the flavour of tobacco.
Mentha aquatica (watermint)	South Africa.	The dried leaves were smoked to treat mental illness.
Michelia champaca (golden champa)	Tamil Nadu.	The dried flowers were burned by the Nilgiris hill tribes at night, to repel mosquitos.
Myrica gale (sweetgale)	North America.	The Potawatomi burned sweetgale as a smoke smudge to repel mosquitos.
Myroxylon balsamum (balsam of Peru)	Amazon.	The powdered bark was burned as incense, and to treat earache.
Nardostachys grandiflora (spikenard)	Nepal.	The dried leaves were burned as incense.
Nardostachys jatamansi (muskroot)	India.	In the Sikkim Himalayas the roots were burned to drive away evil spirits.
Nicotiana rustica (wild tobacco)	Nicaragua.	Tobacco is smoked by the *sukyas*, native healers (shamans) in large quantities, to communicate with the spirits about healing.
Peganum harmala (African rue, Syrian rue, wild rue, harmala)	Ladakh, India.	In the Ladakh region the leaves are burned as incense and the seeds were smoked to 'induce a feeling of exaltation' and for exorcisms; they are also a traditional intoxicant and sexual stimulant, prevalent at wedding ceremonies. The subspecies *stenophyllum* was smoked and inhaled by the Garisia tribe of Rajasthan to relieve toothache.
Petunia violacea (shanin petunia)	Ecuador.	The dried herb was smoked to induce visions of flying.

Botanical species	Location	Incense or shamanic use
Peucedanum officinale and other species (hog's fennel and silverwort)	Ancient Egypt.	Used as incense and to repel insects.
Picea abies (Norway spruce)	Norway.	The resin was burned as incense with artemisia, juniper and yew at Christmas celebrations. Its resin was smoked by Siberian shamans.
Picea rubens (red spruce)	Iceland.	The cones were burned over coals to 'make a man happy'. Resin from the bark was used as winter incense.
Pimenta dioica (allspice)	Jamaica.	The wood was used to smoke jerked foods.
Pinus species	North America.	The smoke from the needles was used as a decongestant and to revive unconscious patients, and as incense; some species were smoked to bring luck in hunting. The sap of some species was collected for use as incense and to treat mental illness; it was also used by shamans in herbal mixtures to protect homes and possessions, and, if mixed with tobacco, it could produce hallucinations.
Pistacia lentiscus (chios mastic tree)	Cyprus, Sardinia. Iran.	The smoke was used to flavour meats. In Iran it was used as incense.
Pistacia terebinthus (terebinth)	Iran.	Smoke from the burning fruits was used to treat sore eyes.
Pogostemon hortensis (patchouli)	Java, Indonesia.	The leaves were used in the preparation of incense.
Polygonatum biflorum (King Solomon's seal)	North America.	The Meswaki heated the roots over hot coals to revive the unconscious. The Chippewa burned the scented roots to promote sleep.

Polygonatum pubescens (hairy Solomon's seal)	North America.	The dried and powdered roots were mixed with cedar leaves and twigs and burned as a smudge; the smoke was thought to revive a dying person. The Menomini believed the smoke would bring the dying back to life.
Populus balsamifera, and other spp. (balsam poplar)	North America.	The bark and inner bark had many uses: insect repellent, smoking fish, smoking buckskins, smoke for pleasure with or without tobacco, used in kinni-kinnick mixtures.
Protium attenuatum (ensens)	West Indies.	Oleo-gum resin burned as incense.
Protium carana (carana)	Colombia.	Shamans added the resin to tobacco or coca leaves, and this was burned as ceremonial incense.
Protium copal (copal)	Central America.	The tree was sacred to the ancient Maya. Prized by the ancient Maya as incense, specifically at ritual offerings, when communing with gods, and ceremonies such as funerals. Its smoke was used therapeutically too – for stomach pain, fright, dizziness. The smoke was thought to stop heavy rain. Copal resin was also used by the San Andréas of Petén in Guatemala to expel sickness, and by the latex harvesters to ward off evil spirits.
Protium crenatum and *P. decandrum* (kurokai, copal capsi and other species)	Caribbean.	Church incense.
Protium icicariba (breu)	Brazil, the Amazon region.	The fragrance of the resin is of commercial importance; it is burned as incense.

Botanical species	Location	Incense or shamanic use
Rhazya stricta (harmal)	Oman.	In the Dhofar region the smoke was inhaled to relieve headaches and chest congestion, and its leaves were burned on campfires to protect from evil whilst sleeping.
Rhododendron anthopogon (anthopogon oil,[6] koont)	Nepal, Himalayas.	Used in Nepal as incense and to create a sacred space. In Tibetan medicine it is called *balu* or *sunpati*; an infusion of its leaves is used to aid digestion and sooth sore throats.
Rhus aromatica (fragrant sumac) and *R. glabra* (smooth sumac)	North America.	The Michaelma, Creek, Chocktaw and Lakota and (many others) use the red leaves (gathered in the fall) to give a pleasant aroma to tobacco; when mixed in equal proportions this was also used in peace pipes. The Oklahoma Delaware use the leaves and roots with tobacco for ceremonial use.
Rosa arkansana (prairie rose) and *R. woodsii* (wood's rose)	North America.	Native people smoked the inner bark with or without tobacco; the wood of *R. woodsii* was used to make pipe stems.
Rosmarinus officinalis (rosemary)	Ecuador, Belize.	Incense. Burned with copal resin to ward off evil spirits and envy.
Ruta graveolens (common rue)	North America.	Mixed with tobacco and smoked as a sedative, and to relieve neuralgia.
Ruta species	Morocco.	Mixed with other incense materials or rosemary to ward off the evil eye and to 'cure the bewitched'.
Salix humulis (upland willow) and *S. lucida* (shining willow)	North America.	The bark was used by Native Americans as a tobacco substitute. The Ojibwa toasted the bark and added it to kinni-kinnick smoking mixtures.

---

6   Anthopogon essential oil from Nepal has an earthy balsamic odour. It is dominated by α- and β-pinene, limonene, and δ-carene. It has anti-inflammatory, antimicrobial and anti-cancer activities (Innocenti *et al.* 2010). Its odour is said to aid meditation.

Salvia apiana (white sage)	California.	Used in traditional Chumash healing, dating back at least 13,000 years. More recently used as a healing smudge accompanied by prayer; the smoke would carry the prayers to God. The Cahuilla used it in sweat lodges for healing.
Salvia divinorum (sage of the diviners)	Mexico.	A hallucinogenic sage, used by shamans of the Sierra Mazateca in Oaxaca as an entheogen.
Sambucus nigra (European black elderberry)	Europe.	Although the smoke had uses in traditional folk healing practices, according to Celtic folklore the smoke was said to draw evil and bring bad luck.
Santalum album (sandalwood)	India, China, Egypt, Greece, Italy.	Widely valued as incense.
Saussurea lappa (costus root)	Tibet, India.	Smoked as an opium substitute. Incense; also as part of a mixture whose smoke would cause blindness in enemies and kill animals as far as the wind carried the smoke. The mixture included *Semecarpus anacardium* (marking nut tree), *Veronia anthelmintica* (ironweed) and unspecified animal parts.
Scopolia carniolica (nightshade)	Latvia, Lithuania.	The dried plant was smoked as an aphrodisiac and a psychoactive love potion.
Selinium tenuifolium (Cambridge milk parsley) and *S. wallichianum* (cow parsley)	India.	The Himachalol Hill people burned Cambridge milk parsley as incense in religious ceremonies. The Kumoan used the powdered roots of cow parsley in incense sticks, and in the Sikkim Himalayas the smoke from the roots was used to drive away evil spirits.
Senecio graveolens (strong-scented groundsel)	Chile.	The pre-Altiplanic people burned the leaves and stems as incense. The Navajo in Arizona smoke groundsel species in ceremonies.

Botanical species	Location	Incense or shamanic use
Shorea robusta (saul tree, sara)	India, Pakistan.	The smoke of the resin is an insect repellent and also used therapeutically. The resin is known as *dammar*, and was used as incense.
Sida acuta (axocatzin) and *S. rhombiflora* (common sida)	Mexico.	In coastal regions and the Gulf smoked as a cannabis substitute.
Solidago species (goldenrod)	North America.	The Ojibwa and others use the flowers in mixtures that were burned to simulate the odour of deer hooves, to attract deer. The Navajo call this 'blue lizard tobacco', smoked for pleasure.
Spartium junceum (Spanish broom)	Tuscany.	On Christmas Eve the smoke of burning branches was used to drive away the evil eye. Elsewhere the yellow flowers were smoked for their psychotropic effects.
Stachytarpheta cayennensis (*verveine*)	Central America.	A sacred herb of the ancient Maya; used to avert evil. In Belize used as incense.
Styrax species	The Americas, Java, Brazil, Paraguay, Cyprus.	The latex sap is burned as incense. The fumes of some species such as *S. tessmannii* may be psychoactive.
Tagetes lucida (sweet marigold)	Mexico.	The Aztecs used its smoke to dull the senses prior to execution, and in ceremonies. Mixed with wild tobacco for psychotropic effects, to induce visions.
Taxus baccata (English yew)	Europe.	Burned in shamanic incense mixtures and at Nordic Christmas celebrations.
Trichocereus pachanoi (San Pedro cactus)	Peru.	In Las Aldas remains of cigars have been found; probably smoked for psychoactive properties.
Tsuga dumosa (Himalayan hemlock)	Nepal.	The leaves were burned as incense.

Turnera diffusa (damiana)	Unspecified location.	The dried leaves were smoked for relaxation and for their pleasant aroma.
Valeriana hardwickii (Indian valerian), *V. jatamansi* (mushkbala), *V. wallichii* (valerian)	India, Nepal.	The leaves and roots are burned as incense and in magic-religious rituals. In India, mushkbala is a sacred plant, also known as *samyo*; it has an intense aroma.
Vetiveria zizanoides (vetivergrass)	Java.	The roots were burned as incense.
Virola species (virola)	South America.	The inner bark of some species was smoked as a hallucinogen. Also used by Brazilian shamans for its psychoactive properties.
Xanthorrhoea latifolia (mudigan), *X. preissii* (balga)	Australia.	The Arawaka of Byron Bay burn these 'grass trees' in campfires, for their pleasant smoke and insect repelling properties.
Ziziphus mauritiana (Indian jujube)	Somalia.	Used by Somali women to fumigate and perfume their hair.

Incense in ancient times

Anthropologist Brian Moeran (2009) writes that incense was used by most ancient civilisations, including, in alphabetical order, Assyrian, Babylonian, Buddhist, Chinese, Egyptian, Greek, Hebrew, Hindi, Japanese, Mayan, Minoan Cretan, Parthian (an ancient civilisation in northern Iran), Phoenician and Roman. In early Christianity, and until the fourth century BCE, incense was not used, not only to differentiate it from pagan or Jewish worship but also because at the time incense offerings were compulsory in Emperor worship. As Christianity grew, and its religious practices became more elaborate, incense use became part of normal worship (Harvey 1998). However, in time, incense reacquired its pagan associations, and was ultimately banned in Christian rites of worship by the reformers of the sixteenth century (Morris 1984).

Morris (1984) mentions the aromatics important to the Mesopotamians. Cedar of Lebanon was highly valued, and he comments that the name 'Lebanon' is derived from the word for incense, *lubbunu*. The Babylonians also favoured the conifers and their resins, especially pine, cypress and fir. Myrtle, which has a fresh, conifer resin-like scent, was also important, and sacred to their sun god Shamash, as were the fresh, piney-scented juniper berries and the intensely green galbanum. Morris also suggests that the Jewish incense cult, which began when the Jews were released from Babylonian captivity, was inspired by the Mesopotamians and not by Moses. On the Assyrians, Sumerians and Babylonians, Lawless (1994) writes that, apart from encouraging divine favour and protection, incense had an important role in purification (a practice still used in Buddhism).

The demand for incense ingredients, especially frankincense and myrrh, became considerable, and for over a thousand years the incense trade became of great economic importance. Pliny the Elder (23–79 CE), the Roman philosopher and natural historian, describes the Arabian incense trade at its peak, where caravans, with thousands of camels, the 'ships of the desert', transported the resins across Arabia to Alexandria in Egypt. The resins were processed in Alexandria before being taken to Greece, Rome and Mesopotamia (Pennacchio *et al.* 2010).

Gilman and Xun (2004) estimate that incense use began five or six thousand years ago. Julia Lawless (1994) conducted her literature research at the Warburg Institute in London, which specialises in classical antiquity and its influences on western culture (Steele 1994), and from this suggested that the earliest use of incense was in ancient China, followed by the Hindus, who would have created the first incense trail to Arabia and Egypt.

She also mentions that the use of incense in Egypt dates back to almost prehistoric times (Lawless 1994). The earliest written evidence would suggest that *sntr*, which translates as the word 'incense', was known from the Early Dynastic times, 2920–2575 BCE onward. This is the first mystery we are confronted by – we do not know the botanical identity of *sntr*. It is often juxtaposed with the word *'ntyw*, which led to the widespread belief that the ancient texts were referring to what we now call frankincense and myrrh. However, these core incenses are resins that were not indigenous to Egypt, and so this mystery has led to collaborative research between archaeologists and botanists. Frankincense and myrrh are gum-resins associated with Arabia, and it was thought that the ancient Egyptians imported their incense from Punt. Inscriptions on the temple of Queen Hatshepsut at Thebes indicate that she attempted to bring back 'incense trees' from Punt. The location of Punt is not clear, but is might have been the land between the eastern Sudan and the northwestern Ethiopian highlands, now modern Eritrea, where frankincense and myrrh trees still grow. Later, New Kingdom texts (1558–1085 BCE) make reference to *sntr* being imported from Syria and Palestine, but frankincense trees do not grow here, and myrrh is rare in this region. So, it has been suggested that *sntr* was the resin of a species in the genus *Pistacia* (which contains the familiar pistachio nuts), as originally proposed by Loret (1949) and later confirmed as *P. atlantica* in 1984, after examination of archaeological artefacts found in the cargo of a New Kingdom shipwreck (Serpico and White 2000).

Ancient Egypt and kyphi

The ancient Egyptians were renowned for their use of aromatics in many aspects of daily life, but especially in ritual and ceremony. This is not surprising, since they believed that fragrance had divine origins, having emanated from the eyes or bones of the deities, including the eye of the sun god, Re (Manniche 1999), and that scent was the sweat of the gods that had fallen to earth (Stamelman 2006). Incense and scent became a means of communication between the humans and the gods, and was of particular importance in ensuring a safe passage to the afterlife; hence its prominence in mortuary, funerary and temple rites. For example, each temple had a god or goddess who resided in their statue within an innermost sanctuary, and was the link between the divine and the earthly. Manniche (1999) quotes the Greek writer Plutarch (50–125 CE) regarding the daily rites performed in the sanctuary, not least the use of incense. At sunrise the sanctuary air would be purified and revived with the smell of resin, possibly frankincense, and at noon myrrh would be burned because its heat 'loosens and disintegrates the turbid and muddy mass which gathers in the atmosphere' (Griffiths 1970). At sunset the best-known of Egyptian incenses, *kyphi*, was burnt before the shrine was sealed again until sunrise. It was thought that the smoke from the incense would reach the god or goddess, even though they were not visible. Kyphi was also used to heighten awareness and the senses at other ritual ceremonies (Lawless 1994; Manniche 1999).

The actual ingredients of kyphi vary depending on the author. Manniche (1999) gives a comprehensive analysis not only of the evolution of various recipes for the incense and its spiritual effects, but also of its uses as a remedy to be ingested for various ailments. Here, perhaps for the first time but certainly not the last, we see how a perfume also has therapeutic and medicinal uses for body and soul. In the case of kyphi, its earliest therapeutic uses (circa 1500 BCE) were to prevent halitosis and perhaps to protect against malevolent gods, demons or spirits. Headaches were treated by anointing the forehead with kyphi. Kyphi would be consumed, perhaps mixed with wine, as an elixir for youth, but also as a treatment for epilepsy, ear problems, stomach and liver disorders and skin disease.

Given its prominence as incense, and the fact that it was not a single substance like myrrh or frankincense, but a complex mixture, it is worth looking at a few of its ingredients. There were several components – a base, gums and resins, herbs and spices. Some of these are familiar to us, while others are not; some are even difficult to identify because of changes in name and botanical language. Even in any one era, there would have been variants – for example, the sun and moon versions of kyphi. The base, however, was always a mix of ingredients that would hold and bind the aromatics, whilst perhaps imparting some fragrance of its own; typically raisins minus their skins and seeds, wine and honey. Gums and resins varied; 'resin', bdellium (from a species of *Commiphora* and similar to myrrh), myrrh, frankincense, mastic (from the shrubs *Pistacia terebinthus* and *P. lentiscus*) and pine resin (from *Pinus halepensis*, the Aleppo pine) are found in both the early and later formulae. The herbs included camel grass (possibly lemongrass, *Cymbopogon citratus*), sweet flag (probably the reed-like *Acorus calamus*), cyperus grass (the rhizomes of *Cyperus longus* are still used in perfumery), saffron, spikenard (a member of the Valerian family), aspalathos (true identity unknown, but possibly thorny trefoil, or a broom-like shrub), juniper berries (from *Juniperus oxycedrus, J. excelsa* and *J. phoenicea*), mastic tree flowers, mint, pine kernels (*Pinus pinea*), seseli (translated as 'hartwort'), lanathos (perhaps sorrel), and, in the oldest formula from 1500 BCE, inektun-herb. Manniche does not elaborate on this; presumably it is unknown to us. Finally, the spices: early formulae specify cinnamon, which was well known and also used in mummification, while later versions suggest that cardamom could substitute for cinnamon. As a matter of interest, cardamom would have been imported from India, so perhaps it was not available in earlier times. Cassia was sometimes included along with cinnamon, but again, not in the earliest formulae (Manniche 1999). This Egyptian cinnamon was not the familiar spice of our times, but was probably obtained from the bark of *Amyris kataf* from Ethiopia (Morris 1984).

Unfortunately there are no detailed odour descriptions to help us understand what the kyphi-permeated atmosphere must have been like – one can only imagine sweet, typically incense-like smoke, with resinous, pine-like notes, warm tones, earthy notes, minty herbal tones, perhaps fruitiness from the raisins, and spicy, cinnamon-like notes.

In 2002 the perfumer Sandrine Videault 'recreated' kyphi, but is quoted as saying 'kyphi will never be sold because some of the ingredients are illegal substances. In any case the smell is probably too pungent for the modern world.'

The Far East – China and Japan

Lawless (1994) writes that incense has been an important part of Chinese culture since early times. Here the archaeological evidence – bronze incense burners – suggests that it was used during the Shang Dynasty (1600–1030 BCE). Chinese medicine also includes many aromatics, some of which were used as incense, including sandalwood, cinnamon, cassia and styrax gum. Important native aromatics are camphor wood and musk, which is obtained from the abdominal glands of a species of small deer found in the area around the Tibetan massif and other mountainous areas. The secular uses of incense were to purify the atmosphere around the sick and in public places, where the air would be scented with jasmine; and for perfuming the environment. However, China had to import many aromatics from India and Arabia, as it was not blessed with an abundance of aromatic plants. However, in the early part of the first millennium it had sufficient wealth to import aromatics, and then became an important player in the trade until the Ming Dynasty (1368–1644 CE), originally using the relays of the Silk Route and then building ocean-going junks that sailed the Southern Seas (Morris 1984).

Around 4 BCE, philosophers Lao Tze and Chuang Tze developed the way of life that became known as Taoism. This is a vitalistic philosophy, centred on the concept of a current of life, the *Tao*, which permeates and connects everything. Incense containing entheogens and the alchemical minerals lead, sulphur and mercury was very important in Taoism. The censer, the *hsiang lu*, was central to the temple and all ceremonies – 'the ancestor and begetter of the alchemical furnace that linked the worlds' (Needham 1974, cited in Dannaway 2010, p.489). When lit, the solid incense transformed into scented vapours, mirroring the transmutation from the physical, mortal state to that of energy or spirit – the *Tao*. In addition to the scented botanicals, cannabis was sometimes used in the censers (Jiang *et al.* 2006), so apart from the symbolism of incense, and its evocative perfume, psychoactive ingredients could also produce altered states of consciousness.

The arrival of Buddhism in China introduced more ways of using incense in ceremony. Purification of the self and the atmosphere by means of incense was important; and the traditional use of joss sticks in Buddhist temples persists. Three sticks are lit and held, and the individual blows over them three times before placing them before the image or effigy of the Buddha or bodhisattvas, followed by a bow with palms pressed together (Morris 1984).

Buddhism and incense had been introduced to Japan by Zen monks and trade contacts, and via the Korean peninsula by the sixth century CE (Morita 1992); but the ideas, concepts, philosophies, practices and customs were adapted and modified and transformed until they became part of the Japanese way. The aromatic species, however, are not indigenous to Japan, and were imported (Morris 1984; Morita 1992). Many of the practices remained similar, such as the use of incense in temples, the scenting of clothing with scented smoke, and the planting and veneration of camphor trees. The Japanese invented devices such as *fusegos* to scent kimonos, and *kohmakuras* to scent the hair with incense. They elevated incense clock design and uses; various versions could tell the time according to what part of the clock the incense smoke was coming from, or how much time had elapsed by the fragrance emitted by incense sticks with differently scented segments. Geishas were paid according to the number of incense sticks used during their encounter with a client (Morris 1984).

The indigenous religion of Japan was Shinto, and Shinto rites and rituals were part of state and court ceremonies. During the period 710–794 CE, known as the Nara period, political power was held by supporters of Buddhism, and so Buddhist purification rituals were incorporated into state ceremonies; this persisted until 1868, the time of the Meiji Restoration, when government was returned to the emperor. Then, incense use returned to its original form – offerings to the Buddha, and in temples and at graves. It is believed that fragrance invokes the Buddha's presence and peace. There was also a distinction between incense used purely for pleasure, such as scenting garments and domestic rooms, or welcoming guests to the home, and incense used in the ritual context. *Soradaki*, meaning 'empty burning', referred to the former and *sonae-koh* indicated an offering to Buddha (Morita 1992). Morita also discusses the aromatics that composed Japanese Buddhist incense. Early mixtures that were simply sprinkled on burning charcoal included *jinkoh* (agarwood), sandalwood, cloves, cinnamon and camphor. Eventually the use of readymade blended incense became commonplace, and there are many forms: *shokoh* (a chipped mixture), *nerikoh* (blended balls, bound with honey or the flesh of plums), *senkoh* (joss sticks, including the temple versions), *ensuikoh* (cones) and *nioi-bukuro* (sachets, not intended for burning, but used to scent a room and protect from ill-fortune).

What distinguishes incense culture in Japan from the rest of the world is *koh-do*, the 'way of incense'. This has its origins in the Muromachi period (1336–1573) when some, rather than using *nerikoh*, returned to the practice of burning *jinkoh* (known as incense wood) on its own, and enjoying the scent; this eventually became known as 'listening' to incense, or *mon-koh*. The concept of listening to, rather than smelling, incense is interesting; in Buddha's realm everything is fragrant, including his words. Incense and fragrance are synonymous, and his words are therefore incense which should be listened to. *Koh-do* was established by Ashikaga Yoshimasa, a patron of the arts, his adviser Shino Soshin, and Sanjonishi Sanetaka, a scholar who was in charge of incense at the imperial court. They classified the *jinkoh* and all of the available incenses at the court, and established the protocols and etiquette for incense appreciation, often linking it with literary themes. At the end of the Muromachi period *koh-do* was an established art form, its popularity endured, and it was taught first by connoisseurs, who then established schools headed by professional masters of *koh-do*. In accordance with traditional Japanese practice, the teachings (including the spiritual and philosophical aspects) were kept secret, passed on by word of mouth, and only shared with proficient students. However, its popularity meant that *koh-do* also became like a game, the spiritual element was lost, and its popularity declined as 'westernisation' increased. The *koh-do* revival began in the 1960s, and continues today in its native Japan, the USA and Europe.

India – aromatic abundance

India has an abundance of aromatic plants – possibly more than anywhere else on the planet – because of its geography, spanning the Himalayas in the north to the Indian Ocean in the south. The Indian peninsula can therefore support plants suited to a wide variety of climates. Perfumes have held an important place for thousands of years, making creative use of India's and Greater India's aromatic flora. Here we find the prized and rare agarwood and sandalwood, the roots of vetiver, spikenard, costus, galangal and ginger, gum-resins such as benzoin, the leaves of patchouli, holy basil and davana, aromatic grasses such as lemongrass and palmarosa, spices such as cardamom, and the exotic flowers of jasmine, champaca, screw pine (*Pandanus*) and lotus. India is also home to some widely used entheogens such as *Peganum harmala*; in the Ladakh region its leaves are burned as incense and the seeds were smoked to 'induce a feeling of exaltation' and for exorcisms; the seeds are also a traditional intoxicant and sexual stimulant, hence their prevalence at wedding ceremonies.

There is evidence that incense was used as early as 3000 BCE in the Indus Valley, at the foot of the Himalayas, where figures of the mother goddess still bear smoke stains. Incense plays an important role in Hindu ritual; for example, offerings of frankincense and *Cyperus* species (aromatic flatsedges) are burnt every four hours in temples dedicated to the god Shiva. Sandalwood, combined with cloves, cardamom and curcuma (turmeric) forms the basis of *abir* powder, also important in ritual. Some scents are dedicated to deities. Tulsi, or holy basil, is sacred to Krishna, whose shrine is at Vrindaban; and tulsi is grown in homes too, in his honour. Benzoin resin is burnt before the *Trimurti*, a composite image of Brahma the creator, Shiva the destroyer and Vishnu the regenerator (Morris 1984; Lawless 1994).

What makes Indian incense so interesting from the olfactory perspective is creative combinations of aromatic ingredients. Although the base ingredients are often similar to those of other cultures, such as agarwood, sandalwood and costus, the Indian formulae introduce many other types of aromatics. Indian incense would contain roots, including the indigenous spikenard and linden tree, and the violet-scented *kapur-kachri* obtained from the dried roots of *Hedychium spicatum*. It is often characterised by flowers too, especially jasmine, champaca and rose, herbs such as patchouli, and spices such as saffron, cardamom and cinnamon.

Ancient Greece – Alexander, Theophrastus and the Pythia

Like many of the other ancient cultures, the Greeks used incense in ceremonies and at altars to honour their gods and goddesses; eventually, by circa 6 BCE, incense replaced human and animal sacrifices. The word *thymiamata* meant 'that which can be burnt as incense'. The Minoan culture on Crete (2600–1250 BCE) traded in aromatics and opium with the Phoenicians; archaeological evidence of the use of incense includes censers from Minoan graves from around 1500 BCE. Alexander the Great (356–323 BCE) was a King of Macedon in the north of Greece. He was tutored by Aristotle (384–322 BCE), and by the age of 25 he was not only leader of the Greeks but also an overlord of Asia Minor, Pharaoh of Egypt and the Great King of Persia. Alexander founded 70 cities, creating a vast empire covering Greece, north to the Danube, south to Egypt and east to the Punjab. His rule was characterised by his ability to unite these peoples by the use of the Greek language and culture, but also by adopting elements of their culture and customs. Therefore, during Alexander's time, the use of aromatics increased. He sent expeditions to find and bring back cuttings and seeds of aromatic species from Persia; and as a result Theophrastus (circa 371–287 BCE, a fellow student of Aristotle), who became known as the Greek 'father of botany', established the first botanical garden and identified the many aromatics of Arabia. As Alexander was a renowned military strategist and leader, Theophrastus was a philosopher of great importance. He studied at Plato's school, then became associated with, and eventually succeeded Aristotle. He also wrote the first text about odours and perfume, *De Odoribus* ('Concerning Odours'), part of *Enquiry into Plants*, a collection of ten volumes.

Important aromatics in ancient Greece included myrtle, an aromatic evergreen shrub associated with Aphrodite, and frankincense, myrrh, costus root, cassia, cinnamon and bay laurel, which were often offered to Apollo (Morris 1984; Lawless 1994). It is in ancient Greece that we see a prominent example of the psychoactive vapours of aromatic plants being used for divination – foretelling the future. The Greek historian Herodotus (circa 484–425 BCE) explained that the Oracle at Delphi was the source of the sun god Apollo's advice, and as Apollo was the son and prophet of Zeus, he could also reveal the will of Zeus. The prophesies, warnings and advice of the Delphic Oracle were used by policy makers not only to make decisions about, for example, the creation of institutions, or whether to go to war, or how to ensure smooth running of sanctuaries, or how to conduct rituals, but also to justify or give credence to these decisions. However, Apollo's advice was delivered by the *Pythia* – a medium who transformed the sacred words into language that could be understood, although often the actual meaning could be obscure. Her prophesies were complex, often delivered in verse, often unintelligible, and often open to interpretation. For example, the prophesy which was delivered to King Croesus of Lydia in 6 BCE was ambiguous: he was told that if he went to war, he would destroy a great empire. Consequently, he declared war on his rival Cyrus, ruler of the Persian Empire – but ironically it was his own empire that was destroyed, although his life was spared (Marchais-Roubelat and Roubelat 2011).

The origin of the Oracle at Delphi, on Mount Parnassus north of the Gulf of Corinth, can be explored in reference to the Greek pantheon and beliefs of the times. Ancient cults are always linked to geographical sites. The site at Delphi would have been associated with older gods than Apollo, and the divine presence was due to the sacredness of the site itself. It is said that the Oracle at Delphi first belonged to Mother Earth, who appointed Daphnis as her prophetess. According to myth, Apollo killed a she-dragon at Delphi, and to pacify her spirit, he created the Pythia – a priestess who would act as his voice in the world of mortals. Other priestesses, who had to be virgins born at Delphi, acted as intermediaries that mortals could petition, and then priests would relay the Oracle's responses to the inquirers. The Pythia conducted her divination in an inner sanctum within the Temple of Apollo. It is thought that she would have fumigated herself with the smoke of burning bay laurel leaves, sacred to Apollo, and also perhaps chewed the leaves, to prepare for divination. She sat upon a tripod which was fastened to the *omphalos*, the 'navel stone'. In a chamber below, herbs were burned to produce *pneuma enthusiastikon*, hallucinogenic vapours, which were vented through a hole in the omphalos, shrouding the Pythia in smoke. Although it has been suggested that toxic natural gases, such as ethylene and ethane, which have anaesthetic properties, could have caused her visions, the vapours of the hallucinogenic plants are just as likely to have induced her trance state. The herbs may have included cannabis, *Datura stramonium*, white henbane and mandrake (Pennacchio *et al.* 2010); Dannaway (2010) suggests that thorn apple seeds (from *Datura* species) and *khat* (*Catha edulis*, also known as *miraa*, a stimulant used by Ethiopian and Somali tribes, the Kikuyu and Masai; see Margetts 1967) may have been used too. However, the Pythia was well prepared to receive these visions, and was adept at verbalising her impressions and visions, albeit in the form of obscure verse. She could be seen as a counsellor, revealing otherwise inaccessible insights that would guide the inquirer about their options and the possible consequences of their actions.

So rulers, kings and policy makers consulted the oracle about important matters, and pilgrims would enquire about more mundane matters. They would, using their own free will, either act upon or ignore the message. For example, King Aegeus chose to ignore a message from the Oracle which warned him, on pain of death, not to father a child before his return to Athens. However, he fathered Theseus, who became his downfall – was this fate or free will?

Marchais-Roubelat and Roubelat (2011) quote Delphic Oracle researcher Roux (1976), who said that:

> The oracle played a considerable role in the Greeks' existence, not only because it helped them to find a solution to the practical difficulties of their everyday lives, but because it reinforced the moral and legal thinking upon which the condition and behaviour of the Greek people were founded. (p.1493)

Although it is not explicit, this statement shows the profound influence of aromatic and psychoactive smoke on ancient Greek culture. The site of the Delphic Oracle still exists, as does a technological forecasting system named the Delphi method, although it should be stressed that the latter does not involve aromatically induced trance states or divination.

Rome – from restraint to unsurpassed excesses

The Greeks had a strong influence on the early Roman civilisation; which Morris (1984) describes as 'rough'. From 8–2 BCE the Etruscans brought a 'civilising' influence, including the use of local aromatics in incense mixtures – myrtle, Spanish broom, labdanum (the resinous exudate of rock rose) and pine. Contact with the Etruscans, Phoenicians and Greeks led to incense being imported from Arabia for temple use; and throughout the Republic incense use was 'restrained'. In the imperial period the use of all things scented became excessive. Huge quantities of incense were burned, especially frankincense and myrrh. Most historical accounts mention the spectacular excesses of the Emperor Nero, and incense use was just one example. It is said that he burned one entire year's supply of incense in just one day to mourn the death of his second wife, Poppaea Sabina. This is perhaps in keeping with her equally extravagant lifestyle (Stewart 2007; Pennacchio *et al.* 2010). Apparently the Romans imported 7000 tons of frankincense alone each year, so the expense of her funeral would have been considerable. Lawless (1994) quotes Pliny the Elder, who wrote that:

Arabia's good fortune has been caused by the luxury of mankind even in the hours of death, when they burn over the departed the products which they had originally understood to have been created for the gods. (p.30)

It is fascinating to read the lines of a Roman historian who makes the same distinction as the Japanese, in that incense had now secular and non-secular uses, and 'empty burning' was becoming commonplace.

The incense cults of Israel

It is probable that the incenses used in Persia and Israel contained entheogens. For example, in the Old Testament we see references to *kaneh bosom*, which is possibly cannabis, as an ingredient in the holy or sacred incense (*ktoret*). The Israelites were nomadic, and would use 'holy smoke' in enclosed meeting tents, which would intensify its psychoactive effects. Le Guérer (1994) emphasises the special relationship between the 'blood of the covenant' – the covenant between the God of the Hebrews and His followers, and 'perpetual incense' – the holy incense. Both were governed by strict taboos and laws. Sacrificial blood had to be used in a very specific way; it was said to contain life, and thus purify and atone the priests and worshippers in preparation for divine communication. The formula for holy incense was very important, and given directly to Moses. Rites were conducted at the specifically and especially constructed Altar of Incense, where the burning of 'strange' (foreign) incenses was prohibited, and only the priests, who were descendants of Aaron, could control the incense and the way in which it was offered. If this instruction was violated, and 'unauthorised coals' were burned, the entire community was at risk from the 'fire of the Lord'. Lawless (1994) quotes Exodus 30:37–7 (around 1250 BCE), which gives explicit instructions on how to make and use holy incense, and a dire warning for those who did not adhere to the restrictions:

> Take sweet spices: storax, onycha, galbanum, sweet spices and pure frankincense in equal parts, and compound an incense, such a blend as the perfumer might make, salted, pure and holy. Crush a part of it into a fine powder, and put some of this on front of the Testimony in the Tent of Meeting, the place appointed for my meetings with you. You must regard it as most holy. You are not to make any incense of similar composition for your own use. You must hold it to be a holy thing, reserved for Yahweh. Whoever copies it for use as a perfume shall be outlawed from his people. (p.37)

The Altar of Incense had enormous political significance too, and was at the heart of power struggles between the Levite priest class and the infiltration of aliens as a result of patriarchs marrying foreign women. It was also at the centre of tensions between the kings and the priests, before losing its importance when a monarchy was established and the meeting tents were replaced with temples. By the time of King Solomon the use of incense was reintroduced, this time as *ktoret ha-samim*, 'incense of drugs', possibly influenced by his foreign wives and concubines. It was prophesised that because of this, the Altar of Incense would be destroyed; and indeed it was, by Josiah, because the foreign incense was seen as desecration and idolatry. Josiah instigated a massacre.

Other than what we read in Exodus, the sacred incense ingredients are not all known, but around the time of Jesus, myrrh, cassia, spikenard, saffron, costus, mace, cinnamon and an undisclosed herb were possibly included in the formula (Lawless 1994). It is also speculated that, since the Israelites made their Exodus from Egypt, they would probably have had experience of the temple incenses – which included benzoin resin, cannabis, henbane and wild rue (*Peganum harmala*). *Peganum* is native to India, but it was also used by the ancient Syrians, who called it *besana* (Dannaway 2010). It was sacred to Bes, an Egyptian deity who in the Old Kingdom was a protector of households, mothers and childbirth, when he was accompanied by the female deity Tawaret. Bes was 'exported' to the Phoenicians and Cypriots, and, in the New Kingdom, he acquired cult status because he was associated with driving away evil and the good things in life – music, dance, sex and pleasure. An island associated with hedonism, Ibiza, takes its name from Bes. *Peganum harmala* remains in current use as magical incense.

Mesoamerica – the ancient Maya

The ancient Maya had a shamanic tradition. The rituals and ceremonies usually involved blood sacrifice, the burning of incense, ritual drinking and dance. There would be a fasting and abstinence, symbolic of spiritual purification prior to the ceremony. The ceremonies would follow a pattern: expulsion of evil amongst the worshippers, incensing of the idols, and blood – human or animal – sacrifice. Sacrifice by drowning was made to the rain god, Thaloc. In the postclassic era (900–1500 CE), the sacrificial blood would be smeared on the idols and the priests' hair; some sacrifices were particularly gruesome. Ceremonies were inevitably closed by feasting and drinking (Sharer 1994).

The ancient Maya used intoxicants such as alcohol. Fermented drinks were made from maize and agave; and for ritual use a drink called *balche*, made from fermenting honey and the bark of the balche tree (*Lonchocarpus longistylis*). Entheogen use was widespread – mainly for divination and entering trance states to communicate with the unseen world. Wild tobacco (*Nicotiana rustica*) was smoked to induce trance; this was much more potent than today's commercially available products. The geographical area also supports the growth of several hallucinogenic fungi. *Xibalbaj okox*, which means 'underworld mushroom' was said to transport the user to a supernatural world; its other name was *k'aizalah okox*, meaning 'lost-judgement mushroom'. The ancient Maya are also thought to have used peyote, morning glory, the water lily, and poison obtained from the glands of the toad *Bufo marinus* as hallucinogens. They ingested the hallucinogens, but also delivered them in enemas, thus bypassing the portal circulation and allowing immediate absorption and speedy effects (Sharer 1994; Pennacchio *et al.* 2010).

Mayan ruins give us evidence of early incense use; large censers have been found in the *Gruta de Balankanche* near Chichén-Itzá. The name of the cave means 'hidden throne', referring to the stalagmite which resembles the *ceiba tree*, 'the sacred tree inside the earth' (Sharer 1994; Pennacchio *et al.* 2010). Incense was an indispensable element of every ceremony. The principle incense was *pom* – made from the resin of the copal tree, *Protium copal*. Another resin was called *puk ak*, but its botanical source has not been verified (Sharer 1994). Pennacchio *et al.* (2010) note that the name 'copal' is derived from the Aztec Nahuatl *copalli*, and suggest that copal was also obtained from *Bursera bipinnata*, the same genus as myrrh, and that pine resin may also have been used. In Mesoamerica other conifers such as *Cupressus* and *Pinus* species and strongly scented herbs such as the mints were used in incenses. The *pom* of the ancient Maya was made from the resins of trees especially grown in plantations for this purpose. The incense itself was prized for both personal and ritual use; it was in the form of small, turquoise blue cakes decorated with hatching – hundreds of such incense cakes were found at the Cenote of Sacrifice at Chichén-Itzá. Even today the Lacandon Maya of Chiapas prepare balls of fresh incense, laid out on special boards, just as the ancient Maya would have done. In modern Mayan ceremonies sacrifice is less of a feature, although chickens might be used. In ancient times, if a human or animal heart was not available, the incense would be moulded into a heart shape. The incense would have been burned in pottery vessels decorated with the image of a god; and even today, in remote regions, the modern Maya burn *pom* in similar censers in the temple ruins of Yaxchilan. It has a 'fragrant odour' (Sharer 1994).

This exploration of smoke has focused on scenting the environment for ritual or pleasure. Some, such as the Japanese, would still choose perfuming their environments over personal scenting. Perfumes for personal use have their own history, rooted in ancient times and crossing cultures, right up to the present day, and always giving an insight into their users.

CHAPTER 4

Perfume

The Transcendence of the Sweet Life

Perfume evokes a transcendence (of the world but not in it) – it could be called the transcendence of the sweet life. But because it is perfume (halfway between thing and idea) it almost partakes of the nature of transcendence (otherwise dimly adumbrated in images, musical sounds, vague feelings and desires) while still remaining part of the world. (Gell 1977, p.31)

Gell's words evoke the symbolic nature of perfume and thus its implicit impact on the individual and societies. Stamelman (2006) quotes the nineteenth-century perfumer Eugène Rimmel, who said that 'the history of perfume is, in some manner, that of civilisation' (p.11) and the contemporary perfumer Serge Lutens: 'A perfume, when it is truly a perfume, adheres to a culture… It becomes our shadow' (p.11). In this chapter we will explore the evolution of perfumery, and how it has not only reflected different cultures, but also influenced them.

Aromatics obtained from plants (and a few animals) formed the palette of the early perfumers, so first we will look at the biology of aromatic plants, and their volatile oils.

Aromatic plants and their extracts

A relatively small proportion of plant species are scented; and the aroma of these plants is due to the presence of volatile oils which contain secondary metabolites – plant constituents that are not involved in growth or development, but have other, complex biological and ecological roles, many of which have yet to be defined. Plant volatile oils are found in specialised cells which are located in various anatomical parts of plants. Frequently they are located in the flowers, but they may also be found in leaves, bark, fruit and seeds; also in woody parts such as stems and roots (Williams 1996). These oils can be extracted by physical means, such as expression in the case of citrus peel, maceration in oils or fats, and water or steam distillation, to yield essential oils. In the early days, before distillation was widely known about or used, maceration was the usual practice. Nowadays, solvent extraction yields aromatic products known as concretes and absolutes; this is widely used for the extraction of floral oils such as jasmine. Sometimes ultrasonic extraction precedes solvent extraction – this disrupts the cells, releasing the volatile oils, and thus helps the efficiency of the extraction process. Recent developments in extraction technology are vacuum microwave hydro-distillation (VMHD) which produces essential oils that have not been subjected to thermal degradation, and supercritical fluid extraction (SFE) which produces volatiles very similar to the ones in the plant, because the solvent (usually carbon dioxide) has a near ambient critical temperature of 31°C, thus preventing heat and chemical modifications in the product (Tonutti and Liddle 2010).

Volatile oils are chemically complex; however, the constituents generally fall into two categories – the terpenoids and the phenylpropanoids. The *terpenes* and their derivatives, the *terpenoids*, are named after turpentine, which gives a clue to the origins of some of them – the pinenes found in many conifers are monoterpenes with a characteristic fresh, piney, coniferous smell. Other monoterpenes include limonene, with a zesty citrus odour, found in citrus peel oils. Monoterpenes often are found in the top notes of citrus and pine oils. Larger molecular weight terpenes are the sesquiterpenes, and as these molecules are bigger, they are heavier and do not evaporate as quickly as the monoterpenes; they are often found in base notes. Many of their names reflect their botanical sources, such as the santalenes from sandalwood, or zingiberene from ginger.

The terpenoids are the oxygenated derivatives of both monoterpenes and sesquiterpenes, and they dominate volatile oil chemistry. The *monoterpenoids* include the alcohols, such as the light, mild, floral-woody scented linalool in many oils including lavender; the sweet, rosy geraniol in geranium; citral, an aldehyde with a harsh lemon odour in lemongrass; menthone, the penetrating ketone in mint; and the herbal, fruity, apple-like esters in Roman chamomile. The *sesquiterpenoids* include mild and woody santalols in sandalwood, the faint woody cedrol in Virginian cedar, and the herbal, patchouli-like patchoulol in patchouli – these constituents are all significantly related to the aromas of their volatile oils.

The *phenylpropanoids* are synthesised in a distinct biochemical pathway; this is a diverse group, but all the molecules share a distinguishing feature – the presence of an aromatic ring structure. Although phenylpropanoids are not as numerous as the terpenes, they do have interesting odours and characteristics. Here we have the spicy, clove-like eugenol in clove oil; the pleasant floral rose/hyacinth-scented phenylethanol in rose; and the sweet, ethereal, *trans*-anethole in sweet fennel and star anise. There are also many aromatic *esters*, found in floral oils such as jasmine and tuberose, and the medicinal methyl salicylate of wintergreen oil; and *aldehydes*, such as cinnamaldehyde in cinnamon, and vanillin in benzoin resin and vanilla.

In the minority, but nonetheless important from the odour perspective, there are *nitrogen-containing compounds* such as pyrazines, which give the intense green notes in galbanum oil, and the anthranilates, which can give floral/fruity or fishy notes in mandarin oil. *Sulphur-containing compounds* are present in some – such as garlic and onion oils – which have powerful, diffusive and pungent odours, rendering them unsuitable in perfumery, but useful in flavouring; and they are also antiseptics.

It is generally accepted that the main biological reasons for plant volatile oil production are defence and survival. Examples of defence are abundant – some plants produce volatile oils that repel herbivores or insect pests, or which act as their own antimicrobial defences. Others can produce volatile oils that contain *semiochemicals* (sign chemicals) when they are damaged by, for example, caterpillars. The volatiles are released into the air when the leaves are crushed or torn, and these attract caterpillar predators, thus preventing further damage (Goode 2000).

Allelopathy is a type of competition between plants. Plants must compete with each other in the environment for resources such as light, nutrients, water and space. Some plant volatile oils can inhibit the growth of other species in the immediate vicinity. For example, some species of thyme produce compounds that inhibit the germination of some species of grass. Another example of allelopathy can be seen in arid or semiarid habitats, where *Artemisia* species and *Salvia* species release volatiles that inhibit the germination of other herbaceous plants. In other cases we can even see *autoallelopathy* – some species of pine produce volatile compounds that inhibit the development of their own seedlings (Evans 1989).

Some plants produce volatile oils that attract rather than repel; this serves the purpose of reproduction and ultimately the survival of a species. Pollination is the method of reproduction in plants and is often carried out by insects or animals. Volatile oils may be produced in flowers to attract insect pollinators, such as bees, beetles and moths. Usually the volatile oils are released at a time when their usual pollinator will detect them. This will vary in terms of the time of day and the season, according to the natural cycles of the pollinators, which could be night-flying moths or insects that are abundant on warm days. Animals that serve in pollination, or as vectors for seed dispersal, will also be attracted. It is believed that floral scent plays a key role in reproductive ecology; however, most studies have focused on visual observations rather than olfactory analysis. Goodrich (2012) suggests that this might be partly because 'most humans typically lack a reliable vocabulary with which to characterise odour and communicate its qualities' (p.262). Some volatile oil components are the same as insect pheromones and, for example, include aggregation (trail) signals for the bark beetle, an alarm signal for aphids, sex pheromones that elicit mating in aphids, and sex pheromones for butterflies (Müller and Buchbauer 2011). Incidentally, birds are attracted by colour rather than odour (Shawe 1996).

We can consider an interesting parallel between incense use and perfumery and nature. The volatile oils either repel or attract; some aromatic plants were used to repel evil or negative influences, or destroy the causes of disease, while others were used to attract good influences, or invoke divine presence, heal, or attract a partner. However, the parallel goes a little further. We can see a pattern – the plant scents used to protect, or drive away undesirable influences, were often the coniferous, minty or herbal types derived from plants that exhibit allelopathy, or with antimicrobial activity. The plant scents used for attraction, on the other hand, are often floral, derived from flowers whose volatile oils attract pollinators. Were we aware that we were mimicking nature when selecting aromatics for ritual and social purposes?

The evolution of perfumery

To discover the nature of early perfumes, made from natural ingredients, we need to return to ancient Egypt, Arabia, India, Greece and Rome; but to explore how modern perfumery has evolved, we will focus on Europe. Contemporary perfumery belongs to a very different world indeed; not least because of the diminished role of ingredients derived from botanical sources and the vast array of aromachemicals now available.

Williams (1995a) tells us that the active and deliberate enjoyment of fragrance probably dates back as far as 5000 BCE; in 1953, Henry Lhote discovered ancient murals in the Tassili caves in the northern Sahara, which depict women wearing simple garlands of flowers. Scents for personal use probably were made after the discovery of fire and the scented smokes of some woods, resins, barks and roots – such as agarwood, sandalwood, frankincense and benzoin resins, cinnamon bark, calamus and vetiver roots. These all emit 'heavy', smoky scents when burned – very different indeed from the odours of their volatile oils. Most ancient cultures held the belief that fragrances were created by the gods, and that the gods were responsible for the destiny of societies and individuals. Consequently, scented offerings to seek favour with the gods were an important part of ceremonies and rituals, along with worship, prayer and sacrifice. It is most probable that early perfumes were these scented smokes. The fragrance would linger on the skin and hair, to be enjoyed long after the ceremony.

At some point it was discovered that if an aromatic plant material was soaked in oil or melted fat, its scent would be transferred into the oil, a process called maceration. The scented oil would retain its odour far longer than smoke, so fragrant oils were offered to the gods too, and would eventually have become the first oily perfumes for skin application and personal use. It is the ancient Egyptians who are credited with this development (Morris 1984; Williams 1995a).

Ancient Egypt – perfume for deities, the deceased and the living

In the early days, scented oils and unguents were reserved for anointing statues of the deities – for example, the eyes and mouths were anointed every day in a ritual 're-awakening' of the god or goddess. The aromatic preparations were also used in mummification, and jars of unguents were left in tombs for use in the afterlife. Morris (1984) suggests that it was in the time of the New Kingdom (beginning circa 1570 BCE) and into the Golden Age that the Egyptians began to apply perfumes for personal use. Unfortunately, at the time no records of the perfume formulae were kept, and the sacred perfumes were made in secret, by priests. However, Kaiser (2006) notes that the Ebers Papyrus (circa 1600 BCE) contains the formulae for around 100 aromatic concoctions. So what we do understand of perfumery in ancient Egypt is based on archaeological evidence, the known availability of aromatics at the time, the *Ebers* Papyrus, and the writings of Theophrastus, Dioscorides[1] and Pliny the Elder, who make reference to the aromatics of Egypt (Williams 1995a; Manniche 1999).

It would seem that the ancient Egyptians were fastidious about personal hygiene; bathing and depilation were commonplace, so perfumes were being used not to mask body odours, but to enhance personal care routines. Scented oils and products made from moulded fats were common. Shaving body hair was facilitated by the application of scented oil to the skin. Cones made from fat and aromatics were sometimes placed on top of the head; these would melt slowly, releasing their scent while coating and protecting the hair and skin (Morris 1984; Manniche 1999).

In ancient Egypt perfumes and cosmetics had more than one function. Apart from personal enhancement, often they had apotropaic uses – as magical charms that kept the wearer safe from malevolence – and cosmetic or medicinal uses. The perfumers were skilled, and had a reasonable array of aromatics to work with. These, according to Williams (1995a), included the botanically derived myrrh, galbanum, cassia, cardamom, cedarwood, angelica, benzoin, storax, labdanum and olibanum (frankincense), the orange fruit and flower, and the animal-derived ambergris, musk and civet. Manniche (1999) gives a review of the aromatic plants used in Egyptian perfumery, often referring to ancient Greek texts for information. Please see Table 4.1 for a summary.

---

1   Dioscorides (40–90 CE) was a physician, pharmacologist and botanist, and author of *De Materia Medica* – a treatise on herbal medicine – but since perfumes were used medicinally this also includes information about perfume formulation.

Table 4.1 The ancient Egyptian perfumers' palette

Compiled and adapted from Manniche (1999).

Name	Botanical source	Scent
Aspalathos	A shrub with red, hard, scented roots and white, rose-like flowers. Various sources suggested: thorny trefoil (*Calycotome villosa* or *Alhagi maurorum*), or a shrubby *Convolvulus* or broom (*Cytisus lanigerus*).	A very sweet scent, used in *kyphi*, Hathor unguent, *medjat* and *hekenu*.
Bdellium	*Commiphora erythraea* and *C. africana*.	Stronger than true myrrh, with a hint of turpentine; less expensive too.
Camel grass	*Andropogon schoenanthus*. (*Andropogon schoenanthus* is now named *Cymbopogon citratus* – lemongrass, or gingergrass. *Andropogon* is a synonym for *Cymbopogon*.)	Lemony-rose, with a biting quality; not long-lasting.
Cardamom	The spice *Elettaria cardamomum*.	Sweet and spicy. Some formulae for *kyphi* mention cardamom as a cinnamon substitute.
Cassia	The bark of *Cinnamomum iners*.	Hot and pungent; rose-scented variants.
Cinnamon	*Cinnamomum verum* (probably *C. cassia*).	Typical of the spice. Extensively used in perfumery and also in mummification.
Cyperus grass (*hodveg*)	Sedges – *Cyperus* species, including *C. rotundus* and *C. longus*, which have fragrant roots.	Said to smell like 'nard' (spikenard).
Dill (*imset*)	*Anethum graveolens*	Light, fresh and spicy/caraway-like; dill stems and flowers were used in mummification.

Fir resin (*sefet*)	*Abies cilicica*	Resinous, fresh, reminiscent of frankincense; used in perfumes for funerary offerings.
Frankincense	Whitish resin collected from *Boswellia* species – small shrubby trees.	Aromatic, resinous, sweet and incense-like.
Galbanum (*metopium*)	*Ferula* species.	Green, musty scent. The Egyptians in Dioscorides' time used it in a perfume called *metopium*.
Henna (*cypros*)	*Lawsonia inermis* seeds were boiled in olive oil and crushed.	A sweet scent; used in the perfume *Cyprinum*.
Iris (*nar*)	The dried rhizomes of *Iris* species including *I. albicans* and *I. florentina*.	Probably used in perfumery.
Juniper	The large (*arkeuthos*) and small (*brathy*) berries of *Juniperus* species. *J. oxycedrus* has small berries, other species may have been *J. excelsa* and *J. phoenicea*.	A fresh, penetrating, coniferous scent; used in perfumes including *kyphi*, and in mummification.
Lily	*Lilium candidum* flowers.	Scent heavy and sweet, typical of the flower.
Lotus (*seshen*)	The water lily *Nymphaea lotus*.	The most important scent of ancient Egypt; included in a formula for an 'Opening of the Mouth' unguent.[2]
Marjoram (*sopho*)	*Origanum* species; herb of the crocodile god Sobek.	Typically warm and herbal; used in perfumery and in mummy garlands.
Mastic	*Pistacia terebinthus* and *P. lentiscus* resin.	Sweet-smelling; used in mummification.
Mint (*nkepet*)	Wild *Mentha* species.	Fresh, penetrating, typical of the herb.

---

2   This was a ritual ceremony that involved applying nine unguents to the limbs of a statue of a deity, in preparation for the 'opening of its mouth' and functioning as a divine being.

Name	Botanical source	Scent
Myrrh	Reddish resin from *Commiphora* species.	Typically sweet and incense-like; *stakte* was an oil produced from myrrh and possibly balanos, making the only simple uncompounded perfume.[3]
Pine kernels (*peru shenu*)	*Pinus pinea*	Only faintly aromatic; used in aromatic formulae including some *kyphi* recipes.
Pine resin (from *qed* wood)	*Pinus* species, probably including *P. halepensis* (Aleppo pine).	Fresh, resinous, typically coniferous. An ingredient in *kyphi* and used in mummification.
Saffron	The stigma of the crocus, *Crocus sativus*.	An ingredient in the *kyphi* formula given by Galen; no other uses known.
Spikenard	*Nardostachys jatamansi*.	The leaves were described as fragrant, and the roots as musty. It is an ingredient in the formula for *kyphi* given by Galen.
Sweet flag (*kenen*)	Probably *Acorus calamus*, not indigenous, and imported from India, the Far East or Syria, so it was probably the reeds and roots that were available.	Sweet, aromatic, with a sharp tang.

Morris (1984) highlights several flowers – the blue lotus, *Nymphaea coerula* (see below), the white lotus, lilies (*Lilium candidum* and other species) and henna flowers (*Lawsonia inermis*). He gives special mention to the resin from rockrose leaves – labdanum (*Cistus ladaniferus* and *C. cretus*), which is still used today in perfumery for its softness and tenacity.

In addition to vegetable oils, including olive, safflower, linseed, almond, castor, sesame, lettuce seed, *moringa* (behen) and *balanos* (the date-like fruits of a tree, also used to make 'Balm of Gilead'), they also used a range of fruit pastes and animal fats, such as ox and goose, in the preparation of perfumes, cosmetics and

---

3   A simple, uncompounded perfume is made with just one single aromatic, compared with a compounded perfume which is composed of several or indeed many aromatic extracts.

skin care products. In the case of animal fats, we see an early enfleurage technique for extracting the volatile oils from plant materials. The containers used to store fragranced products were very beautiful, and made of alabaster or earthenware, giving an indication of the inherent value of perfume at the time.

Although the formulae for ancient temple unguents and personal perfumes were not recorded by their makers, thanks to Theophrastus and Dioscorides we do have formulae for the better-known Egyptian perfumes of their time, around the Nineteenth Dynasty and the reign of Rameses II. Obviously these were described from the Greek perspective, and later writers such as the Roman Pliny the Elder also had much to say about the perfume culture and its excesses, certainly typified by Cleopatra. The Greek writers tell us of perfumed oils such as *The Egyptian*, a spicy oil with cinnamon, myrrh, sweet wine and perhaps cardamom, and *The Mendesian*, which had a base of balanos oil with myrrh, cassia and resin. Both would have been heavy and spicy. Pliny and Dioscorides give the ingredients of *Metopion*, which was characterised by galbanum, with bitter almonds, green olive oil, cardamom, camel grass, sweet flag, honey, wine, myrrh, balsamum seed and resin. Some floral perfumes are also detailed, including *Susinum* (lily), which was apparently also worn by men, *Iris* perfume (although there is not much evidence that this was used in Egypt, and it took 20 years to mature), and *Rhodinium* (rose) which could be a simple perfume or with added herbs such as sage and coriander, and aromatic grasses. Herbal perfumes included *Cyprinum* (henna flower) which was light and delicate, and *Sampsuchinum* or *Amaracinum*, which was based on marjoram and was very long-lasting and, allegedly, could provoke headaches. Other significant perfumes were *The Royal*, a spicy scent prepared for the kings of Parthia, and *Megaleion*, a perfume that achieved some degree of fame; it was difficult to make, coloured and expensive, had 'strength and substantial character', and was suitable for women (Manniche 1999). From all of this we can see that the spicy, spicy/sweet and spicy/fruity perfumes were dominant, but there were also the Egyptian versions of the floral class typified by lily, rose and iris, and herbal scents such as marjoram.

Perfumes also had symbolic uses – for love and eroticism and for transcendence or rebirth. Queen Hatshepsut, who was noted for her use of cosmetics and aromatics, had a divine conception – the god Amun was her father, and her mother first noticed his presence in her bed chamber because of his 'divine scent' ('incense land'). Therefore, perfumes were regarded as having erotic value. Feasting, accompanied by alcohol and perfumes, could also help dispel the barriers between mortals, the gods and the deceased (Manniche 1999).

Perhaps the most important fragrant and symbolic flower was the 'lotus', or more accurately, the blue water lily, *Nymphaea coerulea*, known as *sarpat*. It is shown in art as early as the Fifth Dynasty (2494–2345 BCE). It was to be found in long rectangular pools in gardens, and the highly scented blooms were picked for personal decoration. The fragrance is only found in the open flowers, and it resembles hyacinth. Kaiser (2006) describes the scent of the fresh flower as an 'intensely sweet aromatic-floral, yet refreshing, rather hyacinth-like perfume' (p.114). The flower is an important part of mythology. The blue lotus was thought to represent Re, the sun god; it has blue, lancet-shaped petals the colour of the sky, and a bright yellow-rayed stigma in the centre like the sun. Goody (1993) relates the myth that Re was imprisoned in the bud, submerged in the primordial ocean, and that when he was awakened he emerged from the opening flower with the solar disc. The blue lotus flowers between December and March, rising above the surface of the water to open its petals at dawn, and closing them at noon before sinking back into the water. This represented the cycle of death and rebirth and, in later times, the resurrection of Osiris. The deceased were said to be reborn from the blue lotus. Each flower repeats the cycle three times, on three consecutive days (Manniche 1999). Thus, the blue lotus was very special, and it also became symbolic of love.

(*Sushin*, the white lotus, *Nymphaea lotus*, blooms at night, so does not share the symbolism, but it was appreciated for its odour, which was 'piquant' and 'less intoxicating' than the blue flower (Morris 1984). Kaiser (2006) emphasises that Edwards, a famous Egyptologist, observed that in tomb paintings, artworks and relics, cups or chalices representing the white lotus were used as drinking vessels, but that those representing the blue lotus were used only in ritual.)

The highly fragrant flowers of the blue lotus are delicate and beautiful; in artworks we can see that its scent was appreciated in many ways, not least by simply holding the bloom to the nose, or wearing it in the hair, or in garlands around the neck, or even placed on top of unguent cones. It was not just the beauty and symbolism of *sarpat* that made it such an icon of ancient Egypt – it was the effect of the fragrance on the senses. Artwork shows noses buried in the flowers at banquets and ceremonies such as the Feast of the Valley, and depictions of the gods, with clearly dilated nostrils, appreciating its scent. Prolonged inhalation of the volatile oil undoubtedly had a sedative and hypnotic effect, perhaps eliciting an altered state of consciousness.

Manniche (1999) suggests that the narcotic scent, perhaps coupled with another hallucinogen such as cannabis (Morris 1984), and appropriate magical spells would allow transformation into the form of the flower. (Transformation of form is associated with the use of entheogens and shamanism.) Morris (1984) and Kaiser (2006) give us further insight into the blue lotus's psychoactive properties. The plant contains the narcotic and hallucinogenic substances amorphine, nuciferine and nornuciferine, which might have been enough to achieve an altered state of consciousness by simply inhaling the perfume. The Egyptians also prepared a potion by steeping the blossoms in wine; this would certainly have had psychotropic effects, and it became a favourite drink of the Egyptian nobility. Kaiser also suggests that in *Odyssey* IX, 84, Homer is referring to the blue lotus when relating the experiences of Odysseus and his men. When they landed on the island of the *Lotophagi*, or 'lotus-eaters', they ate the lotus flower, as was the native custom. This made them sleep, and they stopped caring about returning home and succumbed to apathy. Eventually, Odysseus realised what was happening and managed to set sail.

The blue lotus and cannabis were not the only mind-altering substances in use – mandrake was also known to the Egyptians. Mandrake, best known for its roots which resemble the human form, is native to the northeastern Mediterranean region. It has been used as a medicine, poison (large quantities induce a catatonic state), aphrodisiac, intoxicant and psychotropic by many cultures, including the cult of Dionysus in ancient Greece, where it was prepared in wine. In New Kingdom artwork, like the blue lotus, mandrake is depicted in images of gardens, and its fruits in scenes of banquets; the two are sometimes mentioned together in poetry. Literature refers to 'sniffing' mandrake fruits (*reremt*), and this, along with some artworks, is sometimes in an erotic context, indicating that the inhaled scent dispelled inhibitions and was an aphrodisiac. The fruit is said to smell musky, or sweet, and not unpleasant.

Tiryac was another psychotropic, multi-purpose remedy; a modern version remains in use in Cairo. The formula was complex – tiryac was composed of a myriad of aromatics, with additional inclusions of serpent skin and spittle, so that it also functioned as an antidote for snake bites. It was consumed, not used as a perfume; however, it was noted for its mind-altering effects as well as its medicinal ones, which seemed to focus on restoring balance and equilibrium. It could elicit several types of responses, such as provoking abnormal, excited states followed by delirium, but it was also said to treat anxiety and improve the memory (Manniche 1999).

Williams (1995a) notes that the Egyptians were accomplished teachers, who imparted their perfumery knowledge to the Assyrians, Babylonians, Chaldeans, Hebrews, Persians and Greeks.

The Egyptian legacy

Jewish perfumery had its origins in the time of the exile in Egypt, and the Bible makes frequent reference to aromatics and perfumes. It is the Song of Solomon, in the Old Testament, and especially the Song of Songs, that contains the most allusions to aromatic plants. The latter is essentially a love poem and contains highly descriptive passages about the intoxicating scents of the lovers, their perfumes and the scent of their environment – a flower garden with lilies and hyacinths, and the cedars of Lebanon. We can also glean understanding of the perfumers' palette from the references to aromatics – frankincense and myrrh, lilies, hyacinths/lily of the valley, saffron, agarwood or sandalwood, spikenard, mastic gum, pine resin, galbanum, and labdanum (*onycha*) from the resin of the rockrose. We also find references to bdellium (a type of myrrh), hyssop (not what we now call hyssop, *Hyssopus officinalis*, but in this case *Marjorana syriaca*) and myrtle (Morris 1984). Lawless (1994) also discusses the use of aromatic oils for purification – for example, the six-month ritual purification of Hebrew women prior to marriage, first with myrrh and then with frankincense and other perfumes.

Early civilisations, such as the Minoans of Crete, had trade links with Egypt; they imported aromatic oils and exported opium, which was used as an analgesic. Artworks (circa 2000 BCE) indicate that both lilies and roses were enjoyed for their scents too. Greek myth attributes the origin of perfume to the gods, even giving some gods and goddesses characteristic scents. It is said that it was Aeone, a nymph associated with Aphrodite (the goddess of desire and beauty) who inadvertently revealed the secrets of perfume to mortals. It is not until around 7 BCE that we see the widespread development of oil-based perfumes in Greece. They were used by both sexes, and common ingredients were indigenous – lilies and roses, orris root, herbs such as marjoram, thyme and sage, and anise.

Herbs and spices were also used to perfume and flavour beverages. It is thought that Hippocrates, when investigating the tonic and digestive properties of 'bitter' herbs such as dittany and wormwood, invented aromatised wine – Hippocratic wine or *vinum absinthium* – from which vermouth is descended (Tonutti and Liddle 2010).

The Egyptian influence became prevalent at the time of Alexander the Great, when Theophrastus established the cultivation of aromatic plants and wrote extensively about all things scented. He documented his explorations to find Arabian incense, and produced the first work specifically on odours (*Concerning Odours*), which covered the raw materials of perfumery, the composition of perfumes and their physiological and psychological effects, olfaction and the links between smell and taste. It is thanks to Theophrastus and others such as Dioscorides, that the practices of the Egyptian perfumers were preserved for posterity.

Cleopatra (69–30 BCE), who was a descendent of the Ptolemies, a family of Greek origin that ruled after the death of Alexander the Great, also represents the cross-cultural links between Egypt and Greece. Her use of perfumes and cosmetics is, of course, the stuff of legends: greeting her Roman lover Antony in a ship with perfumed sails, her extensive use of incense, her chambers strewn liberally with rose petals, and her scented gowns. However, she was also intelligent, shrewd and politically ambitious; her alliance with Antony was fuelled not only by their mutual passion but also by their desire to unite their countries (Morris 1984) – and so the Egyptian legacy of perfume reached Roman culture via the Greeks.

Ancient Rome – wellbeing, therapy, luxury and excess

The perfumes of antiquity played an important part in feasts, seduction, ceremonies, religious rites, funerals and medicine, and ancient Rome was no different. Sites such as Capua, Herculaneum, Pompeii and Paestum have revealed evidence of how and where perfumes were made and traded, and this, along with the writings of Theophrastus, Dioscorides (especially his first-century *De Materia Medica*), Galen and Pliny the Elder has given us an understanding of perfumes of the place and era (Castel *et al.* 2009). Perfumes were part of daily personal ritual in Roman times, and, along with clothes and makeup, were seen to express identity, gender, social status, ethnicity and power. Both sexes wore perfume and makeup, although literary references to men using such products usually implied effeminacy. Socrates maintained that the only perfume suitable for a man was the scent of the oil used in gymnasiums (Le Guérer 1994; Stewart 2007).

Roman perfumes were oil-based scents, made by the process of maceration: the aromatic plant materials would be shredded and steeped in an oil, such as olive (called *oleum omphacium*, freshly extracted from green, unripe olives) or ben (behen) nut oil. The oil would be made astringent by being heated with sedge before being mixed with the aromatics – flowers, woods, spices, herbs and gum resins – and, depending on the aromatics, heat may or may not have been required. Sometimes a resin such as benzoin (*laserpitium*) would be added to act as a fixative, so that the perfume would have greater staying power, and perhaps a colour such as madder root would be added, to make the product more visually appealing. Honey was used, often applied to the hands and mixing vessels when working the product, and acted as a preservative (Castel *et al.* 2009). After a period of time, and a series of cold or warm 'digestions', and once the aromatic molecules had dissolved into the oil, it would be filtered and ready for use. Because of its oily base, and possible content of resins, the perfume would vary in texture; it could be an oily liquid, or a sticky, semi-solid or solid mass, in which case it was described as an *unguentum* (ointment). Sometimes this term meant 'perfume'. The name of the perfume would often reflect its principle aromatic or its source. For example, the very popular *Rhodinum* (rose) was made in Campania in the south of Italy; *Narcissinum* was made from narcissus, while *Delium* came from Delos in Greece, *Assyrium* from Assyria (Stewart 2007), and *Mendesion* from Mendes in Egypt (Castel *et al.* 2009). Natural aromatics used in ancient Rome were the native rose, lily, sweet flag, iris rhizomes, narcissus, saffron, mastic and oakmoss; imported aromatics included pepper, cinnamon, cardamom, nutmeg, ginger, costus, spikenard, agarwood, scented grasses and gum resins (Morris 1984).

Perfumes were used for scenting the person or the environment, or applied as a deodorant; they were used in skin care and personal hygiene routines, or as medicines; so in Roman times, although perfume was undoubtedly used for pleasure and as an expression of identity, it usually had other health benefits. The word *medicamentum* had several meanings: cosmetic, perfume, magic potion, drug, remedy. For some uses of perfumes in medical and personal care, please see Table 4.2. In several of these instances, the ancient Roman use can still be seen in contemporary aromatherapy practices, and sometimes underpinned with sound evidence for practice. Aromatics were present in almost every drug recipe, and aromas themselves were understood to have a therapeutic effect. Tzvi (2011) cites the writer Herodian, who explains the appeal of the town of Laurentium during a time of plague in Rome:

> The doctors thought this place was safe because it was reputed to be immune from infectious diseases in the atmosphere by virtue of the redolent fragrances of the laurels and the pleasant shade of the trees... Some said that if sweet smelling scent filled the sensory passages first,

it stopped them from inhaling the polluted air. If an infection were to get in, they said, the scent drove it out by its greater potency.

Tzvi also draws on the work of Caseau (1994), who investigated the relationship between aromas and medicine:

It came as a surprise to me that medicines were fragrant not because the ingredients had an odour that could not be reduced, but because their power to cure was precisely granted to their odour.

Table 4.2 Roman perfumes and their uses

Compiled and adapted from Stewart (2007).

Name	Principle ingredients	Uses
Abrotenum	Southernwood, probably *Artemisia* species.	Perfume. Cleaning and deodorising wounds. Treatment of cramps and asthma. Soothing balm.
Agollichium	Imported from India and Arabia – a cheaper substitute for frankincense.	Body perfume. As a breath freshener.
Amaracinum	Sweet marjoram.	Perfume. As an anti-inflammatory. Treatment of haemorrhoids. Treatment of gynaecological problems.
Amomum	A 'shrub' (or a Greek word meaning 'spice').	A strongly scented eastern perfume that became a symbol of self-indulgence and excess. To encourage hair growth.
Anethimon	Dill.	Perfume.

Balsamum	Aromatic resin.	Perfume. To encourage hair growth. To counteract snakebites.
Cinnamomum	Bark and leaves of the cinnamon tree.	Perfume.
Crocinum	Saffron.	Perfume. Eye makeup. Used in the body lotion *helenium*.
Erysisceptrum	Thorny shrub.	Perfume. General medicinal uses.
Foliatum	Spikenard oil with myrrh and ben nut oil.	To darken hair colour and encourage growth.
Galbanum	Galbanum resin.	Perfume. As a treatment for boils. To treat aching muscles.
Irinum	Iris (orris root)	Perfume. As a breath freshener and deodorant. To counteract hemlock poisoning.
Kyphi	Complex perfume imported from Egypt.	Perfume. As an antidote to poison. As a laxative. As an asthma treatment.
Labdanum	Resin of rockrose, with bear's fat and maidenhair fern.	Scented skin care. To reduce hair loss.
Megalium	Ben nut oil, balsam, rush, calamus, resin, cassia.	An eastern perfume, named after the perfumer Megallus, a Greek from Sicily.
Melinum	Quince.	Perfume. To improve vision.

Name	Principle ingredients	Uses
Malabathrum	Cinnamon.	Perfume. To counteract poisoning.
Mendesium	Myrrh, cardamom and galbanum in ben nut oil.	Perfume. To treat aching muscles.
Metopium	Bitter almond, juice of unripe grapes and olives, cardamom, rush, sweet flag, honey, wine, myrrh, balsam, galbanum, terebinth resin.	Perfume. To treat dry skin in a body lotion made with almond oil (*amygdalinum*).
Murra	Myrrh.	Perfume. Skin cleanser and hair ointment. As an analgesic.
Narcissinum	Narcissus flowers.	Perfume.
Nardinum	Nard, amomum, myrrh, oil of unripe grapes, ben nut oil, calamus, costus root and balsam.	A perfume that was shipped all over the Roman world in the form of large, medium and small balls. It softened and perfumed the skin and was also used to scent the hair.
Natron	Spikenard.	Perfume. To encourage hair growth.
Olibanum	Frankincense.	Perfume. Deodorant.
Opobalsamum	Balm of Gilead or *balanos* oil was imported from Judea.	Perfume. Eye treatments. As an antidote to poison.

Regalium[4]	Ben nut juice, costus root, *amomum*, Syrian cinnamon, cardamom seed, spikenard, cat-thyme,[5] myrrh, cinnamon bark, styrax resin, rockrose resin, balm, calamus, sweet rush, wild grape, cinnamon leaf, Arabian spice (*serichatum*), henna oil, gingergrass, all-heal (*panax*), saffron, gladiolus, marjoram, honey, wine.	Perfume allegedly used by the kings of Parthia.
Rhodinum	Rose, gingergrass and sweet flag (calamus).	Perfume. Deodorant. Mouthwash. Laxative.
Roseacum	Rose oil	Possibly with sesame oil.[6] Cosmetic, skin care, eye ointment. Laxative.
Sampsuchinum	Sweet marjoram oil.	Perfume. As a treatment for fits and seizures.

---

4 Pliny, in Book XIII of *Natural History*, wrote about the Royal Unguent: 'We will now speak of what is the very climax of luxury and the most important example of this commodity. What then is called the "royal" unguent, because it is a blend prepared for the kings of Parthia, is made of behen-nut oil, costus, amomum, Syrian cinnamon, cardamom, spikenard, cat-thyme, myrrh, cinnamon bark, styrax tree gum, labdanum, balm, Syrian flag and Syrian rush, wild grape, cinnamon leaf, serichatum, cyprus, camel's thorn, all-heal, saffron, gladiolus, marjoram, lotus, honey and wine.'

5 Cat-thyme is also known as marum. Its botanical name is *Teucrium marum* and it is a small shrub, native to Spain. The leaves and young branches emit a volatile aromatic scent which can cause sneezing, so the powdered leaves were used as snuff, taken for 'disorders of the head' (Grieve 1992).

6 Theophrastus noted that 'sesame oil receives rose perfume better than other oils' (Weiss 1997, p.394).

Name	Principle ingredients	Uses
Susinum	Lily roots.	Perfume. To prevent facial wrinkles. To heal facial sores and scurf. As an anti-inflammatory and diuretic.

Note: Castel *et al.* (2009) also mention as common ingredients in Roman perfumery jasmine (*Jasminum grandiflorum* and *J. sambac*), named roses *Rosa centifolia* and *R. damascena*, henna flower (*Lawsonia inermis*), fenugreek (*Trigonella foenum-graecum*), *Juncus odoratus* (*Cymbopogon schoenanthus*), aspalathos (*Alaghi maurorum*) as a thickener and fixative, orcanette root (*Anchusa tinctoria*) for colour, xylobalsamum (Judean balsam tree bark) as a thickener, and spatha (*Phoenix dactylifera* fruit husk) as a fixative and thickener.

The Romans were famous for their public baths. Although their primary function was to promote and maintain the health of the people, they were also important in maintaining and enhancing personal attractiveness. The towns and cities would have had bad smells, just like anywhere else – the toilets were often sited next to kitchens, the sponges used for cleansing were used by all, the sewage system emitted malodours, as would the buckets of urine that were used for cleaning fabrics…so it is not surprising that personal cleanliness was important and that bathing was popular, perhaps up to three times daily. The facilities were often located near natural hot springs, and the bathing process involved several procedures, the latter stages making use of perfume. First, sweating would be induced in the *sudatorium*, followed by a warm bath in the *tepidarium* and then a cool swim in the *frigidarium*. Finally, in the *unctuarium*, scented oils were applied to the skin and then scraped off, along with grime and dead skin, with a *strigil*. Here the ointments and perfumes were stored in large jars, but individuals often brought their own in an *ampulla*, a round container on a chain. The baths would also be the place where other cosmetic treatments were carried out, such as hair removal and massage. The process would end with the application of scent too; and close by the bath-houses, traders would sell cosmetics, oils and perfumes (Le Guérer 1994; Williams 1995a; Stewart 2007).

Perfumes, regarded in the republican times as an honest pleasure, became widely used, and eventually during the imperial period their use became excessive and also associated with orgiastic cults and 'immoral' lifestyles (Morris 1984; Lawless 1994). Pliny the Elder, who was a Stoic and clearly disapproved of an extravagant lifestyle, commented that 'perfumes serve the purpose of the most superfluous of all forms of luxury' (Stewart 2007 p.121). The word *luxuria* meant all manners of excess – overindulgence, expense and pleasure – and encompassed exotic, fashionable, sensual and even immoral nuances. However, Pliny also wrote about trends in perfumery – the rise and fall in popularity of various perfumes. He tells us that *Irinum* of Corinth was very popular but gave way to *Oenanthinum* (vine flower), first from Cyprus, then from Adramytheum. This was superseded by *Amaracinum* from Cos, and then by *Melinum*. So it is clear that in the towns and cities perfumes were not only fashionable but in great demand; they were expensive, and only the wealthy could afford to use them, so perfume was an obvious indicator of social class and status. Perfumes thus had social importance, and the perfume trade was important to the economy (Castel *et al.* 2009).

Perfume makers were known as *aromatarii*. Then, as now, perfumers did not have 'celebrity' status, although a few perfumes were perhaps named after their creators, such as *Megalion* by Megallus. Some towns had streets dedicated to the sale of perfumes, the *vicus unguentarius*. In Capua the Seplasia was renowned for the manufacture and sale of perfumes and cosmetic. In Rome itself there were shops in the Via Sacra that sold luxury goods including perfumes, and the Subura was an area where cosmetics and perfume shops, artisans' workshops, brothels and houses of the wealthy existed in close proximity. It is recognised that perfumes became associated with sexual gratification, including prostitution, and that some prostitutes asked to be paid with perfume, such a pound of the fashionable *Cosmus* or *Niceros* scent (Stewart 2007).

The excesses witnessed in the time of the Emperor Nero surpassed anything before or probably since. Williams (1995a) noted that at the peak of indulgence 'the Romans perfumed themselves, their mansions, their guests and slaves, their dogs and horses. The entire Roman Empire wallowed in perfumistic gluttony and must surely have reeked accordingly' (p.4). Athenaeus' *Deipnosophists* is cited in Le Guérer (1994): 'Strew then, soft carpets underneath the dog…and with Megallian oils anoint his feet' (p.19). Lavish banquets were also a feature of the lives of the wealthy, and scent played an important part in these affairs too. The floors would have been covered in flowers to resemble a 'most divine meadow', the tables would have been rubbed with mint leaves, and the guests wore garlands of aromatic flowers and herbs. It is said that at one of the Emperor Elagabalus'[7] feasts guests suffocated during a floral 'shower', depicted in the 1888 painting by Alma-Tadema. Stewart (2007) gives several other examples of this perfumistic and cosmetic gluttony: the false ceiling in the dining room of Nero's golden house concealed pipes that sprayed his guests with fragrant water; the Empress Poppaea required the milk from five hundred asses for her daily bath, and she bathed her face in asses' milk seven times each day. Morris (1984) suggests that the Romans loved the rose best of all scents, even creating a festival of *Rosalia*. Apparently Nero used about US$100,000 worth at one celebration alone.

So perfumes in ancient Rome were pleasurable 'luxuries', important in health and hygiene, and they had both cosmetic and therapeutic value. However, they were also used in innovative as well as excessive ways, and acquired a variety of associations – with wealth, status, courtesans, harlots and prostitutes. Morris (1984)

---

7   Marcus Aurelius Antoninus, known as Elagabalus or Heliogabalus after the Syrian sun god, became
    Emperor at age 14, in 218 CE, for four years; his outrageous behaviour led to his death.

notes, however, that despite the 'abuses' of perfume, the Romans should be credited with some major achievements – not least the creation of trade routes, the introduction of their perfumes and cosmetics to England (although this was not developed when they left), the development of glassmaking (perfume bottles, often made from alabaster or glass, including blue and green hues, were known as *unguentaria*), and the interest in the senses, finding expression in the works of Pliny the Elder and the physicians Galen and Celsus. Williams (1995a) also highlights that it was Pliny, in his *Naturalia Historia*, who observed the prime requirement of perfumes intended for personal use by females – that they should 'radiate' enough to attract attention, but not be so brash as to elicit inappropriate comments. This is as appropriate today as it was then; the term used now for the radiant quality is *sillage*, meaning the trail of scent left in the air as the wearer passes by.

However, nothing remains of the perfumes, and so an experimental archaeology project – the Seplasia project, named after the perfume area in Capua – aimed to recreate and analyse a perfume, *Iasmelaion*. This was made according to the instructions given by Dioscorides in *De Materia Medica*, and its formula referred to the methods used to make two other perfumes, *Susinum* and *Liliaceum*. The ingredients were sesame oil (*Sesamum indicum* from India), jasmine flowers (*Jasminum grandiflorum* from France), cardamom (*Elettaria cardamomum* from Sri Lanka), cinnamon (*Cinnamomum verum*, also from Sri Lanka), saffron (*Crocus sativus* from Iran) and myrrh (*Commiphora myrrha* from Somalia). Honey and salt were used in the process. The perfume was analysed to determine its volatile composition: the main constituents were ethyl acetate and acetic acid (19.5%), 1,8-cineole (16.3%), linalool (11.8%), α-terpinyl acetate (10.5%), β-myrcene (7.1%) and benzyl acetate (4.6%). Most of the 80 or so constituents could be directly related to the raw materials. However, it is the olfactory appraisal that is exciting, as we can hear a contemporary description of a perfume of antiquity. In the words of an experienced perfumer, *Iasmelaion* was described as giving:

> …a very pleasant jasmine note, quickly hidden by strong spicy notes (cinnamon, clove, pepper). The perfume also provided terpenic notes and a persistent styrax bottom note, making it recall as the ancestor of Opium™ (Yves Saint Laurent). Although cinnamon was predominant, this floral composition was surprising and interesting. (Castel *et al.* 2009, p.333)

Morris (1984) comments that the Romans were also part of a very significant development in perfumery – that is, the use of distillation to extract the volatile oils from aromatic plants. This took place in the second century CE, in Alexandria, a multicultural centre where the philosophy of alchemy was explored. Amongst other endeavours, the alchemists sought ways to find and extract spirit from matter, and the still was developed to extract the *quintessence*, or spirit, from scented plants. Alcohol was another product of distillation, and this too was to have a significant impact on the future of perfumery. An Alexandrian text, *The Gold-Making of*

Cleopatra, has a depiction of a still invented by Maria Prophetissima, who was also known as Maria the Jewess.

The Roman Empire began to disintegrate under the invasions of the 'barbarians' – a word used by the Romans to refer to the Germanic tribes, the Celts, Iberians, Thracians and Persians. The Empire collapsed in 476 CE, and the Roman ways, including those of perfumery, came to an end. However, the Byzantine part of the Empire, in the east, continued to thrive until the fall of Constantinople in 1453, and so, as northern Europe entered the 'Dark Ages', Islamic culture in the East continued to develop the arts and sciences. Both Morris (1984) and Lawless (2009) emphasise that it was through Islam that all the knowledge of the Greco-Roman world was consolidated, translated, refined and spread over Asia, northern Africa and southern and eastern Europe, thus linking antiquity and the classical world to the modern world.

Islamic influences on perfumery

The prophet Mohammed, born in Mecca, which was the centre of the spice trade, held pleasant smells in high esteem. Perfumes were regarded as both hygienic and therapeutic, they could strengthen the senses, and the use of perfumes and cosmetics could distinguish Muslims from Jews and Christians. The period circa 600 CE is noted for the rise of Islam. Mosques were constructed – some with musk mixed in with the mortar.

Some notable individuals and groups had a major impact on perfumery. These include Al-Razi, the alchemist and herbalist, Jabir ibn Hayyan ('Geber'), who wrote about and publicised the process of distillation, Yakub al-Kindi who wrote the *Book of Perfume Chemistry and Distillations*, and Ibn-Sina (Avicenna), the philosopher. Distillation apparatus was refined and improved, partly because of the advances in glassmaking; they made glass that could withstand high temperatures. They did not, however, manage to extract ethyl alcohol from wine with any consistency, possibly due to the lack of efficient cooling technology to condense the vapours.

In the Arab world the trade in aromatics was considerable – including incenses, balsams, saffron, jasmine ointment, sandalwood, cassia, mastic, agarwood, cinnamon, pepper, cloves, nutmeg and camphor, and the animal-derived musk, ambergris and civet. It was via this trade network that the West came into contact with the East – India and China (Morris 1984; Williams 1995a; Lawless 2009).

The archetypal scents were rose and musk; the rose is to Islamic culture as the blue lotus was to the ancient Egyptians. For the Sufis, the rose was a symbol of spiritual attainment. Distillation of the flowers produced the *attar of rose* – the essential oil – and highly scented rosewater, although the early perfumers referred to both products simply as attar. Attar production was important in southern Iran and Syria, and as well as supplying the home market it was exported to India and China. Attar of rose was also used to scent guests, for flavouring, and for perfuming gloves. Other important symbolic scented flowers were the narcissus, where the 'eye' in the centre represented awareness of the divine glory in the world; the violet, which represented adoration; and the hyacinth, which sustained the soul.

In an exploration of the use of perfume in premodern traditional Muslim societies, Hirsch (2013) suggests that perfumes served as 'a device for separation into gendered spheres of smell'. The Arabic language has an extensive vocabulary to describe the various forms and uses of perfume – such as hair and body oils for personal care and adornment – which in itself indicates the cultural importance of scent. Body oils include *al-ban* (from *Moringa* species, behen oil) and *babafsaj* (violet); these had stronger scents than hair oils and were said to enhance attractiveness. However, the public–male and private–female domains were separated, and personal appearance was strictly controlled. Perfume, although not visible, was considered part of outward appearance, and so perfumes became gender-specific. Men could wear perfume in public and private. Male scents and oils had to be colourless, but could have strong odours. Some types of perfume were prohibited for use by men, such as the saffron-based *khaluq* and *za'fran* (saffron), because saffron is yellow and the wearing of this colour was prohibited. Female perfumes, although they could be coloured, had to be light in fragrance, so that only their husbands or concubines' masters could detect the scent. Women were forbidden from leaving their home wearing perfume, lest they attract attention from men – indeed, a perfumed woman near a group of men would be considered an adulteress. Females wore *khaluq*, and also some male fragrances. Those who did not have a clear gender identity – the *mukhannathun* – occupied a space between male and female. To preserve the patriarchal society, with its strict definitions of acceptable outward appearances, both male and female prohibitions were imposed on the *mukhannathun*; however, there are records which suggest that they used *khaluq* and *za'fran*.

By the tenth century, we can see that perfumes had acquired a considerable element of status. The *zurfaa*, the Baghdad aristocrats, would not wear *bakhur* (frankincense) because it was used by the common people, nor *ghaliya*, a perfume worn by concubines and slaves. Perfume is also mentioned in the *Qur'an* – two kinds of precious perfumes are a heavenly reward for living a life in accordance with its principles (Hirsch 2013). So it is clear that early traditional Muslim societies valued perfume, which became integrated into their customs and daily lives, not least by reinforcing important gender distinctions and restrictions.

We have already seen that all of the ancient cultures used perfumes as medicines and for healing. In the Middle East this became an integral part of Unani Tibb medicine, which is the forerunner of modern western herbal medicine. Please see Chapter 12 to explore this facet of perfumery.

India

Indian perfumery developed alongside incense, utilising the myriad of indigenous aromatic plant species. Although the Persian Avicenna is credited with the invention of steam distillation, the basic concept was known as early as 3000 BCE. In 1975

Professor Paolo Rovesti of the University of Milan, who had been investigating the psychotherapeutic effects of essential oils, led an expedition to Pakistan, where he found a terracotta distillation apparatus in the archaeological museum at Taxila. Attars are still the traditional perfumes – based on the archetypal Indian fragrance of sandalwood – co-distilled with flowers such as rose, jasmine, champaca, tuberose and narcissus. While attars are plant-based, the glandular secretion of the civet was first used in India as a perfume; musk and ambergris were also known (Williams 1995a).

The early Dravidian and Aryan cultures were noted for their use of aromatics in bathing, personal care rituals and personal adornment. Literature describes these rituals and scented products in detail. For example, the Sanskrit *Manasollasa* (circa 1130) gives the ingredients of a perfumed body oil: sesame oil with jasmine, coriander, cardamom, holy basil (tulsi), costus, pandanus, agarwood, pine, saffron, champaca and clove – showcasing many of India's beautiful natural ingredients. Sesame oil was a common carrier for the fragrances – it does not readily oxidise and become rancid. Sesame was used in a form of enfleurage to extract scent from the raw materials – for example, *chameli ka tel* was a hair dressing made from sesame and jasmine flowers.

In India, and the lands to the south and east that were influenced by Indian culture, perfume was very important. The old epic, the *Mahabharata*, tells us that the highest goddess described herself as the 'Scent of Earth'. Mogul period paintings reinforce both the gods' and mortals' love of flowers and scents. One such painting depicts the Princess Sumbawati in a paradisiacal garden in the southern Himalayas, where those who rested would be healed by the beautiful scents (Kaiser 2006). So perfume was not only important in the worship of gods but also for human pleasure and wellbeing; and after death the soul would pass to the *gandhamadana* or 'fragrant mountain'. The Hindu heaven is perfumed by the *camalata* or 'flower of heaven'. The *Gandhasara*, a text dated between 500 and 1000 CE, suggests that perfume leads to the attainment of the three aims of human life, namely religious merit, worldly prosperity and sensual enjoyment. Even the valued elephant was the recipient of the gift of perfume – the ritual of *abhyanga* involved washing, then anointing the female elephant with perfumed oil to encourage the passion of the male, and ensure future progeny.

The *gandhika* (perfume dealer) therefore enjoyed an important role in society, trading in aromatics for incense and vegetable oil-based perfumes. The range of available aromatics was extensive and included woods – sandalwood (*chandana*), agarwood; roots of vetiver, costus, *Hedychium spicatus*, galangal, ginger and spikenard; resins and gums of benzoin, frankincense and pine; spices such as cardamom, saffron, cinnamon, nutmeg, clove and pepper; leaves such as patchouli and holy basil; grasses such as lemongrass and palmarosa, gingergrass and citronella; flowers such as jasmine, champaca, rose, tuberose, pandanus and lotus. All of these were, and still are, used in perfumery and also in aromatherapy.

Indian culture, like the Egyptian, enjoyed the scent of fresh flowers at ceremonies; garlands (*rasamala* or *mala*) were not only decorative but fragrant (Morris 1984). Flowers were important in early Hindu society, where their use was secular. The *Rāmāyana* refers to personal floral decorations used by women, including the use of lotus or jasmine flowers in the hair, and men wore floral garlands, especially in the bedroom. The use of fresh flowers was also associated with perfumes and bathing. Garlands and perfumes were common gifts during courtship, while exchanging garlands was found in some forms of marriage ceremony (Goody 1993); so there was a sexual, erotic and affectionate aspect of flowers and scent too. Lawless (1994) discusses the importance of perfume in the Tantric 'Rite of the Five Essentials', where sex was a means of spiritual realisation and accomplishment via the male–female energetic exchange. In this ritual jasmine oil is applied to the woman's hands, her cheeks and neck are anointed with patchouli, her breasts with amber, her hair with spikenard, her genitals with musk, her thighs with sandalwood and her feet with saffron. The male's forehead, neck, chest, navel, arms, thighs, genitals, hands and feet are anointed with sandalwood oil. The 'Scripture of Love' – the *Kama Sutra* – also reveals much about the significance of scent in this particular context.

Flowers and scents were even more important in religion. In Buddhist practice the basic offerings of the flower, the candle and incense had symbolic meaning. The flower represented impermanence, the central teaching of the Dharma; the candle symbolised the light of the wisdom discovered by the Buddha; and the incense symbolised the fragrance of the pure life of those who practise the Buddha Dharma, which touches everything that grows, enabling us to reach our full potential. Although Hinduism became dominant, the use of flowers as offerings was influenced by both Buddhism and, later, Islam. Hindu gods were associated with particular flowers – for example, the lotus (*Nelumbo nucifera*) signified Vishnu, Krishna and Lakshmi; it is central to Indian culture and symbolic of many things, including the birth of the divine, and purity. However, it is of note that although flowers were symbolic, or used in metaphor, one text, the *Dhammapāda*, placed emphasis on their scents, suggesting that their colours were more likely to deceive. There was some ambivalence about flowers and scents, however – because of their secular use they were also regarded as a luxury, or as objects of temptation, and so were rejected by purists. Goody (1993) suggests that this may be one of the reasons why Buddhist monks will not cut a living flower (which also demonstrates the principle of nonviolence) or wear garlands or perfumes. The monks are not allowed to smell a flower either – possibly because of the belief that devas dwelled in flowers, and that nothing should be taken that is not freely given, and so smelling a flower would take away part of its essence. However, cut flowers are considered suitable offerings in a religious context, because they are then being given to the divine or semi-divine. To this day, flowers and garlands play an important part in daily life, representing the divinity within us all. The most common garland flowers are all highly scented – red roses, spider lilies, frangipani and jasmine.

So far, we have explored the development of perfumery in the ancient world, where perfumes were made first by enfleurage or maceration of aromatic plants, and sometimes animal secretions, in oils and fats. Later on, essential oils were extracted from plants by a primitive form of distillation, and then Avicenna invented steam distillation (circa 1000 CE), thus improving the process. Perfumes remained oil-based until after the 'discovery' of alcohol with the invention of the water-cooled condenser in Europe, around 1150 CE. This is significant in the history of European perfumery, when things started to take a very different direction indeed.

The origins and rise of European perfumery

Between 1190 and 1370, European perfumery was in its infancy. Perfumes were first made in Italy, influenced by the East, and then in Spain under the Arabic influence. From the Middle Ages until the Renaissance, Italy led the way. Venice had monopolised the spice trade, and the city was renowned for its elegance, styles and customs, and use of perfume – on persons, clothing, and even coins. Pendants that held musk or ambergris were worn on sleeves, and herbal potpourris were very popular. Because of the prevalent cultural influences and trade routes, with later the discovery of America, Italy and Spain became prosperous countries with access to a wide range of aromatics, around which their styles of perfumery evolved. The climate allowed citrus trees to flourish, and Sicily became the most important centre for citrus oils, while Calabria was renowned for bergamot oil. Spain was noted for its citrus and also wild sage, rosemary and thyme.

France borders both countries, and because of its proximity and cultural exchanges, perfumery practice had spread to the regions in the south by the latter part of the thirteenth century. It is possible that Catherine de Medici of Italy sent an individual named Tombarelli to Grasse, with the intent of establishing a perfume industry there, because of its alliance with the Republic of Genoa. The climate in the south of France was also perfect for growing scented flowers such as jasmine, rose, mimosa, jonquil, tuberose and, of course, lavender – all important aromatic materials in early European perfumery. Philippe August granted a Perfumers' Charter in 1190, which officially recognised the status of the perfumer, and then, around 1200, a perfume was brought to Europe from Cyprus by a returning Crusader. This was known as *eau de Chypre*.

Perfumery in northern Europe developed very slowly over the following century, during which we see the use of scented pomanders by the aristocracy and royalty in France and England, and the Grasse perfume industry starting to emerge. It was during this period that distillation was used to concentrate alcohol, which at the time became regarded as a panacea, with names such as 'admirable water', the 'soul of heaven' and even 'quintessence' – the fifth element. Ethyl alcohol was used therapeutically at the medical school in Salerno, south of Naples, and from there travelling scientists spread the art of distillation across Europe, where it was used in alchemy, to prepare paints and lacquers, jewellery and metals, cosmetics and medicines, and alcoholic beverages (Antoninetti 2011).

From the fourteenth century until the end of the seventeenth century, pandemic plagues occurred regularly. The pathogens were carried by rats, but at the time this was not known. All manner of causes were suggested, such as astrological forces and even dogs, because plague outbreaks tended to occur in the summer, when Sirius, the 'dog star', rises and sets with the sun. Despite such theories, the prevailing belief was that the cause of the plague was its stench; those who carried the plague emitted a stench similar to rotting meat, and the putrefying bodies of victims had an overpowering, very foul odour. This in turn inspired various elaborate hypotheses, associating planetary or geological influences, or evil spirits, with the foul smell. It was also thought that the spirit or 'life force' was similar in nature to odour: tangible but invisible. Therefore, if the cause of the plague was the malodour, the means of prevention was scent. The pomander prototype – an orange studded with dried cloves – became a popular accessory, posies of aromatic flowers were carried, handkerchiefs were saturated with perfume, and doctors wore nose-bags filled with herbs and spices. The plague thus stimulated consumption of aromatics; however, the Black Death in Europe (1348) was responsible also for an increased interest in alcohol, as it was recognised that, unlike water, it did not deteriorate or become tainted. Alcohol was also known as *eau ardente* or 'burning water' and was used to combat illness, becoming known as *aqua vitae*, or in France as *eau de vie* – the 'water of life' (Tonutti and Liddle 2010).

The first commercial production of alcohol was in 1320 at Modena. In 1370 the first known alcoholic perfume was made. The formula was given to Queen Elizabeth of Hungary by a hermit, who assured her that it would preserve her beauty – and allegedly it did! This simple formula of rosemary and alcohol, with a later addition of lavender, became known as *Eau de la Reine de Hongrie* – 'the Queen of Hungary's water', and later simply as 'Hungary water'; its popularity persisted for five centuries, and it is said to be the forerunner of *Eau de Cologne*. Around the same period, in 1379, the lesser known *Eau de Carmes*, or 'Carmelite water', was made for Charles V of France, by the nuns of the Abbaye St Juste. This too was a herbal scent, containing lemon balm, angelica and other herbs (Morris 1984; Williams 1995a; Williams 1996). Another perfumed product of the time was *lavender water* – this was liqueur-like and used internally as well as externally (Morris 1984). At the time it was believed that bathing was harmful to body and soul. These early aromatic waters, with their fresh aromas and antioxidant and antiseptic properties, would certainly have been helpful in combatting body malodours that developed as a consequence of poor personal hygiene. The demand for aromatic herbs grew, and areas such as Montpellier and Grasse in the south of France became firmly established as growers of herbs and flowers, and producers of aromatic waters.

A landmark discovery was that the small amounts of oily liquid – long considered impurities in the distilled waters – were in fact the source of the scent of the waters; these became known as essential oils, but their recovery was not viable. However, in 1420 the coil-type condenser (or 'worm') was invented, and this development eventually, by the beginning of the sixteenth century, allowed the large-scale distillation of essential oils. By 1560 citrus oils were being produced, and Grasse became known for its essential oils as well as aromatic crops. A further important development was the independent 'discovery' of alcohol by the alchemist Basil Valentine in 1450 – this marked the beginning of alcoholic perfumery and the production of herbal tinctures. Over the next century, perfumes based on herbal and floral essential oils, citrus oils including bergamot, and the animal-derived musk and civet became popular with the French aristocracy; their use declined under the reign of Henri IV, and was revived later by Louis XIV (1643–1715). He was apparently very odour-conscious, and had a personal perfumer who was challenged with creating a different perfume for each day. In 1658 Louis XIV reviewed and renewed the Perfumer's Charter, so that to become a perfumer and gain entry to the company of French Master Perfumers, a four-year apprenticeship and a further three years as a 'companion' were required (Morris 1984; Williams 1995a; Williams 1996).

Meanwhile, in England, the Elizabethan aristocracy (1558–1603) were using lavender and rose waters, pomanders and perfumed gloves, and scenting their wigs with fragrant powders. Glove scenting was a common practice; it masked the bad smell that resulted from the leather tanning process; shoes were scented for the same reason. Homes were perfumed too, to cover up the foul smells caused by the burning of tallow candles, basic sanitation consisting of simple chamber pots, soiled rushes covering floors, and the accumulation of years of filth. Floor coverings could be replaced regularly, and homes could be fragranced by 'strewing herbs' that would release pleasant smells when walked upon. This may also have helped stop the spread of disease – thought to be carried by, or inherent within, malodours – while repelling evil, supposedly another source of disease and epidemics. (As an aside, it is very interesting to note that, even in modern times, people exposed to malodours report that they have been adversely affected in terms of task performance, mood, and perceived health; see Knasko 1993.) Common strewing herbs were representative of the aromatic plants that thrive in the English climate, and included bay laurel, sweet flag, lemon balm, lavender, marjoram, rosemary and thyme; Elizabeth I favoured meadowsweet as a strewing herb. Nosegays were used for similar reasons; wallflowers, sweet william and marjoram were popular. These were small bouquets of flowers carried or worn by men and women, not only to mask bad smells but also to offer protection from the diseases believed to be carried by the smells. Scented herbs such as lavender and rosemary would be grown in pots in the home, and dried and hung from the ceilings. These flowers and herbs were found in the traditional walled gardens of the times – Frances Bacon wrote an essay on gardens in 1625, and mentioned the pleasure of scented flowers such as violets and roses, and herbs such as burnet, thyme and water mint. Clothing and linens would be washed, or 'dry cleaned' by rubbing with herbs. However, despite the efforts made to keep homes smelling fresh, the belief that personal bathing was harmful to wellbeing prevailed. This was possibly because it was considered to be decadent, and because dirt was considered to be a sign of holiness. Moreover, water was thought to weaken the physical body by making it soft and vulnerable (Classen *et al.* 1994). The dreadful personal hygiene situation was not helped by Charles I, who in 1630 imposed an excise duty on soap. This has been blamed for the rise in the lavish use of perfumes to mask personal malodours, and the fashionable gentlemen of the time also began to use the faecal-smelling raw civet. In England, around 1660, we can also see another example of the connection between perfumery and pharmacy: pharmaceutical chemists distilling aromatic herbal waters such as lavender, elderflower and rosemary, which were then sold alongside 'heavier' perfumes such as the civet types with their animalic accords, and cosmetics. Later, with the advent of the 'art' of perfumery, fashion changed and the heavy perfumes were replaced by 'single flower' perfumes, where the perfumers strove to imitate nature.

We return to Italy to learn about the evolution of Hungary water into *Eau de Cologne*, the best-known of all toilet waters. This was a somewhat murky process, and the finer details are lost. In 1690 Jean-Paul Feminis, who was allegedly a perfumer in Milan, gained access the formula for Hungary water via a Florentine convent. He experimented with the addition of Italian neroli essential oil, bergamot and orange, to create the new toilet water. The formula was then passed on to his nephew, Jean-Antoine Farina, who subsequently moved to Cologne, where it was manufactured, named *Kölnisch Wasser* and first sold. *Eau de Cologne* was also credited with therapeutic properties, apparently being good for the skin, the gums and the stomach, and even for use on animals. Farina's name appeared on the bottles, so he is often, but most probably erroneously, given credit as its creator. *Eau de Cologne* was brought to France in 1763 by soldiers returning from the Seven Years' War and became very popular, partly because of the patronage of the Emperor Napoleon Bonaparte (circa 1800). Its success was such that it spawned many imitations, and many false 'Farinas' too. *Eau de Cologne* is still made, and now belongs to the house of Roger and Gallet. It has no 'staying power', and thus is not considered a true perfume (Morris 1984; Williams 1995a).

The early eighteenth century in France is known as the Rococo period, when the fashion for pomp and ceremony was replaced by informality and an emphasis on 'good taste'. This change was reflected in personal care, hygiene and perfumery too; the industry was influenced by individuals such as the Marquise de Pompadour and Marie Antoinette, who popularised the use of perfumes, potpourris and scented fans. The court of Louise XV was called *la Cour parfumeé*, where a different scent would be worn each day of the week. To maintain this custom the King's lover, Madame de Pompadour, allegedly spent a million francs to create a 'perfume bank' (Le Guérer 1994). Perfumes of the Rococo period included rose, orange blossom and lavender waters, and *mille-fleur*. Nevertheless, Versailles and eighteenth-century Paris stank. The writer Louis-Sebastian Mercier suggested that it was the only the

Parisians' familiarity with 'a thousand putrid vapours' that allowed them to live in their 'filthy haunt' (Classen *et al.* 1994).

The French Revolution of 1789 had an enormous impact on the use of luxuries such as perfumes; the industry declined and did not recover until 1835, with the help of Napoleon Bonaparte, who was made Emperor in 1802. Under Napoleon talent, research and technology were fostered and rewarded. He was renowned for his obsession with good hygiene and scents, but it was his consort Josephine who revived the Rococo spirit, establishing her own 'Empire' style. She dressed in white, sleeveless gowns, reminiscent of classical Greece, and wore Kashmiri wraps and shawls made from fine Tibetan goat wool. These would have been scented with dried patchouli leaves, added to preserve the garments. As a result patchouli fragrance became popular, as did rose, which was Josephine's favourite flower and scent. It is said that she also enjoyed musk, but Napoleon disliked it enormously, and when Josephine was replaced by Marie-Louise, she took her revenge by 'saturating' their personal apartments with the long-lasting odour of musk. After Josephine, fashions changed again, her exotic and sensual styles and scents being replaced by something more restrained, demure and modest; perfumes had to be light – and certainly not the sensual and powerful patchouli or musk (Morris 1984).

In France, alcoholic perfumery was firmly established by the early 1800s, and from this point onwards we see the rise of fragrance 'houses' including some well-known names such as Houbigant, Lubin, Charabot et Cie, Farina and, arguably the most famous of all, the House of Guerlain, founded by Pierre François Guerlain in 1828. The Empress Eugénie (1826–1920), wife of Louis Napoleon, was dressed by the English couturier Charles Frederick Worth, who gave his clients perfume as gifts; *Dans la Nuit* became a big success. She also patronised the house of Guerlain – *Eau Impériale* was created for her in 1861. Meanwhile, in Britain, Queen Victoria, by contrast, was not actively encouraging perfumery. By this time France completely dominated the European perfume industry. Louis Napoleon passed a law that required all pharmaceuticals to have their ingredients listed on the label, and so perfumes and medicines parted company, because the perfumers would not reveal their formulae. Thus was perfumery separated from pharmacy completely, coming to be regarded as a creative art, and a profession and industry in its own right (Williams 1995a).

Compared with modern perfumes, these early ones were not sophisticated. Their structure was relatively simple, and loosely based on the molecular weight and volatility of the ingredients. Perfumes consisted of top notes (constituents responsible for the initial impact), merging with middle notes (the heart of the perfume) which in turn merged and faded with the least volatile constituents (the base notes).

In 2010 Alec Lawless was commissioned by the makers of a television documentary to research English perfumery of the Victorian era and create a perfume in the style of the period.[8] Lawless (2010b) explains that in the early Victorian era there were around 40 pharmacist/perfumers working in London, comparable to Paris. He commented that Victorian pharmacists would produce alcohol by redistilling French brandy to separate the ethyl alcohol, which was collected in the first fraction. There was a fairly large palette of aromatics to choose from, thanks to the Dutch spice traders and the expanding British Empire. Often the crude raw materials would be macerated in alcohol (brandy) and water in a large glass container that was sealed and kept warm for several days – courtesy of fresh horse manure, which released heat as it decomposed. Then the contents would be distilled, and the distillate returned to the container with a fresh charge of aromatics, and left to macerate as before. If in turn distilled, this would produce a 'double essence' – and a 'triple essence' if the process was repeated for a third time. By the end of the Victorian period this procedure was replaced by much more sophisticated methods.

For the TV documentary Lawless created a perfume which he named *Empress of India*, to give an impression of a perfume of the late Victorian era. The base consisted of typical oriental materials – sandalwood, vetiver, frankincense, vanilla, opopanax and patchouli. The heart was floral, with tuberose, jasmine (*J. grandiflorum* and *J. sambac*), and rose and orange blossom absolutes. Finally, the top notes were given by neroli, bergamot, green mandarin, rose otto, orris root and coriander. It is interesting to smell this representation of scent from a bygone age, not only for its evocative effect but because it also represents a type of fragrance that can be created by contemporary artisan perfumers working with plant-derived ingredients.

The advent of aromachemicals and couturier perfumes

> One has to rely on chemists to find new aromachemicals creating new, original notes. In perfumery the future lies primarily in the hands of the chemists. (Ernest Beaux, cited in Fortineau 2004, p.45)

Until the mid-nineteenth century, perfumes consisted solely of natural plant and animal extracts. It was thought that the scents (belonging to the large family of hydrocarbons) had been made in the cells of living plants, and that 'life force' or a 'vital force' was necessary in this process. However, in 1845 Kolbé synthesised acetic acid from the elements carbon, hydrogen and oxygen, and as a consequence the vital force theory was abandoned. The first laboratory-synthesised 'aromachemicals' were benzyl acetate by Cannizaro in 1855, and methyl benzoate by Carius in 1859, although they were not immediately used in perfumery (Williams 1995a). As solvent extraction technology advanced, products such as concretes and absolutes became available to the perfumer. Then, as organic chemistry and analytical methods

---

8   *Victorian Pharmacy* (Producer Cassie Braben, for Lion Television) was a four-part historical documentary first broadcast by the BBC (on BBC Two) between 15 July and 12 August 2010. The topic of perfume was addressed in episode four.

continued to develop, fragrance compounds were isolated from these extracts, and examined from the olfactory perspective (Kaiser 2011). The first 'isolates' were coumarin from tonka beans, by Wöhler in 1856, and vanillin from vanilla pods, by Gobley in 1858 (Williams 1995a).

The impact on perfumery was massive. The change began in 1868, when the aromachemical coumarin, a naturally occurring component of tonka beans, was synthesised by Perkin and Graebe. At the time it was not known that this first synthetic coumarin was in fact toxic. Parquet, an owner and perfumer at Parfums Houbigant used this synthetic coumarin in combination with natural ingredients to make a scent for the toilet soap *Fougère Royale*, launched in 1882. Despite his innovation and success, which ultimately led to a class of perfumes known as fougère ('fern'), the prevalent attitude amongst perfumers at the time was one of resistance, and indeed most synthesised aromachemicals were viewed with suspicion, and not used until their presence had been established in natural extracts. However, Parquet continued to use synthetics and produced *Le Parfum Ideal*, while his protégé Robert Bienaimé created *Quelque Fleurs*; these are now considered to be the ancestors of *Chanel No.5* (Williams 1995a). Eventually the use of aromachemicals with naturals became part of creative perfumery, and the evolution of this hybrid form accelerated, with entirely new types of scent, albeit based on the traditional floral and floral/balsamic format. Companies that synthesised and supplied aromachemicals as well as natural extracts flourished to support the industry, including Haarmann and Reimer, Givaudan et Cie, Roure Bertrand Dupont, Robertet et Cie and Charabot.

The final years of the nineteenth century and beginning of the twentieth century – a period known as *la Belle Époque* – is often said to be the 'golden age' of perfumery. Prominent figures in perfumery, such as François Coty (1873–1934), embraced *Art Nouveau* and collaborated with the glass-maker René Lalique in catering for the rich and famous as well as the less affluent. Paul Poiret (1879–1943) linked his luxuriant, fluid and colourful fashion designs with exotic fragrances, and some 'classic' fragrances were introduced. Caron's *Narcisse Noir* was composed by Daltroff, based on the narcissus, an oriental spring flower, and *L'Heure Bleue*, composed by Jacques Guerlain, contained resins, labdanum and synthetics.

Until the beginning of the twentieth century perfumes were produced by the large perfumeries, notably Coty, Houbigant and Piver, who employed 'in-house' perfumers. However, in 1921, the couturier Coco Chanel, noted for her sombre use of colour and pared-down *garçonne* ('boy-girl') style, launched *Chanel No.5*. Composed by the perfumer Ernest Beaux, this was destined to become a well-known and enduring fragrance, but it was also a 'first' in two ways. Although the formula had a traditional construction, with a resinous/rosy wood base of olibanum (frankincense), labdanum and guaiacwood, and a floral heart with gardenia and ylang ylang, the predominant top notes were entirely new and different. They were synthetic, given by aromachemicals known as fatty aldehydes, with aldehyde C_{12} in relatively large proportions. This spawned a new 'aldehydic' perfume style, which was characterised by radiance, power and persistence. Williams (1995a) suggested that *Chanel No.5* was 'artistically a brilliant innovation rather than a great perfume, commercially a superlative success' (p.11).

The second point is that the launch of *No.5* marked the ingress of the world of fashion into perfumery as Chanel was followed by D'Orsay in 1925 with *Le Dandy*, by Lanvin in 1927 with *Arpège*, and Worth in 1932 with *Je Reviens*. Many others designers followed – Balenciaga, Grès, Jean Patou, Christian Dior, Yves Saint Laurent – and this trend has continued to the present day. Indeed, some of the couturiers are better known for their fragrances than for fashion; paradoxically their contribution is in the design and packaging, not the perfumes. These perfumes are composed by the in-house perfumers of the aromachemicals and natural extracts industries, and not the by the traditional perfumeries, as in the early part of the century.

As the synthetics began to dominate, manufacturing companies were formed that employed chemists to synthesise new aromachemicals, and perfumers to create fragrances and perfume 'bases' for incorporation into product lines. Consequently, scented cosmetics, personal care products and household products became widely available – fragranced largely with synthetics to make them more attractive to consumers. As a result of the commercialisation of fragrance, the world of perfumery has changed beyond recognition. According to Turin (2006), there are now six billion-dollar multinational perfumery firms (Firmenich, Givaudan, IFF, Quest Symrise and Takasago) and many smaller ones.

The vast majority of perfumes today contain high proportions of aromachemicals in relation to naturals, and this is not simply because they are better or cheaper. A synthetic aromachemical has one characteristic scent that does not change over time, while a natural extract has a complex scent made up of many aromatic constituents, giving a changing odour profile as it evaporates. Some novel aromachemicals are very expensive, and others are very cheap. 'Captives' are novel aromachemicals created and owned by the parent company, and are not for sale. Some natural extracts are hugely expensive, and there is the additional aspect of variable quality. This all has an impact on the cost of a perfume. Turin (2006) writes that in the second half of the 1990s, a fine fragrance would cost US$200–300 per kilo, but ten years later just US$100 was considered expensive. A more sobering statistic is that the fragrance in the bottle (the 'juice') represents only 3 per cent of the cost of a perfume – the rest being packaging, advertising and margins. The end result is that many fragrances are very poor indeed, although Turin lists 'slavish imitation, crass vulgarity, profound ignorance, fear of getting fired and general lack of inventiveness and courage' (p.13) as additional contributing factors. This is a strange and sad state of affairs indeed.

So what have synthetics contributed to modern perfumery? As well as offering new scents for the perfumer's palette, some allow the inclusion of scents that are very difficult to obtain from natural sources. For example, to produce just one kilogram of violet flower oil, 33,000kg of blossoms are needed. However, ionones are aromachemicals with a violet odour. They were first synthesised in 1893, and have revolutionised perfumery (Fortineau 2004). The perfumer René Laruelle maintains that 'synthetics are the bones of the fragrance, naturals are the flesh' (Turin 2006, pp.189–190). In other words, a better structure or 'scaffold' can be achieved with synthetics, but the naturals give character, complexity, interest and depth.

One of the main criticisms of perfumes constructed entirely with naturals is that they lack coherence and structure; however, an entirely synthetic perfume can be somewhat one-dimensional. So what is meant by perfume structure, and how can we recognise it? First, there are different approaches to perfume construction, giving rise to different styles and structures. Calkin and Jellinek (1994) commented that 'all art depends upon form and structure' (p.84). A perfume at the beginning of the twentieth century would have been influenced by the earlier *Eau de Cologne*. Fresh citrus top notes, essential oils and floral absolutes enhanced by synthetics and natural isolates, with animal and balsamic fixatives, represent this traditional approach to construction, as in Guerlain's *Shalimar* (1925). Such fragrances evolve on the skin, over time. As more synthetics became available, they became the main inspiration, rather than used to support the naturals, and the naturals were used to provide richness or 'the flesh'. An 'accord' is a simple or complex formula of naturals and/or synthetics that gives a particular effect or style. Jean Carles developed the system of creating three accords – a base, middle and a top note – and then exploring the different effects by varying the ratios of each in the final composition. Calkin and Jellinek (1994) suggest that this type of structure gives 'transparency and texture', which leads us directly to the heart of the fragrance; we can smell this in fragrances such as Nina Ricci's *L'Air du Temps* (1948). However, in more recent years, a different approach to construction has become popular, typified by the work of Sophia Grojsman. Here, a very simple synthetic accord constitutes up to 80 per cent of the composition, and additional bases and naturals provide complexity and identity. This style of perfume is characterised by trace amounts of powerful materials that replace fresh top notes; the heart of the fragrance is revealed from the very beginning, and it will remain essentially unchanged on the skin over the duration. Lancôme's *Trésor* (1990) is typical of the genre.

Another factor has influenced the way modern perfumes are constructed. The International Fragrance Research Association (IFRA) guidelines and European Union (EU) regulations have resulted in restrictions on the use of several of the most important naturals, including citrus oils, which provide classic top notes; rose and jasmine, which are at the heart of most florals; and oakmoss, a base note crucial for the chypre genre, as well as some aromachemicals – because they are suspected of being allergens. For several reasons, many perfumers and perfume-lovers take the view that some of these restrictions are over-zealous or even unsound, and that some might be based on insufficient evidence. Citrus, rose, jasmine and oakmoss have been used in perfumery for millennia, but they are complex materials containing many constituents, any one of which might be an allergen. The perfumers' palette has thus become diminished, especially in terms of the naturals. Many staple synthetics have also been restricted – for example, hydroxycitronellal and benzyl salicylate. The bans and restrictions have also meant that some of the earlier 'classic' fragrances have had to be reformulated, often to their detriment, according to critics. Luca Turin comments that 'it is a crying shame that regulatory pressure is destroying so much of fragrance's already fragile heritage' (Turin and Sanchez 2009, p.261). Thierry Wasser of Guerlain has suggested that perhaps some perfumes could be given 'cultural heritage' status so that they could be exempt from the anti-allergen guidelines. However, this does not seem likely, partly because of the secrecy regarding formulae. In a 2012 interview, perfumer Fabria Pellegrin (creator of *Volute* for Dyptique and *Womanity* for Mugler) was asked about his views on the subject. He commented, 'If we tried today to recreate a real, original Guerlain, I think it would be impossible.'

Roman Kaiser of Givaudan (2011) notes that by 1970 we knew of literally hundreds of extracts and in excess of 1000 synthetic fragrance and flavour compounds. In 2004 Fortineau had estimated that out of the 3000 available perfume ingredients, fewer than 5 per cent came directly from natural sources. Calkin and Jellinek (1994) make the important point that there is a 'grey area' between naturals and synthetics, first because the so-called naturals are not really natural, because the extraction process has already changed them, so we should view them instead as products of natural origin. (Indeed, the most useful naturals are the terpeneless (or concentrated) essential oils. These are made by removing the terpenes from essential oils by fractional distillation under vacuum, leaving only the significant aroma compounds which are characteristic of the botanical source. The terpeneless oils are less likely to cause solubility problems; they have more 'body', and are less prone to deterioration over time; see Jouhar 1991.) Second, some of the isolates, such as vanillin obtained from vanilla, or geraniol from palmarosa, are also of natural origin. However, geraniol can also be synthesised from pinene, an isolate of pine oil, and this would be described as synthetic. Geraniol, whether of natural origin or not, is a monoterpene alcohol that can be modified to become an ester called geranyl acetate, and this would also be described as synthetic. Third, many natural extracts are further modified to produce 'derivatives' that behave as naturals in perfume compounding.

Kaiser (2011) suggests that as analytical systems become more sensitive we will find many more aromachemicals and that their synthesis will be more efficient and environmentally friendly; eventually we should be able to recreate most natural odours. If we consider that some important natural extracts come from unsustainable sources, and that the fragrances of natural extracts are influenced by the extraction process, we can view the use of synthetic aromachemicals in a different light. Kaiser's work on the vanishing aromatic flora has allowed him to prepare odour profiles of well over 200 rare and endangered species, and a few that are now extinct. He has used sensitive electronic devices that non-destructively collect micro-samples of scents directly from living plants, so that their true scent, as perceived by our nose, is preserved. This has already allowed the reconstruction of many rare plant scents

– so that even if these plants become extinct, we may still smell them. Theophrastus and Dioscorides would surely have approved.

Classic and contemporary perfumes, their creators and critics

Just as in ancient times, the last few decades have revealed some distinct trends in western perfumery; and these trends are reflected in both fashion and social behaviour. Morris (1984) gives a very detailed account of the development of perfumery from the 1920s to the 1980s – the following analysis is structured around his account. For a summary and explanation of the different perfume types mentioned, please see Appendix A.

In the early 1930s the couturier Elsa Shiaparelli promoted fashion that celebrated female curves and was colourful and flamboyant (especially 'shocking pink'), in complete contrast to Coco Chanel. She associated herself with the Surrealists – Salvador Dali designed the bottle for her fragrance *Roi Soleil*. Her perfumes, such as *Shocking* (1937), containing patchouli and hyacinth, reflected her attitudes and the times. France, like many other countries, went through the Depression in the 1930s, so many of the perfumes echoed the indomitable spirit of the people. *Vol de Nuit* (Guerlain 1933) was inspired by the fascination with air travel and was named after a popular novel; the glass bottle was decorated with the shape of the French Air Force wings. The scent itself included spices, orris root, woods, oakmoss and aldehydes. Perfumes by Dana (a Spanish company) such as *Twenty Carats* (1933) also show us how dreams of wealth counteracted the austerity of the era. Jean Carles created *Tabu* for Dana in 1931 – a rich oriental scent. Jean Patou, a couturier who had enjoyed success in the 1920s, worked with the perfumer Jean Almeras (and others) to develop a line of fragrances, the most successful and enduring being *Joy* (1931). The ethos behind *Joy* was to be free of all vulgarity, regardless of the cost – it was known as 'the world's most expensive perfume', containing expensive rose, jasmine and synthetics. Despite the cost, it was an instant success.

It was not fashionable for men to wear fragrance, other than 'Bay Rum' hair dressing or perhaps *Eau de Cologne* and lavender water. However, in America, in 1938, William Schultz launched a clove-scented aftershave lotion called *Old Spice*. This became a massive success, and marked the return of 'masculine' fragrances. The perfume industry grew with the cosmetic and personal care industry in America – names such as Elizabeth Arden (founded by the Canadian nurse Florence Graham), Helena Rubinstein (originally of Krakow in Poland), Charles of the Ritz (Charles Jundt), Avon Products Inc. and Revlon (Charles Revson) were all established by the 1930s, and survived the Depression years.

After the Second World War, Christian Dior, with financial backing to help the recovery of the couture industry, introduced the 'New Look' – a backlash against the austerity and rationing of the war years – with glamour, defined curves, sweeping fabrics and full skirts. The British were appalled by this excess; the government demanded a boycott of the style, and the early liberationists considered it a retrograde step for women. However, the next two decades were prosperous years, and Dior thrived. The perfumer Edmond Roudnitska was responsible for many of Dior's successful fragrances, advertised with elegant posters financed by the champagne producer Moët. Roudnitska's notable perfumes of the time included the 'classic' *Diorama* and *Diorissimo* – which remain successful fragrances, albeit reformulated. The 1940s also saw the introduction of two important 'green' perfumes – Carven's *Ma Griffe* (1944) and Balmain's *Vent Vert* (1945) – both now reformulated and sadly unrecognisable. The actress Audrey Hepburn, whose distinctive and elegant appearance continues to fascinate, was dressed by Givenchy, and was the inspiration behind *L'Interdit* in the 1950s. This was possibly the first 'celebrity fragrance', although it should be said that Hepburn was in the role of the muse, not the creator of the perfume brief.

The late 1950s and 1960s were also prosperous years, but the 60s were marked by youthful rebellion against authority and convention, and the formation of countercultures. Perhaps it is the popular music and style of the era that is best remembered, but this marked the decline of the couturier houses and their fragrances as the demand for 'ready to wear' clothing grew. Dior died suddenly in 1957, leaving Yves Saint Laurent in charge of his business. After a short time Yves Saint Laurent severed his relationship with the company; it is said that he did not cope with the stresses; however, he survived the decade and emerged as a designer rather than a couturier. The American company Estée Lauder Inc. was formed in 1946, and had its first major success in 1953 with the oriental fragrance *Youth Dew* – originally it was a bath oil, not an alcohol-based perfume. It was powerful but affordable – part of the key to its enormous success.

In the 1960s the hippie counterculture emerged, originating in America but spreading to Europe, along with a 'back-to-nature trend'. Accordingly, the scents of the era were persistent, oil-based single notes called simply *jasmine, sandalwood, musk, civet,* and so on. Paradoxically, many of the perfumes were synthetic rather than natural, and some of the scents bore no relation to their names. Musk perfumes were probably the most popular, although many versions actually smelled of blackberries; and Williams (1995a) suggests that we should be very thankful that the civet representations were also inaccurate.

New men's fragrances were introduced in the late 1960s and 1970s too. These were variants of the 'chypre' type, which was first created by Coty in 1917 and simply named *Le Chypre*. This type is less gender-specific than the florals and aldehydics, and can be varied with the addition of 'masculine' tobacco, leather, green and herbaceous notes. Popular fragrances were Fabergé's *Brut* and, at the top end of perfumery, the critically acclaimed *Eau Sauvage*, composed for Dior by Roudnitska, and originally intended for both men and women. In America, Lauder launched the successful male fragrance *Aramis* in 1964.

The 1970s saw the rise of lifestyle and fantasy perfumes, perhaps mirroring what many people were aspiring to. For example, the low cost *Charlie!* by Revlon (1973) was advertised in such a way as to imply that its female wearers would be made to feel confident, successful, assertive and independent. The perfume itself was quite complex and instantly recognisable – powerful and sweet, with a green citrus top, an aldehydic floral heart and musky base. *Charlie!* has since been a victim of reformulation and has changed beyond recognition.

The success of *Charlie!* was followed by others, such as Lentheric's *Tramp*. Other perfumes alluded to a fantasy or an exciting or glamorous place rather than a lifestyle, such as Yves Saint Laurent's *Rive Gauche* (1971) and Rochas' *Mystère de Rochas* (1978). Other well-established perfume houses produced fragrances that are now considered to be classics, notably *Chanel No.19* (1971), *Diorella* (1972) which was derived from *Eau Sauvage*, and Lauder's *White Linen* (1978). The phenomenally successful *Opium* (Yves Saint Laurent) was launched towards the end of the decade, in 1977, and this heralded a trend that continued through the 1980s. As its name suggests, it was inspired by the scents of China, and is an oriental fragrance dominated by spices and balsams, and with formidable sillage and persistence.

The 1980s, at least in the West, were characterised by consumerism and the acquisition of wealth and possessions, and fashions were big and bold. As always, fragrance trends paralleled the times. Many of the perfumes launched in the 1980s were powerful and impossible to ignore. Success is copied, so there were others in the *Opium* genre, such as the slightly more subtle *Cinnabar* (Lauder 1978) and later *Samsara* (Guerlain 1989). Other fragrance types were launched, especially in the floral/aldehydic class, often featuring tuberose, and several were considered so overpowering that some establishments even 'banned' the wearing of these strong and diffusive perfumes. Examples of the particularly 'huge' and diffusive type are Giorgio Beverly Hills' fruity-tuberose *Giorgio* (1981), Dior's syrupy-tuberose *Poison* (1984) and Givenchy's soapy-tuberose *Amarige* (1991). (Turin and Sanchez (2009, p.284) suggest that we can see a parallel between the excesses of the 1980s and the days of Tiberius, Caligula and Nero in ancient Rome, while the 1990s were more like the Emperor Claudius school of fragrance – 'pinched, mean and full of sour probity'.)

There is no doubt that fragrance preferences changed again as the bold fashion statements of the 1980s came to be seen as vulgar and dated. Mugler's *Angel* (1992), Calvin Klein's 'unisex' *cK One* (1994), *Comme des Garçons* (1994), Chanel's *Cristalle* (1993), Dior's *Dune* (1992), Gucci's *Eau de Gucci* (1993) and Issey Miyake's *L'eau d'Issey* (1992), all launched in the first half of the decade, illustrate the new trends: the sweet, candy-floss *Angel*, the beautifully constructed and subtle transparent-floral-spicy *Comme des Garçons*, the unusual, orris-dominated, sombre and interesting *Dune*, and the crisp-citrus-chypre *Cristalle* were all innovative and different from anything that had gone before. *L'eau d'Issey* popularised an aquatic, melon-like note provided by the ubiquitous aromachemical 'Calone' – a trend that persisted. We can also see light, clean floral and sometimes 'aquatic' fragrances coming to the fore with *Acqua di Giò* and numerous others – a popular antidote to the excesses of the previous decade, but strangely incongruous with the styles espoused by the Goth and Grunge countercultures...

Since the turn of the century, we continue to observe perfumes mirroring popular culture. In the early 1990s a few film actresses and actors launched their 'own' fragrances – for example, Elizabeth Taylor, Priscilla Presley and Omar Sharif. There is no doubt the public fascination with the rich and famous and the cult of 'celebrity' has grown, and now we have countless examples of their fragrances – some hailed as good examples, whilst others have been harshly criticised by perfume writers and critics.

The perfume world has been changed forever by the internet, where there are sites dedicated to fragrance and numerous perfume blogs and 'communities of people clustered around this single obsession' who can discuss fragrance in complete freedom, and review and critique perfumes without commercial bias (Turin and Sanchez 2009). The internet has also contributed to the rise of niche perfumery – small perfume houses with a focus on creativity rather than commercialisation. This is a healthy change. Thanks to expanded interest and freedom of information, we are finally seeing perfumers being given credit for their fragrances, rather than being hidden behind a name on a bottle. Before the advent of the internet, and the increasing number of popular books on the subject, only those studying perfumery would have heard about the fragrance composers and their work.

There has also been an increased interest in ecology and the natural world, and consequently a rise in personal care and household products that claim to be 'green' in various ways – for example, by containing naturally derived and/or organic ingredients, and being free from various 'chemicals'. As a further consequence, natural and organic perfumes are more available. (The first were made by Aveda in the late 1970s.) An extension of this trend can be seen in the growing numbers of natural perfumers, in America at first, but reaching the UK in recent years. Courses in artisan natural perfumery became available; however, in the UK, insurance and issues of product safety testing make its practice expensive, and bespoke natural perfumery virtually unaffordable. In America the 'Guild of Natural Perfumers' is a flourishing organisation that offers support and insurance to its members.

Since the early days of simple plant- and oil-based perfumes, perfume has undergone a radical transformation, and at every stage has reflected the peoples and the times. Perfume – invisible, tangible and transient – is at the heart of a vast industry, which has developed because of our desire to fragrance ourselves and our environment for pleasure. Perfumes in various forms, and which can be delivered in a wide range of ways – from simple atomiser bottles and diffusers to sophisticated electronic devices – are used mostly for pleasure and for mood enhancement, and for creating a pleasant or congruent ambience. Occasionally scent is used as therapy, or to enhance therapeutic practices, or to facilitate meditation or promote wellbeing. Scent is an integral part of our daily lives – whether we are conscious of this or not. Are we all aware of its enormous yet subtle impact, and that perfume is indeed the reflection, or perhaps the shadow, of our culture?

CHAPTER 5

The Psychology and Sociology of Fragrance

In this chapter we will explore motivations and behaviours that shed light on our relationship with fragrance, and why we are attracted to particular scents and choice of perfumes. There have been many attempts to provide a structure and context for this, to assist analysis of the phenomenon by formulating a philosophical and then a scientific framework with both therapeutic and commercial importance. The psychology of perfumery also emerged from attempts to align fragrance types and characteristics with personality traits. However, recent research has revealed why it is so difficult to match fragrance with personality, and suggests that our fragrance preferences also arise from underlying biological origins.

Fragrant motivations

It has been observed that many types of terrestrial mammals deliberately rub on, or roll in, aromatic materials. Laska, Bauer and Hernandez Salazar (2007) investigated self-anointing behaviour in free-ranging Mexican spider monkeys. In 250 hours of observation, two males rubbed their sternal and axillary areas with a mix of saliva and aromatic plant material on 20 occasions. They used just three aromatic plant species – *Brongniartia alamosana*,[1] *Ceropia obtusifolia*[2] and *Apium graveolens*[3] – and there was no correlation between the anointing behaviour and other factors, such as time of day, weather conditions, season, presence of insects or presence of skin infections or infestations. All three plant species emitted an intense aromatic scent when crushed by biting and chewing. The two males who scented themselves were adult, and high ranking within their group, and it was suggested that this behaviour was in fact a form of social olfactory communication. It is known that spider monkeys have a highly developed sensitivity to aromatic plants (Hernandez Salazar, Laska and Rodriguez Luna 2003, cited in Laska *et al.* 2007) and also to

---

1   The beautiful Mexican pea tree, with vividly coloured (often deep cerise) sweet-pea-like flowers; known as *palo piojo*.

2   The 'trumpet tree', or *guarumo*; used in Native Amercan Indian medicine for heart problems.

3   Celery.

odorous steroids which might act as pheromones (Laska, Weiser and Hernandez Salazar 2005, 2006, cited in Laska *et al.* 2007), so self-anointing with aromatic plant materials might be either a sign of social status or an attempt to increase sexual attractiveness, or both. In our exploration of perfume in Chapter 3 we discovered many instances where humans used scent for exactly the same reasons. We also use scent to mask malodours – in the form of underarm deodorants, air fresheners and cleaning products. In many western societies body odours are usually regarded as offensive, and although we know now that our body odour is determined by our genes – making it our biological 'signature' – many of us go to great lengths to stop it forming, and to replace it with fragrances of our own choosing (Schilling *et al.* 2010).

Fragrance use and appreciation is a global human phenomenon, and can give a great deal of pleasure. For example, we can stop to smell a favourite rose in a garden, taking time to actively enjoy its scent and 'just be'; or we might spend a few moments each morning appreciating the aroma of the shampoo or shower gel that is part of our self-care ritual. We might also select a fragrance to match the season, or modify our mood, or to reinforce our social olfactory signature, or to help us project a facet of our personality, thus consciously or perhaps unconsciously attempting to influence our social interactions.

Whatever our motivations might be, in some cultures fragrance use is much more sophisticated than this. Classen *et al.* (1994) made a very pertinent observation:

> Fragrance, in the cultures we have studied, is never simply a matter of dabbing oneself with a sweet-smelling liquid out of a bottle. Rather, fragrance is at the centre of sophisticated rites designed to make full use of the aesthetic and attractive forces of perfume within the bounds of social norms. (p.129)

In Middle Eastern culture, and from India to the Far East, perfumes have, for centuries, played an important part in ritual and cultural practices; in some cultures fragrances are symbolic, or are even used to mark the seasons (Moeran 2007). In western societies not all who use fragrance treat it with this degree of respect, and many simply spray on some perfume without much thought at all. However, here is the paradox: in the West, despite this superficially casual attitude, a great deal of money is spent on fragrances. In 1999 estimated sales in the fragrance and flavour industry were US$12.9 billion, and by 2010 this had risen to US$22 billion (Lenochová *et al.* 2012).

Scented strategies

There is evidence that we behave more confidently when wearing a pleasing fragrance; and so it has been postulated that perfume-wearers can modify their nonverbal behaviour through the positive mood changes that fragrance can elicit. In 2005 Higuchi *et al.* conducted a study which showed that wearing perfume inhibited nonverbal behaviours that project negative impressions, such as touching the hair or nose, or shifting posture, and that the perfume-wearers in the study appeared more confident than the no-perfume participants. However, what makes this study most interesting is that those who were evaluating the behaviours were watching recordings, so that they were unaware of the scent, and indeed unaware of the fact that the effect of perfume was being investigated. Most of the studies explored in this chapter are concerned with the effects of fragrance not only on the wearers but also on the affective responses of others. Lenochová *et al.* (2012) cite another study (Roberts *et al.* 2009) which suggested that deodorant use contributed to self-confidence. This had a similar design, but looked at the perceived attractiveness of men introducing themselves to an imagined woman. The evaluators watched mute recordings of the participants, and those who were wearing commercial deodorants were rated as more attractive than those wearing the placebo deodorant. It was suggested that the commercial deodorant changed the wearer's self-perception and self-confidence, and that this in turn had an impact on the observers.

Commercial fragrances are usually advertised as having some type of positive social impact – usually in the attraction of a romantic partner. The use of perfume has always had romantic connotations, and even pleasant ambient scents can facilitate compliance to solicitation or courtship (Guéguen 2012). Fragrances are also marketed to appeal to us in other ways, such representing a style that resonates with us, or a style that we aspire to, or representing confidence, success, desirability; they may help us to be colourful and bold, or dark and mysterious, sophisticated or sporty, approachable or aloof…or even to identify with a 'celebrity'. If we base our choice on the advertisement rather than the fragrance itself, we might find that it does not have the intended and expected effect! Stamelman (2006) wrote that 'if seduction is a game, like bridge, then perfume is the trump card, an advantage one must use with *savoir-faire* and tactical skill' (p.267). He explores the view (taken from the 1930s to the 1960s) that a woman who mistakenly wore a perfume that clashed with her appearance or personality could be 'victimised by the scent'; he quotes the poet, novelist and social commentator Louise de Vilmorin (1902–1969), who suggested that in such cases 'her cause [is] lost, the perfume…has taken its revenge' and that 'there are no perfumes without consequences' (p.267). So it has been observed for some time that it is important to make the 'right' perfume choices. In 1988, when drawing conclusions from a range of studies that had investigated the impact of perfume on managing social situations, Baron (1988) confirmed that the use of scent can indeed affect the impression that we make on others, and that scents can extend the character of our personal style, but not always to positive effect. For example, even if most people agree that a scent is pleasant and attractive, not everybody who likes it will be equally impressed when evaluating a wearer (Baron 1983). The mechanisms that underlie these findings are highly complex, and perhaps a reminder that odour perception is derived from multimodal integration, where visual, auditory and tactile cues play an important role, as do semantics and hedonics.

The influence of cross-modal associations

Most odours are perceived in the context of everyday activities – for example, the smell of exhaust fumes goes together with traffic sounds. However, there is a deeper, biological phenomenon that may link odour with sound. Wesson and Wilson (2010, cited in Seo and Hummel 2011), discovered that, in mice, single units of the olfactory tubercle not only responded to odours but also showed tone-evoked activity, with either enhanced or supressed responses to the simultaneous presentation of odours and tones. Seo and Hummel (2011) then explored auditory–olfactory integration in humans, taking into account two factors – congruency and the 'halo/horns effect'. The 'halo' effect is where something is perceived more positively due to other positive sensory influences, and the 'horn' effect is the opposite. They demonstrated, for the first time, that congruent sounds can enhance perceived odour pleasantness to a greater degree than can incongruent sounds, but that congruency is dependent on the judgement of the individual, which is a cognitive and semantic function. Furthermore, the halo/horns effect was also demonstrated where *pleasant* sounds were shown to enhance perceived odour pleasantness, and the reverse was observed with *un*pleasant sounds.

This is perhaps not entirely unexpected; however, Crisinel and Spence's 2012 study, which investigated cross-modal associations between odours related to wine and musical pitch revealed new layers of complexity. Not only did they demonstrate that there were consistent cross-modal associations, but also that some of the odours were preferentially matched to specific musical instruments. For example, the piano was associated with blackberry and raspberry, while vanilla was paired with both woodwind and piano. They found that fruity odours – apple, lemon, apricot, raspberry, pineapple, almond and blackberry – were associated with high pitches, apple being the highest, and that smoky, musk, dark chocolate, hay and cedar were associated with lower pitches. Honey, liquorice, pepper, mushroom, caramel, green pepper, vanilla and violet occupied the middle ground. The piano, which was associated with pleasant odours, was not matched with more complex odours, and intense or less pleasant odours were paired with brass instruments. Generally, woodwind was associated with low intensity floral, fruity and spicy odours, and strings with the same, only not to the same extent. Crisinel and Spence hypothesise that more complex food stimuli could be matched with more complex musical stimuli, such as chords or even pieces of music; because music can activate brain mechanisms related to semantic processing, they suggest that it could also prime taste words or phrases.

It has also been demonstrated that shades and intensities of colours impact on our perception of odours (Gilbert, Martin and Kemp 1996; Kemp and Gilbert 1997; Schifferstein and Tanudjaja 2004), in the same way as visual stimuli (Gottfried and Dolan 2003), symbols (Seo *et al.* 2010) and odours affect our perceptions of touch (Demattè *et al.* 2006).

So how do these cross-modal associations impact on the way that fragrances are portrayed and on presented to us, and our responses? In 1997 Gilbert suggested that when designing scented products, a multisensory perspective was very important. Fifteen years later, the subject is still being discussed. In relation to the connections between scent and colour, Burns and Harper (2012) suggested that alignment of colour with a fragrance is probably the most important branding decision, because specific colours and intensities shape our olfactory expectations. For example, light yellow suggests that a fragrance will be stimulating and uplifting, while navy blue is consistently described as masculine or soothing, and deep purple as soothing and feminine. Images, shapes and symbols on the packaging will all have further associations for us, and even the texture and feel of the boxes and bottles will give suggestions about what to expect: here we see how a colour can suggest a mood and gender, and that congruent packaging reinforces our expectations well before a fragrance is sampled, and perhaps purchased.

In order to explore how we make choices about fragrance, we need to remain aware of these multisensorial aspects, and look at fragrance preference from a wider stance, beginning with the philosophies of our ancestors.

The evolution of a fragrance philosophy

The ancients recognised that fragrances could elicit various types of feelings, and in the twentieth century the first investigations into psycho-aromatherapy were made. These studies demonstrated quite clearly that odours could act on the nervous system and influence mood. Very soon odour types were linked to specific effects. In 1949 the perfumer Paul Jellinek, who did not underestimate the psychological impact of fragrances, produced a model that had similarities to the ancient Greek concept of the 'Four Elements', and which attempted to explain the psychotherapeutic effects of odour types (Tisserand 1988).

The origins of Four Element philosophy

Empedocles was a Greek philosopher who, in his 'Doctrine of the Four Elements' (*Tetrasomia*), circa 5 BCE, proposed that all matter was comprised of the elements of Air, Fire, Earth and Water, and that they have both physical and spiritual manifestations. His work is clearly influenced by the Greek mystery traditions, including the Brotherhood of Pythagoras and the cult of Dionysus. Empedocles associated the

Four Elements with the gods and goddesses. Hades, the ruler of the underworld, represented Fire, and Zeus, the ruler of the gods and unfaithful husband of Hera, was associated with Air. Hera, the goddess of women and marriage, represented the Earth element, and Water was represented by Nestis, a consort of Hades, and queen of the dead, who later became known as Persephone. So here we have Fire and Air – masculine, outward-reaching forces – represented by two powerful gods, and Earth and Water – feminine, inward-reaching forces – represented by their consorts. The elements were equal yet opposite in gender and direction, and their relationships were characterised by love, as seen in the marriage aspect, and conflict. Hera was angry with Zeus's womanising and infidelity; he was also the god of philandering; and the relationship between Hades and Nestis/Persephone began with her abduction and subsequent confinement to the underworld for half of the year!

The dynamic of 'Love' and 'Strife' is at the heart of Empedocles' treatise on the Four Elements: an ongoing cycle of joining and dissolution, known as the 'Vortex', that can be witnessed in all aspects of existence. He suggested that in the beginning all was 'Love', and that the elements were distinct and equal, but held as one in a 'Sphere' divided into quarters. In time 'Strife' dissolved the sphere and then became the dominant force. However, in turn, Love became stronger and the elements were gathered again under its influence, eventually re-forming the Sphere – and the cycle would be repeated (O'Brien 1969). This represents the dynamic interplay of the Four Elements and what they symbolised, in the natural world and in human nature.

The concept presented in *Tetrasomia* was developed by the philosopher Aristotle and the physician Hippocrates. Aristotle proposed a fifth element, *Aether*, a divine substance, which gave form to the stars and planets. He also added the dimensions of hot, cold, dry and moist to the Four Element philosophy; moistness was fluid and flexible, and thus able to adapt, and in contrast dryness was rigid and less flexible, and more structured and defined. Aristotle suggested that Air was hot and moist, Fire was hot and dry, Earth was cold and dry, and Water was cold and moist. Hippocrates developed the concept in the context of physiology and medicine. He viewed the elements as 'humours', or bodily fluids: Air was associated with yellow bile and an irritable personality, the *choleric* type; Fire was associated with blood and an enthusiastic personality, the *sanguine* type; Earth was associated with phlegm and an apathetic personality, the *phlegmatic* type; and Water was associated with black bile and a pensive personality, the *melancholic* type. The 'Four Humours' were, then, constitutional types with associated personality traits.

Hippocrates then applied the principle termed 'the remedial power of opposites', according to which the predominant humour denoted a predisposition to particular afflictions, so that if one of the humours was out of control, remedies related to its opposite element would counteract the consequences. If a patient had an excessively choleric temperament, a Water remedy would be prescribed;

a melancholic temperament would indicate that an Air remedy was required; the sanguine afflictions would be treated with an Earth remedy, while a Fire remedy would be used for phlegmatic afflictions.

This philosophy explained the nature of the universe, our planet and mankind, and had an extensive influence over the centuries, eventually being rejected by science but embraced in alchemy, astrology and many spiritual traditions.

The Greek Four Elements have also been used to symbolise aspects of the psyche, personal growth and transformation. Carl Jung (1875–1961), the Swiss psychotherapist and psychiatrist and founder of analytical psychology, used the symbolism of the Four Elements in his classification of eight personality types. This combined the polarities of introversion and extroversion with the qualities of thinking (Air), intuiting (Fire), sensing (Earth) and feeling (Water). Stephen Arroyo, an astrologer and psychologist, also suggested that the four elements represent specific areas of consciousness and perception, and the ability to relate to different realms of life experience and vitalising forces (Arroyo 1975).

An ancient philosophy and the psychology of perfumery

Initially, Paul Jellinek, in *The Practice of Modern Perfumery* (1949), proposed that there were eight mood effects, linked to odour types and characteristics (cited in Williams 1996), and in 1951 he proposed a model for perfumers that could explain these odour effects (Jellinek 1997b). Essentially this was a map based on two axes, marking quadrants, with odour effects marked on the inner aspect, and odour correspondences on the outer aspect. On the vertical axis 'erogenous' was the polar opposite of 'anti-erogenous' (meaning 'refreshing'), occupying the top position; and the horizontal axis was portrayed at right angles to this, with 'narcotic' (left) and 'stimulating' (right) being the polar opposites. He suggested that the space (the upper left quadrant) between narcotic (identified with sweet, floral and balsamic odours) and anti-erogenous odours (acid, green, watery and resinous) was occupied by calming odours (fruity). In the upper right quadrant, between anti-erogenous and stimulating odours (which are bitter, woody, herbaceous, mossy and burnt), we find refreshing effects, typified by camphoraceous, minty and spicy odours. The lower right quadrant, the space between stimulating and erogenous (alkaline, rancid, cheesy, urinous and faecal odours) is occupied by exalting effects denoted by dusty odours. Finally, in the lower left quadrant, between erogenous and narcotic, we find sultry effects, which can be given by honey-like odours.

Tisserand (1988) noted that Paul Jellinek made no mention of the Greek philosophy of the Four Elements. He too developed a model, which he called the 'mood cycle' that suggested correspondences between essential oil aromas, moods, the Greek Four Elements and the four personality types suggested by Mensing and Beck (1988): introvert and extrovert; emotionally stable and unstable. Although this cycle was developed independently, and before his knowledge of Jellinek's work, Tisserand too identified eight positive moods, and opposing negative moods that we can all experience at different times.

For an illustration of fragrance types and their relationships with Four Element philosophy, please see Appendix C. The hypothesis that distinct odour types could elicit specific responses in humans became the focus of much enquiry, observation and research, much of which has already been presented in preceding chapters. This, of course, had significance in aromatherapy practice and commercial implications in the fragrance industry.

Mood profiling and fragrance mapping

Fragrance research in the late 1970s and 1980s, using mostly physiological parameters, had established that fragrance-evoked mood changes were small but measurable. It was also known that fragrance could reduce stress, but that if the subject was already relaxed, this response would be minimal; and that the changes elicited by many fragrances were nonetheless beneficial and enhanced wellbeing. In the early 1990s, on the basis of this, fragrance researchers Warren and Warrenburg (1993) developed the 'Mood Profiling Concept' (MPC) as a tool to classify the typical effects of fragrances. The MPC used psychological self-reporting to measure subjective mood changes that were evoked by fragrance. Again, eight mood categories were identified, four positive and four negative. The positive moods were described as stimulation, sensuality, happiness and relaxation, while the negative ones were stress, irritation, depression and apathy. Warren and Warrenburg found that exposure to different fragrances elicits either increases or decreases in these categories, and so profiles of the effects of specific fragrances could be constructed and presented in graphical format. In 1993 they reported their results with four 'living flower' reconstructed fragrances. The profiles of the four fragrances are included in Table 5.1 along with those of clementine and vanilla. In 1995 Warrenburg reported that a 'mood mapping' tool, which can measure the mood associations of aromas, had been developed. This was being used in consumer research, and from it, a global data base was constructed – the 'Consumer Fragrance Thesaurus'. Apart from the commercial application of this information, Warrenburg was also exploring the stress-relieving aspects of fragrance, and found that certain relaxing fragrances identified in mood mapping also produced a specific physiological response: that of significantly reducing tension in the trapezius muscles, as measured by electromyogram. He suggested that fragrance is certainly powerful enough to counteract stress during performance tasks.

Table 5.1 Fragrances: the Mood Profiling Concept and mood mapping

Compiled and adapted from Warrenburg (1995) and Warren and Warrenburg (1993).

Fragrance	Mood Profiling Concept	Descriptive analysis
Muguet	Increased happiness, relaxation and stimulation. No effect on sensuality. Decreased irritation, depression, and especially apathy. No effect on stress.	This shows an increase in three positive moods and decrease in three negative moods. However, it also indicated both relaxation and stimulation, suggesting a heightened sense of calm and increased awareness and energy. This state was described as 'calm vitality'.
Douglas-fir	Increased happiness and relaxation. No effect on sensuality or stimulation. Decrease in irritation, stress, depression and apathy.	This shows an increase in two positive moods and a decrease in all negative categories. It was described as qualitatively similar to taking a warm bath or meditating.
Osmanthus	Increased stimulation and happiness. No effect on sensuality or relaxation. Decreased irritation and stress, and prominently decreased depression and apathy.	This shows an increase in two positive moods and a prominent decrease in all four negative moods. This profile highlighted the fragrance's stimulating qualities.
Hyacinth	Increased all four positive moods; prominently in the case of happiness, relaxation, stimulation, and slightly less so with sensuality. Irritation and stress were decreased, while depression and apathy were prominently reduced.	This was the only fragrance tested that showed an increase in all four positive moods and a decrease in all four negative moods. This would appear to be a complex fragrance, with a broad spectrum of mood effects.
Clementine	Significantly increased happiness, increased stimulation, and slightly increased relaxation and sensuality.	This profile emphasises stimulation/arousal rather than relaxation. This is not surprising for a citrus aroma.

Fragrance	Mood Profiling Concept	Descriptive analysis
Vanilla bean	This significantly increased relaxation and also happiness, and produced a smaller increase in sensuality, and a slight increase in stimulation.	This profile emphasises relaxation rather than arousal.

In 2009 Chrea *et al.* studied the verbal labels that were being used in fragrance research and developed the Geneva Emotion and Odour Scale (GEOS), which measured the feelings elicited by odours; their work was introduced in Chapter 2. Their vocabulary took into account three aspects of the *emotional* response: the cognitive element, such as nostalgia or romantic feelings; the *physiological* responses, such as shivering and salivating; and the *motivational* element, such as 'feeling attracted'. The GEOS was adapted for commercial flavour and fragrance development by Porcherot *et al.* (2010).

After statistical analysis of the results, Chrea *et al.* were able to identify very clear differences in the feelings elicited by the different odours, and that these were not always related to a simple 'liking' judgement. Six perfumery oils – basil, cumin, jasmine, mandarin, pepper and vanilla – were investigated. It was found that the odours of basil and cumin were given significantly higher scores on the 'disgusted – irritated – unpleasantly surprised' feelings, and the odours of jasmine, mandarin and vanilla were given significantly higher scores on 'happiness – wellbeing – pleasantly surprised' feelings. Mandarin also received high scores for 'energetic – invigorated – clean' feelings, while vanilla scored highly in relation to 'nostalgic – amusement – mouthwatering' and 'relaxed – serene – reassured' feelings. The findings for mandarin (a citrus fragrance not dissimilar to clementine) and vanilla both correlate well with Warrenburg's (1995) observations, summarised in Table 5.1. Mandarin was also compared with jasmine; the two oils were equally liked by the participants, but mandarin was given significantly higher ratings in both the 'energetic – invigorated – clean' and 'romantic – desire – in love' dimensions than jasmine.

The GEOS was also adapted to explore feelings in relation to fine fragrances, classed as oriental-vanillic, citrus-aromatic, floral-muguet, floral-fruity green variants (two versions) and oriental-floral. Here it was found that although one of the two floral-fruity-green fragrances and the oriental floral did not differ significantly in terms of being liked, their emotional effects were quite different. The floral-fruity-green fragrance scored higher on 'energetic – invigorated – clean' feelings, and lower scores in 'nostalgic – amusement – mouthwatering' feelings, compared with the oriental-floral fragrance. The two floral-fruity-green fragrances were also explored to reveal any differences between two fragrances that belonged to the same family. They were rated by the participants as equally liked. However, one evoked significantly higher scores in relation to 'nostalgic – amusement – mouthwatering' and also 'romantic – desire – in love' feelings than the other. Although it was suggested that the scale could be further adapted to meet the needs of fine fragrance development, the findings are nonetheless an important contribution to our understanding of the emotional effects of scents.

An eastern, vitalistic perspective

From the western perspective, the influence of odour on mood is usually explained in terms of the biological and behavioural sciences. Eastern philosophies, however, are founded on the concept of a vital energy, and this offers an alternative way of thinking about our responses to scents. Holmes (2001) described this vital energy, which is known in Chinese medicine as *Qi*, in Ayurveda as *prana*, and was known in ancient Greece as *pneuma*, as 'the principle or dynamo that runs life and so connects all life-forms in a living web of interconnections' (Holmes 2001, p.18). He developed a philosophical approach, which he named 'fragrance energetics', to explore the effects of scent, and from this he constructed a working model which helps us to understand the potential effects of scent on the psyche.

Holmes (1997) proposed that the inherent nature of a fragrance – that is, its tone, intensity, note and characteristics – is responsible for its specific psychotherapeutic effects. These fragrance parameters and suggested effects have been borne out by observation, and align well with Jellinek's and Tisserand's thinking, and also with contemporary research. Holmes has also integrated clinical and energetic approaches to aromatherapy; his work has undoubtedly influenced contemporary aromatherapy practice. This might be because many aromatherapists already embrace vitalistic approaches.

Aromatherapy is a comparatively recent practice; its underpinning philosophies are constantly evolving, and the evidence base is small but growing. Perhaps because of this, it is still viewed by many, including some in the fragrance business, as an eclectic mix of pseudo-science and nineteenth-century vitalism. However, vitalistic eastern philosophies, which are based on thousands of years of observation about the nature of the world we live in, and our interactions with it, can only enhance our understanding about fragrance, because they offer us another way of thinking. This alternative perspective is not incompatible with western science, but because it is holistic rather than reductionist, it can give us important insight into the reason why the effects of fragrance cannot always be predicted: we are dynamic, not static, beings.

Perfume preferences

Much of the research explored thus far has been based on the reactions to fragrances delivered by, for example, ambient evaporation, pen-delivery or 'Sniffin'Sticks'. Fine fragrances, however, are designed to be worn on the skin, as are our personal care products such as deodorants. In an early but extensive analysis of perfume preferences, involving hundreds of users, Byrne-Quinn (1988) made an important point at the very outset, which was that 'smell marks people'. Women in particular are very concerned with the 'messages' they broadcast about themselves when they use perfume. However, when asked about why they used it, the response was often hedonistic and simple: 'I like it.' Byrne-Quinn acknowledged that this was most certainly because they enjoyed the sensations that arose from the olfactory stimulus, but also because perfume was being used for a purpose – to convey a message that could give the wearer a level of biological, psychological and social gratification. Perfume can give the wearer confidence that this gratification will be achieved, and this is a direct response, gratification, for the user. However, marketing focuses on the effects that the fragrance will have on others – that is, the perfume's 'message'. We have already discussed how scent can help identify the somatic self, and this olfactory message can be broadcast, establishing an individual's actual and aspirational sense of self.

Olfactory messages and perceptions

Within this broad context, there are many variables. We do not necessarily all perceive scent in exactly in the same way, and, indeed, 'in-nose' biotransformation of odorous materials may well modify the quality of the compounds and, as a result, how we receive and interpret these olfactory signals (Schilling *et al.* 2010). This will ultimately be down to our genetic makeup, as are our eye and hair colour, and components of our immune systems. Other variables are our social, economic, geographical, cultural and experiential backgrounds. For example, Ayabe-Kanamura *et al.* (1998) conducted a Japanese–German cross-cultural study investigating differences in odour perception, and concluded that cultural experience influences even basic perception of odour intensity. In 2011 Seo *et al.* conducted another cross-regional study that investigated attitudes to olfaction, this time looking at age (21–50), gender and culture (Mexican, Korean, Czech and German). They found that in all of the regions investigated, women had a higher degree of interest in smell than men, and that there was a positive correlation between the individual's self-rating of olfactory sensitivity and general attitude towards olfaction. Additionally, there were significant cross-regional differences. The Mexican culture is classed as a 'contact culture', unlike the others in this study, and the Mexicans had more odour-related emotions and memories, which they use in daily activities and decision making, than the other cultures.

Generally, non-contact cultures, which maintain a greater interpersonal distance, are characterised by a lower involvement of sensory cues in social settings. However, it is not simply this one factor that influences attitudes to olfaction, because earlier studies (Schleidt, Hold and Attili 1981) showed that there was little difference between two European cultures – Italian (a contact culture) and German (a non-contact culture). Seo *et al.* (2011) found that regional influences shaped general and affective attitudes. For example, Mexicans rated 'social relationship' odours as pleasant and 'civilisation' odours as unpleasant more frequently than the other cultural groups, whereas the Czechs and Germans reported that 'nature' odours were pleasant more frequently than the Koreans and Mexicans. The results may also have a genetic influence, because previous studies (reviewed by Hudson 1999) had indicated that genetic differences in human olfactory receptors are related to olfactory performance. Knaapila *et al.* (2008) investigated genetic factors in twins from Australia, Denmark and Switzerland, in relation to the evaluation of odour pleasantness and intensity. They suggested that the genetic factor accounted for 21 per cent of variance in pleasantness ratings of the odour of cinnamon, and the non-shared environmental factor accounted for 79 per cent of the variance. There is a wide range in affective response to, and attention to odours, which extends across all sensory domains (Wrzesniewski, McCauley and Rozin 1999), and it is important to bear this in mind when exploring fragrance preferences.

Perfume choice: some hypotheses

Although we now have a lot of information about the likely effects of specific odour types and characteristics, and we also have some well-developed theories about how and why these effects occur, it remains difficult to match individuals to fragrances with any accuracy. Mensing and Beck wrote, in 1988, that there were three prevalent views concerning the physical and psychological factors that influenced perfume selection. One was that perfume choice was non-rational, and therefore difficult to explain in terms of psychology, and another, proposed by Paul Jellinek in 1951, was that physical characteristics such as hair and eye colour influenced perfume selection. At that time the third view, that individual personality motivated fragrance preference, prevailed. The original concept refers to the link between personality and fragrance preference and Corbin's 1996 exploration of odour and the social imagination in *The Foul and the Fragrant*. It was seized upon, investigated, and, based on the evidence, this theory was applied to fragrance sales and marketing.

The 'Colour Rosette Test' was a tool that was developed from Mensing and Beck's research in the mid-1980s, which focused on almost 1000 German female perfume users, and investigated the relationship between scent and personality. This is summarised in Mensing and Beck (1988). In the first series of studies, 270 women were asked to use four preselected fragrances,[4] and then assessed to establish their emotional characteristics, using both questionnaire and colour tests. The data allowed Mensing and Beck to establish that *extrovert* users, who look for stimulation, had a significant tendency to prefer fresh fragrances; *introverted* individuals preferred

---

4   These were *Ô de Lancôme* (fresh citrus), *Nahéma* (rosy, floral-powdery), *Shalimar* (ambery oriental) and *Parure* (chypre).

oriental fragrances; and *emotionally ambivalent*[5] users liked floral-powdery scents. *Emotionally stable*[6] perfume users did not display any significant tendency towards any one type of fragrance. It was also suggested that colour preferences are linked to this. Extroverts, who seek stimulation, preferred stimulating colours such as red or orange, while introverted characters tend to prefer softer colours such as violet. Emotionally ambivalent users preferred black and white; emotionally ambivalent with extroverted tendencies liked bright pastel shades, while emotionally ambivalent with introverted tendencies preferred dark green and violet. Emotionally stable extroverts preferred, deep greens, turquoises, deep pinkish reds and oranges, and the emotionally stable introverts favoured single colours, blues, yellow and silver grey. In a second series of studies, 600 women sampled 'blind' fragrances,[7] they were then asked to describe their 'ideal' fragrances using a list of 50 adjectives, and their personalities were examined using five psychodiagnostic tests. Sociobiographical data was also collected. Analysis of the data allowed Mensing and Beck to identify three significant relationships: *extroverted* perfume users had the highest average mean for fresh perfumes, *introverted* users had the highest average mean for oriental fragrances, and *emotionally ambivalent* users had the highest average mean for floral-powdery fragrances. These three user groups were identified by the letters A, B and C respectively. However, an analysis of subfactors allowed the additional inclusion of four subgroups. These were D (emotionally ambivalent but with extroverted tendency), E (ambivalent with introverted tendency), F (emotionally stable with extroverted tendency) and G (stable with introverted tendency). A further 'cluster analysis', controlled by cross-validation which took personality, colour and fragrance factors into account, allowed the researchers to place 81 per cent of the participants in the seven groups. Other variables were also considered and explored. These included the subjective experience of the perfumes, the matching of fragrances to desired lifestyles, age group factors,[8] seasons and atmospheric humidity. A summary can be found in Table 5.2.

---

5   This term indicates individuals who experience varying moods, which can change readily; and this is not experienced as being a negative trait.

6   This term indicates individuals who experience and show balanced moods and feelings, and can adapt their moods to current demands.

7   These were chypre (*Miss Dior, Parure* and *Mitsouko*), oriental-floral (*Must de Cartier, Jicky, Oscar de la Renta*), oriental (*Opium, Shalimar, Cinnabar*), floral-fruity (*Valentino, Fidji, Anais Anais*), floral-powdery (*Nahéma, Rive Gauche, Tosca*), fresh-green (*Ô de Lancôme, Eau de Courrèges, Eau de Guerlain*), and aldehydic-floral (*Chanel No.5, Chamade, Madame Rochas*).

8   In mid-life, women undergo endocrine, somatic and psychological changes, and men also undergo biological and psychological transitions, although the interrelationship between biological and psychological factors is not fully understood. Pleasant fragrances can improve moods at this stage of life (Schiffman *et al.* 1995a and 1995b). The full repercussions on fragrance preference have not been established.

Table 5.2 The Colour Rosette Test

Compiled and adapted from Mensing and Beck (1988).

Group	Personality characteristics	Possible dimensions	Preferred colours	Preferred fragrance types
A	Extroverted mood tendency.	Search for stimulation, readiness to take risks, sociability.	Single colours. Orange and yellow.	Fresh, green scents had an activating effect. In Group A 'fresh' means 'active', 'clear' and 'green'. Oriental fragrances were perceived as too heavy and sweet.
B	Introverted mood tendency.	Less need for stimulation. May seek individual/ alternative lifestyle. Narcissistic tendency. Younger users.	Single colours, especially dark blue and violet.	Oriental fragrances were preferred and described as having a characteristic harmonious note. Fresh-green scents were perceived as one-dimensional and uninteresting, 'lemon-water'. In Group B 'fresh' meant a new and interesting top note, not a green impression. The concept of 'erotic' meant 'deep', 'warm', 'sensitive', 'sensual' and 'mystical'.
C	Emotionally ambivalent mood tendency.	Romanticism. Fashion- oriented.	Single colours, black and white.	Floral powdery fragrances were preferred and described as soft, rounded, rosy and appealing, and were associated with a dreamy experience. This group disliked chypre perfumes which they found to be too hard, too intensive and too strong.

Group	Personality characteristics	Possible dimensions	Preferred colours	Preferred fragrance types
D	Emotionally ambivalent with extroverted mood tendency.	Flexibility, contentment and satisfaction with life. Idealistic and cheerful. Younger and older users.	Bright colours.	Floral-fruity fragrances. For Group D the term 'erotic' meant 'light', 'playful', 'romantic' and 'tender'.
E	Emotionally ambivalent with introverted mood tendency.	Need for security and a well-ordered life-style. Materialistic values.	Warm colours. Dark green and violet.	Oriental-floral fragrances preferred.
F	Emotionally stable with extroverted mood tendency.	Conservative. Socially active. Family orientation. Older age groups.	Dark red, green, orange.	Chypre fragrances preferred.
G	Emotionally stable with introverted mood tendency.	Well-mannered. Classic values.	Single colours. Blue, yellow and silver grey.	Aldehydic-floral fragrances preferred.

Notes

It was found that:

1. The emotional perfume preference was sometimes suppressed to comply with the criteria and norms of the environment, so some women used several fragrances.

2. Some people liked two rosettes. An affinity to Groups E and C preferred oriental-floral or powdery florals, such as *Poison* and *Oscar de la Renta*. An affinity to Groups B and C preferred fragrances such as *Chlöe* and *Ysatis*. Affinity to Groups F and A preferred, for example, *Armani* or *Miss Dior*.

3. These preferences were expressed following experience of the perfume, rather than knowledge of perfume notes.

4. The popularity of some fragrances was dependent on the season. For example, *Mitsouko* was preferred in cooler seasons.

5. Humid conditions dulled the perception of heavy oriental fragrances.

6. The appeal of the chypre perfume *Parure* was stronger for perfume users over the age of 30.

The Colour Rosette test that emerged from these extensive studies has been used in perfume consulting and sales, and also as an accurate orientation aid in fragrance marketing. Mensing and Beck (1988) claimed that the test can predict fragrance preference with 80 per cent accuracy and fragrance rejection with 90 per cent accuracy. However, since the 1980s aesthetic trends have changed – perfumes have gradually become less gender-specific, new aromachemicals have allowed an expansion of the types of fragrances that are available, new fragrance classifications have been proposed, and fashions and trends have emerged and receded. Nevertheless, the Colour Rosette test has historical significance, not least because of the rigorous research that underpinned it, and the body of evidence that now shows the relationship between colour and our sense of smell (Maric and Jacquot 2012).

Perhaps the most comprehensive and current tool for sales and marketing is Michael Edward's 'Fragrance Wheel' (Edwards 2010). Although first impressions may suggest that, because of the use of colour, this might a variant of the Colour Rosette, a closer examination reveals that it comes from a very different angle, that of perfume classification. It also shows the relationships between the fragrance types. It does not, however, make any attempt to match fragrances to personality or biological types. For an interactive illustration, go to www.fragrancesoftheworld. com/external/wheel/index.html

Fragrance and gender

Donna (2009) discussed the gender classification of fragrances, with reference to Zarzo and Stanton's (2009) and Edwards' (2008) proposals. In traditional classification schemes, floral fragrances are usually feminine and woody fragrances are predominantly masculine, as are fresh, water and marine fragrances. Donna notes that sweet and dry ('not sweet') characteristics suggest feminine and masculine respectively. So, it is possibly not the actual odour *types* that imply gender, but just two *characteristics*. She also suggests that odour types that fall into a gender-ambiguous category are citrus and green, besides the classic chypre based on oakmoss, and that the 'fresh' term is the one most likely to be misused by the general public. This particular misinterpretation of an odour characteristic had earlier been noted by Mensing and Beck (1988).

Lindqvist (2012) explored how perfume preferences were related to gender classifications of fragrance. At the outset, she acknowledges that perfumes are important in human social interactions, and that it would appear that women and men aim to increase their gender-specific attributes with fragrance. This study was 'gender-sensitive' – that is, gender was not regarded as a 'solid attribute' – and it encompassed the many social and cultural influences that lead to expected differences between men and women. Previous studies had indicated that women and men have similar gender associations with perfumes, and that preferences for different scents are learnt within a social or cultural context (Classen 1992; Ayabe-Kanamura *et al.* 1998). Moreover, Martins *et al.* (2005) had conducted a study which indicated that, when making preferential judgements about body odours, sexual orientation and gender had an influence. This might suggest that sexual orientation could affect gender-related fragrance associations.

The participants in Lindqvist's study did not have any experience in the perfume industry, had no particular experience in evaluating fragrances, and were heterosexual. This study showed that the twelve perfumes[9] were not separated into two distinct clusters, but that there was considerable overlap, and that self-preference and partner-preference were positively correlated with each other, and also with perceptions of pleasantness. In other words, if a participant liked the perfume, they wanted to use it and they wanted their partner to use it too. This is incongruent with the notion that women and men have different preferences concerning the fragrance used by their partners, and indeed with Milinski and Wedekind's (2001) observation that the odour preferences of a prospective partner differ between men and women. Lindqvist acknowledges that in her study, the small panel of 18 naïve participants could have affected the results. Donna (2009) suggested that, despite an increase in fragrances marketed as 'shared' scents, perfumes probably did have a gender. The message here is that as we learn more, we realise just how much we still do not know – but the process of investigation is always stimulating.

Can fragrance resonate with and amplify biological and energetic signatures?

It might also be significant whether an individual selects their own fragrance, rather than having the choice imposed upon them; this could also have an impact upon self-perception and the way a person is perceived by others. It is during adolescence, a phase of physiological and psychosocial change, that commercial fragrances usually become incorporated in daily routines, and Freyberg and Ahren (2011) conducted a preliminary investigation of the impact of fragrance on social interactions in adolescent females. Twenty-seven participants wore their favourite perfume or an alternative on two separate days over a period of two weeks. The alternative was rated as less pleasant, but it did not have a direct effect on social behaviours. However, in comparison with the favourite perfume, the alternative was associated with reduced social enjoyment, and reduced use of words that implied intimacy in their narratives. This would suggest that at a superficial level, perfume choice is perhaps not perceived to have a major impact on social activities, but that at a deeper level, an imposed as distinct from a chosen fragrance can reduce the quality of social interactions. Perhaps in this group, the wearing of a less pleasant scent yielded less personal gratification, and as a consequence affected the persona projected, which in turn would have an impact on the quality of social interactions.

---

9   The fragrances in Lindqvist's study (2012) were Escada's *Incredible Me, Desire Me* and *Ocean Lounge*; The Body Shop's *Vanilla*; Dior's *Eau Sauvage, Higher Energy, Homme* and *Fahrenheit*; DKNY's *Be Delicious*; Gaultier's *Gaultier 2*; and Dali's *Laguna*.

Or perhaps others responding to the girls less favourably than when they wore their favourite perfume, because their olfactory signature was different, at both a superficial and biological level.

The anthropologist Jan Havlíček suggested that there is a strong interaction between perfume and individual body odour, and that individuals select fragrances that complement their own odour. He found that when people apply self-selected fragrances, the effect is rated as more pleasant than when they apply a scent chosen by someone else (Gray 2011; Lenochová et al. 2012). The view that self-selected perfumes can work with body odours to enhance their signal was shared by Milinski and Wedekind (2001). So rather than 'replacing' our biological olfactory signature by applying a fragrance, perhaps we are indeed reinforcing, amplifying and complementing it?

Lenochová et al. (2012) reported the results of a study that was designed to test this hypothesis. The study was conducted in both Vienna and Prague, so that cultural factors could be taken into account. The hedonic ratings (for odour attractiveness, pleasantness and intensity) of perfumed and non-perfumed axillary samples, obtained from the same group of male donors for each experiment, were compared. A further experiment compared ratings of axillary samples collected when the donors were wearing either a self-selected perfume or an assigned perfume. Lenochová et al. found, in the first study, that perfume had a positive effect on the perception of axillary samples. They acknowledged that in European cultures there is a prevalent negative attitude toward untreated body odours, so this result was not surprising. However, they also noted that the impact of the perfume varied amongst individuals, suggesting that there was interaction between body odour and perfume rather than a simple masking effect. It was suggested that this interaction creates an individually specific odour mixture. A second experiment demonstrated that if an individual chose their own perfume, their body odour was rated as more pleasant than if they were wearing an allocated fragrance. There was no perceived difference in the pleasantness of the perfumes per se. These findings support the hypothesis that we choose perfumes that interact positively with our own body odour, and could explain why our perfume preferences are highly individual.

This leads to another phenomenon regarding the interface between our biology and fragrance. Most of us will have noticed that a fragrance does not smell the same on the skin of different individuals; for example, a simple combination of essential oils of rose, sandalwood and citrus might smell very sweet on one person, and more vibrant or woody on another. Fragrances change, too, certainly over time as the different notes emerge, but the change can also sometimes happen very quickly and unexpectedly. It is more difficult to explain this in terms of fragrance construction or 'skin chemistry', simply because of the speed with which this happens. In aromatherapy practice, the phenomenon of sudden and incongruous changes in odour characteristics has been noted. To illustrate this, two examples are presented here. On one occasion a therapist was carrying out an aromatherapy massage with a blend of essential oils, the most dominant of which was Roman chamomile, which has a fresh, apple-like and diffusive nature. However, while performing massage to the back, she was astonished to perceive, quite suddenly, what she described as a 'wet dog' smell. This disappeared before she had completed the back massage, and she did not mention it to the recipient of the massage. In discussing this with her mentor, it transpired that the smell was more like 'wet springer spaniel' or 'Labrador retriever'; and owing to the oily undercoats in these breeds, the odour could be classed as 'rancid'. On another occasion a woody-scented cypress blend became noticeably 'scorched' and shortly after 'damp, like stagnant water', and these changes were noted by both the therapist and recipient. In the light of the research that started with Milinski and Wedekind in 2001, and most recently of that carried out by Lenochová *et al.*, perhaps our genes are responsible? Perhaps these transient olfactory impressions are manifestations of body odour interacting with an imposed odour? This has interesting implications for aromatherapy practice, where usually essential oil blends are prescribed for an individual; it is rarely left to the individual to design the scent of their treatment. Or is the imposed odour facilitating and amplifying the expression of our own odour, as it shifts and changes under the influence of the touch and massage elements of the therapeutic intervention, or indeed, the client–therapist interaction?

Chinese Five Element theory can give us another way of looking at this phenomenon. The elements – Earth, Metal, Water, Wood and Fire – have corresponding odours (Hicks *et al.* 2011). The rancid odour perceived in the first example above is associated with the Wood element, and the recipient of the back massage did indeed appear to have an 'imbalance' in this element, according to Five Element diagnostic criteria. In the second example the Fire element is, unsurprisingly, associated with a scorched odour, while the stagnant, putrid odour corresponds to the Water element, and both of these were imbalanced in the second case. Even more noteworthy was the nature of the second case, where the essential oil blend was being used in conjunction with manual stimulation of Fire and Water meridians (pathways) when these changes arose. Instances like this suggest that the energetic approach, where odours can be perceived as both real and symbolic manifestations of our dynamic energetic signature, deserves further consideration and investigation.

PART II

A Natural Palette of Aromatics

CHAPTER 6

The Language of Fragrance

Fragrance, when directly experienced, is a pure form of sensory communication, and can express all manner of ideas, feelings and impressions. Gell's words capture the essence of what perfume is:

> Perfume is symbolic, not linguistic, because it does what language could not do – express an idea, an archetypal wholeness, which surpasses language while language remains subservient to the more or less worldly business of communicating... (Gell 1977, p.30)

Herein too lies the art of the perfumer, who can create this phenomenon from an inspiration or by interpreting a perfume brief. Nevertheless, in order to communicate how fragrance manifests within our senses and psyche, we need language. The vast majority of people are not aware of the vocabulary that pertains to odours, and consequently are unable to communicate effectively in this realm.

The ability to put into words, describe and evoke an odour is a skill that needs to be cultivated and developed. The average person with normal olfactory capabilities will probably struggle to characterise and describe an odour, other than by using a word to indicate the perceived source, perhaps coupled with a few adjectives. Others, with no less normal olfactory senses, will be completely at a loss, especially if confronted by an unfamiliar or complex smell. The odour psychologist Tyler Lorig suggests that this is due, in part, to competition between the brain's mechanisms for odour and language, if we are asked to smell and describe an odour simultaneously, since it is thought that the perceptual and cognitive aspects of odour recognition are carried out in the brain's right hemisphere, while the language aspect is in the left hemisphere. However, Lorig maintains that it is also because, especially in the industrialised west, we are not encouraged to use or develop this ability (Glaser 2002).

In the English language there are no words that are exclusive to the description of smells – odours do not have names. Usually, when describing an odour, we refer to its actual or supposed source, such as a flower – a *flowery* scent; or an animal – a *doggy* smell. This is usually qualified by some supporting adjectives, such as a *rich* flowery scent or a *sweet* flowery scent, a *wet* doggy smell or a *strong* doggy smell. So the language of odour uses words and expressions that are normally applied in other contexts. In perfumery the vocabulary is adapted from that of the other senses, and from arts such as music. For example, perfumers refer to *notes, chords* or *accords*, and even the traditional furniture that houses a perfumer's aromatic raw materials and aromachemicals is known as the *perfumer's organ.*

It is not just perfumers who need an odour vocabulary – we all use odour expressions on a regular basis. For example, when describing smells, we often use expressions related to taste, such as *sweet* or *sour*, or touch and textures, such as *harsh, soft* or *sharp.* Our visual sense also contributes to odour description – we use expressions such as *rounded* and even colours are used to describe smells. Sometimes we will also use more abstract terms related to feelings and sensations, such as *mellow, heady* or *harmonious.* In this way, when relating the experience of a smell, it is possible to incorporate all of the senses, bringing a meaning to the experience that can be shared with all who will listen. These cross-modal associations – smell and sound (Seo and Hummel 2011; Crisinel and Spence 2012); smell and touch; smell and colour (Maric and Jacquot 2012), and smell and shape – are quite widespread, and have been the subject of many studies.

A quick look on the internet will reveal that perfume is written about extensively. Dr Claus Noppeney of Bern University investigated how bloggers and journalists write about fragrance – that is, use words to describe something that can only be experienced subjectively, which requires olfactory competence. He commented that writing about artistic perfumery is actually part of the creative process, and gives perfume a trans-sensual significance (Das Gupta 2012). However, we do need to use odour terminology to convey meaning that is consistent and acceptable to our audience, besides finding words to describe what it evokes in us.

When evaluating the odour profile of, for example, essential oils and absolutes, odours are first described according to their type, followed by their characteristics, comments about their volatility (top, middle and base notes), their intensity, how they change over time and the nature of that change, and their ability to diffuse and persist. Personal preferences (neutral, like/dislike, love/hate) are not appropriate or even relevant; objectivity is more important. For example, using this evaluatory approach, jasmine absolute could be described as a floral odour type, with *floral, fruity, green top notes* (initial impact), *heavy floral, fruity, animalic body notes,* and *floral, fatty, heavy, animalic dryout notes* (Williams 1996). Lawless (2009) gives a similar description, but also comments on its intensity and its heady character, and its long dryout period – implying that the scent of jasmine is persistent as well as diffusive. However, Aftel (2008) infuses her description of jasmine with its effect on the senses. She describes it as a narcotic (sultry and calming) scent, rather than using the terms 'heavy' or 'heady', and as having the ability to 'seize the senses and the imagination' (p.111).

Please refer to Table 6.1 for an exploration of the fragrance types and characteristics found in plant aromatics.

Table 6.1 Odour types and characteristics encountered in plant fragrances

Compiled from Lawless (2009), Williams (1980, 1996) and author's observations.

Abbreviations: e.o. – essential oil; res. – resinoid; abs. – absolute.

Odour type	Associated characteristics	Examples
Anisic – a scent reminiscent of aniseed.	Often sweet, or ethereal.	Anisic notes can be found in star anise, tarragon and sweet fennel e.o., also in tulsi e.o. (exotic basil). They are often conferred by a group of constituents called phenolic ethers.
Balsamic – a vanilla-like scent with a soothing effect, often found in base notes. Sometimes there is a resinous subsidiary note.	Sweet and/or warm, smooth.	Balsamic notes can be found in benzoin res., labdanum res., opopanax res., Peru balsam, tolu balsam, vanilla abs.
Camphoraceous – an odour reminiscent of camphor, somewhat medicinal, and may have elements of menthol or eucalyptus.	Medicinal, pungent, harsh.	A typical camphoraceous example is white camphor e.o.; however, many others including the 'paperbark trees' have camphoraceous notes such as niaouli, cajuput and tea tree. Camphoraceous notes are also found in herbal oils such as spike lavender e.o. and some eucalyptus and rosemary oils.
Caramel – a scent reminiscent of burnt sugar, with balsamic characteristics.	Sweet, warm.	Tuberose abs., although a heavy floral, has subsidiary caramel notes.
Cineolic – eucalyptus-like.	Medicinal, diffusive.	Most of the 'pharmaceutical' eucalyptus oils are dominated by the constituent 1,8-cineole, an oxide that imparts the characteristic odour.

Citrus – the scent of citrus fruit peel. Also, lemony notes fall into this category.	Fresh, light, crisp, sometimes bitter in subsidiary notes. Lemony notes can be sweet and fruity, rosy, or harsh and coarse.	Typical citrus notes are found in the top notes of citrus peel oils – bergamot, grapefruit, kaffir lime peel, lemon, lime, mandarin, orange (bitter and sweet), tangerine. Lemony notes are found in *Litsea cubeba* e.o. (sweet, fruity), *Eucalyptus citriodora* e.o. and citronella e.o. (harsh rosy-lemon), lemongrass e.o. (harsh, coarse), lemon verbena e.o. and ginger e.o. top notes.
Coniferous – the fragrance of coniferous trees, their needles, resins and cones and berries; subsidiary camphoraceous, green and resinous notes.	Fresh, invigorating, but can be disinfectant-like because of associations with this particular application.	The coniferous trees all share this note – but most notably the fir, spruce and pine e.o.'s. The disinfectant-like note is imparted by the constituents α- and β-pinenes. Atlas cedar is warm and camphoraceous with soft floral notes, while Virginian cedar is mild, dry and woody/balsamic. Cypress and juniper are more resinous.
Earthy – the smell of damp soil; fresh, but with a vegetation/fungal nuance.	Rich, damp, musty adjectives can be applied.	Several e.o.'s have earthy characteristics, including spikenard, patchouli and vetivert.
Faecal – the smell of excrement.	Although in its unadulterated form this is disgust-provoking, traces may be found some e.o's and absolutes.	Trace amounts of faecal-smelling compounds can be found in some of the 'indolic' floral oils such as jasmine abs., orange flower abs. and white champaca abs., giving a 'natural' element to the odour profile.

Odour type	Associated characteristics	Examples
Floral – suggestive of flowers, either a single flower or a bouquet. Subsidiary types include rosy, indolic (white blooms), jasmine-like, tropical, hyacinth, lily-like, violet-like. Subsidiary notes include green, fruity, spicy, citrus, herbal, caramel, honey, waxy.	As the category is so wide, many adjectives are used to describe floral characteristics. These include sweet, soft, rich, intense, heady, heavy, light, delicate, and fresh.	*Rosy* – rose e.o. and abs., rose geranium e.o. and abs. *Indolic* – jasmine abs., jasmine sambac abs., neroli e.o. and orange blossom absolute, tuberose abs., white chamapaca abs. *Tropical* – ylang ylang e.o., red champaca (fruity floral) abs., tiaré abs., frangipani abs. *Violet-like* – violet flower, orris root (also floral, woody).
Fruity – a sense of edible fruits, and not restricted to citrus. Subsidiary types include dried fruit, raisin, pear, plum and apple.	Sweet, sour, sharp, smooth, mellow, fresh.	Fruity notes can be detected in jasmine abs., frangipani abs., tagetes e.o., lavender e.o., clove bud e.o. Dried fruit, raisin, and plum notes are in the floral osmanthus abs. Apple-like notes are in Roman chamomile e.o. Blackcurrant bud abs. is fruity, but with dominant green notes.
Green – reminiscent of crushed green leaves, fresh peas in the pod, cucumber, cut green bell peppers.	Fresh, cool, light, sharp.	Violet leaf abs. is typical; so is galbanum e.o. and resinoid (also musty, earthy notes). Green notes are also in many herbal oils, especially mint e.o.'s. Geranium e.o. and abs. are floral/rose with green/minty subsidiary notes.

Hay – the scent of hay drying in the sun, reminiscent of the countryside; typical of the agrestic family. Subsidiary notes include coconut, green.	Warm, mellow, sweet.	The hay note is imparted by a constituent of grass, clover and tonka beans – coumarin (a synthetic version is available in perfumery). Hay abs. is typical. Tonka bean abs. is balsamic (vanilla) with hay notes. Lavender, immortelle, genet and oakmoss absolutes have subsidiary hay notes.
Herbaceous – the scent of aromatic culinary and medicinal herbs. Subsidiary notes often include green and woody, sometimes floral, minty, anisic or tabac.	Sharp, pungent, penetrating, fresh, light.	Thyme e.o. and abs., artemisia e.o. and abs., clary sage e.o. and abs., rosemary, marjoram and lavender e.o.'s are typical herbaceous scents. Rosemary and marjoram e.o.'s are fresh, pungent. Lavender e.o. is a light herbaceous with floral and woody notes. Thyme abs. and clary sage e.o. have warm subsidiary tabac notes. Lemon myrtle has a lemon subsidiary note. Laurel abs. is herbaceous with green and anisic subsidiary notes.
Honey – a sweet odour reminiscent of honey; may have floral undertones.	Sweet, smooth.	In perfumery, honey notes are derived from beeswax abs. (which is sweet, smooth and honeyed, but waxier in character than honey). Subsidiary honey notes can be detected in some florals such as tuberose abs., white ginger lily abs., linden blossom abs. and immortelle abs.

Odour type	Associated characteristics	Examples
Minty – the odour of mint. Green, herbaceous and mentholic subsidiary notes are often present.	Fresh, penetrating, sharp, refreshing, light.	Spearmint and peppermint e.o.'s are typical, with sharp and penetrating characteristics. Mint abs. may have a smoother quality. Minty notes are also found in herbal oils such as pennyroyal e.o., and florals such as geranium abs.
Mossy – reminiscent of the forest floor and its vegetation. Green, fungal, earthy and woody notes can be present too.	Deep, rich, natural.	The botanical sources are lichens (a symbiotic association of an alga and a fungus) that grow on the bark of oak trees and conifers, yielding oakmoss and treemoss absolutes – the archetypal mossy scent of perfumery essential in chypre and fougère fragrances.
Oily – this is often accompanied by the word 'fatty', although there are subtle differences. An oily note is reminiscent of fixed vegetable oils, such as linseed.	Faint, not dominant.	Oily notes are present in lemongrass e.o., Atlas cedar e.o.; fatty notes (smoother and with more body) can be detected in jasmine abs.
Peppery – reminiscent of freshly ground black peppers; a woody/spicy odour.	Warm, dry, fresh.	Black pepper e.o. is typical. Peppery, almost effervescent notes are also present in the citrus oil of bergamot, this effect possibly conferred by the shared constituent terpinen-4-ol. Coriander seed e.o. also has peppery notes.

Resinous – the scent of tree resins and exudates. Subsidiary notes include balsamic and coniferous.	Fresh, sweet, clean.	Frankincense e.o. is resinous, with a typical coniferous, pine-like note and fresh lemon notes in the top note. Myrrh is resinous but also sweet, spicy and somewhat medicinal. Benzoin resinoid is typically balsamic, yet has a resinous quality. Juniper berry e.o. is coniferous, sweet, fresh and resinous, without the pine disinfectant note. Most of the conifers have resinous notes.
Rosy – a scent reminiscent of roses, but not necessarily sourced from the rose. Subsidiary notes are floral, herbal, green, spicy and woody.	Sweet, light, mild, rich.	Rose otto (e.o.) is typical; this has waxy top notes. Other rosy-scented aromatics are geranium (green, rosy), palmarosa (a scented grass with rosy herbal notes), immortelle (rich, sweet rosy, honey), rosewood (floral, rosy, woody and mild) and guaiacwood (woody, smooth, mild, balsamic).
Smoky – the odour of smouldering woods and leaves, when smelled from a distance.	Deep, fragrant.	Cypress e.o. is woody, resinous and balsamic with smoky notes. Vetivert e.o. is earthy, woody, rooty and green, with smoky undertones.
Spicy – the scents of aromatic culinary spices. Sometimes woody subsidiary notes.	Pungent, warm, dry, sweet – although there is enormous variety in the spicy characteristics – see the examples opposite.	Caraway seed (sweet), cardamom (cineolic top), cinnamon bark and leaf (strong, sweet, warm, floral or fruity notes), clove bud (fruity, woody), coriander seed (light, woody), ginger (lemony, warm, woody, pungent), nutmeg (warm, pine-like, ethereal), pimento berry (sweet, warm, clove, herbaceous).

Odour type	Associated characteristics	Examples
Tabac – the odour of semi-dried pipe tobacco. Subsidiary notes include hay and green nuances.	Sweet, pungent, rich, warm.	Tobacco leaf abs. is typical. Also detected in the dry oil notes of German chamomile e.o. and the middle notes of clary sage e.o.
Waxy – a note reminiscent of paraffin wax, or beeswax. Usually a subsidiary note.	Soft, rich, warm.	Beeswax abs. has a waxy note, but this is also found in the dryout of jasmine abs. and the top note of rose otto.
Wintergreen – the medicated scent of wintergreen oil.	Strong, penetrating, diffusive	Wintergreen e.o. is typical, so is sweet birch. The medicated scent is conferred by the main constituent, methyl salicylate. This is present in much smaller amounts in the intensely floral, diffusive ylang ylang; however, you can still detect the medicated wintergreen note.
Woody – the scent of the woods of exotic trees. Balsamic, resinous, floral and camphoraceous are possible subsidiary notes in this category. Many spice and root oils have a woody note.	The woody category has many associated adjectives – soft, mild, sweet.	Arguably the most important woody oil is that of true sandalwood (soft, sweet and warm; some will detect a faint urinous note). Guaiacwood and rosewood are sweet, balsamic and mild and have floral/rosy notes.

Classification

Once the odours of aromatic materials have been described, using a consistent and accepted terminology, it then becomes possible to classify them. Classification is simply the grouping together of the aromatics according to their sensory similarities, and then it becomes possible to look at their interrelationships – essential for the cultivation of the sense of smell, and indeed the understanding of perfumery.

Although the concept is simple, the process is not. Gilbert (2008) cites the *Encyclopaedia Britannica*, which states that 'no satisfactory classification of odours can be given' (p.1). However, there have been many attempts at classifying odours since the first one proposed by Aristotle (384–322 BCE), where smells were simply classed as sweet, harsh, astringent, pungent and rich. Since then, several notable individuals have proposed classification schemes. These include Carl von Linné, also known as Linnaeus (1756), the well-known botanist and taxonomist; Eugene Rimmel (1865), the famous perfumer whose name persists in cosmetics today; and Septimus Piesse (in the nineteenth century) who first suggested the analogy between perfume notes and musical notes and scales. The most widely used scheme was developed by Marcel Billot (1948), a perfumer of note, although it is generally acknowledged that the most comprehensive classification of natural materials to date is that of Steffen Arctander (1960), which also includes odour descriptions and defines the relationships between 88 groups of over 400 aromatics (Williams 1995b). Such classification schemes are thought-provoking, and of importance to the perfumer. The focus of this book, however, is on the impact of plant aromatics on wellbeing, and the relationship we have with these fragrances.

Fragrance groups

As will be apparent, some plant aromatics almost defy categorisation – such as patchouli essential oil and blackcurrant bud absolute – whilst others fall neatly into their groups, with just some overlap. The main categories are *woody, coniferous, resinous, balsamic, spicy, herbaceous, green, agrestic, floral, citrus* and *fruity*. If we group these according to botanical sources as well as main fragrance characteristics, we can consider them in the following way.

WOODY, CONIFEROUS, RESINOUS AND BALSAMIC

This group includes *woods* such as the prized exotic agarwood, sandalwood, camphor; *conifers* such as the cedars, junipers, cypresses, pines and firs; and *resins* from the 'torchwood' family – the small shrubby trees that yield frankincense and myrrh. Myrrh is at the very far end of the resinous spectrum, and with a balsamic character too, so this large category can be extended to include the sweet, warm *balsamic* scents of vanilla, cacao, benzoin, labdanum, tonka bean, opopanax, and balsams of Peru and tolu.

SPICY

The spice group is just as diverse in terms of botanical origin, but perhaps easier to populate because of the dominant culinary aspect. The spices are all flavours which elicit varying sensations of warmth and pungency when tasted. Important aromatics in this category are black pepper, caraway, cardamom and coriander seeds, cinnamon, clove, fennel seeds, nutmeg, pimento, saffron and star anise.

HERBACEOUS, CAMPHORACEOUS, CINEOLIC, GREEN AND AGRESTIC

This group is defined by its botanical sources – the medicinal and culinary herbs – and also by their scents which, although broadly *herbaceous* and often pungent, also include *camphoraceous, green* or *minty* notes, which include the familiar rosemary, marjoram and thyme, the sages and the artemisias. The eucalypts and paperbarks with their *cineolic* odours are also in this category, which can be extended to include the *agrestic* scents that are reminiscent of the countryside in one way or another – drying cut grass (hay), leafy green and crushed green leaves (violet leaf), green and musty (galbanum resin), earthy and damp (vetiver), sweet/honey earthy/woody (oakmoss), green/fruity (blackcurrant bud), complex earthy/woody (patchouli and rich, intense tobacco leaf).

FLORAL

This fragrance family is easily defined – it comprises solely fragrances derived from flowers. While the scents may have this in common, there is a very wide range of floral fragrances, from rich, heavy and sombre tuberose through to sweet, delicate and ethereal genet. Even individual floral scents such as rose and jasmine will vary considerably according to the particular species and country of origin. Others, such as geranium, are not overtly floral but will have rose-like and green/minty elements. Beginning with the use of flowers for personal decoration in the form of garlands, and throughout the history of perfumery, the floral scents have been the most widely exploited.

CITRUS AND FRUITY

Citrus comprises the smallest group of fragrance types, and is easily defined as fragrances derived from citrus peel, or aromatics from other sources that have a distinct and dominant lemon note, such as *Litsea cubeba*. Citrus peel oils are all distinct, but they do share a light, fresh character. Some (such as bergamot) have *floral, peppery* notes, while others (such as lime) have *sweet, fruity* notes.

   In the following chapters a selection of the plant scents that have had a significant impact on our wellbeing will be discussed. The exploration of our sensory relationships with plant aromatics will begin with the woods and resins. These are often base notes, but they were probably the first incenses, and so have been with us since the very beginning.

CHAPTER 7

Woody, Resinous, Balsamic and Coniferous Scents

Aromatic woods of antiquity

It seems fitting to commence our exploration of the woods with the rare and costly agarwood, sandalwood – inextricably associated with India – and camphor, which is the most important aromatic in China. From the incense as well as the perfumery perspective, we must include here the resins produced by trees of the torchwood family – frankincense and myrrh – and also benzoin and the 'balsams', and the sweet-scented vanilla and sweet, coumarin scent of tonka bean. We will then turn to the cedarwoods, which have importance in many ancient cultures, but are of special significance to the northwest and Pacific Native American Indians. We will also explore other aromatic conifers and their impact on wellbeing, as in the Japanese practice of *shinrin yoku*, or 'taking the forest air'. Throughout, woody, resinous and balsamic scents in perfumery and aromatherapy will be highlighted.

Agarwood (aloeswood, eaglewood)

Agarwood, when lit and left to smoulder, produces an unforgettably fragrant smoke – exotic, deep, enveloping, warm and persistent – that can transport us through time and space to an imagined antiquity, or even into a trance state. Agarwood was, and remains, the most costly and sought-after aromatic wood – not only for incense production, but also for its aromatic oil. So, apart from the inevitable allure of the rare and exotic, why should this be so?

Agarwood is sourced from the heartwood of Indomalaysian flowering trees – *Aquilaria* species of the Thymelaeaceae family – which have become infected with fungi after natural damage to the bark, perhaps caused by gnawing insects or browsing elephants. The fungal species responsible is *Philalophora parasitica*. As a response to the infection, an oleoresin containing secondary metabolites is produced, and over a period of several years the heartwood fibres become congested with this aromatic resin. From the tree's perspective, this is to limit the spread of the infection within the wood. Uninfected, healthy wood is odourless and light in colour, unless it is very old, when a mild woody odour is present, but infected wood becomes dark in colour and highly aromatic. The infected heartwood is known as *gaharu*, and in Arabia it is called *oud, ood* or *ud* (Kaiser 2006; Pennacchio *et al.* 2010). The oleoresin increases the bulk and density of the infected parts of the wood, so it becomes heavier and sinks in water; the Chinese call it *ch'en hsiang*, 'the sinking incense wood', and the Japanese call it *jinkoh*, meaning 'wood that sinks' (Kaiser 2006; Morita 2006; Naef 2011). It is estimated that only 7–10 per cent of *Aquilaria* species contain agarwood – see Table 7.1 for a summary of the main species, and their geographical sources.

Table 7.1 Agarwood species and geographical origins

Botanical name	Country	Notes
Aquilaria crassna	Cambodia, Laos, Thailand, Vietnam.	In Japan high-quality agarwood imported from mountainous areas of Cambodia and Vietnam is known as *kanakoh* or *kyara*; lower grades are known as *jinkoh* (Naef 2011). In Japan there are six categories of *jinkoh*, classed according to the country of origin and the scent, using flavour terminology: *kyara* (from Cambodia and Vietnam, has a gentle and scent with slight bitterness; the word is Sanskrit for 'black'); *rakoku* (from Thailand, is sharp, pungent and sandalwood-like); *manaka* (from Malacca, is light and enticing); *manaban* (from the Malabar coast of India, is sweet, but coarse and unrefined); *sumotara* (from Sumatra, is sour at the beginning and the end); and *sasora* (probably from western India, is cool and sour) (Morita 2006). In Vietnam and Laos there is ongoing research into the cultivation of *Aquilaria* trees and agarwood (Naef 2011).
Aquilaria filaria	Philippines.	This species has been commercially exploited in more recent years (Naef 2011).

Aquilaria malaccensis (variant *A. agallocha*)	Northeastern India, Burma.	In India there are four grades: Grade A – *black* or *true agarwood*; Grade B – brown *bantang* wood; Grade C – *butha* (where 50% is uninfected and free of the resin); Grade D – *dhum* (yellow wood) (Naef 2011).
	Malaysia, Sumatra, Borneo, Philippines.	In Malaysia good-quality agarwood is called *kalambak*; lower grades are known as *gaharu* (Naef 2011).
Aquilaria sinensis	China, Hainan Island, Hong Kong	This species is the subject of whole-tree agarwood-induction technology to produce agarwood within 20 months (Zhang *et al.* 2012).

The main commercial use of agarwood is as an incense ingredient. Traditionally, agarwood was used in Buddhist, Hindu and Islamic ceremonies, and was a common incense ingredient, either alone or with other aromatics. The Hindi word for incense is *agarbath*. In Indonesia, especially Java, agarwood incense was used to aid communication with the deceased. It was also burned in India and China, notably on Hainan Island. In Japan, agarwood-based incense is used in the *koh-do* ceremony, an organoleptic art form. The best odour profile of burning *kyara* (the highest quality agarwood) is given by Kaiser (2006), who describes the initial fragrance as 'very sweet-balsamic, woody-floral, and reminiscent of α- and β-vetivone and related compounds'. Then the smoke becomes 'more woody, incense-like with a characteristic spiciness, and shades of vanilla and musk', followed by 'deep noble woody, incense, ambery shade', and after nine to twelve minutes the scent is 'deep woody with phenolic note of castoreum, sweet vanilla note' (p.63).

Agarwood also yields an essential oil via distillation. Naef's (2011) review of agarwood discusses its odour, which is described as 'warm, unique, balsamic notes with sandalwood-ambergris tonalities' (p.73). This paper also looks at the odour of some of the essential oil constituents, which vary according to botanical species as well as geographical sources. Agarwood is extremely complex from this perspective; it is dominated by a huge range of constituents known as sesquiterpenes, and other important chemicals are agarol, agarofuranes, agarospirol and chromones, amongst many others. Some of the constituents have very interesting odours in their own right, all of which will have an impact on the overall agarwood odour profile. Some constituents are fresh, sweet and floral, herbaceous/minty, smoky sandalwood, amber-like, woody with vetiver character, powerful, long-lasting, sweet woody, spicy and peppery woody, and even green and galbanum-like. In Turin and Sanchez (2009), Turin states that 'good agarwood has something unique in its weird combination of honeyed sweetness and woody freshness' (p.430).

The essential oil is difficult to obtain. Alec Lawless, who was involved in the essential oils trade for many years, commented that 'I have yet to come across oil that I believe is genuinely distilled from infected agarwood' (Lawless 2009, p.2). Naef (2011) observed that that adulteration of both the wood and its essential oil is common practice, and that poor quality oils could fetch US$100/kg and pure material up to US$100,000/kg.

Agarwood oil is a valued perfume ingredient, albeit more important in the East than the West, although it has developed a cult following in western artisan perfumery. Agarwood is a traditional *attar* in India, where it is co-distilled with sandalwood. It is also a key ingredient in the traditional Arabian scent known as *oud*. In modern western perfumery, agarwood, or more likely its synthetic copies, can be found in 'masculine' fragrances. Quoting Turin and Sanchez again, 'real *oud* is a complex material, with honey, tobacco leaf, minty-fresh and castoreum animalic notes all together' (p.365). Notable western *oud* fragrances are *M7* (Yves Saint Laurent); *Oud Cuir d'Arabie* (Montale), where it is paired with leather; *Black Aoud* (Montale), where it is paired with rose and is very much in the style of Omani perfumery; and *Oud Wood* (Tom Ford).

Like most plant-derived aromatics, agarwood has a role in traditional healing – in this case, in Chinese, Ayurvedic and Tibetan medicines. It has a wide range of therapeutic properties. Perhaps unsurprisingly and probably related to its fine odour, it is said to be an aphrodisiac, and also a sedative. However, it is also used as a cardiotonic, carminative, for stomach problems and as an anti-emetic, as well as for coughs, rheumatism and fever (Pennacchio *et al.* 2010; Naef 2011; Zhang *et al.* 2012). Naef (2011) cites a few studies that have attempted to identify the pharmacologically active compounds present in agarwood. Some compounds such as *jinkoh*-eremol, and agarospirol and spiro-compound can have effects on the central nervous system, which might help explain the sedative effect. Antimicrobial effects have been investigated, including activity against methicillin-resistant *Staphylococcus aureus*, and *in vitro* studies with human gastric cancer cell lines showed cytotoxic potential.

Today, the main importers of the oil are the United Arab Emirates (UAE), Saudi Arabia, China and Japan, and the major exporters are Malaysia and Indonesia. The UAE is also a re-exporter to the Middle East. The international trade in agarwood dates back to the thirteenth century, and today the main centre for the agarwood trade is Singapore; Kaiser (2006) gave the annual value of the export as US$1.2 billion. Because of its rarity, its enduring value as a unique scent and the constant demand for it in the incense and perfumery industries, it is not surprising that agarwood trees have been over-exploited and become even scarcer; some are extinct or are approaching extinction (Pennacchio *et al.* 2010). Wild trees are now seriously depleted, due to both indiscriminate harvesting, since there are no outward signs that the wood contains the resin, and over-harvesting, as they are considered to be a 'botanical gold mine' (Kaiser 2006). In 2010 seven of the 18 agarwood-producing tree species in Malaysia were at risk of global extinction. The high market value of agarwood has resulted in organised groups of illegal harvesters spending long periods in protected forest areas. Between 1995 and 2002 there were almost 200 arrests, in spite of which less than half of the agarwood exported from Malaysia had the required permits (Al Bawaba 2010).

The highest yield of agarwood is from trees that are 75–80 years old, so there have been numerous research programmes to establish an alternative way of producing agarwood to satisfy demand and help conserve the wild trees. *Aquilaria* plantations have been established in Indonesia, Cambodia, Thailand, Vietnam (on Phu Quoc Island) and China. The young cultivated trees are intentionally damaged, using axes and nails, and inoculated with fungi that have been isolated from naturally infected agarwood. To increase the chances of successful infection, these artificial wounds are encouraged to stay open. In addition, the ferric oxide in the iron nails promotes a desirable dark colour in the wood fibres. It appears that agarwood takes 15–20 months to form under these conditions. Low-grade agarwood results, but the yields are poor (Naef 2011; Zhang *et al.* 2012). However, in China, 'whole-tree agarwood induction technology' has been developed. *A. sinensis* trees are injected with a degradable chemical solution that is claimed to induce agarwood production within 20 months. Agarwood produced this way has been assessed as being of high quality, with a strong scent of honey or concentrated sugar (Zhang *et al.* 2012). It remains to be seen how viable this method is in terms of satisfying the demand for agarwood, but anything that helps to protect and conserve the wild *Aquilaria* trees must be seen as a step forward.

Sandalwood

Like agarwood, sandalwood is one of the oldest known aromatic woods. It is a tropical hardwood, with a deep, soft, smooth, sweet, woody scent (Weiss 1997; Lawless 2009). Sandalwood is the archetypal fragrance of India; it is mentioned in Vedic literature such as the *Nirkuta* dated circa 500 BCE, and the *Vinaya Pitaka* of 400–300 BCE (Weiss 1997), and also the *Mahabharata*, the *Ramayana*, the *Arthashastra* and the *Dhammapada* (Morris 1984). Sandalwood's collective Sanskrit name is *chandana*; the white type is known as *srikhanda* and the yellow is *pitachananda*. It acquired other names through the aromatic trade; it was named *santal* by the Arabs, hence the European name of sandalwood (Weiss 1997). The aromatic wood and its oil have been used for over 2500 years, and before that it certainly would have had ritual and ceremonial uses. Sandalwood fragrance has been used to induce a calm state of mind by all of the Indian spiritual traditions; the wood, incense and perfume are a feature of Brahmin, Buddhist and Hindu religious rituals, and Hindu erotic arts (Morris 1984; Weiss 1997). The wood itself is fragrant and attractive; it is close-grained with the best quality having small marks known as 'bird's eyes'; because of these characteristics it is perfect for carving. Traditionally, wood carvers would create small religious statues, prayer beads, ornate caskets and furniture, and even temples – the scent would last indefinitely, and the wood is resistant to termites. The chippings and sawdust were made into incense, such as the blend used to honour Vishnu.

The scented oil obtained from sandalwood has many important cultural associations and applications (Morris 1984; Erligmann 2001; Lawless 2009; Baldovini, Delasalle and Joulain 2011). The yogis maintain that sandalwood is the scent of the 'subtle body', and in tantric practice it is used by males to awaken *kundalini* energy and transform this into an enlightened mind (Lawless 1994). Sandalwood oil was, and still is, used in traditional perfumery; when combined with rose otto it made a purification fragrance known as *aytar*, which was used at the end of the Hindu year to symbolically remove past influences and prepare for a fresh start. It is also the base of the attars, where it is co-distilled with other aromatics to make traditional perfumes. In Ayurvedic medicine, sandalwood is classed as bitter, sweet, astringent and cool, and is used to control the *doshas*, but has more physical effects on *pitta*. It is also used to lighten and concentrate the mind (Svoboda 2003). Other cultures place a high value on sandalwood too. Sandalwood reached China when the Buddhist monks travelled the Silk Road, bringing sandalwood incense sticks. In China sandalwood became known as *tanheong*, the 'scented tree', and by the Ming dynasty it had found its way into most aspects of daily life; carved sandalwood fans were highly valued. Lawless (1994) mentions the Japanese, who burn sandalwood with agarwood at Buddhist shrines, and at Shinto ceremonies. In Tibetan medicine it is used with other aromatics as a massage oil or incense for insomnia and anxiety. In Islam sandalwood is used in aromatic incense that is placed in a censer at the feet of the dead, to carry the soul to heaven.

Sandalwood is part of the botanical family known as the Santalaceae, which contains around 30 genera, including the fully parasitic mistletoe, *Viscum album*. The genus *Santalum* contains around 20 tropical, evergreen, semi-parasitic trees and shrubs (Weiss 1997). Within this genus, the most important species is *Santalum album*. The Latin name translates as 'white sandalwood', but in the essential oil trade it is often called 'East Indian sandalwood' to differentiate it from other species, whose oils are considered to be inferior in terms of scent. This species is indigenous to India, the islands of Timor in Indonesia, where it is known as *haumeni*, and Sunda, where it is called *sandal*. Sandalwood spread over Indonesia, where it is called *cendana*, and also Sri Lanka. It is now being planted on a large scale in northwest Australia, for future essential oil production.

S. album is an evergreen tree that can reach 12 metres in height at maturity, at around 60 years of age. The heartwood and roots contain the volatile oil, which acts as a 'preservative' so that the wood and roots do not rot or decay. The sandalwood tree has an unusual way of growing and surviving. It is described as an 'obligate root parasite' or as having a 'semi-parasitic' habit. In its early stages of growth, the seedling's roots contact the roots of other plants, and a structure known as a *haustorium* develops from its roots and acts as a sucker, absorbing nutrients such as nitrogen and phosphorus for the sandalwood from its host. Host trees include teak, clove, bamboo, and guava. Once the sandalwood tree is established, the parasitic habit continues, but becomes less important for survival once its true roots are established. However, the parasitic habit is detrimental to the host trees, which eventually die (Weiss 1997; Erligmann 2001).

Sandalwood trees are felled by uprooting, rather than cutting the trunk. The branches and most of the sapwood are removed, leaving a small covering to protect the heartwood. Traditionally, the felled trees were left for ants and termites to eat away at the sapwood, leaving the fragrant heartwood and roots – the parts where the volatile oil is most abundant. Traditionally, sandalwood oil was obtained by water distillation of the heartwood and roots, which would have been reduced to a coarse powder and soaked in water for two days. One charge could be distilled several times. However, nowadays the essential oil is obtained by steam distillation of the powdered heartwood and major roots, at modern state-owned or private plants (Weiss 1997).

Due to over-harvesting, exploitation and fraud, white sandalwood is now very scarce – at least in accessible areas. The main production areas are Mysore and also Madras, in India. Sandalwood harvesting is now officially controlled in India; however, trees are more than 30 years old before they contain significant quantities of the volatile oil, and so the availability situation is not likely to change for a considerable time – even with an intensive planting programme. Some producers of the essential oil have persistently undermined the government's sustainability measures, and this, coupled with the rising price of the oil, has fuelled the attractiveness of harvesting young trees, and adulterating the product with essential oil distilled from imported woods of *Eucaria spicata* from Australia or *S. austrocaledonicum* from Vanuatu. In other cases the sandalwood oil has been extended with coconut oil. Lawless (2009) commented that this type of problem is 'endemic'.

Only two other species of sandalwood are harvested for essential oil production. These are *S. austrocaledonicum* and *S. spicatum*. *S. austrocaledonicum* is found only in the New Caledonian and Vanuatu archipelagos in the South Pacific. Vanuatu has been producing the oil, on a small scale, for over 200 years. Because the trees have not been over-harvested, and the seeds are tough, natural regeneration has maintained the balance. Harvesting is controlled by the government, in contrast to some of the other New Caledonian islands, where over-harvesting and the absence of a regeneration programme has terminated the industry. The essential oil from Vanuatu is usually rectified – it is distilled twice, and the top and bottom fractions of the second distillation are discarded. Although this reduces the yield, it improves the odour (Lawless 2009). *S. spicatum* is found in the arid regions of southwest Australia. The wood is extracted initially with solvents, followed by vacuum distillation of the residue (Erligmann 2001). Because the extraction process involves solvents rather than steam or water distillation, this is not a true essential oil, so now the technique is being progressively abandoned, despite the good odour of the product (Baldovini, Delasalle and Joulain 2011). Another species, *S. insulare*, is closely related to *S. album*; this is native to the islands of eastern Polynesia, but is not exploited for its essential oil, as the trees are not abundant enough to sustain production. Other so-called sandalwood oils are West Indian sandalwood from *Amyris balsamifera*, East African sandalwood from *Osyris tenuifolia*, budda wood or false sandalwood from *Eremophilia mitchellii* and red sandalwood – a natural red dye from *Pterocarpus santalinus* (Weiss 1997; Baldovini *et al.* 2011).

East Indian sandalwood essential oil has a soft, mild, fatty, balsamic, sweet-woody odour. Some individuals detect a faint urinous quality. It has virtually no top note, and is remarkably persistent. Its main chemical constituents are the sesquiterpene alcohols known as α- and β-santalols (Bowles 2003). The α-santalols confer the woody, cedar-like attributes of the fragrance, while the typical warm-woody, milky, musky, urinous and animalic characteristics are contributed mainly by the β-santalols and traces of 2-α-*trans*-bergamotol, a sesquiterpenoid. The constituent responsible for the tenacity is β-santalene, and trace constituents such as phenols (eugenol and *para*-cresol), monoterpene alcohols (such as linalool) and ketones (nor-α-*trans*-bergamotone) also have a subtle impact on its odour profile (Erligmann 2001; Baldovini *et al.* 2011). *S. spicatum* has a soft, woody, extremely tenacious, balsamic, sweet odour with a dry spicy resinous top note (Valder *et al.* 2003). It contains over 70 constituents and, like *S. album*, it is dominated by sesquiterpenes. *S. spicatum* contains levels of β-santalol similar to *S. album*, but much less α-santalol. However, it contains a sesquiterpenol that is not found in *S. album*, II-farnesol at over 5 per cent. This same compound is found in rose and ylang ylang essential oils. A sesquiterpenoid known as dendrolasine may be present at up to 2 per cent, and this is only found in trace amounts in *S. album*. So, given the differences in some major, minor and trace components, the oil does smell different from that of *S. album* – it has a top note, floral notes and green notes. Erligmann (2001) classifies *S. album* as amber-like, and *S. spicatum* as resinous. In the case of *S. austrocaledonicum*, less is known about its constituents and their contribution to the odour profile. However, we do know that the main chemical constituents are similar to *S. album*, but that it also contains compounds called lanceols, which have a weak odour, and lanceals, which are more powerful and sandalwood-like (Baldovini *et al.* 2011).

In aromatherapy, sandalwood essential oil is used as a general tonic, an antidepressant and a sedative; its antimicrobial properties are indicated for genito-urinary tract infections, and bronchodilatory actions indicate its use in respiratory infections. It is also used in skin care for maintaining skin health and alleviating acne, dermatitis and eczema; many phytocosmeceuticals contain sandalwood oil for these reasons. It has been suggested that sandalwood oil is possibly a diuretic, and a lymphatic and venous decongestant. Some of these uses reflect its traditional medicinal uses. Research has also suggested that some of sandalwood's constituents have antitumour activity, and that that *S. album* could be included in topical drugs for the treatment of human papillomavirus (HPV) skin infections, and the prevention of pre-cancerous skin lesions (Viroxis 1999 and Haque and Haque 1999, cited in Baldovini *et al.* 2011).

Despite the reputation of sandalwood as an aphrodisiac, probably due to traditional erotic poetry and its use in the Tantric 'Rite of the Five Essentials', there has been no research that specifically supports this use. However, some contemporary research has supported the topical use of sandalwood essential oil to elicit both relaxation and behavioural activation simultaneously (Hongratanaworakit, Heuberger and Buchbauer 2004), and it is possible that this effect, in appropriate circumstances, could be conducive to sexual arousal. A further study conducted by the same team of Heuberger, Hongratanaworakit and Buchbauer (2006) investigated the effects of inhalation of α-santalol, a component of sandalwood oil, and *S. album* oil compared with an odourless placebo. In this study, *S. album* oil had an activating effect – increasing pulse rate, skin conductance, and systolic blood pressure – compared with the α-santalol and the placebo. However α-santalol produced higher ratings of attentiveness and mood than the essential oil or the placebo. It appears that such effects on arousal and mood are related to perceived odour quality. Both studies support the use of *S. album* as a relaxing, antidepressant oil.

Sandalwood maintains a very important place in perfumery. Natural and synthetic versions are said to be present in up to 250 fragrances launched on the international market each year (Baldovini *et al.* 2011). This is because it is so very versatile, it supports and enhances other aromatics, contributing soft, woody, powdery notes to the dryout of a fragrance, and acts as an excellent fixative (Aftel 2008). Lawless (2009) maintained that sandalwood 'priced itself out of commercial perfumery years ago, but remains one of the most useful of all perfume materials' (p.68). Turin and Sanchez (2009) agree with Lawless, commenting that 'natural sandalwood oil is, because of restrictions due to overharvesting, missing from the perfumer's palette' (p.492). Conversely, Baldovini *et al.* (2011) suggest that despite the shortages and steadily rising cost of sandalwood essential oils, they are widely used in fragrance compounds at high levels of 2–3 per cent, despite the availability of cheaper synthetic alternatives. However, it should be remembered that it is common practice to say that a perfume contains notes of a particular kind, such as sandalwood or jasmine, even if the genuine extract is absent.

Because 'sandalwood' is ubiquitous in modern commercial perfumery, and because it contributes to numerous base accords in both feminine and masculine scents, it is impossible to give examples of 'typical' sandalwood fragrances. Some are named after sandalwood, such as Serge Lutens' *Santal Blanc* and *Santal de Mysore*, and Maître Parfumeur et Gantier's *Santal Noble* – all receiving decent reviews from Turin and Sanchez (2009), despite the important missing element of white sandalwood, and the presence of synthetics and Australian sandalwood. A few others could be said to have a prominent, although not dominant, element of sandalwood. These include Lauder's *Sensuous*, where it is combined with lily and vetiver, and Guerlain's *Samsara*, where it forms an accord with jasmine. In the earlier versions of *Samsara* (1989), genuine East Indian sandalwood was featured, underpinned by the potent synthetic known as 'Polysantol', but *Samsara's* sandalwood content would now appear to be completely synthetic. Turin and Sanchez (2009) suggest that 'a moratorium should be put on all sandalwoods until they find a reliable supply of the real stuff' (p.487). The situation is not quite as bad as that of agarwood, but it is unfortunate that such an important aromatic is all but absent from contemporary perfumes.

Camphor

Perhaps the defining aromatic plant for China is the majestic camphor tree. This is in fact native to Japan, and the true camphor tree is *Cinnamomum camphora*, known in Japan as *hon-sho*. Camphor trees growing in other countries are considered to be sub-species, but botanically they are very similar. In China, it is known as *yu-sho*. *C. camphorum* is a tall evergreen tree, with a dense and spreading head. There are small fissures in the rough bark, and from these camphor oil exudes and solidifies. This is easily collected, and the exudate can be encouraged by making slits in the bark – and this would have been the original way of harvesting camphor. Its yellow-brown wood is hard, with a fine texture. It carves and polishes well, and has a very long-lasting, pleasant fragrance, so it is widely used for cabinetmaking, especially camphor chests. (The Chinese will not store silk fabrics in camphor chests, however; they maintain that the scent causes deterioration of the fibres.) The large, leathery, bright green leaves have the sweet, clean, fresh scent of camphor. The camphor tree produces insignificant yellow flowers, but the seeds smell like cardamom and are the source of an aromatic fat used in soap making (Weiss 1997).

The camphor tree does not grow in the north of China, so it was not used by the earlier dynasties, but eventually it was highly valued as a building material and for making lattice filigrees for temples, as well as for cabinetmaking – like many aromatic woods, it is insect-resistant and long-lasting. Morris (1984) mentions its use in the construction of covered arcades, where the scent would enhance meditative walks, and for carving effigies of the Buddha for temples such as the massive one at the Spiritual Grove Temple at Hangchow, and the even larger one at the Temple of Universal Peace at Ch'eng-te. He also tells us that individual trees of great antiquity are still growing at Taoist and Buddhist shrines throughout Szechwan and the Yangtze valley.

Natural camphor or pure camphor (*d*-camphor) is a transparent or whitish crystalline solid. It has a distinctive and characteristic camphoraceous odour that is penetrating and pungent, clean, fresh and sharp. It consists of a ketone named camphor, which is a derivative of a dicyclic terpene (Weiss 1997). Natural camphor is capable of sublimation – that is, it changes in form from solid to gas without going through the liquid phase. It was part of the old formula for mothballs, as the smell repels insects, moths and worms. Lawless (1994) comments that it was worn in a pouch around the neck to ward off infections, and that the Arabs used its scent to lessen sexual desire. Camphor was also useful to calm hysteria, as an analgesic for nerve pain, and as a cardiac stimulant. In China, camphor was also a medicine; it is mentioned in the sixteenth century herbal known as *Pun-Tsao-kang-mu* where its main use was for gastric stimulation – because it is slightly water-soluble, it was used in teas. It has traditional culinary uses too – the leaves are used in steaming liquors. Outside of China camphor was known in European medicine by the twelfth century. The German abbess Hildegarde von Bingen called it *ganphora*, and suggested that it should be used topically as a counter-irritant for the treatment of rheumatism and arthritis (Weiss 1997).

So we can see that the scented wood was culturally important, and that natural camphor had medicinal attributes – but camphor oil never became a significant player in the fine fragrance world; it simply does not have an odour that is particularly attractive in this particular context! Moreover, seduction was an important facet of early perfumery, but the scent of camphor was considered the opposite of an aphrodisiac, again rendering it undesirable in perfumery. Nevertheless, a camphor accord can be found in a few contemporary fragrances. Heeley's *Esprit du Tigre* has top notes of a subtle wintergreen and camphor, with a heart of cardamom and dry down of vetiver and cinnamon. Turin and Sanchez (2009) suggest that this is reminiscent of Tiger Balm (or Tiger Balsam), a traditional healing liniment that contains camphor, eucalyptus and cajeput. They also mention a camphor effect in *L'Eau Neuve* (Lubin), a 'camphor chypre' that occupies a middle ground between 'medicine and cologne'.

Nowadays the essential oil obtained from camphor is the most important camphor product, although demand has diminished due to the availability of cheap synthetic camphor. The entire tree is felled, including the roots, the wood is chipped and then steam or water distilled, and sometimes the leaves are distilled. This produces the essential oil, which contains some crystallised camphor. This crystalline component is removed by filter pressing, to produce what is known as crude camphor oil. This is further rectified under vacuum, and further fractionation yields oils of different specifications. White camphor is the lightest fraction, brown the medium fraction, and blue camphor the heavy fraction. White camphor, which contains 1,8-cineole (an oxide dominant in eucalyptus oils), is used as a solvent in varnish and paint manufacture, and for scenting detergents. Brown (or red) camphor contains safrole and terpineol; safrole is the base for some important fragrance derivatives such as heliotropin and vanillin. Yellow camphor is a by-product when sassafras oil is derived from brown camphor. Blue (or green) camphor is dominated by sesquiterpenes, and is of little significance (Weiss 1997). Because of the fractionation, camphor oils are incomplete and are not classed as true essential oils.

Only white camphor is used in aromatherapy, and then only rarely and with caution, because of potential convulsant and neurotoxic hazards due to the camphor content of around 30 per cent. The safrole content of the other fractions is high, at 80 per cent in brown camphor and 20 per cent in yellow. Safrole is a very toxic compound, and is associated with genotoxicity and carcinogenicity (Tisserand and Balacs 1995).

Perhaps camphor is a scent best enjoyed in its natural state, in the wood, leaves and seeds – this is where we see its finest effects on wellbeing.

Rosy-scented woods

There are two aromatic woods that yield scents that have rosy characteristics. They are both obtained from tropical trees – rosewood and guaiacwood – and both have been valued for carving, furniture making, incense and perfume.

Rosewood

Rosewood is obtained from members of the genus *Aniba*, tropical evergreen trees belonging to the Lauraceae family, which also contains *Cinnamomum* species. The rosewoods are forest trees, native to French Guyana and the Amazon basin. The bark of *Aniba canelilla* has a cinnamon-like scent, hence its name 'cinnamon of the Amazon'. The bark of this species is used locally to make a tea, and to scent stored clothing (Weiss 1997). In Guyana *A. canelilla* has medicinal uses – the smoke of the burning stems and twigs is inhaled to relieve diarrhoea (Pennacchio *et al.* 2010). The wood of other species – *A. duckei*, *A. parviflora* and *A. rosaeodora* – is chipped and softened in hot water, then steam-distilled to yield rosewood essential oil. In the trade, rosewood oil is known as *Bois de Rose Femelle*, most of which comes from *A. rosaeodora* in the northern parts of Brazil (Jouhar 1991), but overharvesting has threatened the species, and there are also major concerns about deforestation. Santana *et al.* (1997) noted that sustainable management plans had been implemented, and legislation requires companies to re-plant in proportion to the number felled, but Burfield (2004), cast doubts on the actual relevance of these initiatives, because they were not supported by an independent audit of the natural resources. Nevertheless, rosewood is widely used and has many commercial applications, such as the flavouring of tobacco, soft drinks and confectionery.

Bois de Rose Femelle from Brazil is a yellowish, slightly oily liquid – the yield is highest from the yellowest wood. Jouhar (1991) suggests that the true oil is characteristically viscous and has a floral odour, reminiscent of rose, orange and mignonette. Weiss (1997) comments that *Bois de Rose Cayenne* from Guyana has a finer scent, but that only small quantities are available, finding use in fine perfumery and toiletries. Chemically, rosewood is characterised by the presence of the ubiquitous monoterpene alcohol *d*-linalool at up to 85 per cent, and even at 97 per cent in the Cayenne type. According to Burfield (2004), the linalool content is typically in the region of 84–93 per cent and is a racemic mix of *d*- and *l*-linalool. Rosewood oil is therefore a source for the isolation of linalool (Williams 1995c). The rosy odour is partly due to the presence of the rosy-scented alcohol named geraniol, at around 2 per cent.

Rosewood essential oil is used in aromatherapy as an anti-fungal agent to combat *Candida* infections, and for its stimulating and tonic qualities that can aid in cases of debility and stress. In perfumery, the terpeneless oil is used; this is around three times the concentration of the essential oil. This is often part of lilac and lily types of perfumes, and is used as a modifier in May blossom (*Cratageus oxycantha*) and *Corylopsis* types of scents (Jouhar 1991).

Guaiacwood

The botanical source of guaiacwood is *Bulnesia sarmientoi*, of the Zygophyllaceae family. It is native to Argentina and the jungles of Paraguay. In northwest Argentina it is known as *palo santo*, and here it has therapeutic uses. The Criollos[1] burn the wood chips in combination with the leaves of fringed rue (*Ruta chalepensis*) and blow the smoke into the ears to alleviate otitis. It was also used in a therapeutic smoking mixture, along with *yerba maté* (*Ilex paraguariensis*) and the feathers of *Rhea americana*, a flightless bird (Pennacchio *et al.* 2010).

Guaiacwood essential oil is sometimes called champaca-wood oil, and is produced by steam distillation of the waste wood. The wood itself contains guaiac resin, which causes the cut wood to develop a greenish-blue colour on exposure to air. The oil is solid, melting at 45°C. The distilled oil is used to produce guaiacwood acetate – a sweet, delicate-woody-rosy derivative for use in perfumery. Guaiacwood has a sweet, balsamic odour that is said to be reminiscent of tea roses, so it is often used in rose and violet formulae. However, its odour profile also makes it a potential adulterant of otto of roses and sandalwood oil (Jouhar 1991). Lawless (2009) suggests that guaiacwood is a 'clean' middle note that acts as a fixative in woody and floral compositions, and can also be used in delicate florals. It appears to play a supportive rather than a dominant role in compositions, such as providing woody notes that support the rose in *Chanel No.19*, a green floral fragrance launched in 1970–1971 (Calkin and Jellinek 1994).

The torchwoods

The Burseraceae family includes some of the shrubs and trees known as 'torchwoods', that exude fragrant oleo-gum resins which were burned as incense in ancient times, and remain important incenses today. Frankincense and myrrh have been closely associated since early times. Morris (1984) quotes Theophrastus, who in 'Enquiry into Plants' wrote about the flora of the regions now known as Yemen and Oman. He noted that:

> The trees of frankincense and myrrh grow partly in the mountains, partly on private estates at the foot of the mountains; wherefore some are under cultivation, others not; the mountains, they say, are lofty, forest-covered and subject to snow, and rivers from them flow down into the plain. The frankincense tree, it is said, is not tall, about five cubits high, and is much branched... The myrrh tree is said to be still much smaller in stature and more bushy. (pp.75, 76)

The myrrh of ancient times was actually what we now call oponapax. Finally we will explore aromatic *Amyris* species – also traditionally known as torchwoods.

---

1   The Criollos were the decencants of the Spanish and Portuguese settlers who arrived in the sixteenth century. The word 'Creole' is derived from Criollo.

Frankincense

The modern name for frankincense is derived from the mediaeval French *franc*, meaning free, pure or abundant, and the Latin *incensum*, meaning to set alight. Its trade name is olibanum, and this is derived from the Hebrew *lebonah* (Lawless 1994). An ancient Egyptian legend tells that frankincense was first brought to Egypt in the talons of a bird that built its nest from the twigs of frankincense trees; in time this bird became the mythical phoenix of later legends (Miller and Morris 1988, cited in Pennacchio *et al.* 2010). From the very beginning, frankincense has inspired mankind. We have already explored its role in all of the ancient cultures, where it was used as incense, and in perfumes and medicines. So perhaps we can view frankincense as the 'archetypal' incense, with a cultural presence throughout the Middle and Far East, India, Africa, the Mediterranean, and eventually in Roman Catholic churches, along with benzoin and storax (Lawless 1994).

Dannaway (2010) refers to research which shows that frankincense provokes psychoactivity (Moussaieff *et al.* 2008), and there is also the phenomenon of 'olibanum addiction' to the mild narcotic properties that can be observed in its ritual use (Martinetz, Lohs and Janzen 1989). Frankincense was indeed used in incense mixes intended for use as entheogens – a possible clue to its enduring importance in that particular context. The resin and incense smell sweet, balsamic, dry and resinous with a fresh, slightly green element.

The botanical sources of frankincense oleo-gum resin are small, shrubby (multi-stemmed) trees belonging to the *Boswellia* genus, which thrives on stony, soil-less, arid ground. Please see Table 7.2 for a summary of the main species, and their geographical sources and uses.

Table 7.2 Frankincense species and geographical origins

Compiled and adapted from Pennacchio *et al.* (2010).

Botanical name	Country	Uses
Boswellia ameero	Island of Socotra, southeast of Yemen.	Oleo-gum resin harvested and burned as incense.
Boswellia bhau-dajiana	Northeastern Africa.	Known as *mohr-add*, the oleo-gum resin was burned as incense and traded as frankincense.
Boswellia carteri	Middle East, including Iran and Iraq; Somaliland.	Known as frankincense or olibanum, prized in Mediterranean regions; burned as incense. Also sold in markets at Jima (Ethiopia) – the main trading place for frankincense, where it was called *k'eyi it'an*.

Boswellia dalzielii	West Africa.	Known as the frankincense tree; the resin was burned to fumigate and scent clothing.
Boswellia frereana	Mediterranean and tropical Africa.	Oleo-gum resin harvested and burned as incense.
Boswellia glabra	Middle East.	According to Avicenna, the oleo-gum resin was burned to produce smoke for the treatment of skin diseases.
Boswellia hildebrandtii	Kenya.	The Pokot burned the resin (*songoluwo*) on their fires to repel insects. The Rendille and the Turkana also used the dead wood (known as *ekinyate*) as incense for ceremonies and home use.
Boswellia macrophylla	Nigeria.	The oleo-gum resin was burned to fumigate rooms and clothing; it was exported as frankincense.
Boswellia neglecta	Liban (Ethiopia).	Farmers generated income from this species; the oleo-gum resins were burned as incense, but also used in perfumery, food and beverage flavouring and traditional medicine.
Boswellia ogadensis	Liban (Ethiopia).	As *B. neglecta* (above).
Boswellia papyrifera	Ethiopia, East Africa and northeastern Africa.	This species is known as the 'elephant tree', and it is now endangered due to over-harvesting and insect infestations. The oleo-gum resin was burned to produce smoke to control fever; it also had a tranquilising effect. The smoke was also used to ward off evil spirits.
Boswellia sacra	Middle East, Oman.	In Oman the oleo-gum resin was harvested and burned to perfume clothes, hair and houses. It was the major source of Arabian frankincense in the classical world.

Botanical name	Country	Uses
Boswellia serrata	India.	Known as Indian frankincense, this had many uses, including as incense for magico-religious ceremonies to hasten recovery of the sick, in the hope that the deities would drive away evil. It is considered sacred, and burned in houses as incense during ceremonies. In the Gwalior Forest division of Madhya Pradesh, the smoke was inhaled through a censor – a *chilam* – to relieve gastric pain and flatulence.
Boswellia socotrana	Island of Socotra, southeast of Yemen.	Oleo-gum resin harvested and burned as incense.
Boswellia species	Southern Oromia, Ethiopia.	Women of the Borana tribe would burn the smoke in sauna-like chambers, to perfume and cleanse their bodies.

The woody tissue of these trees contains specialised, elongated resin ducts, where the oleo-gum resin is formed. If incisions are made in the bark, the milky white resin exudes and then hardens into tear-shaped, amber-coloured drops. Pliny the Elder, in his *Naturalia Historia*, says that in ancient times it was only found in Saba (Sheba), a remote area of Arabia. Harvesting frankincense was a privilege reserved for certain men from sacred families, who observed restrictions to maintain this honour, such as refraining from sexual intercourse with women, or attending funerals. The harvested frankincense was transported by camels to Sabota, where one gate opened to receive the consignment; if anyone turned from the road, they were sentenced to death, such was its value. Sales were prohibited until the priests had taken one tenth of the load for their god Sabin (Aftel 2008). In later times, although the oleo-gum resin was still greatly valued, harvesting was no longer the preserve of the chosen few, and the frankincense trade became economically important. The oleo-gum resin became known as the 'tears of frankincense', which were once used as currency; Lawless (2009) points out that the town of Petra in Jordan was built with wealth generated by the frankincense trade. In ancient times frankincense was a valued commodity, as well as having religious significance. This is probably why it was one of the gifts, along with myrrh and gold, given to the baby Jesus by the Three Wise Kings. (Watt and Sellar (1996) suggested that these 'kings' were possibly Zoroastrian astrologer-priests from Babylon, who believed that Jesus was the great leader prophesied in Micah 5:2, in the Old Testament.)

Nowadays the oleo-gum resin is usually exported to Europe or America, where it is either steam-distilled to yield an essential oil called olibanum oil, or extracted with solvent to give a resinoid; an absolute is also produced. These products are used in perfumery. The essential oil is a pale yellow liquid that has a spicy, pine/resinous, woody odour, with lemony top notes and a balsamic dryout (Williams 2000). The fresh, pine-like scent is conferred by the presence of its dominant constituent, α-pinene. Mertens, Buettner and Kirchoff (2009), in an extensive review of the volatile constituents, identified the main constituents common in most species, and also another complex carbon structure named verticilla-4(20),7,11-triene. So far this has not been found in any other naturally occurring resin, so it could be a 'marker' for frankincense products. Despite this, no compound has been found that is typical of frankincense odour. Olibanum absolute is more incense-like, with a less dominant pine note.

In aromatherapy, frankincense essential oil is used as a respiratory decongestant, and as an immunostimulant. Its odour is usually used to calm and uplift, and alleviate anxiety and depression. This aligns with the views of both Avicenna, who used frankincense to 'strengthen the wit and understanding', and the herbalist Culpeper,[2] who suggested that it helped with depression, poor memory and strengthening the nerves (Lawless 2009). Holmes (1998/1999) observed that frankincense encompasses four main categories of scent – spicy, sweet, woody and green. There is, therefore, an inherent polarity, because the spicy element imparts an uplifting and clarifying effect, while the sweet, woody and green aspects exert a calming, grounding and balancing effect. Therefore the scent of frankincense creates a dynamic balance, but the net balancing effect is provided by the sweet and green notes.

Holmes (1998/1999) also described frankincense as 'the rainbow bridge' – 'the olfactory link that binds the long history of the West into a single tapestry' (p.156). Just as frankincense was important in perfumery in ancient times, it now plays a role in modern perfumery, as a fixative and in base accords, where it is diffusive rather than heavy. It is present in numerous fragrances, especially orientals and florals, including *Chanel No.5*. When reading modern perfume descriptions, it is often referred to as 'incense' – and a few fragrances have an incense theme. Czech and Speak's *Frankincense and Myrrh* does not smell like incense smoke; it is more musky and lemony. However, *Gucci pour Homme* (Gucci) features frankincense, and started a trend for masculine incense fragrances. The niche perfumer Andy Tauer created two variants – *Incense Extrême* and *Incense Rosé* – and Annick Goutal created *Encens Flamboyant*, described as 'cigarette incense' because frankincense's citrus and pine notes evoked the sense of smoking a cigarette in the woods on a cold day (Turin and Sanchez 2009).

---

2   Nicholas Culpeper studied medicine at Cambridge, but gave up and served a long apprenticeship with a London apothecary. He published *The Complete Herbal* in 1649. He considered that the works of Gerard (1597) and Parkinson (1640) were not accessible to the people as they were in Latin and included many imported herbs. *The Complete Herbal* is still in print.

Myrrh

The name 'myrrh' is derived from the Arabic word *murr*, which means 'bitter' – it has an astringent and bitter taste. Myrrh has mythical origins. In *Metamorphoses*, Ovid relates the Greek legend of Myrrha, who, as a result of a 'curse' by jealous Aphrodite, fell in love with her own father, Cinyras, the King of Cyprus. She did not realise that he was her father, and when he discovered her identity and realised the incestuous nature of their relationship, he threatened to kill her. Myrrha escaped, and Cinyras then killed himself. Myrrh was formed from her tears, hence the expression 'tears of myrrh', and she was transformed into a small tree. Myrrh is often associated with frankincense, because of their common habitat and botanical similarities. This undoubtedly led to their similar cultural uses, and consequently the many references in literature to 'frankincense and myrrh'. Along with frankincense and gold, myrrh formed part of the magis' gift to the baby Jesus. It was not as valuable as frankincense, and was symbolic of suffering and death. At the crucifixion Jesus was offered wine with myrrh – a traditional way of easing suffering and elevating consciousness – and myrrh with aloe was used to anoint his body after it was removed from the cross. This led to the practice of anointing Christian martyrs with myrrh before burial (Watt and Sellar 1996).

Myrrh has long been a dominant incense ingredient; it was present in the ancient Egyptian *kyphi* and the Hebrew holy incense. Many cultures included it in their perfumes, such as *stakte*, the simple uncompounded perfume of ancient Egypt, and several compounded therapeutic perfumes of ancient Rome such as *Mendesium*, which was also used to ease aching muscles, and *Metopion*, which was used to treat dry skin. A myrrh perfume, called *Murra*, was valued as a skin cleanser and hair tonic. Myrrh has a long association with purification – ritual anointing practices included the purification of Hebrew women prior to marriage, and it was also used to anoint corpses before burial. The fragrance was also used to purify (deodorise) the atmosphere. Theophrastus noted its fixative property and persistence. Myrrh has an important place in many traditional medical practices – usually as an analgesic or for healing the skin and treating wounds and ulcers.

Myrrh is an oleo-gum resin that exudes from small, shrubby trees of the *Commiphora* genus, which is widespread in the Arabian Peninsula and Red Sea region. (Refer to Table 3.1 on page 59 for some of these *Commiphora* species and their uses.)

Like frankincense, these trees have specialised resin ducts, and the harvesting method is similar. There are two types – *heerabol*, which forms reddish-brown, hard, roughened 'tears', and *bisabol*, which is dark yellow and forms softer tears. The oleo-gum resin can be steam-distilled to yield an essential oil with a sweet, spicy, slightly medicinal scent. It is a liquid when fresh, but becomes sticky and resin-like upon exposure to air; the aged oil becomes softer and mellower, losing the sharp medicinal element. An alcohol extract – a tincture – is also made, and this is sometimes used in oral hygiene practices and the treatment of inflammation and mouth ulcers. Myrrh essential oil is dominated by the group of constituents known as sesquiterpenols, which have anti-inflammatory effects, and a ketone known as curzerenone. The essential oil also has antiseptic qualities, and in contemporary therapeutic practice it is indicated for urinary tract infections, as a respiratory tract expectorant, for healing the skin and cleansing sores and ulcers; it is perhaps the most widely used herbal antiseptic (Lawless 1992; Bowles 2003; Price and Price 2007). Although the ancients used the resin, which also contains commiphoric acids and heerabo-myrrhols, rather than the essential oil, we can see similarities in its current usage.

Myrrh resinoid and absolute from species such as *Commiphora molmol* is produced for the perfumery industry. Myrrh's warm, spicy scent is considered to be 'at the far end of the balsamic spectrum', finding a place in oriental, woody and chypre compositions (Lawless 2009). Contemporary myrrh fragrances are Serge Lutens' *La Myrrh* (1995), which was created by Christopher Sheldrake and does not go down the predictable oriental route but is, instead, a successful resinous aldehydic; Annick Goutal's *Myrrhe Ardente*, where myrrh is dominated by a woody-amber element; and Keiko Mecheri's *Myrrhe et Merveilles*, which takes the same approach as Sheldrake, but is sweeter and amber-like (Turin and Sanchez 2009). However, myrrh does not have the importance in modern perfumery that it enjoyed in ancient times.

Opopanax

Opopanax is an oleo-gum resin from another member of the *Commiphora* genus – this time *C. erythraea*. In ancient times and in the classical world, this was in fact the main species of 'myrrh' that would have been used in incenses, unguents and perfumes. Opopanax resin was also used by the Borona women of southern Oromia in Ethiopia. They would enter sauna-like chambers to cleanse and scent their skin and hair with the smoke; it was also burned to clean and perfume clothing. The wood and bark of a subspecies, *C. erythraea* var. *glabrescens*, was widely used as incense in Somaliland (Pennacchio *et al.* 2010).

Opopanax oil has a sweet, balsamic, resinous, warm and slightly spicy scent, without the slightly medicinal character of fresh myrrh essential oil. Like myrrh, it thickens into a sticky mass upon exposure to the air. Tisserand and Balacs (1995) suggested that opopanax oil is characterised by *cis*-α-bisabolene and α-santalene – both closely related to anti-inflammatory essential oil constituents found in German chamomile and sandalwood; however, anti-inflammatory action has not been specifically related to opopanax, and the ancient cultures may inadvertently have exploited this property by including it in their medicinal perfumed unguents. Unfortunately a 1977 report on phototoxicity testing (Forbes *et al.* 1977) indicated that opopanax carried this risk, so it has not been the subject of wider investigations, nor is it used in aromatherapy. Başer *et al.* (2003) published an analysis of opopanax, or 'scented myrrh', obtained from *C. guidottii* from Ethiopia and Somalia, citing earlier studies that confirmed the presence of *cis*-α-bisabolene at 22.2 per cent, and α-santalene at 15.8 per cent, and also furanodiene. However, their analysis indicated that β-ocimene was present also, at 33 per cent. The first reported chemical composition of *C. erythraea* essential oil was in 2009, where Marcotullio *et al.* revealed that it was rich in sesquiterpenes, particularly furanosesquiterpenes at around 50 per cent.

In perfumery, opopanax is used as a fixative and to impart its smooth, slightly floral, balsamic character to base notes in oriental fragrances such as Guerlain's *Shalimar*, and it plays a minor role in the base notes of some sweet florals, including Dior's *Poison* and Lauder's *Spellbound* (Glöss 1995).

Amyris (torchwood)

Two aromatic species are commonly known as 'torchwood'. They are *Amyris balsamifera*, also known as West Indian sandalwood or balsam torchwood, and *A. elemifera*, simply called torchwood. *Amyris* species belong to the large Rutaceae family, which also contains citrus trees.

A. balsamifera is a small, bushy tree that thrives in tropical areas, especially Haiti, where it is called 'candle wood', and is used as a torch and for making furniture. The wood has a high aromatic oil content, and it is burned as incense all over Latin America (Lawless 1992; Pennacchio *et al.* 2010). An essential oil called amyris oil is obtained, and this has a mild, cedar-like scent that resembles sandalwood, but it is much less persistent. It cannot substitute sandalwood in fine perfumery, but does find a role in low-cost perfumes, and soaps (Jouhar 1991).

A. elemifera does not have a commercial value, but it does have cultural significance on the Island of Montserrat in the Caribbean, where its resin is harvested for use as incense and in voodoo ceremonies (Pennacchio *et al.* 2010).

The balsams
The true balsams

The balsams are aromatic, oleo-resinous exudates that have had a role in folk traditions and perfumes since early times. Here we will explore two of the most important ones – Peru balsam and tolu balsam.

Peru balsam

Myroxylon pereirae is a large forest tree of Central America. The entire tree is aromatic. It tree produces an oleo-gum resin when the trunk is wounded, and as this is a response to injury, it is correctly described as a pathological exudate. To encourage the production and flow of the balsam – an amber-coloured, sticky mass that resembles treacle – the wood is cut, and strips of the bark are removed. The balsam is harvested after the last rains in November and December. The crude balsam is a skin sensitiser, but an essential oil can be produced by distillation of the balsam and this is used in perfumery. Ironically, traditional uses of the balsam were to treat skin problems, including itching and wounds. It was also used for rheumatic pain and respiratory disorders. Peru balsam is still used in tropical medicines and cough syrups.

In the Amazon region the bark was powdered and burned as incense, and the seeds were burned to produce a smoke that was used in the treatment of earache (Pennacchio *et al.* 2010). The essential oil is dominated by the esters of benzoic and cinnamic acids, with small amounts of vanillin, and has a sweet, balsamic, vanilla-like scent, which has soothing qualities (Jouhar 1991; Lawless 1992).

In perfumery, Peru balsam can be found in the balsamic, ambery, sweet and warm base notes of Yves Saint Laurent's *Opium* (Glöss 1995).

Tolu balsam

The botanical source of tolu balsam resinoid and oil is a tall tree native to Central and South America – *Myroxylon toluiferum*. The balsam is harvested in the same way as Peru balsam, except that the trees are 'bled' for eight months of the year. The exudate becomes hard and brittle as it dries out (Jouhar 1991). Like Peru balsam, it has traditional uses in the treatment of respiratory and skin problems, including damaged skin. The resin of a related species, Brazilian balsam (*M. peruiferum*), is used in Bolivia, where the resin is burned and the smoke inhaled to treat *susto*, 'fright illness' (the reaction provoked by a shock). Again, this is suggestive of comforting, reassuring odour effects. A resinoid and absolute are produced by solvent extraction and an essential oil by distillation. Like Peru balsam, tolu balsam is dominated by the esters of benzoic and cinnamic acids, with the presence of vanillin. It has a warm, balsamic odour, which Jouhar (1991) suggests is reminiscent of hyacinth. In perfumery it is used as a fixative and in heavy, spicy orientals and florals such as Lauder's *Youth Dew* and *Cinnabar*, where it imparts warm, balsamic base notes, and Guerlain's *Vol de Nuit* (Glöss 1995).

Other balsamic aromatics

Several other species yield aromatic products that are described as having 'balsamic' odours. Here we will look at the versatile labdanum, with reference to its role in imparting the character of the unique ambergris in perfumery, the sweet balsamic scents of poplar bud, benzoin and vanilla, and then cocoa and tonka bean.

Labdanum

Labdanum (also called rockrose) is mentioned in the writings of all the ancient cultures. Lawless (1994) tells us that it was an ingredient (*onycha*) in the holy incense of Moses, that it was widely used by the Egyptians as incense an in cosmetics, and that it was probably sacred to Aphrodite and burned at her altars on Cyprus, her mythical birthplace. Dioscorides mentions labdanum among the ingredients of the 'Royal Unguent', as does Pliny in *Natural History* (see footnote 4 on page 103). Labdanum remains an important raw material of perfumery, not least because it can impart long-lasting balsamic and 'ambergris' elements to a composition.

Labdanum is obtained from *Cistus ladaniferus* and *C. creticus*, perennial shrubs belonging to the Cistaceae family ('rockrose'), which are widely distributed in the rocky regions of southern France, Spain, Portugal and North Africa, and also on the islands of Corsica, Crete and Cyprus. *Cistus* secretes an oleo-gum resin from glandular hairs, which are specialised structures on the leaf surface, and this coats the leaves and stems. Lawless (2009) tells us that Herodotus, in the fifth century BCE, observed Arabs combing the resin from the beards of goats that had been browsing among the bushes; Herodotus also regarded labdanum as one of the principal perfume ingredients from Arabia. In Crete and Cyprus, the oleo-gum resin is collected with a *ladanisterion* – an instrument resembling a double rake, with leather thongs instead of teeth. This is used like a whip, and the resin is scraped off the thongs when they are fully charged (Jouhar 1991). Several products can be obtained from the oleo-gum resin – cistus resinoid, concrete and absolute via solvent extraction, labdanum gum or oleo-resin by boiling the plant in alkaline water, and labdanum essential oil via steam distillation of the gum.

Some traditional medical uses of the gum were for the treatment of catarrh, diarrhoea and dysentery, and to promote menstruation; it was also used externally in plasters (Lawless 1992). However, it is undoubtedly its scent that is responsible for its place in aromatic history and modern perfumery. It has a complex odour, usually described as rich, sweet, slightly herbaceous-balsamic (Lawless 1992); or powerful, sweet, and recalling ambergris (Jouhar 1991); or as having a sweet, rich, balsamic amber character with warm, dry, woody back notes (Lawless 1994). Williams (1996) wrote that cistus oil has powerful, warm, ambra-like top notes, and the body is rich, warm, ambra and balsamic, with a dry, balsamic dryout. He described labdanum resinoid as lacking a top note, with a sweet, balsamic, herbaceous, ambra body and a dry, woody, ambra dryout. The term '*ambra*' means ambergris-like – a scent that is difficult to define but is complex, rich, musty, musky, earthy and ambery, and reminiscent of the sea. Ambergris is a unique aromatic, derived from the pathological secretion of the sperm whale, and thus falls outside the scope of this book, but, given its importance, a profile can be found in Appendix B.

The chemical composition of labdanum has been the focus of several investigations since 1912, when two compounds were identified – acetopheneone and 2,2,6-trimethyl-cyclohexanone. Ohloff (1994) suggested that labdanum oil contained around 250 compounds, 75 of which had been identified, including 25 phenols, 9 lactones and 8 acids. Weyerstahl *et al.* (1998) attempted to assign labdanum's odour characteristics to some of the constituents. Dihydroambrinol contributes a powerful woody-amber, with an ambrinol-like nuance, while α-ambrinol is strong, amber and woody, having an exceptionally strong odour of damp earth with a crude civet subnote, which on high dilution gives a warm animal amber scent. Drimenone is described as powerful tobacco and amber, and various other components give soft, warm, woody amber notes, sometimes with animalic or resinous variations. Weyerstahl *et al.* (1998) also reported the isolation of another ketone – 6,6,10-trimethyldecal-2-one – which they describe as 'strong woody – dominant tonality – with a distinct note of damp earth, cellar, geosmin'.

The scent of labdanum has a place in aromatherapy as an uplifting, comforting, soothing agent. Lawless (1994) quotes Fischer-Rizzi (1990) who suggested that:

> Its essential oil conveys a warmth that deeply affects the soul. Rock rose is favoured for treating patients who feel, usually after a traumatic event, cold, empty or numb... Rock rose incense aids meditation and centring as well as visualising spiritual experiences and bringing them to consciousness. (p.159)

Labdanum is an important element in the classic chypre accord. Calkin and Jellinek (1994) mention its presence in the original formulae of *Femme* (Rochas 1942), *Ma Griffe* (created by Jean Carles for Carven in 1945), and *Miss Dior* (1947). Williams (1995c) stresses its value as a good fixative, blender and sweetening agent for chypre, fougère, modern *eaux de cologne* and masculine fragrances. Turin and Sanchez (2009) mention two fragrances where labdanum is a prominent raw material: Le Labo's *Labdanum 18* created by Maurice Roucel (describing it as a pleasant 'hippie amber'), and the green resinous *Mystra* (Aesop) where it forms an accord with frankincense and mastic.

Poplar bud

Populus balsamifera is the balsam poplar. It has sticky, resinous, aromatic buds and its bark contains salicylin, a glycoside that is the precursor of salicylic acid, or aspirin (Mills and Bone 2000); both the bark and the buds have a long tradition of use in North America and Alaska. The bark is used in Native American folk medicine as an analgesic, anti-inflammatory and febrifuge. Its smoke is used by the Inuktitut Eskimo to repel mosquitoes, and the leaf galls are smoked for pleasure, with or without tobacco. The Dena'ina and the Montana use the wood for smoking fish, and the Montana also use the inner bark in *kinni-kinnick* mixtures. In Alaska the dried, rotten wood was used to smoke animal skins, and the Shuswap of North America used the inner bark for this purpose (Pennacchio *et al.* 2010). The resin from the sticky buds was used as a salve, and it is also used in contemporary herbal medicine as an expectorant.

Poplar bud absolute is an opaque, golden, viscous substance, with a tenacious, sweet, cinnamon-like, balsamic odour, with resinous and coumarinic undertones (McMahon 2011a). Research has also demonstrated that poplar bud absolute showed strong inhibitory activity against an enzyme that is present in the skin, human leukocyte elastase (HLE), *in vitro* (Baylac and Racine 2004). This enzyme is important in the pathophysiology of inflammation, and is involved in the degradation of the matrix proteins collagen and elastin. UV exposure will stimulate HLE activity, hence the ultimate visible effect of sun damage to the skin, including wrinkles and loss of elasticity. Poplar bud is used to a limited extent in aromatherapy as an anti-inflammatory, but does not appear to be used in phytocosmeceuticals or perfumery, despite its very pleasant odour profile and therapeutic potential.

Benzoin

The family Styracaceae is composed of small trees and shrubs that are native to tropical and subtropical regions. The shrubs and trees in the genus *Styrax* produce aromatic resins or gums in response to injury. Benzoin gum, sometimes called gum benjamin, is a balsamic resin obtained from *Styrax* species. In Mexico, 'silver styrax' from *S. argentum* is burned for its aromatic smoke, as are *S. benzoin* in Java, *S. ferrugineum* in Brazil and Paraguay, and *S. ovatus* and other species in the Americas. It is thought that some of the fumes of *Styrax* species, such as those of *S. tessmannii* of the Americas, may be psychoactive (Pennacchio *et al.* 2010). *S. officinalis* is a deciduous shrub found only in the Mediterranean region, although for some time it was believed that it also grew in California, but this is now recognised as a distinct species. Its resin, known as 'storax', was used in traditional medicine in the Mediterranean basin as an antiseptic and for the treatment of respiratory diseases. In Cyprus, where it was known as *steratzia*, it was burned for its scented smoke (Tayoub *et al.* 2006; Pennacchio *et al.* 2011).

The name 'benzoin' is derived from the Arabic *luban jawi* (meaning 'incense of Java'), which was corrupted to '*banjawi*' and eventually 'benzoin' and 'benjamin'. In ancient times the gum was an important incense; in India benzoin was offered to the Trimurti, and in Malaysia benzoin was used generally to repel evil, and specifically at the rice harvest ceremony (Morris 1984). Benzoin, along with agarwood, sandalwood and patchouli, is burned by Muslim women in religious ceremonies; when burned at the feet of the deceased its scent was thought to raise the soul to heaven. The Greeks and Romans used the resin not only as incense, but also in perfumes and cosmetics, and in later times benzoin resin was powdered and used in pomanders – it is said that Elizabeth I of England carried a pomander of benzoin and ambergris (Lawless 1994).

Benzoin resin is a pathological exudate; that is, only trees that have sustained damage to the cambium will form resin ducts that produce and secrete the resin. The main botanical sources are *Styrax benzoin*, *S. paralleloneuris* and *S. tonkinensis*. These are tall, rapidly maturing, birch-like trees native to tropical Asia. When trees are around seven years old, the trunk is hacked, usually with an axe; the liquid resin collects just under the bark, and exudes from the cuts. It is believed that the finest benzoin is produced in the first three years, after that the resin is known as 'the belly', and eventually the tree is felled and the final yield scraped out, and this is called 'the foot'.

Two types of product are available, depending on the geographical and botanical origins. Siam benzoin gum originates from *S. tonkinensis* in Laos, Vietnam, Cambodia, China and Thailand, while Sumatra benzoin gum is from *S. benzoin* and sometimes *S. paralleloneuris* in Sumatra, Java and Malaysia. Although they are both aromatic resins from closely related species, the two products appear and smell distinct. Siam benzoin occurs in brittle 'tears' that are yellow or reddish-brown on the exterior and white inside, while Sumatra benzoin is a milky, resinous sap which hardens into a dull red or grey-brown resin before it is scraped off the bark. This is formed into rectangular blocks, which break into 'almond'-shaped pieces. Siam benzoin resin has a sweet, balsamic, vanilla and chocolate-like scent, and Sumatra benzoin resin is warm, sweet and powdery – more styrax-like (see below) than vanilla-like (Jouhar 1991; Lawless 1992; Fernandez *et al.* 2006).

The name benzoin relates to the resin, while benzoin extract is a further extraction of the resin, and it is these extracts that are used in perfumery and aromatherapy. Benzoin resinoids are brown, thick and sticky, and chemically are dominated by aromatic esters and acids. Siam benzoin resinoid is dominated by coniferyl benzoate, and also vanillin, hence its characteristic odour. Sumatra benzoin contains coniferyl cinnamate and traces of vanillin (Jouhar 1991; Lawless 1992). Grieve (1992) notes that Siam resin contains up to 38 per cent benzoic acid, and that Sumatra resin has nearer 50 per cent benzoic acid, and also about 20 per cent of cinnamic acid, which is absent in the Siam variety.

Benzoin has a well-established tradition of medicinal use. Grieve (1992) comments that it was used externally in tincture form to sooth irritated skin, as it has stimulant and antiseptic properties. When taken internally it acts as a carminative, expectorant diuretic and urinary antiseptic. The compound 'tincture of benzoin' can be inhaled with steam to alleviate laryngitis and bronchitis. It is also present in pharmaceutical preparations for the gums and skin, as a component of tinctures to aid the respiratory system. Like poplar bud, it was investigated for ability to inhibit HLE; it was found to be a good inhibitor, and so has anti-inflammatory potential. This type of study helps to support benzoin's traditional uses. Benzoin resinoid is also used in aromatherapy, primarily used for its calming, comforting scent. Marguerite Maury (1989), a pioneer of holistic aromatherapy, commented that 'this essence creates a kind of euphoria; it interposes a padded zone between us and events' (p.96). Very often the scent of benzoin can aid sleep. It is sometimes used for skin problems and respiratory problems (Lawless 1994), but with care, as it does have a reputation as a skin sensitiser.

In perfumery Sumatra benzoin is a useful fixative that is often added to soaps and detergents – it is more robust that the Siam type. It is also used as a tobacco flavour (Fernandez *et al.* 2006). An alcoholic extraction of the Siam type, which is known as 'benzoin resinodour', is preferred in fine perfumery; it is said that this can give 'body' to almost any perfume (Jouhar 1991). Williams (1995c) commented that if certain resinoids such as benzoin are used to excess in a fragrance, they will seriously suppress it, and Lawless (2009) concurred, suggesting that it is a useful fixative in light floral compositions, if used sparingly. The classic floral aldehydic fragrance *Chamade* (Guerlain 1969) contains a benzoin accord in the base notes; here it is combined with vetiver, sandalwood, tolu balsam, vanilla and Peru balsam (Glöss 1995). Benzoin is also notable in an amber accord with patchouli, vetiver and rose in Histoire de Parfums' *Ambre 411* (Turin and Sanchez 2009).

Styrax, storax and sweetgum

In the past there has been much confusion regarding 'styrax' and indeed 'storax', common names which have also been used to refer to the balsamic resinoids obtained from *Liquidambar orientalis* and *L. styraciflua* – trees of the family Hamamelidaceae, native to Asia Minor, Honduras and Guatemala. Their exudates are sometimes called sweetgum. In Cyprus the wood, known as *xylon tau Aphenti* ('wood of the Lord'), was burned in a significant religious rite. The resin was also burned in the Americas; the Aztecs used it as incense and also mixed with tobacco, and later the American tobacco industry used it to flavour cigarettes (Pennacchio *et al.* 2010). Styrax gum is not used in perfumery because it is a skin sensitiser; however, the products obtained by alcohol extraction or steam distillation can be used as fixatives. They have pleasant balsamic scents with hyacinth-like characteristics. Styrax is useful in hyacinth and lilac accords (Jouhar 1991; Williams 1995c).

Vanilla

The Aztecs of Mexico used vanilla – the dried bean of *Vanilla planifolia* – to flavour *chocolatle*. According to Morris (1984), 'vanilla', the name originally used by the Spanish conquistadors, is derived from *vaina*, meaning 'bean'. Although it is native to Mexico, vanilla is now grown in other regions specifically for the flavour and fragrance industry, and there are three species that yield vanilla: *Vanilla planifolia*, the original Aztec species, yields Bourbon or Réunion vanilla, which is considered to be of the best quality; Tahiti vanilla is from *V. tahitensis* and West Indian vanilla is from *V. pompona*.

Vanilla is a member of the Orchidaceae, the orchid family. It is a perennial, herbaceous vine, with an epiphytic habit – sometimes described as an 'air plant'. It has dark green, tough leaves, and produces pale green-yellow or white flowers that occur in large racemes of 20 or more blossoms. In its native Mexico, the flowers are pollinated by hummingbirds and *Melipona* bees; however, the plants that were transported to Réunion need to be hand-pollinated. This has become the preferred method of pollination now, even in Mexico. After fertilisation the flowers produce fruits. The long, green, slender, capsule-like fruits, known as pods, are harvested while immature. They are filled with an oily mass containing numerous small, black, shiny seeds. The pods are cured over a period of six months, and treated by solvent extraction to yield a resinoid and absolute, or sometimes by percolation in an aqueous alcohol solution. Vanilla has therapeutic uses; medicinal preparations are said to be tonic, cephalic, diuretic, decongestant, a blood purifier, a digestive aid, and stimulant of childbirth (Hossain 2011).

Vanilla absolute is a brown viscous liquid with the characteristic sweet, rich, deep, balsamic odour of vanilla. It is chemically very complex. Vanillin, a phenolic aldehyde, is present at around 2 per cent (Jouhar 1991), and other constituents include hydroxybenzaldehyde, acetic acid, *iso*-butyric acid, caproic acid, eugenol and furfural (Klimes and Lamparsky 1976; Lawless 1992).

Vanillin was first isolated by Gobley in 1858, but its chemical structure was not confirmed until 1870, by Carles. Vanillin itself is not found in the fresh beans – it is formed from the precursor glucovanillin, found in the interior of the bean, during the curing process. Because of the scarcity of natural vanilla, vanillin is now synthesised using lignin from wood as a starting point, or from petrochemical sources. Natural vanillin, isolated from vanilla pods, costs in the region of US$2000–3000 (Hossain 2011).

Many derivatives of vanillin have its characteristic odour, and these are found in, for example, wines aged in French oak barrels. The esters ethyl vanillate and iso-amyl vanillate, along with phenolic compounds, contribute to the vanilla aroma in such wines (Kaiser 2006).

Vanilla is a familiar and widely used food flavour, and it also finds applications in perfumery, where it has good tenacity and adds richness and sweetness to heavy floral, floral/woody and oriental scents. However, as synthetic vanillin is much cheaper and readily available, this is what will be found in many fragrances.

The early versions of synthetic vanillin were sweeter and creamier than natural vanilla.

Turin and Sanchez (2009) relate the role of vanillin in two Guerlain fragrances (*Jicky* and *Shalimar*), and this illustrates its impact in perfumery.

Jicky, first launched in 1889, is one of the oldest perfumes in continuous existence. Its creator, Aimé Guerlain, used a combination of natural and synthetic vanillin with lavender essential oil, citrus, herbs and civet. The synthetic vanillin contained traces of impurities – smoky-scented phenols – and in modern *Jicky*, rectified birch tar is now added to retain that specific effect. At the time, other perfumers such as Ernest Beaux were challenged by the use of vanillin, which could confer an undesirable *crème anglaise* effect. It could be said that *Jicky* is the ancestor of *Shalimar* – the sweet, vanilla/amber oriental with citrus top notes, which retains *Jicky's* woody, smoky, animalic nature.

Several more recent perfumes are characterised by vanilla. L'Artisan Parfumeur's *Vanilia* (1978) is described as a 'candyfloss vanilla' by Turin and Sanchez (2009), the vanilla being combined with ethylmaltol to give the candyfloss characteristic – possibly one of the effects that Ernest Beaux was trying to avoid! A more sophisticated use of genuine vanilla absolute can be seen in Hermès' *Vanille Galante*, where it is used with ylang ylang and jasmine. Vanilla also figures in the classic 'ambreine' accord, which is widely used in oriental ambery fragrances including *Shalimar*, and also in *Must de Cartier* (Cartier 1981) and *Obsession* (Calvin Klein 1985). The ambreine accord is formed between bergamot, vanillin (or ethyl vanillin), coumarin and civet, with woody and rose notes (Calkin and Jellinek 1994).

Possibly vanilla's contribution to chocolate is more memorable and accessible to many – but cacao, the core ingredient of chocolate, also has a role in ritual, medicine, perfumery and skin care.

Cacao

The botanical source of cacao is a tree, *Theobroma cacao*, native to the Americas. The tree reaches four to five metres in height; its wood is light and the bark brown. It bears bright green leaves and small, reddish flowers which produce smooth, flesh-coloured pods with a white pulp. When the seeds (known as 'beans') within are ripe, they rattle when the capsule is shaken. Each pod contains around 25 seeds, and although the entire tree has value, it is the seeds that are used as 'cacao'. When cacao is cultivated, the trees are grown in the shade of other trees, such as the banana, and the pods are produced continuously. When ripe, the pods are slit open, and then allowed to ferment slightly before being dried for use (Grieve 1992).

Cacao has a long tradition of use in both Mesoamerica and South America. The name originated in the Olmec vocabulary, where it was called *kakaw*. The Mayans developed a detailed *cacao* vocabulary, and in the Aztec language it is known as *cacahuatl*. Traditional knowledge of cacao was passed down in many ways, oral tradition, stonework and codices. Mayan myth tells us that the god known as Sovereign Plumed Serpent gave cacao to humans after they were created from maize. It is clear that, from the very beginning, cacao was highly valued. The cacao god, Ek Chua, had an annual festival held in his honour. Cacao was made into a beverage, and its intoxicating nature was discovered early on. For this reason, it was only consumed by adult men who held important positions, such as priests, those in government and the military; but it was also offered at sacrifice mixed with the priests' blood. At the festival of Huitzilopochtli, the god of war and the sun, cacao beverage was given to the sacrificial victims – allegedly to bring 'comfort'. High doses of green cacao beverage made from fermented cacao seeds would produce a drunken, dizzy state, but moderate consumption was 'refreshing and invigorating' (Sharer 1994; Batchelder 2004). The smoke of burning cacao beans was also used in Panama. According to Pennacchio *et al.* (2010), during female puberty rites, two burning cacao beans were placed on the ground, and the participants would inhale the smoke. The Cuna of Panama would also burn cacao beans with red peppers to treat malaria, and in Aligandi the smoke was used to drive away evil spirits.

Knowledge of cacao reached Europe via Christopher Columbus, who observed that cacao seeds were used as currency (circa 1502), and Hernando Cortéz was offered cacao beverage and a chocolate feast at Montezuma's court. It is said that Montezuma (or Moctezuma) consumed nothing else. The Spanish conquistadors introduced cacao to the Spanish court, where it rapidly became a popular luxury. According to the Florentine Codex (1590), which was compiled by the priest Bernardino de Sahagún, the Mexican culture used chocolate on its own or in combination with other botanicals, such as vanilla, to treat a wide variety of ailments, from digestive complaints to fever, shortness of breath, faintness of heart and fatigue. A compound medicine known as *atextli*, made with cacao, maize, *mecaxochitl* (*Piper sanctum*) and *tlilxochitl* (vanilla) was formed into a paste to excite the 'venereal appetite' – this is the first mention of cacao's aphrodisiac effects.

Along with coffee, tea and sugar, cacao was seen as a highly desirable, mood-altering, exotic novelty, and trade routes between the New World and Europe opened up for these new commodities. The French established cacao plantations in the Caribbean, and the Spanish in the Philippines. In 1753 the naturalist and taxonomist Linnaeus gave it the Latinised name *Theobroma cacao*; 'theobroma' means 'food of the gods'. Very soon cacao found its way into the European pharmacopeia, where it was used for weight gain, poor appetite, and to stimulate the nervous system, amongst other uses. Cacao oil or 'butter' was used, along with its flowers, leaves and bark, to treat burns, cuts and skin complaints; this remains an important ingredient in phytocosmeceuticals. Linnaeus noted that chocolate helped wasting due to lung and muscle diseases, hypochondria and haemorrhoids, and that it was an aphrodisiac, while others noted that it was capable of 'repairing the losses due to work, pleasures and staying up late at night' (Batchelder 2004, p.106). It is interesting that cacao was originally valued as a pharmaceutical. However, it was the use of chocolate as a vehicle and binder for bitter medicines that was the original inspiration for the thriving chocolate confectionery industry. Only later, thanks to its agreeable taste (not to mention its psychoactive and aphrodisiac properties), did it come into favour in the West as the popular beverage and food we know (and often crave) today. In 1842 cacao was found to contain theobromine, a unique psychoactive compound (Jay 2010), which certainly explains its psychotropic effects. The aphrodisiac effects of chocolate are possibly due to the presence of phenylethylamine and N-acylethanolamines, which are pharmacologically active compounds (Salonia *et al.* 2006, cited in Melnyk and Marcone 2011). Afoakawa (2008) reported that phenylethylamine could induce pleasurable sensations and affect serotonin and endorphin levels in the brain, as well as raising blood pressure and heart rate, and heighten sensations. This in turn can improve mood and increase sexual desire. N-acylethanolamines might also activate cannabinoid receptors, or increase endocannabinoid levels, thus increasing sensitivity.

It is, however, good to know that the traditional uses of chocolate continue to thrive in many Mesoamerican and Colonial communities, and that it remains a principal food in Oaxaca. Its oils are used to treat bronchitis, as an antidote to scorpion, bee or wasp stings, and to treat *espanto*, an illness of fright. This is done by feeding the earth at the location of the fright with cacao.

According to Grieve (1992), the seeds contain 2 per cent theobromine and 40–60 per cent solid fat; the shells also contain theobromine at 1 per cent. Theobromine is a xanthine alkaloid related to caffeine, and resembles caffeine in its actions. However, theobromine has less impact on the central nervous system and more pronounced effects on the muscles, kidneys and heart. It has a diuretic effect, useful especially if there is fluid accumulation due to cardiac failure. Theobromine can also dilate blood vessels and can be used to treat high blood pressure.

So it could be argued that cacao is one of the most important botanicals from the perspective of human wellbeing. Despite this, it is less well known as an aromatic and fragrance. A dark brown absolute can be obtained by solvent extraction of the seeds; it has a rich, warm, balsamic scent that is certainly reminiscent of chocolate, but minus the vanilla. It has fixative properties, and is used in base accords; Lawless (2009) suggests that it imparts 'edible' (gourmand), exotic effects. He uses it along with tobacco and vanilla absolutes to add intrigue and depth to his *Kuan Yin* fragrance, which is constructed around the scent of osmanthus. Cacao finds a role in gourmand fragrances such as the mainstream *Blue Agava and Cacao* (Jo Malone) and the niche natural fragrance *Cacao* (Aftelier), where it is paired with citrus and orange accords. A chocolate and rose accord can be found in the niche S-Perfume's *100% Love*. Turin and Sanchez (2009) describe Serge Lutens' *Borneo 1834* as 'virtual chocolate'; this fragrance has an oriental structure, with a 'skilful juxtaposition' of patchouli and chocolate. Cacao plays a role in several masculine fragrances too, such as *Dior Homme Intense*, which also has spiced apple notes.

Tonka bean

Tonka bean (or tonquin bean) is obtained from *Dipteryx odorata* of the Leguminosae family. It is a forest tree native to Brazil and British Guiana, where it is known as *rumara*. Tonka beans have a characteristic odour of coumarin, which is soft, smooth, sweet and reminiscent of coconut and hay. This compound also occurs in sweet clover (*Melilotus* species; see Chapter 9), and related grasses. In traditional medicine, tonka bean was used as a cardiac tonic and narcotic. A fluid extract was used to treat whooping cough, 'but it paralyses the heart if used in large doses' (Grieve 1992, p.819). The fatty portion of the seeds is known as 'tonquin butter'.

Tonka bean is an important aromatic in perfumery. Trees for tonka bean production are cultivated in Africa, eastern Venezuela and South America. Two distinct species are grown: *D. odorata* for its 'angostura beans' and *D. oppositifolia* for the smaller and less valuable 'para' beans. The beans contain about 3 per cent coumarin. The pods are harvested, and the beans are removed and dried. They can be immersed in rum, placed in casks and covered in strong alcohol for 24 hours before being air-dried. This process causes them to shrink, and crystals of coumarin cover the exterior. The dried tonka beans can be solvent-extracted to yield a concrete and absolute. Tonka bean can be used to flavour pipe tobacco, but its main use is now in perfumery, although it has largely been replaced by synthetic coumarins (Jouhar 1991).

The absolute is dominated by coumarin. According to Williams (1996), its top notes are rich, sweet, warm and herbaceous; the body is also warm and sweet, with hay-like notes, and the dryout is hay-like and coconut-like. Lawless (2009) classes it as a balsamic odour, but it is certainly not typical of the genre. Its hay-like nature could also place tonka bean in the agrestic category. Lawless also comments that it has both vanilla and herbaceous characteristics and is delicate and subtle. Jouhar (1991), however, describes its odour as 'pleasant and herbaceous with slight caramel and coumarin undertones' (p.330). It seems that it is classed as a balsamic because of the rich, sweet and warm characteristics, reminiscent of both caramel and vanilla, at the expense of the coumarin hay-like facet of the odour which could place it in the agrestic class. As well as imparting a sweet, powdery accord to fragrances, tonka bean is also used as a fixative, and it can be found in the base notes of many fragrances. Calkin and Jellinek (1994) describe its role in the classic *Madame Rochas* (1960), a floral aldehydic fragrance, where it is used along with natural vanilla to complement the rose, jasmine and tuberose accords. Tonka bean is also important in the fougère category, where it typically forms an accord with lavender and oakmoss. Tonka bean can be found in numerous masculine fougère fragrances, including Calvin Klein's *Calvin* and Yves Saint Laurent's *Jazz* (Glöss 1995). Tonka bean is often paired with vanilla, where it can give a coconut-like drydown; this effect can be found in Serge Lutens' *Un Bois Vanille*. Tonka bean is also in the base notes of Dior's *Fahrenheit*, along with amber and leather accords. Hence it is a versatile aromatic that plays a subtle part across a wide range of fragrances. See also Appendix A.

Some woods produce resins that have balsamic scents; however, the woody tissues and leaves of conifers contain resins and oils with a very different and distinctive type of scent which has been favoured by many diverse cultures, such as the ancient Egyptians and Greeks and the Native Indians of the Pacific Northwest.

Conifers

Three hundred million years ago, the first aromatic plants appeared on the planet. These were the coniferous trees. These trees generally grow at high altitude in northern latitudes, most showing a pyramidal growth pattern, with simple leaves, needles or scales. Most are evergreen and they all produce cones which contain the seed. The conifers are widely distributed, resilient, and able to survive in cold climates. Some of the conifers have a lifespan in excess of 1000 years. The Pinaceae and Cupressaceae families include several essential oil bearing species, including sequoias (redwoods), spruces, pines, thuja, cypresses, Chamaecyparis, cedars and junipers.

In conifers, the aromatic oils are produced in *schizogenous* glands. These are enlarged intercellular spaces known as *lumina* and *lacuna*, enclosed by intact cells that have separated during development, and lined with specialised secretory cells. These cavities join up to form ducts known as resin canals, which can reach ten centimetres in length, and each needle-like leaf can have up to seven ducts. Ancient literature makes many references to these species, but the earliest references to coniferous trees mention cedars.

Lebanese, Atlas and Himalayan cedars

These are the true cedars from the genus *Cedrus* of the Pinaceae family – many other species that are referred to as 'cedars' belong to other genera and a different botanical family.

Lebanese cedar

Cedrus libani is the Lebanese cedar; it also grows wild on Cyprus. The cedar of Lebanon was valued as incense by the Mesopotamians; it was brought to the cities of the Tigris and Euphrates Valley from the forests of Marduk in Lebanon. It could be argued that the oil from the Lebanese cedar was one of the earliest aromatics used by mankind. The wood was also used to build palaces like that of Sargon II at Khorsabad (722–705 BCE), and Solomon imported it to build his temple in Jerusalem. In 586 BCE, the original temple was destroyed and the peoples deported to Babylon, where another temple was built, again using the cedar of Lebanon. It was restored, yet again, with Lebanese cedar in 20 BCE (Morris 1984). Lawless (1994) notes that Solomon's chariot was also made of this wood. Apart from being suitable for construction, the main appeal of this cedar was because of its high proportion of volatile oil, which imparted long-lasting fragrance and rendered the wood resistant to decay and infestation. In ancient Egypt cedar wood was used to construct temple doors and build ships, and cedar oil was used in mummification, medicines (including the well-known and widely used antidote to poison known as *mithridat*) and perfumes. The Epic of Gilgamesh, written in 12 BCE, but referring to 28–27 BCE, describes how Utnapishti, the father of all men, burned cedar and myrrh to give thanks for his rescue from the Flood (Kaiser 2006). The Lebanese cedar came to symbolise fertility and abundance, and also spiritual strength – the name 'cedar' is derived from the Arabic word *kedron* which means 'power'.

Many other cultures valued the ability of cedar to preserve. Ancient Greek and Roman manuscripts mention the preservation of books with its oil, the storage of valuable documents in cedar chests, and its ability to prevent putrefaction of dead bodies, calling it 'the life of him that is dead' (Lawless 1994). According to Avicenna, in Iran, the smoke of the wood was used to induce abortions, and elsewhere it was mixed with other herbs and resins and burned as incense (Pennacchio *et al.* 2010).

The essential oil of the cedar of Lebanon is no longer available, but its close relative, the Atlas cedar, produces an essential oil.

Atlas cedar

The Atlas cedar, *C. atlantica*, is a tall evergreen tree with a highly aromatic, hard wood. It is native to the Atlas Mountains of Algeria. Most Atlas cedarwood essential oil is from Morocco, extracted from the woodchips and sawdust left over from wood used for construction and furniture. Atlas cedar oil has a woody, warm, slightly camphoraceous odour. Burfield (2002), in a review of cedar oils, suspects that many of the 'cedar' oils sold to aromatherapists are not genuine, and are probably adulterated with the cheaper and readily available Chinese cedar *Cupressus funebris*.

Burfield (2002) states that the sesquiterpenes α-, β- and γ-himalchenes constitute almost 70 per cent of the oil; other components include α- and γ-atlantone isomers at 10–15 per cent. These have sweet woody odours (especially the *d*-α-atlantone) that make a significant contribution to the odour profile. Because of its camphoraceous element, Atlas cedar is not widely used in fine perfumery, but it does have therapeutic uses. In traditional medicine in the East, and in Tibetan medicine, it was used to treat bronchial and urinary tract infections. In contemporary aromatherapy practice it is used as an antiseptic for skin problems and for the urinary tract, as a mucolytic for the respiratory system and as an antipruritic when combined with bergamot (Price and Price 2007). Holmes (2001) suggests that the scent, which is sweeter and woodier than the other conifers, can help ground and calm the mind.

Himalayan cedar

The Himalayan cedar, *Cedrus deodara*, is also closely related to the Lebanese cedar. This tree grows on the Himalayan slopes of northern India, Afghanistan and Pakistan. In India it is used for external structures such as railway sleepers, and, like the cedar of Lebanon, it has now been over-exploited. Himalayan cedar oil is used in Ayurvedic medicine for intestinal worms, and the treatment of ulcers and skin diseases. The leaves and twigs were also dried in the sun and soaked in ghee (clarified butter) and then smoked to relieve asthma (Pennacchio *et al.* 2010). Burfield (2002) describes its essential oil as having a 'dirty', slightly crude note, woody and also with sweet, resinous and urinous notes; rectified oils which have a more pleasant odour are used in aromatherapy.

Burfield considers that the aromatherapeutic uses of Atlas and Himalayan cedarwood oils, based on their sesquiterpene and sesquiterpene derivatives, are broadly confirmed by a few studies. For example, himachalol and other sesquiterpenes from *C. deodara* were shown to have spasmolytic activity (Kar *et al.* 1975; Patnaik *et al.* 1977, cited in Burfield 2002), and *C. deodara* was also shown to have analgesic and anti-inflammatory activity in animal studies (Schinde *et al.* 1999a, 1999b, cited in Burfield 2002). Baylac and Racine (2003) confirmed that it might have anti-inflammatory activity, as it was an inhibitor of the enzyme 5-lipoxyoxygenase, which is involved in the production of inflammatory agents. Like Atlas cedar oil, Himalayan cedar is probably more valued for its therapeutic potential than for its scent. It is not used in fine perfumery; however, it is used in soap perfumes, and perfumes for household cleaning products (Williams 1995c).

Yellow, incense and Virginian cedars

There are several other 'cedar' oils that have played significant roles in various cultures. These belong to the Cupressaceae family and include the yellow cedar, incense cedar and Virginian cedar.

Yellow cedar

The yellow cedar is *Thuja occidentalis*, also called *arbor vitae*, the 'tree of life'. This is one of the tallest conifers, reaching up to 20 metres in height, and it belongs to the Cupressaceae – the cypress family. Thuja is native to the northeast of North America, but there are many other closely related cultivated varieties that are widespread. These include *T. plicata*, the western red cedar or Washington cedar, *T. orientalis*, the Chinese or Japanese cedar or 'oriental *arbor vitae*', and *T. articulata*, the North African cedar. The name 'thuja' is a Latin derivation from a Greek word that means 'to fumigate', and *thuo*, meaning 'to sacrifice' (Grieve 1992; Lawless 1992). This gives a clue as to its ancient and traditional uses. The wood of *T. occidentalis* was burned by many cultures in Canada and North America for its fragrant smoke, but also as a purification agent, either to disinfect homes or in smudging ceremonies, when participants and sacred objects would be fumigated. *T. orientalis*, the oriental *arbor vitae*, was used in China as well as North America for incense. In North America it was used in sweat baths, and as a perfume in purification rites. Its smoke was also used to revive unconscious persons and to exorcise evil spirits (Pennacchio *et al.* 2010).

The wood of the yellow cedar is durable but also soft, finely grained and light, conferring pliability, and so it is used not only in construction of buildings but also for boats and furniture. Its branches make good besoms (brooms), which have the additional attraction of its pungent and balsamic scent. Traditional therapeutic uses of thuja made use of its astringent property, but it was also used as a diuretic and an abortifacient, because it can produce severe gastro-intestinal irritation. Tincture of thuja was also injected into venereal warts to make them 'disappear'. Its essential oil contains ketones such as fenchone and thujone, both of which are cardiac stimulants; however, the oil is highly toxic to the nervous system and produces convulsions (Grieve 1992). Thuja oil, therefore, is not used in aromatherapy. It is dominated by α-thujone at around 60 per cent, and contains around 10 per cent β-thujone. Thujone is one of the ketones that may not only cause convulsions but also inflict liver and central nervous system damage. Even small doses can result in nausea, hallucinations and coordination difficulty (Bowles 2003). Schnaubelt (1999) suggests that it can be used externally in small amounts, citing its use on warts, perhaps inspired by the practice of tincture injections for venereal warts; however, he does comment that there is insufficient evidence to support this practice. Grieve (1992) suggests that *T. orientalis* has the same properties, but that its wood yields a yellow dye, and that it is resistant to humidity. *T. articulata*, the North African cedar, produces a resin known locally as *sandarac*. This was used therapeutically in the form of ointments and plasters, and in India to treat haemorrhoids and diarrhoea. In tincture form it treated 'low spirits'. Thuja oils do not have a role in perfumery, mainly because of their toxicity, but also because, although the trees have a wonderful scent in their natural state, their oils are very pungent and camphor-like.

Incense cedar

Calocedrus decurrens (also known as *Libocedrus decurrens*) is the incense cedar. It is native to Oregon and California, and it is often referred to as the Californian incense cedar. It is a tall tree, sometimes reaching 60 metres in height, and is drought tolerant. Its wood is decorative and durable, but its main use is in the manufacture of pencils; it is easy to 'sharpen'. The incense cedar is used in Native American smudging. In 2011 Veluthoor *et al.* reported research which revealed that incense cedar essential oil may have significant biological activity against fleas, ticks and mosquitoes, and also against *Phytophthora ramorum*, the fungus responsible for 'sudden oak death'. Analysis of the essential oil revealed that the main constituents were thymoquinone and carvacrol, both of which would explain its bioactivity. Carvacrol is also found in essential oil of thyme and oregano, both of which are well-established antimicrobials and antioxidants with insecticidal or repellent actions. Thymoquinone is also found in black cumin, and has an impressive array of biological actions – antioxidant, anti-inflammatory and perhaps anticancer – so it is of potential importance in human and animal health. Additionally, thymoquinone, along with *para*-methoxythymol, *para*-methoxycarvacrol and β-thujaplicin, which are also found in the oil, accounts for the antifungal activity. Veluthoor *et al.* suggested that in the light of this research, the incense cedar might be the source of a new biocide and repellent that is safe for the environment and for people.

Virginian cedar

Although it is commonly called red cedar, Virginian cedarwood essential oil is obtained from a species of juniper – *Juniperus virginiana*. This particular species is significant in northwest/Pacific Indian tradition. According to the Cherokee, cedar wood holds powerful protective spirits. Pieces of cedar wood are placed in medicine bags, and also above the doors of homes to ward off evil spirits. Cedar wood was also used to make totem poles and ceremonial drums. In ceremony and prayer, cedar is burned – and in sweat lodges, cedar wood is used along with sage and sweetgrass, for purification. The Pacific and northwest tribes maintain that cedar brings in good energies whilst driving away evil and negative influences. Its smoke was inhaled to relieve head colds, or neck cramps, and to relieve anxiety and bad dreams, and the Native Ozarker of the Midwest burned the twigs as an inhalant in purifying baths to relieve bronchial asthma. The smoke is also said to counteract the itching caused by contact with poison ivy (*Toxicodendron* species). The needles of the '*virginiana*' subspecies were used by the Kiowa, who burned the needles as incense during peyote prayer meetings; and the leaves of the '*silicicola*' subspecies were used as a fumigant by the Seminole, for eagle sickness, fawn sickness[3] and ghost sickness. These are culture-bound syndromes; ghost sickness is a psychotic disorder characterised by loss of appetite, feelings of suffocation, nightmares, and feelings of terror in relation to death and the loss of someone. They also used all parts of the tree in whole body fumigation for insanity (Pennacchio *et al.* 2010).

The wood of *J. virginiana* has an attractive red colour and it is very durable; it can withstand exposure to the elements, including very wet weather. The heartwood is very fragrant because of the volatile oil. Because of these characteristics, the wood is

---

3   Eagle sickness was characterised by a stiff neck and back, while the symptoms of fawn sickness were swollen legs and face. The Seminoles also used *Juniperus virginiana* var. *salicola* to treat hog sickness (unconsciousness), mist sickness (eye problems, fever and chills), opossum and racoon sicknesses (where children dream about these animals), rainbow sickness (fever, stiff neck and back ache) and thunder sickness (fever, dizziness, headache and diarrhoea). Decoctions as well as the smoke were used (Austin 2004).

a valuable commodity. Its main use is in the manufacture of lead pencils, but also for household utensils and boxes. The traditional 'cedar chest' is made from Virginian cedarwood; the wood imparts its fragrance to the contents, and it is also an insect repellent and useful for preservation of fabrics. Virginian cedarwood essential oil is distilled from the waste powdered wood from sawmills. The essential oil has a light, fresh, soft, resinous woody scent that is reminiscent of pencil shavings – clean, woody/oily. Its dominant constituents are α-cedrol at up to 15 per cent, α- and β-cedrene, thujopsene, β-caryophyllene and γ-eudesmol (Burfield 2002). In aromatherapy, its scent is used to anchor the emotions and focus the mind; it is also possibly analgesic and anti-inflammatory, and so useful for muscular and joint pain. Like its smoke in Native American medicine, its oil is supportive of the respiratory system.

Virginian cedarwood essential oil is used widely in the fragrance industry – it is stable in soaps and widely used as a soap fragrance. It is sometimes used as an extender of sandalwood and vetiver oils, as an adulterant of the fragrance chemical ionone (violet scents), and for the isolation of cedrol, a white crystalline solid that is also used as a fragrance ingredient. The essential oil is used to impart woody notes, to form the basis of violet fragrances and 'cold cream' scents, and act as a fixative in fragrances (Jouhar 1991; Williams 1995c). Fragrances that include cedar accords are the masculine fougère/fresh *Boss* by Hugo Boss and Davidoff's *Cool Water* (Glöss 1995). The floral-aldehydic feminine fragrance *Rive Gauche* (Yves Saint Laurent) owes much of its impact to a cedarwood and kephalis (a woody-amber synthetic with good tenacity) accord (Calkin and Jellinek 1994). Serge Lutens' *Bois de Violette* is a woody oriental with a violet theme (Turin and Sanchez 2009) that perfectly illustrates the synergy of cedar and violet accords, in this case with methyl ionone. Of all the cedars, Virginian cedar fragrance is the one that has crossed cultures and transcended time, with as much relevance today as in ancient Egypt.

Juniper, cypress and Douglas-fir

The Cupressaceae family also includes important *Juniperus* species, cypress, the iconic tree of the Mediterranean, and the majestic Douglas-fir.

Juniper

The genus *Juniperus* includes many trees and shrubs that have played a role in cultures across the globe (some of them are summarised in Table 3.1). For example, *Juniperus communis*, the common juniper, has been used by the ancient Greeks, the inhabitants of the Inner Hebrides in Scotland, rural France, Tuscany, North America and Alaska, and its subspecies were used in both India and North America.

There are another 20 or so juniper species of importance in addition to those already mentioned. Common aspects of its use include incense and fumigation, prayer, ritual, ceremony, ritual purification, driving away evil, protection from natural elements, producing smoke signals, deterring insects and pests, and relief of conditions such as asthma, headaches and vertigo. In Britain, on the eve of May Day, a branch of juniper with its berries would be hung on doors to protect against witchcraft. Juniper also had a culinary role – *J. drupacea* was burned by the ancient Egyptians to grill and smoke their food, and the Ramah Navajo of North America flavoured their tobacco with the fruits (berries) of *J. communis* var. *montana* (Lawless 1994; Pennacchio *et al.* 2010). One species, *J. procera*, commonly known as East African cedarwood, or African juniper, was used as incense during ceremonies, and in Kenya it was distilled to produce an essential oil that was used in perfumery. It has a dry, woody, earthy, slightly smoky odour, and was used in woody and oriental perfumes and as a fixative in soap perfumes, and also for the isolation of cedrol (Williams 1995c).

The berries of the common juniper have also played an important role in health, the flavouring of foods and beverages, and in perfumery too. The common juniper is a small shrub found all over Europe, North America, North Africa and North Asia. The berries take two or three years to mature, so each plant will bear berries in various stages of ripeness, from the immature green berries to the ripe blue ones. Only the ripe berries are harvested, then partially dried, which develops a more black coloration. The berries are eaten by animals such as sheep. In traditional medicine, infusions and oil of juniper, made with the green berries, is used as a diuretic, digestive aid, and to treat 'dropsy', although its ability to irritate the urinary tract was also noted. In France juniper berries were used to treat chest complaints. Culpeper maintained that juniper berries strengthened the brain and nerves, and the infusion was also believed to restore youth (Grieve 1992; Lawless 1994).

Juniper berries can be distilled to yield an essential oil which has a fresh, resinous, woody aroma. The needles and twigs also yield an essential oil that has an 'inferior' turpentine-like odour. Juniper berry oil is dominated by monoterpenes; it contains a significant amount of α-pinene and also myrcene, both of which are thought to have pain-relieving properties, and β-farnesene. Two monoterpene alcohols formed in the same biosynthetic pathway, terpinen-4-ol and α-terpineol, are also found; these are said to have diuretic action. In contemporary aromatherapy, juniper berry oil is considered to be a useful analgesic, used externally for muscle and joint pain, also as a urinary antiseptic and for acne and weeping eczema (Bowles 2003; Price and Price 2007).

Juniper is a well-known flavouring in gin. François de la Böe (1614–1672), also known as Franciscus Sylvius, was a German physician employed at Leyden University in Holland. It is thought that he was the first to prepare the distilled spirit aromatised with juniper berries, to combat tropical fevers suffered by the Dutch colonisers of the West Indies. This ancestor of gin was called 'Dutch courage' as it helped in difficult situations! The soldiers of Charles II brought gin to England in the late sixteenth century; and the seventeenth-century ban on alcohol actually contributed to the production of gin-type spirits. As distillation technology advanced, and the 'patent still' was introduced by Aeneas Coffey, the quality of gin improved immensely. *Distilled gin* is made by the distillation of alcohol and water with juniper berries and other botanical flavourings, usually including coriander and angelica. The botanicals may be included in the still, or contained in baskets through which the distillation vapours pass. Water is added at the end of the process. The quality of the product is highly dependent on the type of still and the amount of copper in the apparatus. *Compounded gin* is made by solubilising the essential oil of juniper and others in neutral alcohol and water; this method of preparation does not produce a product of the same quality as the distilled type. There are many recipes for gin, each with different combinations of botanicals, and the ultimate quality will be highly dependent on that of the botanical ingredients and even their geographical sources. Apart from juniper berries, angelica and coriander seed, botanicals can include lemon peel, cinnamon bark, cassia bark, liquorice root, cardamom seed, orris root, fennel seed, aniseed, caraway seed, and sweet and bitter orange peels. Quality and consistency with the individual brand characteristics is assessed by sensory analysis, where a range of characteristics will be evaluated. For example, sensory evaluation will consider pungent, sulphury, solvently, juniper, citrus, herbal, floral, fruity, spicy, aniseed, sweet, buttery, oily, soapy, sour and stale tastes and aromas (Tonutti and Liddle 2010). Juniper berries have long been used as a culinary ingredient, and are now becoming more popular again after a long period of relative obscurity. In modern British cuisine they are often paired with game such as venison and pheasant, and winter seasonal vegetables – typically red cabbage.

Juniper berry essential oil is used in the fragrance industry, although its terpenes do present solubility issues, and the oil does not keep well. Its duration is short to moderate, and juniper derivatives are used as a modifier in chypre, fougère and masculine fragrances (Williams 1995c). Examples include *Herrera for Men* (Herrera), a fresh fougère fragrance, where it is present in the fruity green top note, and *Lauder for Men* (Lauder), an animalic fougère, in its green, herbaceous top note (Glöss 1995).

Cypress

A few species of cypress have played important roles in human culture. The Arizona cypress (*Cupressus arizonica*) was burned by native North American Indians for its fumes, which aided childbirth and helped expel the afterbirth, and for shrinking the womb; also as a diuretic. *Cupressus lusticana*, commonly known as the cedar of Goa, was used in parts of Uganda to ward off spirits, and the Himalayan cypress was burned as incense in Nepal (Pennacchio *et al.* 2010). Kuiate *et al.* (2006) investigated the essential oil of *C. lusticana* that had been introduced in Cameroon during the colonial era. Their aim, apart from elucidating its chemical composition, was to establish its suitability for treating skin diseases. In the western highlands of Cameroon the leaves are used to protect stored grain from insect infestation, and the leaves are used to cure skin diseases caused by dermatophytes – fungi that can invade keratinised tissue and produce dermatophytosis. The research revealed that the leaf oil has antidermatophytic properties, probably due to the constituents acting in a synergistic manner, and by disrupting the fungal cell walls and membranes. This supported the traditional practice of treating some skin diseases with the juice from the leaves.

Best known is *Cupressus sempervirens*, the iconic cypress tree of the eastern Mediterranean. It is a tall, graceful, evergreen tree with long, slender branches and a neat conical habit. The Greek legend of Kyparissos explains its mythical origins and cultural associations. Kyparissos was a boy loved by the sun god Apollo (although some versions suggest it was Sylvanus, the god of the woodland), reflecting the social custom of pederasty. Kyparissos was given a tame stag, symbolising the hunter's prey, which he came to love dearly – but one day, when out hunting, he accidentally killed it with his javelin as it lay sleeping in the woods. He was inconsolable, and so Apollo transformed him into the cypress tree – which became a classical symbol of mourning. Ovid elaborates on this myth within the story of Orpheus, who was the inspiration of a cult. When Orpheus the musician failed to retrieve his wife Eurydice from the Underworld, he was so griefstricken that he forsook love of women in favour of boys. He played his lyre, and even the trees were moved to grief, the cypress, with its tears of sap on the bark, marking the sadness and metamorphoses of Kyparissos. So the cypress became inextricably associated with grief, mourning and the Underworld, but also with transition and transformation. The species name, *sempervirens*, translates as 'always living'. It is still planted in graveyards.

The Mediterranean cypress was widely used as incense in ancient Egypt and Greece, and the Tibetans still use it as purification incense. An essential oil is obtained from the needles and twigs, and occasionally the cones. It has a lingering, fresh, sweet, slightly balsamic and smoky scent; Jouhar (1991) notes that it resembles ambergris as it dries down. It has a complex chemical make-up, as might be expected with such an interesting odour; the monoterpenes α-pinene, δ-3-carene and the sesquiterpenol cedrol are its major constituents (Bowles 2003). The aromatic oil has astringent qualities which are reflected in its application in traditional medicine to stop excessive loss of fluid; Culpeper maintained that its cones were 'drying and binding' (Lawless 1992). In aromatherapy the essential oil is used as a nerve tonic to help with debility; as a tonic/decongestant for the venous and lymphatic systems, aiding fluid accumulation, varicose veins and distended capillaries; and as an antispasmodic in bronchial conditions (Valnet 1982; Schnaubelt 1999; Price and Price 2007). Some aromatherapy writers such as Davis (1991) clearly consider its mythological symbolism and associations with transition, in suggesting that its scent is helpful during times of grief and transition or fear.

In perfumery, cypress is used in amber accords (Jouhar 1991). Calkin and Jellinek (1994) explained its role in the structure of Dior's *Poison*, where fresh top notes are more or less eliminated and replaced with the 'somewhat narcotic' effect of cypress in an accord with the rose-like aromachemicals rose oxide and α- and β-damascones.

Douglas-fir

The hyphen in the common name indicates that this is not a true fir. *Tsuga* is the hemlock genus, and the botanical name of the Douglas-fir is *Pseudotsuga*, meaning false hemlock. There are two notable species: *P. menziensi* of British Columbia, Canada, and *P. taxifolia*, also known as the Oregon Douglas-fir, or the Oregon balsam. The Douglas-fir is widespread across western North America, where it can reach a height of over 100 metres. It rarely reaches this height in the UK. (It was introduced to Britain, first to Scone Palace near Perth in Scotland, by the Scots botanist David Douglas, in 1827.) It has soft, flat, linear leaves that completely encircle its branches, and produces pendulous cones with persistent scales. The cones are distinctive in appearance in that they have a three-pointed bract that protrudes above each scale. This bract resembles the back half of a mouse's body with two hind paws and a tail. A Native American folk-tale explains that this is because the tree provided sanctuary and sustenance in its cones for mice during severe winters and forest fires. The wood of the Douglas-fir is resilient, with high tensile strength, and so it is valued for structures that need to bear heavy loads. Apart from construction, the Thomson of British Columbia burn the rotten wood to smoke-cure animal hides (Pennacchio *et al.* 2010).

A very fragrant essential oil is distilled from its leaves, and sometimes the resin. It is dominated by geraniol at 31–32 per cent, and also bornyl acetate and traces of citral (Jouhar 1991). It is unusual to encounter such high levels of geraniol, a rosy-scented monoterpene alcohol, in coniferous oils. The scent of the oil is also distinct from that of all of the other conifers – it has a slightly lemony, pineapple-like odour, with a very slight floral characteristic. Research conducted by Warren and Warrenburg in 1993 reported that the fragrance of Douglas-fir had significantly relaxing effects, said to be similar to those brought about by meditation. Holmes (2001) describes Douglas-fir as having an appetite-stimulating lemony note, which can counteract mental and emotional confusion. Surprisingly, it is not widely used in fragrances or aromatherapy.

Pine, spruce and fir

Returning now to the Pinaceae family, there are three other important genera to consider – *Pinus* (pine), *Picea* (spruce) and *Abies* (fir).

Pine

The Pinaceae family is very large, comprising around 100 species, mainly in the northern hemisphere, but also in lowland equatorial areas such as Sumatra. They are very tolerant trees, showing resistance to adverse conditions such as dryness, salt air and cold winds, and so are planted for protection against erosion due to tides and sand, and as windbreaks. They have various other uses, as fuel, in construction, and for their resins and seeds.

The high resin content confers a degree of water resistance too, so they are used for bridges and shipbuilding (Kurose, Okamura and Yatagai 2007). In this family, volatile oils are produced in the resin canals that extend from the wood to the needles and cones. Resins that exude through the bark can also be collected and used.

Various species of pine and various parts of the tree have been used for thousands of years, for a myriad of purposes. For example, pine resin was used to help preserve mummies in ancient Egypt; the American Indians stuffed mattresses with dried needles; the kernels were eaten as food by the Egyptians and Romans, the young twigs were brewed in beer, the twigs were burned as incense and the cones were fertility charms. Pine barrels were, and still are, used to store a type of Greek wine – *retsina* – that has a characteristic pine-like, resinous aroma and flavour. Pine also had medicinal uses – for example, as a respiratory aid and for exhaustion and debility. Culpeper maintained that pine had a softening, healing and purifying functions, and pine sawdust poultices were a panacea for rheumatism, joint and bone diseases and debility. Pine smoke also had a major role in some societies, especially the North American Indian cultures. Please refer to Table 3.1 for more information.

Aromatics from the pines, and to a lesser extent the spruces and firs, are widely used – they have a range of applications from scenting household products and as disinfectants, to therapeutic and medicinal uses. In aromatherapy the main applications of the pine essential oils are to aid the respiratory system as expectorants and antiseptics, to aid convalescence and to help in cases of general debility. The pine oils are also used as analgesics for articular and muscular pain, and are also indicated in cases of urinary system infections. In short, all of these applications mirror the traditional external uses. Spruce and fir oils are less frequently used, despite their very pleasant, typical conifer fragrances; their principal therapeutic application is to aid the respiratory system.

Sources of pine oils include the dwarf pine (*Pinus mugo* var. *pumilo*), the longleaf pine (*P. palustris*), which produces an oleoresin that is steam-distilled to yield turpentine (although the leaves and twigs yield an oil that has therapeutic applications), and the Scots pine, *P. sylvestris* (also sometimes called the Norway pine). This species is named after Scotland, where it forms part of the ancient forests. Scots pine essential oil has a somewhat harsh, strong, coniferous, fresh odour that is perhaps less like disinfectant than that of *P. palustris*, but it does have turpentine characteristics too. This is the oil preferred in aromatherapy (although they all have the potential to irritate the skin). Scots pine oil is dominated by monoterpenes, notably α- and β-pinene and δ-3-carene. These constituents are said to be mucolytic, but they may also be irritating to the respiratory tract (Bowles 2003). If they irritate and stimulate the goblet (mucus-producing) cells, these cells will produce more mucus, and as a consequence the mucus will be less viscous. The same constituents are said to be analgesic, hence their use for muscle and joint pain. Schnaubelt (1999) suggests that Scots pine is also an endocrine stimulant which can be used for adrenal support.

In perfumery the oil from the dwarf pine is preferred, as it has a sweet, balsamic, woody odour, with a slightly spicy character. Although the chemistry is similar to that of the other pines, its higher phellandrene content might be at least partly responsible for this. (Phellandrene itself has a fresh, citrus, woody and spicy odour; see Williams 2000.) Pine needle is sometimes used to impart resinous middle notes in masculine fragrances, usually of the aromatic fougère type such as Paco Rabanne's *Paco Rabanne pour Homme* (Glöss 1995).

Spruce

There are several scented, essential oil-yielding spruces, which have aromatherapy and traditional uses. The essential oil of the black spruce, *Picea mariana*, is thought to have uses as a bronchial decongestant and endocrine stimulant – even more so than Scots pine. Schnaubelt (1999) suggests that it can be used in conjunction with the absolute of blackcurrant bud in cases of severe and prolonged stress. According to Holmes (2001), its scent gives a feeling of endurance and stamina, especially if used in combination with grand fir (*Abies grandis*) or Scots pine. White spruce cones (*P. alba* or *P. glauca*) were used in the Yukon region of Alaska to fumigate moose hides. *Picea abies* is the Norway spruce. Its resin was burned as incense, along with common juniper, common mugwort and yew during Nordic Christmas festivities. The Flambeau Ojibwa of North America use the smoke of the Canadian white spruce (*P. canadensis*) to alleviate respiratory disorders. In Iceland the cones of the red spruce (*P. rubens*) are burned on coals, and the smoke, when inhaled, was said to 'make a man happy', while also 'moistening the body' and treating blood illnesses. Resin was collected from the bark of this species for use as winter incense (Pennacchio *et al.* 2010).

Fir

In comparison, the firs (*Abies* species) appear to have a greater range of both traditional and perfumery uses. Pennacchio *et al.* (2010) highlight some traditional uses of fir smokes. The pacific silver fir (*A. amabilis*) was used to treat colds and sickness by the Ojibwa of the upper Midwest and the Nitinaht of British Columbia. The balsam fir (*A. balsamifera*) was used as incense in Iceland, in Native American sweat baths, and even as a frankincense substitute in Paris. The grand fir, already mentioned in conjunction with black spruce, was used by the Nitinaht to prevent sickness. The smoke of the Rocky Mountain fir, *A. lasiocarpa*, is that which appears to have the most significant part to play in Native American culture. For example, the Crow use it in ceremonial incense; the Blackfoot use it as a smudge to treat headaches, unconsciousness and tuberculosis, facial swelling due to venereal disease, and sick horses; the Cheyenne used the incense to help those afraid of thunder, and for driving away evil, while the Nez Perce use it in sweat lodges. In Nepal the Himalayan fir, *A. spectabilis*, makes pleasant incense.

Fir essential oils are obtained from the young shoots. Generally they have fresh, typically coniferous scents, sometimes with a lemony aspect, and lacking the resinous base notes of the pines and junipers. Typical constituents are α- and β-pinene, limonene and bornyl acetate. In aromatherapy several species, but typically the balsam fir, are used primarily to alleviate respiratory conditions, muscular aches and pains, cystitis and depression, and to support the immune system (Lawless 1992). The scent of fir is also said to promote mental clarity (Holmes 2001). Studies have demonstrated that Siberian fir is a useful antimicrobial, and that in traditional Siberian medicine it is used to maintain good health during the adverse winter weather. Matsubara *et al.* (2011) demonstrated that it can also be used to maintain health in a contrasting contemporary environment. Prolonged use of a visual display terminal use can lead to problems such as mental fatigue, sleep disorders and anxiety – and inhalation of Siberian fir is not only pleasant, but can prevent these problems without affecting task performance. Another species that has been investigated with regard to its therapeutic potential is *A. sachalinensis*, which is found in Hokkaido in Japan. Satou *et al.* (2011a) conducted a study using mice, and found that inhalation of *A. sachalinensis* could elicit an anxiolytic-like response, which was probably mediated by brain concentrations of its constituents and possibly the olfactory sense. This study would support the aromatherapeutic use of *A. sachalinensis* for alleviating anxiety.

In perfumery *A. siberica*, the Siberian fir, is the one preferred for its powerful, fresh, coniferous fragrance. It would appear to play a supporting rather than dominant role imparting freshness in the middle notes of fougère and chypre masculine fragrances.

Possibly the most striking example of the role of the firs in wellbeing can be seen in Japan where scent and the natural environment together have a powerful effect. For many, coniferous forests are special places; some are considered sacred, and they are also associated with wellbeing. Being surrounded by trees, with the sounds of the air moving through the branches and leaves, or absolute stillness, can be a profoundly relaxing experience, and the diverse and complex scents of forest and woodland undoubtedly contribute to this feeling. Walking and/or staying in forests to promote health are a recognised form of relaxation in Japan. *Shinrin-yoku* translates as 'forest bathing', or 'taking in the forest atmosphere', and the practice has been shown to have numerous and measurable health benefits. In 2007 Morita *et al.* evaluated the psychological effects of *shinrin-yoku* in a large number (498) of participants, and identified the factors related to the effects. They found that acute negative emotions, including hostility, depression and anxiety, which are all implicated in the risks of coronary heart disease, are improved by taking part in *shinrin-yoku*. They also demonstrated that the improvements in negative emotions were caused not simply by exercise or taking part in favourite activities but by the forest environment. Moreover, the forest environment enhanced positive emotions, and this directly benefits the immune system. Even simply reaching the forest had positive effects on wellbeing. This could also suggest that the visual impact of seeing green trees can improve emotions, and the type of forest or even the duration of the stay did not seem to alter this. However, it did appear that those who were chronically stressed, or those with poor mental health, received the greatest benefits.

Tsunetsugu, Park and Miyazaki (2010) have been focusing on the 'Therapeutic Effects of Forests' project for several years now. They have been investigating the physiological effects of exposure to the 'total environment' of forests, including deciduous broadleafed forests as well as conifer-dominated ones, and also the effects of certain elements (such as the odour of the forest, as well as some essential oils derived from forest species, the sound of running streams, and the scenery) in relation to their physiological effects (including central and autonomic nervous system activity and biological stress markers). Their work has confirmed that *shinrin-yoku* can reduce stress, reduce blood glucose levels in diabetic patients, increase natural killer cell activity and immunoglobulins A, G and M, reduce feelings of hostility and depression, and lower blood pressure. They suggest that *shinrin-yoku* is 'forest medicine' and that the practice makes a significant contribution to human health.

There seems to be little doubt that forests and woods are therapeutic landscapes, but we still do not know if this is due simply to their scenic beauty or whether other factors are involved. However, our senses do not work in isolation, and it could be said that they have a synergistic effect on our psyche. As Tilley (2006) suggested, it is the multisensorial aspects of gardening that reconnect us with the natural world, and so it is very likely that this is what happens with *shinrin-yoku*, where scent closely underpins the visual impact.

Yews

We will conclude this chapter with a look at the yews, aromatic trees and shrubs that have indeed had an impact on wellbeing, but are often overlooked, and more associated with toxicity.

The yews belong to the genus *Taxus* of the Taxaceae family; these are slow-growing, evergreen trees or shrubs which are widely distributed in Europe, North America, North India, China and Japan. The smaller, shrubby types are common garden plants, planted for their attractive foliage and scarlet berries. Three species in particular have had an impact on wellbeing, and so are included here.

Taxus brevia

In 1971 Wani and Wall discovered the novel anticancer drug Taxol from *T. brevia*. This heralded a great deal of research into several species of yew – investigating their needles, bark, shoots, seeds and heartwood – and identifying over 300 chemicals in the class of 'taxoids'. This research also elucidated the presence of other potentially important groups of constituents, such as the ecdysteroids which cause insect moulting; the red-coloured rhodoxanthin; pro-anthocyanidins, which are amentoflavones that bind to nervous system receptors; and biologically active lignans (Khan *et al.* 2006). The other important yews are the English and Himalayan types.

English yew

The English yew, *Taxus baccata*, formed part of European shamans' incense, along with fir species, black henbane, common mugwort and creeping thyme, and also in an incense mixture burned at Nordic Christmas ceremonies. This species contains the toxin called taxine. All parts of the tree, apart from the fleshy aril (the red fleshy cup surrounding the seed), are poisonous, a property which has been exploited since the time of Julius Caesar. However, some tribal peoples would eat the aril as a digestive aid and as an expectorant, and *T. baccata* is also thought to be the source of the drug *zarnab* in Unani Tibb medicine. Extracts may also be used in cosmetic and hair lotions and dentifrices (Khan *et al.* 2006; Pennacchio *et al.* 2010).

Himalayan yew

T. wallichana is the Himalayan yew, found in the temperate Himalayas and the Meghalaya and Manipur hills. Unlike the other yews it does not contain taxine, and it does have a history of cultural and medicinal use. It was burned as incense, and the Brahmins used a red paste from the bark to mark a small red dot on the forehead, between the brows, to symbolise the 'third eye'. Tinctures were made from the young shoots to treat headache, giddiness, weak pulse, coldness of the extremities, diarrhoea and biliousness. The leaves are also used for treating various complaints such as hysteria and epilepsy; and research has indicated that an aqueous leaf extract has indeed a tranquilising effect. Leaf extracts can also inhibit fertility and prevent pregnancy.

Khan *et al.* (2006) investigated the constituents of the volatile oil of the Himalayan yew, finding the main components to be (*E*)-2-octen-1-ol (also found in fruits such as apple, blueberry, melon, grape; also in potato, cognac, rum, black tea, mushroom and kelp); *n*-pentacosane (also found in cardamom, melon seeds, *Ginko biloba* leaves and poplar buds); caryophyllene oxide (common in many essential oils but also in orange juice, lime, cranberry and cinnamon, and used in beverages, icecream, meat products and tobacco products); 1-octanol (also in citrus essential oils and in green tea), hexanoic acid, which smells of rotting flesh, cheese and rancid butter; and (*Z*)-3-hexenol, which smells of green grass and leaves and is an important flavour and fragrance material. Other constituents that will be more familiar to perfumers and aromatherapists were geraniol, anisaldehyde and pinene. Khan *et al.* concluded that most of these major constituents potentially have a wide range of applications in the flavour and fragrance industry.

CHAPTER 8

Spices

A spice is usually defined as a seasoning that imparts a pungent flavour and sometimes a sense of heat to food. However, spices can also contribute to the visual appeal of foods in terms of colour or garnish; consider the yellow colour of saffron, or a garnish of cracked black pepper, and the difference that this can make to the appeal of a dish. Spices also have medicinal value, and considerable aromatic value (Figueiredo and Miguel 2010). Spices have had an enormous cultural impact – mainly because of their value, which is directly related to their importance as modifiers of flavours, their role in defining cuisines, their medicinal attributes and role in perfumery. A few words about the 'spice trade' can help to illustrate this. For millennia civilisations have traded; as early as 10 BCE, Neolithic peoples would have been trading commodities such as spices and precious minerals and gems. The spice trade originated in Asia, northeast Africa and Europe; the trade in aromatics between Egypt and Punt is one of the earliest examples. Spices such as cinnamon, cassia, cardamom and ginger had high commercial value, so much so that when these commodities from Asia reached the Middle East, the traders did not reveal their true sources, and many fantastic stories were told to embellish their exotic origins. Spices became more valuable than other commodities, such as silks. The Greeks and Romans became active players in the spice trade; they used the established incense route and created new routes between the classical world and India. Consequently, India, Ethiopia and the Red Sea became important, but in the seventh century CE the rise of Islam resulted in the closure of the overland 'caravan' routes through Egypt and Suez. Arab traders then dominated, via Levantine and Venetian merchants; the Republic of Venice had also become a major player in the trade. The trading routes were cut again, this time by the Ottoman Turks, in 1453. From then until the early modern period, Muslim traders dominated the seas, trading throughout the Indian Ocean to the Persian Gulf and Red Sea, then overland to Europe, but during what has become known as the European 'Age of Discovery' (when, for example, Columbus inadvertently discovered South America while actually trying to reach India by travelling west) the European nations – Portugal, Spain, France and Britain – entered the trade. A new sea route was established from Europe via the Cape of Good Hope to India, pioneered by the Portuguese explorer Vasco de Gama in 1498. Channels such as the Bay of Bengal were also important cultural bridges, but because of the by now huge economic importance of the spice trade, nations struggled and fought to gain control along all of the routes.

The Dutch found yet another route to circumvent the problems, this time from the Cape of Good Hope to the Sunda Straight in Indonesia. The Dutch East India Company was formed and was very successful, and this was followed by the British and French East India Companies. However, continual attempts to gain monopoly persisted – first the Portuguese dominated, then the Dutch, marked by the capture of the Portuguese Moluccas. This was followed by a protracted and bloody struggle, and destruction of plantations to control supplies; entire native communities were destroyed and islands depopulated. Eventually the British gained dominance, thus weakening the hold of the Dutch East India Company. So, as well as enriching lives and being at the heart of cultural exchanges between many diverse civilisations, spices were also at the very centre of some of the bloodiest conflicts and acts of destruction during the height of the trade.

Here we will explore their traditional and more contemporary uses in incenses, foods, perfumery and healing, and for pleasure. Specifically, those significant in ritual, folk medicine, contemporary herbal medicine, ceremony and perfumery will be considered. Using a concept borrowed from western herbal medicine, we will start with the 'aromatics', followed by the 'pungent' spices, loosely grouped according to their odour characteristics, and finally, in a class of its own, the unique and subtle saffron.

The aromatic spices

This group includes the aromatics of traditional western herbal medicine – the remedies that were used to treat colic and flatulence, irritable bowel, congestive dyspepsia, and catarrh and bronchial congestion (Mills and Bone 2000) – including the seeds of angelica, caraway, carrot, celery, coriander, cumin, dill, fennel, star anise – all from the same botanical family, the Umbelliferae, the 'carrot family'. All its members have specialised ducts which secrete and store volatile oil, and such ducts are found in the fruits ('seeds') of caraway, aniseed, fennel, dill and coriander. Many of the spices in this family are reputed to be digestive aids, with decongestant, diuretic and depurative (blood-cleansing) properties. The aromatics also include cinnamon, cassia, clove and nutmeg.

Warm and sweet

Caraway
The botanical source of caraway is the seeds of *Carum carvi*, a large biennial herb belonging to the Umbelliferae family. In past times caraway root, which resembles a small white parsnip, was eaten as a vegetable, and, when mixed with milk and made into bread, or *chara*, it provided sustenance for Valerius' soldiers in Julius Caesar's

army. It is said that the seeds were first used by the ancient Arabic peoples, who called it *karawaya*, although Pliny maintained that the name came from Caria in Asia Minor. Dioscorides suggested that the seeds should be consumed by 'pale faced girls' (Grieve 1992, p.157). Caraway seeds were, and still are, added to bread and baked goods, and also to vegetable dishes – its flavour is particularly compatible with cabbage. In Germany it is also used in sauerkraut and *Kümmel* – a caraway liqueur. In Britain, during the time of Shakespeare, caraway was very popular, making an appearance in most meals. In Shakespeare's *Henry IV Part 2* there is a reference to the popular pairing of pippin apples with a dish of caraways, possibly referring to a caraway sauce or candied seeds; this custom is continued at Trinity College in Cambridge. In England, caraway seed cake was served at celebrations hosted by farmers following wheat sowing. North of the border, in Scotland, buttered bread was dipped into a dish of caraway seeds, and this was known as 'salt water jelly'. Apart from these varied culinary uses, caraway seeds were made into tinctures to treat flatulence, hiccups and headaches. According to Culpeper, 'caraway confects, once only dipped in sugar, and a spoonful of them eaten in the morning fasting, and as many after each meal, is a most admirable remedy for those that are troubled with wind' (Potterton 1983, p.37). In early times in America, hiccups were viewed as a conflict between the flesh and the spirit, and so caraway seeds, along with dill and fennel, were given to children in churches, so that they would not hiccup during sermons (Gordon 1980). Grieve (1992) relates a superstition about caraway, telling us that it 'was deemed to confer the gift of retention' (p.157), which meant that it prevented the theft of any object that contained it, or held the thief in custody. This apotropaic custom was extended to include the prevention of infidelity, hence the inclusion of caraway in love potions such as *l'huile de Venus*, and to prevent livestock from straying. Grieve makes the interesting observation that if tame pigeons are given caraway bread or cake in their dovecot, they never stray from home.

Caraway was first cultivated for its essential oil in Holland, around 1815 (Jouhar 1991). Caraway essential oil is obtained from the dried, ripe seeds and is often rectified to improve the odour. The rectified oil has an intense, warm, sweet, spicy odour that resembles that of the dried seed. The dominant constituent is *d*-carvone; carvone is a ketone with two chiral forms that are mirror images of each other. The *d*-carvone molecule has the odour of caraway, while the *l*-carvone molecule smells minty. It also contains limonene and small amounts of the related ketone *cis*-dihydrocarvone, myrcene and others (Bowles 2003). According to Lawless (1992), its main uses in aromatherapy are for the respiratory system – the dominant ketone might confer mucolytic properties (Bowles 2003), and the digestive system.

In perfumery, caraway is used in small amounts, because of its intensity, to complement jasmine or cassie (*Acacia farnesiana*), and in tabac and fougère fragrances such as Azzaro's *Azzaro pour Homme* (Glöss 1995). It is used as a 'mask' in insecticides. Caraway is also used to add an aromatic character to soap, and in the flavouring of mouthwashes (Morris 1984; Jouhar 1991).

Dill

Anethum graveolens, or dill, is also a member of the Umbelliferae; it is a hardy annual that is native to the Mediterranean region and the south of Russia, and has much in common with caraway. The whole plant is strongly aromatic, and both the leaves and seeds are used. The tiny seeds are in fact flattened fruits. Dill is considered to be a sweet herb, and its young, feathery leaves are used to flavour sauces and pickled vegetables, and fish. Dill seeds are used to flavour vinegars, pickled cucumber, sauces and pastries. Its original Greek name was *anethon*, and it was well known in the classical world. The physician Galen commented that 'dill procureth sleep, wherefore garlands of dill are worn at feasts' (Gordon 1980, p.69). The modern name comes from the Old Norse word *dilla*, which means 'to lull' – alluding to its widespread reputation for soothing colicky babies. Like caraway, it was used to cure hiccups and 'expel wind, and the pains preceding thereof...' (Culpeper, cited in Grieve 1992, p.256). During the Middle Ages dill was hung at doors and windows to protect against witchcraft, and it was also used in spells, including love potions.

Dill essential oil is obtained from the seeds and it has a light, fresh, spicy, slightly minty, caraway-like odour. Like caraway, dill seed oil contains a substantial amount of *d*-carvone. According to Lawless (1992), its main uses in aromatherapy are to alleviate colic, dyspepsia, flatulence and indigestion. In soap perfumery, it is used as a substitute for caraway seed oil (Jouhar 1991).

Coriander

Staying with the Umbelliferae, *Coriandrum sativum*, or coriander, is a small annual herb that produces spherical aromatic seeds. It is now widely distributed, and was well known as a spice and medicine the East, Egypt, all over the Mediterranean, Africa and Peru. It is thought that coriander was introduced to Britain by the Romans. Coriander may well be one of the first culinary herbs, and nowadays its leaves and ripe seeds are important in many cuisines, especially those of Asia and the Middle East. The seeds are a common ingredient in curry, and are also used as flavouring in gin. The medicinal uses of coriander seeds as a stimulant and carminative have been known since early times; it was used by Hippocrates and is mentioned by Pliny. The Chinese maintained that the seeds could confer immortality.

In 1551 the British herbalist Turner[1] suggested that coriander seeds could be used in bread or barley meal to combat St Antony's Fire (Grieve 1992): this was a disease caused by the consumption of rye that had been infected by the fungus *Claviceps purpureum* ('ergot of rye') which causes the fatal disease ergotism. This disease is caused by alkaloids produced by the fungus, and is particularly unpleasant, being characterised by both convulsive and gangrenous aspects. It was reputed to have been cured by the intervention of St Antony, hence the common

---

1   William Turner (circa 1508–1568) was a natural historian and herbalist; he published 'A New Herball' in 1551.

name at the time. In North America the symptoms of ergotism were thought to be a sign of bewitchment, so it was also implicated in the Salem witch trials.

The unripe seeds are said to have a very unpleasant odour, but this recedes as they ripen, and when dried they have a very pleasant fragrance. Coriander essential oil is distilled from the seeds and has a sweet, aromatic, slightly woody aroma, with faint fresh floral-citrus undertones. The dominant constituent of the oil is *d*-linalool, sometimes called coriandrol, a monoterpene alcohol. It is a useful aromatherapeutic essential oil with a wide range of applications, including supporting the digestive system and as an analgesic for osteoarthritis and rheumatic pain. Coriander seed oil is also an appetite stimulant, and can impart a sense of euphoria (Schnaubelt 1995; Price and Price 2007). In perfumery, coriander can impart freshness in the top notes of fragrances. Calkin and Jellinek (1994) discuss its role in *Coriandre*, a fragrance that heralded a new direction in the chypre family. It was launched by Couturier in 1973, and had a coriander and ylang ylang top note, while the main theme had a strong emphasis on patchouli with a dominant rose accord. However, Turin and Sanchez (2009) comment that although the current version retains its rose-chypre structure, the original was a much better fragrance. *Le Feu d'Issey* (Issey Miyake) is an example of a very innovative fragrance with a dominant coriander element in the top note. It was short-lived, and discontinued. Turin and Sanchez suggest that '…if you can find it, it should be in your collection as a reminder that perfume is, among other things, the most portable form of intelligence' (2009, p.262).

Cardamom

Cardamom (*Elettaria cardamomum*) is a robust, perennial, reed-like plant that belongs to the ginger family, the Zingiberaceae. Like ginger, it grows from a rhizome, but in this case it is the aromatic seeds rather than the rhizome that are used. The fruits are pale green or yellow capsules that contain dark brown seeds. The aromatic volatile oil is produced in single secretory cells in the seed coats. Cardamom has been valued for millennia; Weiss (2002) notes that an ancient Sumerian clay tablet makes reference to it; Lawless (1994) explains that the oldest medical text in existence is recorded on two clay tablets, from Sumer, a city state of Mesopotamia around 3500 BCE. At the time Sumerian society was based on matriarchal principles, and their goddess Ninlil was, amongst other things, the protector of plants. Females healers were either shamanic *ashipu* or herbal practitioners called *asu*. The *asu* probably used distilled plant essences – we can suggest this because a clay distillation vessel dating back to 5500 BCE was found at a Sumerian grave site. From this we can begin to see how aromatics such as cardamom, through the Sumerians, became used by all of the other cultures that they influenced.

Cardamom featured in ancient Egyptian rites and perfumes, and consequently *cardamomum* was used by the Greeks and Romans – for example, in the *Metopion*. Greek myth tells us that Hecate, a goddess of the Underworld, had two sorceress daughters, Medea and Circe; this powerful triad was well acquainted with the magical uses of herbs and spices, especially cardamom, which was also regarded as a powerful aphrodisiac.

In early Arabic cultures, cardamom was indeed used as an aphrodisiac, and can be found in a formula endorsed by Shaykh Nafzawi, the author of *The Perfumed Garden of Sensual Delight*, along with cinnamon, cloves, nutmeg, pepper and gilliflowers, which could be any of several scented flowers, especially carnation, clove pink or wallflower. It was an important spice in its native India, where it was used as a flavour, fragrance and in Ayurvedic practices. Here it was known as *elattari, ilachi* or *ela*, and it was used as an aphrodisiac and incense. *Abir* is an aromatic powder, used in Hindu ceremonies, which contains cardamom, curcuma (turmeric) cloves and sandalwood (Jouhar 1991). The sweet and pungent taste of cardamom flavours many dishes, and it is also added to coffee to counteract acidity – a practice adopted by other Middle Eastern cultures, which remains popular.

Another current practice with ancient origins – that of chewing betel – also involves cardamom. In Indonesia, the *quid* is composed of the nut of the areca palm, wrapped in the leaf of the betel pepper that has been spread with lime ash paste. The paste helps release alkaloids in the nut and leaf, so when the quid is chewed a sensation of alertness, relaxation and euphoria is experienced. Digestion is aided, but the saliva is stained red, which can cause damage to the teeth and gums, but nonetheless is seen as a mark of beauty. Often, in order to freshen and sweeten the breath, costly spices will be added (Jay 2010) – cardamom, nutmeg, cloves, musk and camphor are all used.

In the mediaeval west, cardamom retained its aphrodisiac reputation and became known as the 'fire of Venus'; as might be expected, it was often found in love potions. Its medicinal properties were also noted, although it was used more as an adjunct in formulae for indigestion and flatulence, colic and 'disorders of the head'. In more modern times in the West, the emphasis has returned to its use as a flavour. In Russia, Sweden, Norway and Germany, cardamom is used to flavour cakes and liqueurs, and in the East it is used as a condiment (Grieve 1992).

Cardamom essential oil is obtained from the dried fruits; the main producer of the oil is India (Weiss 2002). The aroma is warm and spicy, with a slight camphoraceous note due to a major constituent, an oxide called 1,8-cineole. This has a fresh, camphoraceous, eucalyptus-like odour which is described as 'cineolic'. Good-quality oil should not have a strong cineolic quality – the aromatic, warm and spicy character is much preferred. Cardamom essential oil has a role in contemporary aromatherapy, unsurprisingly as a digestive aid, and to combat mental fatigue and nervous strain. It is also tonic and stimulating, antispasmodic, anticatarrhal and expectorant (Franchomme and Pénoël 1990), possibly due to its 1,8-cineole content. Cardamom plays a role in modern perfumery too. Aftel (2008) suggests that it gives spicy, warm notes in floral fragrances, while Jouhar (1991) states that it plays a role in both masculine and feminine fragrances, and often in lily of the valley types. *Femme* (Rochas) is a chypre fragrance, whose underlying warmth comes from an accord with cardamom, cumin and carnation (Calkin and Jellinek 1994).

There are few spices that have such an exotic and colourful history and reputation; perhaps the Australian company Aesop was inspired by this in the creation of the 'all-natural' *Marrakech*. This is a spicy, resinous fragrance where cardamom forms an accord with clove and sandalwood, described by Turin and Sanchez as 'an archaic fragrance of biblical directness and beauty' (p.372).

Nutmeg

The last aromatic in the warm and sweet group is *Myristica fragrans* – nutmeg – a spice central in the conflicts of the spice trade, and with unusual psychotropic effects. *Myristica* species, of the family Myristaceae, are evergreen rainforest trees which produce yellow, fleshy drupes. (A drupe is a fleshy fruit in which the seed is surrounded by a hard endocarp; examples are plums and cherries.) The fruit is walnut-sized, and when opened a red, net-like covering known as the *arilus* or *aril* is revealed – this is the spice called mace, and the kernel itself is the nutmeg. Nutmeg is native to the Banda Islands, the Malayan Archipelago and the Amboina Islands in the Moluccas; it is also cultivated in India, Penang, the Caribbean (St Vincent, Tobago and Grenada), Brazil and Réunion. Allegedly, the scent of the 'Nutmeg Islands' is so pervasive that birds of paradise become intoxicated.

The use of nutmeg as a medicine, aphrodisiac and spice has a long history; the first mention of it in literature is in the Sanskrit *Susruta Samhita* of 600 CE, where it is called *jai phal*. It was not known in ancient Greece or Rome, nor is it mentioned in the Bible. The next mention of nutmeg is in 540 CE, by Actius of Constantinople. It is thought that Arab traders brought nutmeg to Europe from the Moluccas via India, but that they kept its source secret, and so the first mention of the Moluccas as the source of nutmeg was not until 1300 CE. It became a valuable spice in Europe, and in 1191 when King Henry VI of Germany was crowned Holy Roman Emperor in Rome, the streets were fumigated with nutmegs and strewing herbs. It was the search for nutmeg and the Spice Islands that prompted Vasco de Gama's voyage and subsequent discovery of a new sea route to the East. Later, when the Dutch eradicated all nutmeg trees except those on Banda and Amboina islands, it was probably fruit pigeons that continued to spread the species. These birds swallow entire seeds, digest the fleshy portion and void the seed with its hard outer coat, and thus distribute them to neighbouring islands (Gordon 1980; Weiss 1997).

The medicinal attributes of nutmeg had long been recognised – it was used as a remedy for appetite stimulation, digestive disorders, flatulence and vomiting, but also for pain reduction, nerve stimulation and mental ailments, and oil of nutmeg was used as a narcotic. Nutmeg kernels were also preserved in sugar syrup, and eaten as a delicacy. In 1576 Lobelius, in a text known as *Plantarum seu Stiripium Historia*, recorded that an English woman had attempted to induce an abortion by consuming 10–12 nutmegs, and became 'deliriously inebriated'. Later, in 1829, a physiologist named Purkinje ate three nutmegs, and likened the effects to cannabis intoxication. So nutmeg's reputation as a narcotic with toxic effects grew, and it was noted that it was freshly grated nutmeg that was most potent. In Bombay in

1883, a *Materia Medica* was published; this revealed that the Hindus used nutmeg as an intoxicant, and that the Ayurvedic name is *made shaunda*, meaning 'narcotic fruit'. It is one of the aromatics used to flavour and enhance the effects of betel nut, and on Zanzibar and Pemba, nutmegs are chewed as an alternative to smoking *bhang* – the local marijuana. The bark extract of the closely related *Virola* species is used to produce a snuff that is used by local shamans to produce hallucinations. So from intoxicated birds of paradise to European ladies and nineteenth-century physiologists, Hindus, and the local residents of Zanzibar and Pemba, nutmeg's narcotic effects are witnessed. Nevertheless, it has never been widely exploited or abused as a recreational drug.

Nutmeg contains constituents known as aromatic (or phenolic) ethers, including myristicin and elemicin, and it is possible that these are responsible for the narcotic effects. It has been shown that, *in vitro*, these are converted into trimethoxyamphetamine (TMA) and 3-methoxy-4, 5-methoxyamphetamine (MMDA), and this is possibly what happens in the body (Weiss 1997). Used in small amounts, the effects are very mild, and really only exploited as a soporific in bedtime drinks! Nutmeg remains a popular flavour in both sweet and savoury dishes, as does mace, which has a stronger taste and is used sparingly (Gordon 1980). The reputed aphrodisiac effects of nutmeg were not scientifically investigated until 2003. Two studies conducted by Tajajuddin *et al.* (2003, 2005) investigated the effects on rats that were fed a 50 per cent ethanolic extract of nutmeg. A dose of 500mg/kg of body weight per day, over a period of seven days, appeared to be most effective for increasing sexual activity (usually occurring one hour after treatment), possibly due to its nerve-stimulating properties (Melnyk and Marcone 2011).

Nutmeg essential oil is highly aromatic, with a fresh top note and warm, spicy middle notes. Its main constituents are monoterpenes, including the pinenes, and the aromatic ether myristicin is present at around 6 per cent. The oil is an analgesic, digestive stimulant and tonic, and of use in diarrhoea, hypertension, rheumatoid arthritis, anxiety, depression and sleep disorders (Tisserand and Balacs 1994). The amounts of the essential oil used in aromatherapy practice are too small to carry the risk of major psychotropic effects such as intoxication or hallucination. Nutmeg is not a dominant ingredient in perfumery, but mace is more common and found in masculine fragrances (Glöss 1995).

Earthy

Angelica

Angelica archangelica of the Umbelliferae family was regarded as a holy plant. Culpeper said that 'some call this an herb of the Holy Ghost; others more moderate called it angelica, because of its angelical virtues' (Potterton 1983). According to folk tradition, its therapeutic properties were revealed to a monk during the time of the plague, by the archangel Michael. The plant is also said to bloom on Michael's holy day, 8 May, and so was believed to protect against evil spirits, spells and enchantment, becoming known as 'the Root of the Holy Ghost'. However, it is clear that angelica has pre-Christian, pagan associations. Grieve (1992) tells us that in Courland, Livonia and East Prussia, in early summer, peasants would gather wild angelica flowers and take them to the towns while chanting ancient songs in the Lettish language. These words and tunes were learned in childhood, and the meanings were no longer understood, but it is thought that they were the remnants of an ancient pagan springtime festival.

Angelica is a native of northern Europe, although some botanists argued that it originated in Syria. It is a highly aromatic biennial that can reach three metres in height, with a hairy appearance, large lobed leaves and bearing huge umbels of green and white flowers. It has been cultivated since the sixteenth century for its leaf stalks, yellow dye, roots and seeds – so clearly it was of value. John Parkinson,[2] apothecary to Charles I, considered it to be the best of all the medicinal plants. Grieve (1992) commented that it has merits as a 'sovereign remedy' for protection against contagion, for purifying the blood, and for curing every conceivable malady. It was used as a tonic and to treat coughs and colds, diseases of the lungs, shortness of breath, colic, amenorrhoea, toothache and ulcers, gout and sciatica. The stems reduced flatulence, and the aromatic root was held in the mouth as a preventative during times of plague. The stems were eaten in much the same way as celery, and the roots and stems were candied as a confection. Angelica is still used in this way, usually for decorating cakes and puddings. It is also a botanical flavour in many alcoholic beverages. In France it flavours Chartreuse, anisette and vermouth, and angelica is also one of the botanicals used in gin.

Angelica essential oil is obtained from the rhizome/roots or occasionally the aromatic seeds. The root oil has a rich, herbaceous, earthy odour, while the seed oil is fresher and spicier (Lawless 1992); Jouhar (1991) describes the root oil as 'pleasantly aromatic, a mixture of musk and pepper with a spicy top note' (p.20). The musky note is due to a musk-like lactone present in the root. Its notable chemical constituents are α-pinene, 1,8-cineole and α-phellandrene (Bowles 2003). Angelica root oil is not toxic or irritating to the skin, but it is strongly phototoxic and so is restricted in therapy and perfumery. The seed oil is not phototoxic. In aromatherapy it is indicated for the respiratory system, circulation and muscles and joints, especially 'toxic accumulations', for the digestive system and also anorexia, and for fatigue and stress/tension (Lawless 1992). Jouhar (1991) commented that a remarkably good fixative is obtained by solvent extraction of the roots, and this is occasionally used in masculine fragrances, while the root and seed oils are both used in flavours for dental products.

---

2   Parkinson was an apothecary and botanist, herbalist to Charles I. He was also known for his work on decorative gardens, and is associated with the birth of horticulture and public medicine. His best known work is *Paradisi in Sole Paradisus Terrestris* (1640).

Carrot

Carrot seed oil is obtained from the seeds of another umbellifer, *Daucus carota*. Grieve (1992) comments that 'from the time of Dioscorides and Pliny to the present day, the carrot has been in constant use by all nations' (p.161). It is a well-known vegetable; however, its seeds are less commonly used. The seeds have medicinal value; like all of the other spices discussed here, they are carminative and stimulant and so have been used to treat flatulence, colic, hiccups, and so on. They were also considered valuable for treating kidney stones, 'obstructions of the viscera' and jaundice. The essential oil has, according to Jouhar (1991), an earthy, woody and root-like odour, while Lawless (1992) describes it as warm, dry, woody and earthy. In aromatherapy it is not widely used, but it does have applications in skin care, for indigestion, loss of appetite, and for arthritis and rheumatism. In perfumery carrot seed oil is used in 'natural type' fragrances, fougères and chypres, such as *Cerruti 1881* (Cerruti) where it is included in the resinous, floral, spicy middle accord (Glöss 1995). Jouhar (1991) suggests that by blending it with cedar wood a 'fairly good imitation' of orris can be achieved.

Celery

Celery seed oil is obtained from *Apium graveolens* of the Umbelliferae family. Like the carrot, celery is a well-known vegetable, and the seed is used as a seasoning. In traditional medicine it was used as a carminative, stimulant, diuretic, tonic, and for promoting sleep. Grieve (1992) said that it also diffused through the system a 'mild sustaining influence'. Lawless (1992) notes that the seed is used for bladder and kidney disorders and digestive upsets, and that 'it is known to increase the elimination of uric acid', making it useful for gout, and neuralgia. She also notes that it is current in the British Herbal Pharmacopoeia for rheumatoid arthritis with mental depression.

As is often the case, the aromatherapeutic uses mirror these traditional ones. Celery seed oil has a persistent, spicy, warm, rich, sweet, celery-like odour; its main constituent is limonene. Lawless (2009) maintained that celery is a useful base note that imparts warmth in heavy floral fragrances, and Jouhar (1991) states that it is used in sweet pea and tuberose accords. According to Calkin and Jellinek (1994), celery seed is found in accords with jasmine absolute (possibly augmenting the celery-like *cis*-jasmone found in the absolute), and a trace of celery seed oil forms an 'interesting accord' with tuberose in the chypre fragrance *Miss Dior* (Dior).

Cumin

The botanical source of cumin is *Cuminum cyminum*, an annual herb closely related to coriander. Like coriander, it was cultivated in early times across Arabia, India, China and the Mediterranean region. It is mentioned by Hippocrates, Dioscorides and Pliny, who wrote that the ground seed was taken with bread, water and wine as both a medicine and a condiment. If the seeds were smoked, they produced facial pallor, which Horace described as *exsangue cuminum* – a complexion that suggested studiousness. The Greeks maintained that cumin symbolised cupidity (greed) (Grieve 1992); in Roman times it represented cheapness, and eating excess cumin was said to make a person 'tight' with money, or a bit mean. For this reason Marcus Aurelius was nicknamed Marcus 'Cuminus'.

Black cumin, *Nigella sativa*, belongs to the Ranunculaceae (buttercup) family and is unrelated, despite its common name. This, too, is well known in the same regions, and cultivated for its aromatic seeds, which have been used since antiquity in traditional medicine, as well as to flavour breads and cheeses, and as a spice in many other dishes (Wajs, Bonikowski and Kalemba 2008). Its essential oil contains a bioactive constituent, thymoquinone, which is anti-inflammatory and antioxidant; this might explain its therapeutic benefits and value as a medicine and food spice.

Cumin seeds were, and are, a widely used spice with a strong aromatic smell and slightly bitter taste, typically found in curry spice blends. Medicinally, cumin was used chiefly as a stimulant, carminative and antispasmodic. It is still used in Ayurvedic medicine for these purposes, and in aromatherapy cumin essential oil can be used to support the digestive system and nervous system, and to aid with 'toxic accumulations' (Lawless 1992). Cumin essential oil is not widely used in aromatherapy – mainly because it is strongly phototoxic. The oil contains a large amount of an aldehyde called cuminaldehyde (Tisserand and Balacs 1995) and has a distinctive, warm, powerful, spicy, earthy fragrance that closely resembles that of the seeds.

The scent of cumin oil provokes extreme reactions. Some find that it is reminiscent of a sweaty body odour, and many appear to be very sensitive to it, detecting even tiny amounts. The remainder find it pleasant or unobjectionable, or without this particular connotation. In perfumery it is used in synthetic cassia compounds, and the isolated cuminaldehyde is used, in traces, in cassia, orris, lilac, lily, mimosa and violet perfumes. Cumin was used in the complex floral accords (tuberose, lily of the valley, jasmine, rose, carnation, coriander, cumin, orris, cedarwood and sandalwood) in the heart notes of the original *Kenzo* (Kenzo 1988). Alexander McQueen's *Kingdom* is a heavy cumin fragrance. *Rose 31* (Le Labo) has a cumin note (although Turin and Sanchez (2009) describe it as 'aldehydic carrot juice'), as does the indolic orange blossom and jasmine fragrance, *Fleurs d'Oranger* (Serge Lutens). Turin and Sanchez comment that here, the 'savoury-sweaty' cumin is reminiscent of 'a poorly ventilated alleyway in some unidentified south east Asian city' (p.273). These comments, and many that can be read on the fragrance websites, show just how divisive the cumin aroma can be!

Fenugreek

Fenugreek is another aromatic spice with a long tradition of use. *Trigonella foenum-graecum* belongs to the Leguminosae family. It is an annual herb that grows up to 0.5 metres in height and produces long, narrow, sickle-like pods that contain brown, oblong, rhomboidal seeds with a deep furrow that divides them into unequal lobes. These taste bitter, reminiscent of lovage and celery. The species name, *foenum-graecum* translates as 'Greek hay', because it was used to fragrance inferior hay and render it palatable for horses and cattle, which apparently enjoy its flavour.

Fenugreek seeds have a very long tradition of use as a culinary spice, medicine and perfume since ancient Egyptian, Arabic, Greek and Roman times. In Cairo it was used in a preparation named *helba*, for the treatment of fever, to aid the stomach and manage diabetes. Fenugreek seeds, when soaked, yield a soothing mucilage that can be used internally for stomach and intestinal problems, and externally as a poultice for abscesses. The ground seeds are used to impart a maple flavour to confectionery. They contain an alkaloid, trigonelline, and a steroidal saponin, diosgenin (Grieve 1992). Fenugreek seeds yield an essential oil by distillation, and a resinoid via solvent extraction. Both have an intense, woody odour (Jouhar 1991); Lawless (2009) commented that the initial impression is overwhelmingly of curry, which gives way to a warm, rich, walnut-like scent. Fenugreek is used, usually very sparingly, in perfumery. In *Patchouli* (Comme des Garçons) it is used in an accord with patchouli (Turin and Sanchez 2009).

Anisic, ethereal and sweet

Anise

Anise, sometimes called aniseed, is the small fruits (called 'seeds') of *Pimpinella anisum*, a small, dainty herb of the Umbelliferae family. It has a long history of use; it was well known to the ancient Egyptians, Greeks, and indeed all over Asia Minor. In ancient Rome anise was used to spice a cake known as *mustaceae* that was served at the end of celebratory feasts such as weddings, along with anise seeds and cumin seeds. This way of using anise reflects its therapeutic value as a carminative and digestive aid; it also freshened the breath. Anise was also highly valued as an expectorant. Its smoke had therapeutic properties; according to Avicenna, in Iran smoke from the burning fruits was inhaled for pain and vertigo (Pennacchio *et al.* 2010).

Anise essential oil is distilled from the dried and comminuted fruits, and has a powerful, warm, spicy sweet odour, very characteristic of the herb. It has a very high proportion of *trans*-anethole, a phenolic ether, at up to 90 per cent. This constituent can produce psychotropic effects when used in high doses, and it also has considerable therapeutic value as an antispasmodic and analgesic. However, high levels such as this mean that in aromatherapy aniseed should be used with caution. It is also a potential skin irritant (Lawless 1992; Tisserand and Balacs 1995).

The scent is so distinctive that it is a recognised odour type – anise. The most important constituent in all anise-scented botanicals, such as anise, star anise (see below) and sweet fennel (also see below), is *trans*-anethole. These botanicals are used as flavours in a class of alcoholic beverages known as 'aniseed aperitifs', which includes *arquebuse, ouzo, tripouro, raki, sambuca* and *pastis*. It was also used in absinthe (see Wormwood, *Artemisia absinthium*, on page 255). *Pastis*, a French aperitif, is flavoured with anise, star anise and fennel, and also with liquorice roots and stolons, which contribute an additional sweetness and their distinctive flavour. *Pastis* has a relatively high alcoholic strength of 40–45 per cent, and so it is usually consumed with the addition of water, which produces a cloudy yellow haze. (In French, this phenomenon is known as *louchissement*.) This is because *trans*-anethole is insoluble in water, and so even at the low level of 1.5–2.0 grams per litre of *pastis*, it forms small (1 micron) droplets in the alcohol and water mix. These scatter light, producing the cloudiness, and they increase in size with time, so that eventually the emulsion breaks down. *Ouzo*, a Greek/eastern Mediterranean aperitif, is produced by the distillation of ethanol with anise, star anise and other botanicals, such as cardamom, the choice being made by the individual producers. *Tsipouro* is a lesser-known Greek aperitif that is made by the distillation of the grape pomace after fermentation. The fermented pomace is then distilled twice with herbs and seeds, including anise. *Tsipouro* is more alcoholic, with a stronger odour and less sweet than *ouzo* (Tonutti and Liddle 2010; Tsachaki *et al.* 2010).

In perfumery anise is used, in small quantities, as a 'toner' in perfumes. Anise derivatives (or their synthetic equivalents) such as anisaldehyde are also used. This has a heavy floral odour, similar to blooming hawthorn, and is used in lilac, mimosa, heliotrope and sweet pea accords (Jouhar 1991; Gimelli 2001).

Star anise

Star anise is the stellate (star-shaped) fruit of a tree of the magnolia family – *Illicium verum*. This is the botanical source of Chinese star anise – a carminative, stimulant and diuretic spice that was used in the East for colic and rheumatism, as well as a seasoning in savoury and sweet dishes.

Chinese star anise should not be confused with the Japanese star anise – a tree which is planted near Japanese temples and tombs, and whose bark is used as incense (Grieve 1992). Japanese star anise is obtained from different species such as *I. anisatum*, *I. religiosum*, *I. japonicum*, *I. shikimmi* and *I. skimmi*. These species are highly poisonous and have been associated with food poisoning – they are not fit for human consumption – because they contain methyleugenol and safrole, both of which are toxic. In 2002 the European Commission imposed strict controls on imports of star anise but they were repealed by 2009, so there is a continued need for vigilance when importing star anise (Tonutti and Liddle 2010).

Chinese star anise essential oil has a warm, spicy, sweet scent that is reminiscent of liquorice. Like anise, it contains a lot of *trans*-anethole (80–90%) and its aromatherapeutic uses and contraindications are similar. In France, where it is used in *pastis*, it is known as *badiane*. Anise is not common in fragrances, maybe because the anise note is very difficult to work with; however, Etro's *Anice* has, according to Turin and Sanchez (2009), anise present in the top, middle and drydown. This has been achieved by using star anise in the top notes, with a fennel seed and fennel–celery-like *cis*-jasmone accord in the heart, and anisic ambrette musk in the base. Turin and Sanchez also compliment Histoires de Parfums on their anisic lavender fragrance *1725*, which uses liquorice and star anise with a lavender and citrus accord linked by heliotropin and cedarwood. *Jazz* (Yves Saint Laurent) is a fresh, masculine fougère that has anise featured in its top notes, as did Fabergé's original *Brut* (Glöss 1995). An example of an anisic woody oriental is *Douce Amère* (Serge Lutens), and apparently *Paname* (Keiko Mecheri) gives the olfactory impression of a glass of *pastis* (Turin and Sanchez 2009).

Sweet fennel

Sweet fennel, *Foeniculum vulgare* var. *dulce*, is a hardy perennial umbelliferous herb that is indigenous to the Mediterranean, and associated closely with Italy and Italian cuisine. The genus name *Foeniculum* is derived from the Latin *foenum* meaning 'hay', although the ancient Greek name was *maraino*, which translates as 'marathon' and means 'to grow thin'. To the Greeks, fennel conferred longevity, strength and courage. The Romans cultivated fennel for its shoots, which were used as a vegetable that often accompanied fish, and the aromatic seeds, which were a seasoning and a medicine. Fennel rapidly acquired the reputation for helping the eyesight, because Pliny observed that 'serpents eat it when they cast their old skins, and they sharpen their sight with the juice by rubbing against the plant' (Grieve 1992, p.294). This association persisted beyond mediaeval times. Fennel, like many other aromatics, was believed to avert the evil eye and witchcraft, and was traditionally hung over doors on Midsummer's Eve. Grieve (1992) mentions that early English herbalists like Gerard[3] (1597) and Parkinson (1640) discussed fennel and its culinary uses, while Coles[4] (1650) reported its use in drinks and broths to combat obesity – no doubt all influenced by the early Greek and Roman beliefs. Traditional medicinal uses exploited fennel seeds' antispasmodic, carminative and expectorant properties. It was used along with purgatives to reduce cramp, and to make 'gripe water'. Another use was as a deterrent of fleas.

Sweet fennel (seed) essential oil has a characteristic fresh, sweet, anise and earthy aroma. According to Bowles (2003), sweet fennel oil contains *trans*-anethole at 80 per cent, limonene at 6 per cent and estragole at 4.5 per cent. A ketone, fenchone, may also be present as a minor constituent; this is dominant in the essential oil obtained from the bitter fennel, *F. vulgare* var. *amara*. In aromatherapy it is used for the respiratory system, the digestive system and the female reproductive system. Sweet fennel seeds were traditionally used to treat dysmenorrhoea; it was thought that this was due to the antispasmodic effect of the volatile oil. Animal studies have demonstrated that sweet fennel oil has a direct, relaxing effect on the uterine muscle; therefore the oil could be used in the treatment of dysmenorrhoea, but may also increase bleeding due to the relaxation effect (Ostad *et al.* 2001, cited

---

3   John Gerard (1545–1611 or 1612) was a botanist and herbalist, known for his herb garden in London and his 'Herball' or *Generall Historie of Plantes* (1597). He was not especially well educated, but had an accessible style and his book was notable for its illustrations, and so was very popular with the literate people of his time.

4   William Coles (1626–1662) was a botanist and herbalist; he wrote *The Art of Simpling* and *Adam in Eden*.

in Harris 2001). Because of the *trans*-anethole content, sweet fennel oil is a useful analgesic too. It has antifungal activity, and could be used in the treatment of fungal nail infections (Patra *et al.* 2002). The inhalation of sweet fennel essential oil can produce a decrease in mental stress, fatigue and depression (Nagai *et al.* 1991). It is not a common fragrance ingredient although it is used in herbaceous-type perfumes and fern-type soaps. *Anice* (see above) contains fennel in the middle notes, along with *cis*-jasmone – a component of jasmine, a fruity and celery seed-like aromachemical that becomes jasmine and cherry blossom-like on extreme dilution (Jouhar 1991).

Warm and fruity

Cinnamon and clove are the last aromatics to be discussed here, before we move on to the pungent spices. It seems natural to group them together, not only because they share a warm and fruity aspect to their aromatic profiles, but also because they share an aromatic history. They are often used together as spices in savoury and sweet foods, as synergistic ingredients in medicinal formulae and also in spicy perfumes.

Both cinnamon and clove have been used for millennia. From early times, they were very important aromatics in the spice trade. As we have already mentioned, the geographical sources of the spices were closely guarded by the traders, but their origins were eventually revealed; for example, the scent of cinnamon wafting out to sea alerted Alexander the Great to its presence on the Arabian shores. Both are mentioned in the Old Testament of the Bible, and both reached Europe because of the returning Crusaders, who had used the spices to enhance the flavour of their unpalatable rations, but were also aware of their medicinal and cosmetic uses.

Cinnamon

There are around 250 species in the genus *Cinnamomum* – including *C. camphora*, the camphor tree of China, and *C. malabatrum*, one of the 20 or so Indian species. The immature fruits of this species are used in *pan*, a masticatory that is a mixture of betel leaf, areca nut and clove buds, and its powdered bark is used as a base in the manufacture of incense sticks (Leela *et al.* 2009). However, because *C. cassia*, Chinese cassia, is most probably the cinnamon of antiquity, this will be explored first.

Weiss (1997) tells us that the bark of Chinese cassia was mentioned in China around 4 BCE in a text entitled *Elegies of Ch'u*, and later in 3 BCE, when it is referred to as *kui* or *kwei*. It is, however, believed that the medicinal uses of cassia bark were known long before recorded history. The Arabs and Persians called it *darchini*, meaning 'wood or bark of China'.

C. cassia is a subtropical forest tree; tall, conical shaped and evergreen, with a coarse, grey-brown bark (Weiss 1997). Grieve (1992) describes it as a very beautiful tree, especially when coppiced and its new flame-coloured leaves and delicate flowers emerge. According to Weiss, it is the inner bark of mature trees that is used – this is brown-red in colour and contains a high proportion of volatile oil-producing cells. The volatile oil contains between 60–98 per cent cinnamaldehyde (Weiss 1997), which is an aromatic aldehyde with a sweet, balsamic, cinnamon-like odour. On the other hand, Grieve (1992) maintained that the best and most pungent bark was obtained from young shoots, when the leaves are red. The wood itself is odourless and used as fuel, and when the bark is removed, cleaned and dried, it curls up to form 'quills'. Like all of the aromatic spices, cassia is a digestive tonic and carminative. Cassia essential oil is a powerful antimicrobial, but also a powerful irritant and sensitiser, and so its use is restricted (Tisserand and Balacs 1995). The oil is also toxic if taken internally. However, cassia is used safely as a spice, although it is considered to be coarser in flavour than cinnamon. Both Chinese cassia and cinnamon bark are used as flavours in gin.

By the time of Theophrastus, Dioscorides and Pliny, Chinese cassia and cinnamon were treated as distinct aromatics. True cinnamon is from *C. verum*, which was previously known as *C. zeylanicum*. In order to maintain their hold on the spice trade, the Arabs generated many fantastic stories about cinnamon, some of which are recorded in *The Thousand and One Nights* (also known as *The Arabian Nights*), a collection of folk tales. The name cinnamon has evolved from the words *chini* meaning 'China', and the Arabic *mama* and the Greek *amomum*, both meaning 'spice'.

Cinnamon production was associated with Ceylon as early as 1275 CE and continued throughout the Portuguese and Dutch eras, when it was a strictly controlled state monopoly, which the British abolished in 1833. By 1850, 16,000 hectares were devoted to cultivated cinnamon. By this time the Dutch had introduced cinnamon to their colonies in the East Indies too, including Java, which is now a major supplier of cinnamon. *C. verum* is indigenous to the wet tropical regions of Sri Lanka, India and Southeast Asia. It is a scented, bushy evergreen, with leathery, red and yellow young leaves which mature into bright green aromatic leaves, and an aromatic bark. The inner bark from the young shoots is removed, cleaned and dried into quills, which are golden brown and have an aromatic scent. The wood is not useful, as it warps and splits easily, but the roots are aromatic, and yield an oil with a camphoraceous character. Cinnamon is a local stimulant, carminative and antiseptic, and has been used since ancient Egyptian times for these purposes. It is often compounded with other medicinal spices, and in modern aromatic medicine it has been demonstrated that when co-administered, cinnamon, clove and coriander essential oils can increase the sedative effects of phenobarbital (Dobetsberger and Buchbauer 2011).

Cinnamon was also used in many of the early perfumes/remedies, such the Royal Unguent. To the Arabs cinnamon was a symbol of wealth, and to the Chinese it was a panacea and burned as incense. In mediaeval Europe, like many of the exotic spices, it was considered to be an aphrodisiac, and so found its way into perfumes and love potions. The spice is widely used in cooking, and can be found in various cuisines, including traditional and modern Greek and North African dishes. It is a traditional spice, along with clove, in Christmas cakes, puddings and dried fruit pies, and seasonal mulled wines.

Two cinnamon oils are available – a bark oil and a leaf oil. The latter is preferred in aromatherapy, as it is less irritating to the skin than the bark oil; however, it needs to be used with caution and at low concentrations. It contains 70–90 per cent *iso*-eugenol, a phenol with powerful antibacterial and analgesic qualities, but is toxic to the liver and inhibits blood clotting (Tisserand and Balacs 1995). Eugenol itself smells warm, spicy and clove-like. Cinnamon leaf oil has a harsh, warm and spicy odour, typical of cinnamon but also reminiscent of clove, with its sweet, fruity characteristics. Cinnamon bark oil is preferred in perfumery; it has a lower eugenol content but contains up to 75 per cent cinnamaldehyde. It has strong, sweet, warm and spicy top notes, sweet, spicy, slightly floral middle notes and warm, powdery base notes. Cinnamon bark oil is restricted in perfumery, but it is found at low, safe levels in oriental fragrances. The original *Shalimar* (Guerlain) contained a spicy cinnamon bark accord that complemented the leather aspect provided by castoreum and a leather base. The dominant spices in *Youth Dew* (Lauder) are cinnamon and clove, in an accord with *iso*-eugenol (Calkin and Jellinek 1994). However, restrictions on *iso*-eugenol probably forced a re-formulation. A more contemporary approach to the use of spices such as cinnamon can be found in the first *Comme des Garçons* fragrance, simply named *Comme des Garçons*, launched in 1994. Here there is a cinnamon, carnation and rose accord in the heart of the fragrance, with a spicy cardamom, mace and pepper top and a balsamic and ambery base (Glöss 1995).

Clove

The clove is indigenous to the Indonesian Moluccas, often known as the Spice Islands, and clove buds were and are an important spice. It is interesting that clove is not mentioned in ancient Egyptian formulae, and instead has its ancient historical roots in China. Its botanical name is *Syzygium aromaticum* and it belongs to the Myrtaceae family, although previously it was classified as *Eugenia caryophyllata* and *E. aromatica*, before that genus was revised. The Myrtaceae family also includes the eucalypts, paperbark trees, pimento and myrtle.

The cultivated clove is an evergreen tree, conical in habit; its young leaves appear in pink flushes and the mature leaves are glossy green and resemble bay leaves; it produces fragrant red flowers and reddish-purple fruits known as 'mother-of cloves'. The flowers are harvested when the buds are full size, but before they open – so the 'clove bud' is composed of the petals and their enclosed stamens. The trees need to mature to nine or ten years before they bear flowers. The buds appear at the beginning of the rainy season. At first they are pale green and as they expand they become peach pink. When the corolla fades in colour and the calyx turns yellow, then red, the embryo seeds are beaten from the trees and sun-dried. Clove trees are long-lived, and can remain productive for 150 years. Apparently they can take up huge amounts of water, so that very little else will grow near them. It is said that the finest cloves are from the Moluccas, where the girls wear its flowers, and children wear necklaces of clove seeds to avert evil and protect against illness. Here the seeds are also used as an aphrodisiac (Gordon 1980; Weiss 1997).

The first recorded use of the clove is in China, circa 220–206 BCE, when cloves were used to freshen the breath in the presence of the Emperor. They were known to the Chinese as *theng-hia*, and to the Persians as *makhak*. It is thought that the clove reached India around the fourth or fifth century CE, and in Sanskrit it was called *lavanga*; oddly, this was what the Tamils called cinnamon bark. In India, like *C. malabatrum*, clove was used in the betel quid, known as *pan pati*.

Between the second and fourth centuries CE, cloves were exported to Alexandria and all over the Mediterranean, and they were known throughout Europe by the eighth century CE. Clove was very important to the Venetian traders, who imported it from the Arabs and exported it throughout Europe. In the seventeenth century, when the Dutch broke the Portuguese monopoly on the spice trade, they destroyed all clove trees except those on Amboina (in the Moluccas) and islands close by. However, because of this, cloves were introduced to other areas, such as islands in the Indian Ocean, including Mauritius and the Seychelles, and also Zanzibar and Madagascar, which then became major producers.

The introduction of the clove to Zanzibar is an interesting tale. An Arab named Harameli bin Saleh had been banished to Zanibar for murder; however, he found work serving a French officer. He obtained clove seeds from Réunion, which he presented to the Sultan, and this act earned him a pardon for his crime. The Sultan recognised the economic value of the clove, and instigated plantations on Zanzibar and Pemba.

Finally, Sir Joseph Banks introduced clove to Britain. Here it became a popular culinary spice used in apple pies, ham pies, marinades and pickles, and in alcoholic beverages such as mulled claret (Gordon 1980; Weiss 1997).

It is probable that the earliest medicinal use of clove was to treat toothache – probably discovered in parallel with the early Chinese practice of chewing cloves to sweeten the breath. It is, in common with its fellow aromatics, a digestive aid and used for flatulence, as an expectorant and as a tonic for the nerves. It is also a very effective analgesic; traditionally, a liniment of clove, camphor, wintergreen and origanum was used for aching muscles.

As might be expected, clove has similar uses in contemporary aromatherapy. Clove bud essential oil contains a substantial amount of eugenol, which has pain-relieving qualities, but carries several cautions regarding its use. Clove oil, in high dilution, would also appear to have anti-inflammatory action (Schnaubelt 1995), and so is very useful for muscular and joint inflammation and pain. Schmidt *et al.* (2009) conducted an *in vivo* study using mice, and demonstrated that clove essential oil had immunostimulant activity, possibly by supporting humour- and cell-mediated immune response mechanisms, so it certainly has further therapeutic potential.

Clove bud essential oil has a scent directly related to the spice; it is spicy, rich, warm, sweet and fruity, with soft woody notes. In perfumery it is used in small amounts, but adds a spicy warmth to fragrances. It is particularly compatible with rose and carnation scents. Clove features in many spicy oriental fragrances, such as Dana's *Tabu*, which was created by Jean Carles and launched in 1931, and by now will have undergone several changes. Clove was dominant in the spicy middle notes, which were expended by the use of spices such as coriander in the top accord. This effect can be seen in Guerlain's *L'Heure Bleue*, with its fresh, spicy top of bergamot underpinned by coriander, and clove dominating the heart along with jasmine, *rose de mai*, ylang ylang and orchid. *Youth Dew* (Lauder) is constructed in a similar way, with clove dominating the middle (along with rose, ylang ylang, cassia, cinnamon, jasmine and 'orchid'), while a fruity spicy accord is also present in the top. Lauder's spicy oriental fragrance *Cinnabar* has a middle note characterised by the spicy notes of clove and cinnamon with an exotic floral accord (Glöss 1995) while Serge Luten's *Serge Noire* has, according to Turin and Sanchez (2009), 'clove in such quantities that you think of dentists' (p.493). A pairing of clove with a fruity plum note (provided by a base called Prunol) can be found in *Kenzo Jungle L'éléphant* (Kenzo). Clove was also present in the 'Mellis accord', which was a widely used base in spicy oriental fragrances including *Youth Dew, Opium* (Yves Saint Laurent) and *Coco* (Chanel). The Mellis accord was based on the relationship between benzyl salicylate and eugenol, with patchouli and hydroxycitronellal (which has a linden blossom-like, sweet, green, radiant odour), spices, woods and coumarin (Calkin and Jellinek 1994). Since then restrictions have been placed on some of these, so it will have been modified.

The pungent spices

Herbal remedies that have warming effects include the pungent spices galangal, ginger, pepper, pimento and turmeric (curcumina). These are indicated for congestive dyspepsia, nausea, colic and diarrhoea, bronchial congestion, poor peripheral circulation, and for joint and muscle pain and inflammation (Mills and Bone 2000). In contemporary aromatherapy their essential oils are indicated for the same reasons, but are externally applied and inhaled.

Warm and pungent

Galangal

The botanical source of galangal is *Alpinia officinarum*, a plant with reed-like leaves and reddish-brown, branched rhizomes. These have an aromatic odour and a pungent and spicy taste. Galangal is a member of the Zingiberaceae – the ginger family. The genus *Alpinia* was named after Prospero Alpino, a well-regarded Italian botanist in the seventeenth century. It is thought that the common name is derived from the Arabic *khalanjan* that loosely translates as 'mild ginger'. Galangal is distributed throughout the East – China and Hainan Island, Indonesia, Thailand

and Japan. A very similar species, *Galangala officinalis*, grows in India. The main use of galangal is culinary: it is used to spice curry dishes, and is an ingredient in many Thai curry pastes; and in Russia it flavours vinegar and an alcoholic liqueur called *nastoika*. It was also popular in Lithuania and Estonia. The dried, powdered root was used as a snuff, and in India it has been used in perfumery for thousands of years (Grieve 1992; Lawless 1992). An essential oil and oleoresin are available, and the typical odour is fresh, spicy and cineolic/camphoraceous.

Literature and research regarding galangal is scant, but an animal study conducted by Satou *et al.* (2011) investigated the potential for anxiolytic effects via inhalation of the essential oil of *A. zerumbet*. The principal chemical constituents were *para*-cymene, 1,8-cineole, limonene, α- and β-pinenes and camphene; an organoleptic evaluation was not given. (*A. zerumbet* is a related species that has been widely used in folk medicine in various subtropical regions, including Okinawa Island, Japan. It has also been used in contemporary herbal medicine specifically for depression, stress and anxiety, including chronic problems associated with female reproductive hormone imbalances.) Satou *et al.* considered time-dependent effects of inhalation, and attempted to elucidate the mechanisms by which this essential oil produced its effects. If an essential oil is inhaled, effects can occur via the olfactory nerve pathway, or via the blood stream. The olfactory route is mediated through rapid neurotransmission, so any effects due to olfaction should show up fairly quickly. The route through the bloodstream is much slower, because the constituents need to be absorbed and then delivered to the brain, but the potential for sustained reaction is increased. In this study, an anxiolytic effect was not observed with short (five minutes) duration of exposure, suggesting that the olfactory nerve pathway makes a very small or negligible contribution to the anxiolytic effect. However, longer exposure did produce an anxiolytic effect, which supports the bloodstream pathway and a pharmacological response. If the exposure continued for 150 minutes, no anxiolytic effect was observed, possibly because the olfactory receptors had become fatigued or habituated, or because receptor desensitisation in the brain was caused by more than the tolerable amounts of the constituents. The researchers concluded that an appropriate essential oil inhalation time is required with a particular dose to elicit anxiolytic-like effects. However, this research was conducted with mice, not humans, and so it was impossible to evaluate the influence of hedonic valence and the many other factors that could affect a human response to this essential oil aroma.

Ginger

In contrast, ginger has been well documented and researched. *Zingiber officinalis* grows from a horizontal rhizome that lies near the surface of the soil. In spring, green, reed-like stalks emerge, along with narrow, lance-shaped leaves. The stalk eventually bears a white or yellow flower. The rhizome itself is firm, and has a corky and scaly skin which can be buff-coloured, dark brown, or even black. The interior of the rhizome, the cortex and pith, contains secretory cells that produce the volatile oil.

Ginger is native to tropical India, Southeast Asia, Australia and Japan. It was naturalised in America by the Portuguese, and was introduced to Spain from the East Indies. Ginger is also associated with Jamaica and the West Indies, which have become significant producers (Grieve 1992; Weiss 1997). It has been used for thousands of years. The Chinese made a ginger tea to aid dyspepsia and loss of appetite, Hippocrates used it medicinally, and the Romans made use of it in cooking. The herbalist Gerard quoted Dioscorides: 'Ginger, as Dioscorides reporteth, is right good with meat in sauces and otherwise in conditures, for it is of a heating and digestive quality' (Gordon 1980, p.82).

Ginger essential oil is obtained from the unpeeled, dried and powdered rhizomes; it has a lemony, spicy top note, a warm, spicy and woody body, with a spicy, balsamic dryout (Williams 2000). The oil is dominated by sesquiterpenes such as zingiberene and α-curcumene, and sesquiterpene alcohols, but it is thought that monoterpenes and aldehydes influence its distinctive aroma. Several studies investigating the therapeutic effects of ginger have demonstrated that topical application and inhalation can mitigate nausea and vomiting (Geiger 2005; de Pradier 2006) and that it can support the humoural immune response (Schmidt *et al.* 2009). The effects of ginger on the psyche were explored by Holmes (1996), who maintained that the fragrance of ginger combined 'the potential for increased willpower and clarity' (p.19), and so is indicated when there is loss of motivation, apathy, indecision and disconnection. Ginger has a powerful aroma; according to Jouhar (1991), ginger is used as a toner in perfumery, and its odour is very difficult to imitate. Gucci's *Envy for Men* has a dominant ginger note, as does Serge Lutens' *Five o'Clock au Gingembre* which Turin and Sanchez (2009) describe as 'salty gingerbread' (p.265).

Pepper

There are many species that are commonly known as pepper, including the betel pepper (*Piper betle*). Its leaf is spread with slaked lime paste and used to wrap a sliver of the areca nut (*Areca catechu*) and other aromatics, forming the *quid* (also called the *pan*) which is chewed for its narcotic qualities. However, here we will explore black pepper, which is possibly one of the oldest trade commodities of the East, and possibly one of the main stimuli for world exploration. *Piper nigrum* is a perennial climbing vine that is native to the hills of western India and cultivated in the East and West Indies, Malaysia, Thailand and India (Weiss 1997); it has been said that the best black pepper comes from Malabar (Gordon 1980). The plant is very attractive, with dark green, heart-shaped leaves and spikes of white flowers which form berries. Unripe berries are green, and ripe ones are red. They are gathered before completely ripe, then dried, when they take on a black, wrinkled appearance – this is the black pepper that we use as a culinary spice. In ancient times it was very valuable; in 408 CE allegedly Attila the Hun asked for 3000 pounds of black pepper as part of the ransom for the city of Rome.

In ancient Greece and Rome it was also used as a medicine, and its use became widespread. Traditionally, black pepper (in addition to being used as a digestive stimulant and carminative) was used to treat many conditions such as gout and rheumatism, and to stop bleeding from wounds and reduce fever. Infectious diseases such as smallpox, scarlet fever, typhus, dysentery, cholera and even the bubonic plague were treated with black pepper (Gordon 1980; Grieve 1992). Writing about the uses of black pepper from an aromatherapy perspective, Maury (1989) commented on the ability of black pepper, which 'has its own personality and past' (p.89), to confer strength and endurance, adding that 'the mendicant monks of India, who cover daily considerable distances on foot, swallow 7–9 grains of pepper a day. This gives them remarkable endurance' (p.90).

Black pepper essential oil has a fresh, dry, spicy top note, and a spicy, woody middle and dryout. Williams (2000) classes it as a base note, but Lawless (2009) maintains that it is used in top notes. Its composition can vary widely according to its source, but typical constituents include limonene, the pinenes, phellandrene and caryophyllene, the clove-scented sesquiterpene. It is possible to detect a clove-like note in black pepper, and, like clove, it is used in carnation bases. Many masculine fragrances have pepper accords; however, Calkin and Jellinek (1994) discuss the use of black pepper with coriander to impart a dry, spicy note in the classic feminine chypre, *Miss Dior* (Dior). Turin and Sanchez (2009) mention the use of green peppercorn with peony in *Poivre Piquant* (L'Artisan Parfumeur) and also the spicy floral fragrance *Poivre* (Caron). Another Caron classic, *Parfum Sacré*, has a spicy pepper and incense accord in the top note, over a rosy woody heart (Glöss 1995; Turin and Sanchez 2009). In *Wonderwood* (Comme des Garçons) black pepper is noticeable, and used in conjunction with the synthetic sandalwood 'Javanol' and incense (Gilbert 2013).

Pimento

Pimenta species belong to the family Myrtaceae, and are native to tropical America and the Caribbean. Two *Pimenta* species are commercially important, and these are *P. racemosa*, the bay rum tree, and *P. dioica*, the source of allspice. The name comes from the Spanish word for peppercorns, *pimento*, because the berries resemble them.

Pimenta racemosa, the bay rum tree, is an evergreen forest tree that is used as fuel and for carpentry. It has aromatic, leathery leaves, and it is these that yield an essential oil (Weiss 1997), but its fruits are also aromatic. However, the tree is often grown alongside the allspice, and the berries of both are harvested and dried to make a culinary spice. Its leaves can be distilled in rum, and this forms the basis of a traditional hair tonic known as 'bay rum'. The essential oil distilled from either fresh or partially dried leaves is known as bay leaf oil or Myrica oil, or West Indian bay oil, and should not be confused with bay laurel oil from *Laurus nobilis*. Crude oil has a sweet, penetrating, somewhat phenolic odour with spicy, sweet balsamic undertones. It contains monoterpenes and eugenol, and was used in hair lotions, but in recent years terpeneless oil has been preferred: here the monoterpenes have been removed, leaving the sesquiterpenes, and the oil has an intense, sweet, mellow, spicy balsamic odour (Weiss 1997). Absolutes are also available.

Pimenta dioica is widely cultivated in Jamaica, Mexico and Central America. Like the bay rum, it is an evergreen tree, but it branches from a height of one metre, giving a bushy appearance. Its bark is smooth and shiny, and is shed in long strips. It also has highly aromatic leaves, and it produces small, white, aromatic flowers and small fruits. The ripe berries are sweet and spicy, and deep purple or glossy black in colour. These are dried, and become dark brown. They are ground and used as a spice for flavouring and curing meat and baked products. The berries can be crushed and steam-distilled to give an essential oil with a warm, spicy sweet scent. Like West Indian bay, this oil too has a high eugenol content, in the region of 60–90 per cent (Weiss 1997), and both oils are used in aromatherapy, mainly for pain and poor circulation – but always with caution, as eugenol has the potential to be a severe irritant and sensitiser.

Both types are represented in perfumery. *Opium* (Yves Saint Laurent) has an orange spicy top note with a pimento and bay accord, and Shulton's *Old Spice* has pimento, carnation and cinnamon in the spicy middle note (Glöss 1995).

Turmeric

Turmeric is a member of the Zingiberaceae (ginger) family. Its botanical name is *Curcuma longa*, and sometimes it is referred to as curcumin or curcumina. Turmeric is native to eastern India, the East Indies, Madagascar and the Pacific Islands, and is also cultivated in Tobago, Sumatra, Java and Bengal, but Gordon (1980) maintained that the best comes from China.

As with ginger, it is the rhizomes that are of interest – they contain single secretory cells that contain the volatile oil. It has culinary uses as a pungent flavour, and also for adding a yellow colour to dishes. It is found in curry and rice dishes, and also in pickles and chutneys.

Traditionally, the roots were used specifically for bowel and liver complaints and for treating jaundice. In Chinese medicine it is used in combination remedies for a range of complaints such as bruises, ringworm, sores, toothache, chest pain, colic and menstrual problems (Lawless 1992). In Ayurvedic medicine turmeric is classified as bitter, astringent, pungent and hot, and is used to purify and protect, and as an antiseptic. However, the main use of turmeric is as a dye. It is used for body painting in the Pacific Islands, and in India followers of Vishnu use turmeric to make a perpendicular mark on their foreheads. It is also used to colour varnishes and cotton fabrics (Gordon 1980).

Turmeric rhizomes yields an essential oil that has a distinctive yellow colour called curcumin, and it has a fresh and spicy odour, characteristic of the spice. Turmeric oil was used by the Egyptians to perfume the red slippers that were sold in bazaars. The oil contains tumerone and other sesquiterpenes. Tumerone is a ketone, which is thought to be toxic and irritant if used in large amounts. However, in Baylac and Racine's 2004 study which investigated the potential for aromatics to inhibit the human leucocyte elastase (HLE) enzyme that is implicated in inflammation and skin aging, turmeric oleoresin showed the strongest activity of all the aromatics tested. This, along with its antioxidant activity, would suggest that turmeric in its various forms has a part to play in contemporary personal care. Turmeric, and curcumin, its yellow pigment, is notable for its anti-inflammatory activity and potential antitumoural properties; it also has antiplatelet activity and so might be useful for the treatment of cardiovascular degeneration (Mills and Bone 2000).

One of the other uses of turmeric is as a substitute for saffron, one of the costliest aromatics known.

Saffron

Saffron is the dried elongated stigmas and tops of the styles of *Crocus sativus*, a perennial, stemless plant of the Iridaceae family. It has a subtle, sweet, spicy, slightly earthy aroma. Schier (2010) describes saffron as having 'unique sensorial qualities' (p.57). The importance of this spice should not be underestimated; its presence permeates our aromatic history. Ferrence and Bendersky (2004) wrote that 'saffron has been the most pharmacologically active and potent ethnomedicine known for almost four millennia' (p.220). In modern times it is best known as a spice with a vibrant yellow colour and subtle aroma and flavour that is used in dishes such as paella and bouillabaisse. It is also a colour and flavour in Yellow Chartreuse, a sweet liqueur that was developed from Green Chartreuse by monks of the Grande Chartreuse monastery in 1838.

Perhaps the best way to explore saffron is from the historical perspective, tracing its uses as a spice, medicine, psychotropic, aphrodisiac and perfume.

An Aegean wall painting in a building known as Xeste 3 at Akrotiri on the island of Thera (also known as Santorini) depicts a goddess of medicine, the Aegean crocus (*Crocus cartwrightianus*) and saffron. This fresco dates back to the Bronze Age – circa 3000–1100 BCE – and indicates that the Therans of ancient Akrotiri used saffron as a versatile medicine. Akrotiri was destroyed by a volcanic eruption circa 1648 BCE, and the town was buried under pumice and ash. However, this has preserved much for archaeologists and other scholars to investigate. No human remains have been found, so the inhabitants are thought to have escaped, and the frescos are very well preserved. The Xeste 3 fresco, which covers two adjacent walls over two floors, is considered to be one of the best preserved paintings in all of Bronze Age Aegean art history. It has been interpreted with reference to Minoan culture. This is because at the Palace of Minos at Knossos on Crete, the 'Blue Monkey Fresco' depicts a blue monkey wearing a red harness, in a field of crocuses, picking the flowers and placing them in a vase. In the Minoan villa of Hagia Triadha there is another fresco of a kneeling female figure, who is gathering crocuses. However, the

Xeste 3 fresco would seem to suggest that saffron had divine connections, because of the presence of a beautifully dressed goddess, attended by a griffin, while a blue monkey offers crocus stigmas to her. This is interpreted as showing either the goddess bestowing curative powers on the saffron, or that she has given the gift of saffron to mortals. In the fresco the goddess is almost touching the stigmas, and this may well represent the potentiation of saffron as a medicine. This magic of this fresco and the goddess would have had genuine validity, and certainly would have enhanced saffron therapy at Akrotiri (Ferrence and Bendersky 2004).

Saffron, from *C. sativus*, later appears in an Assyrian dictionary of botany written circa 668–633 BCE, where it is indicated for dyspnoea, painful urination, childbirth, menstrual disorders, and 'diseases of the head' (Thompson 1908, 1924, cited in Ferrence and Bendersky 2004). As this would have followed the healing traditions of the Old Babylonians, saffron was undoubtedly used in the seventeenth century BCE or earlier. Subsequently saffron is mentioned in various texts, including the *Hippocratic Corpus* of the fifth to the fourth centuries BCE, and Dioscorides' *Materia Medica* of the first century CE, and in these we can see a growing number if indications for its use, including the treatment of eye infections, corneal disease and cataracts, pain, ulcers and open wounds, throat inflammation, genital ulcers, and as a topical soothing agent. Ferrence and Bendersky (2004) point out that the lower Xeste 3 fresco shows a young woman applying crocus stigmas to her bleeding great toe – an indication that its early uses were prevention of bleeding, and/or as a soothing antiseptic. By this time saffron was also used orally as an aphrodisiac; in India it was especially well regarded in this aspect. Pliny the Elder wrote about saffron and its uses, adding treatment for bladder inflammation, pleurisy, pruritus, the restoration of hair growth, and as a soporific; he also tells us of the ancient Roman custom of using saffron to delay the intoxicating effects of wine. Its scent was also appreciated – Pliny mentions that the benches of public places were strewn with crocus flowers, and their petals were placed in small fountains to scent banqueting halls. Saffron was used in Ayurvedic medicine, which influenced Tibetan medicine. The *Four Treatises*, written in 400 CE, and still used, mentions the use of saffron to treat liver and lung disease, joint pains, nervousness, diarrhoea, indigestion and menorrhagia. Also, in traditional Persian medicine, saffron has been used for depression, as well as menstrual disorders, difficult labour, inflammation, vomiting and throat diseases (Ferrence and Bendersky 2004; Fukui, Toyoshima and Komaki 2011). Over the centuries its use spread, and its reputation grew; by the tenth century saffron was being cultivated in Spain, and by the fourteenth century considerable qualities were being grown in England. In 1728 the area between Saffron Walden and Cambridge was especially noted for the cultivation of *Crocus sativa* (Evans 1989).

The English herbalist Gerard thought that saffron could combat some of the infectious illnesses of the day, such as measles, smallpox and the plague; he suggested that it could also be used to treat St Antony's Fire. He also noted some of saffron's effects on the psyche, suggesting that it could cause euphoria and alertness (in contrast to Pliny, who said that it was soporific). Gerard, in his *Great Herbal* of

1597, wrote, 'But moderate use of it [saffron] is good for the head, and maketh the senses more quicke and liuely, shaketh off heavy and drowsie sleepe, and maketh a man merrie' (cited in Schier 2010, p.63). Recognising the marginal significance of saffron in contemporary western culture in comparison with the Middle Ages and Renaissance, and to explore why this might be, Schier (2010) analysed the use of saffron in medieval nunneries. He describes how in 1249 Archbishop Eudes Rigaud of Rouen visited the Benedictine priory of Villarceaux, and was troubled by his perception that the nuns were leading an extravagant life and enjoying amorous escapades. This was suspected because the nuns wore their hair long (to their chins!) and scented their veils with saffron – a luxurious commodity with multisensory properties. Saffron was noted for the vibrant orange-yellow colour derived from its dried red stamens – which is more obvious than its odour. The public display of this colour sent a social signal that an individual could afford saffron, and yellow became a marker of social segregation. So why did the nuns scent their black veils with saffron? The practice was probably based on the knowledge that saffron was a stimulant and an elevator of mood. The nuns' duties, which included the performance of canonical hours, the Marian mass and memorials, could lead to exhaustion, so to prevent and alleviate fatigue that could lead to the deadly sin of *acedia* (sloth, or boredom), saffron was made available. Its use in convents became widespread, and consumption in some convents was very high indeed – more than could be accounted for as a food flavour and colouring, and in the alcoholic beverages that were also consumed, since, in addition to their dietary intake, saffron was used to scent the veils. This scent, coupled with singing and chanting, could well have produced trance states, hypnosis, or even ecstasy. Schier suggests that 'the intake of saffron was capable of affecting and changing the chanting of the nuns – and this was the firm belief of donors and performers alike; saffron thus enhanced the performance of sung prayers, so "boosting" their impact' (p.67).

It was not just the nuns who were enjoying saffron. In the Middle Ages it was a legal drug that enhanced the feeling of wellbeing: it heightened and altered sensory perceptions and even induced hallucinations, but was socially controlled by its high price and therefore used only by elite members of society. Some of these psychotropic effects have been investigated in several pharmacological studies, including double-blind, randomised, placebo-controlled trials (Akhondzadeh *et al.* 2004, 2005, cited in Schier 2010) which demonstrated that saffron can successfully treat mild to moderate depression without side effects. However, in large doses, saffron is toxic, and can also elicit hallucinogenic effects. A daily intake of more than one gram can result in a chronic level of toxicity – originally noted by Avicenna, who believed that large quantities were 'hurtful to the brain', and Gerard, who observed its intoxicating effects. In the early twentieth century, when attempting to induce abortion, saffron was taken in a lethal dose (in the region of 12–20 grams). The toxic symptoms were gastric pain, blood in the vomit, diarrhoea and urine, vertigo, severe metrorrhagia, brachycardia and tachycardia, convulsions and coma (Blacow 1972; Arena 1973, cited in Ferrence and Bendersky 2004).

By the twenty-first century saffron was being analysed and researched in relation to its biological activities. It was found to contain several carotenoid pigments, volatile constituents such as safranal, bitter principles such as pirocrocin, and dye materials such as crocetin and its glycoside crocin (Fukui *et al.* 2011). Apart from safranal, the essential oil contains over 34 volatiles, mainly terpenes, their alcohols and esters (Evans 1989) and the flavonoid quercitin in the crocus flower. The main component responsible for the characteristic saffron odour is 2-hydroxy-4,4,6-trimethyl-2,5-cyclohexadien-1-one.

Both Ferrence and Bendersky (2004) and Fukui *et al.* (2011) cite numerous studies that have elucidated more of saffron's medicinal and therapeutic properties, and have confirmed and substantiated many of its traditional uses. These have shown that saffron and/or its pharmacologically active constituents have anticonvulsant, anti-inflammatory, antinociceptive, antitumour properties, as well as free radical scavenging activity, learning and memory improving actions, the ability to promote oxygen diffusion through tissues, chemopreventative and protective effects against oxidative stress, and the ability to significantly inhibit the growth of colorectal and breast cancer cells. Quercitin, contained in the flower, is also an antioxidant and free radical scavenger that can reduce the progression of atherosclerosis. Saffron was also demonstrated to lower cholesterol, control hangovers and migraines, and alleviate measles, chronic uterine haemorrhage, diarrhoea and nasal polyps. Crocin has the potential to be used in the prevention and treatment of degenerative brain diseases, as *in vitro* studies have demonstrated that crocin suppresses neuronal cell death (Soeda *et al.* 2001, cited in Ferrence and Bendersky 2004).

This is an impressive catalogue of biological activities that indicates saffron's massive therapeutic potential. However, despite the fact that saffron has been used in ethnomedicine and experimental studies for the treatment of over 90 distinct conditions, there is still a need for more double-blind, placebo-controlled trials. Because of this, its therapeutic effects are often regarded as folk medicine, or inadequately proven by quasi-empirical trials, or the placebo effect, and even sympathetic magic (Ferrence and Bendersky 2004). Nevertheless, interest in saffron endures. In 2011 Kukui *et al.* published their research into the effects of saffron odour on premenstrual syndrome, dysmenorrhoea and irregular menstruation. This is a significant study – it explores the psychological and physiological effects of a fragrance, and it was also a double-blind, placebo-controlled trial, which is believed by many to be the best type of research design. The saffron odour was adjusted to a level where it was imperceptible. In summary, the anti-stress actions were clearly identified; saffron may adjust steroid hormone levels via an odour sensory perception mechanism; and anxiety was reduced, regardless of the stage of the menstrual cycle. As Akhondzadeh *et al.* (2005) had already suggested, saffron has antidepressant effects through a serotonergic mechanism. Sex hormones interact with cholinergic and serotonergic systems and so affect the frontal cortex functions and memory; Kukui *et al.* (2011) suggest that saffron may alleviate PMS by adjusting steroid hormone secretion, and that saffron odour may be effective in the treatment of menstrual distress.

Saffron's renowned aphrodisiacal attributes have also been the subject of recent scientific investigations, albeit without placebo controls. In 2008 Hosseinzadeh, Ziaee and Sadeghi conducted an animal study where rats were fed an aqueous extract of saffron with crocin and safranal. The aqueous extract and crocin had a positive effect on sexual activity within one hour of administration; safranal alone had no effect. The following year, Shamsa *et al.* (2009) investigated the effect of oral saffron (200mg per day prepared from dried saffron stigma, for ten days) on 20 human males with erectile dysfunction (ED), although there was no differentiation between the organic or psychogenic types of ED. This study showed that saffron produced a positive effect on erectile function, sexual desire, intercourse satisfaction and overall satisfaction. In 2010 Safarinejad, Shafiei and Safarinejad conducted a similar study, cited in Melnyk and Marcone (2011), using 30mg per day of an ethanolic extract of saffron over a much longer period, on 346 males. This did not find that saffron had any effect on sexual satisfaction – and so there is a clearly a need for further research in this area.

So far, we have looked at saffron as a spice, medicine, psychotropic and aphrodisiac, and it is clear that the scent of saffron is important. Therefore it is hardly surprising that saffron has a long history as a perfume ingredient. It was enjoyed by the ancient Greeks and Romans, especially in Rome, where it was a single note perfume, a cosmetic, an ingredient in a body lotion called *helenium*; and in the *Regalium* formula for the perfume used by the Kings of Parthia (in Iran). Saffron was an ingredient used in the Seplasia project, where an ancient Roman perfume called *Iasmelaion* was recreated according to the original formula (see page 105). In India, the scent of saffron was enjoyed in perfumes, and also in an erotic context in the tantric Rite of the Five Essentials, where it was used on the female's feet. In ancient and modern Arabic cultures, crocus (*kurkum*) was significant. Saffron, or *za'fran* was used as a perfume on its own, and also in *khaluq*. Classen *et al.* (1994) explored the aesthetics of smell in the United Arab Emirates (UAE). They tell us that there, the most important and popular fragrances are agarwood, ambergris, saffron, musk, rose, jasmine, Arabian jasmine, narcissus, sandalwood, henna (flower) and civet; these are used as oils, sometimes with the addition of ground aromatic seeds and leaves. An Arab woman will use this as her aromatic palette and compose her own scents from this, each of which will be applied to different parts of her body. They give examples that contain saffron: musk rose and saffron for the whole body; ambergris and jasmine for the hair; and a red mixture called *mkhammariyak* (containing agarwood, saffron, rose, musk, and civet) for anointing the ears. Perfume is thus used extensively, and not to mask odours but to make the body fragrant. Nowadays, as in premodern Muslim society, women do not use perfume when in the company of men other than their husbands; it is only used in the private realm. Classen *et al.* (1994) cite Kanafani (1983), quoting of a husband describing his wife's charm:

Her body is rubbed with a paste of [scented oil] and rose petals; her sleeping gown is redolent of beautiful aloewood [agarwood]. Her hair smells of ambergris and saffron oils. We men like all scents used but have a preference for musk, ambergris, aloewood and saffron. (pp.126–127)

The differences between this very beautiful and aesthetic way of using fragrance, and the modern western use of perfume are quite striking. It is also interesting that we do not see the use of saffron in early or modern European perfumery; it simply does not seem to have become part of western olfactory culture. It is rarely found in fragrances; however, the perfumer Olivia Giacobetti has used saffron in two of her compositions. *Safran Troublant* (L'Artisan Parfumeur) is based on an accord of rose, vanilla and saffron. Turin and Sanchez (2009) consider that this is an example of 'high art', and that the saffron 'has a cream-like effect on the other notes and gives this fragrance the caressing, almost moist feel and colour of the best chamois leather' (p.483). *Idole* (Lubin) also has ingredients that are found in Arabic and Indian desserts, such as rosewater, saffron and cardamom. This is described as 'saffron suede'. These impressions penned by Turin and Sanchez give a real sense of the feel and texture of the multisensorial saffron.

CHAPTER 9

Herbaceous, Green, Camphoraceous, Cineolic and Agrestic Scented Botanicals

This is a very wide and diverse group of aromatic plants, so, as before, this chapter will be led by their scents and organised using their olfactory characteristics. We will begin with those that have predominantly herbaceous fragrances, and then progress to the green odour type. The camphoraceous and cineolic odours are also related to herbaceous types, providing a link to the agrestic scents, which evoke the countryside and natural environment in many different ways, from the scent of meadows and damp earth to woodland and even the seashore. During the course of this chapter we will encounter some fascinating uses of these aromatics – from strewing herbs, apotropaics and mood-altering ingredients in beverages, to traditional and contemporary healing and, of course, fragrances.

Herbaceous scents

The botanical term 'herbaceous' refer to plants that die back after flowering, and the word 'herb' refers to plants that have culinary uses, or are used as medicines. When we use the term 'herbaceous' in perfumery, we mean odours that are reminiscent of aromatic herbs. Between the sixth and the eleventh centuries, monks and nuns created cloistered gardens, based on the atria of ancient Roman villas. Scented herbs for medicinal and culinary purposes were cultivated, such as bay laurel, basil, sage, clary sage, lavender, dill, thyme, rosemary, valerian, chamomile, pennyroyal, spearmint and peppermint (Morris 1984). At that time they were not cultivated specifically for their fragrance – that came later, at the beginning of European perfumery. Most of these have herbaceous odours, and we will be exploring many of them in this chapter. Typical herbaceous scents are those of sweet marjoram, rosemary and thyme of the large Lamiaceae family. This family is also known as the Labiateae, and it is often referred to as the 'mint' family. Many essential oil-bearing plants are found in the Lamiaceae; it is one of the ten largest families, comprising some 3200 species of herbs and shrubs. Members of the Lamiaceae are distinguished by their flowers, which have discrete, gaping lips – hence the term *labiate* and the old family name. In many cases the leaves are highly aromatic; the volatile oil is found in glandular trichomes, which are cells or glandular 'hairs' mainly located on the leaves.

There is another botanical family that contain herbaceous-scented species. This is the Asteraceae (also called the Compositae), which is the 'daisy' family. Here we find aromatics such as mugwort, wormwood and tarragon and chamomile.

Herbal bouquets

Several of the above species are included in herbal bouquets which are ritually blessed in churches in Poland on 15 August, Assumption Day. This tradition arises from early days in Poland, where life was strongly tied to the seasons and agricultural activities. Many ritual acts were carried out to ensure the wellbeing of the farms, ensure fertility of the crops and protect against magical or evil influences. When Christianity was introduced to southern Europe in the late tenth to early eleventh centuries, it amalgamated with the older pagan traditions, but it seems that the religious use of plants was linked with the Catholic holidays. Plants were blessed on several days, including Palm Sunday, but the largest number was blessed on 15 August, when herbs and cereals were collected from the wild and the fields, assembled into bouquets and taken to the churches. Most of the herbs included in the bouquets are medicinal or apotropaic (Łuczaj 2011).

Basil

The genus name for basil is *Ocimum*, of the Lamiaceae family. Several species have ritual, culinary, therapeutic and medicinal significance, such as *O. basilicum*, *O. gratissimum* and *O. sanctum*.

O. basilicum is the familiar culinary herb known simply as 'basil'. It is closely associated with Italian cuisine, and well regarded for its ability to complement the flavour of tomatoes; it is also prevalent in North African, Greek and French cuisines. The name 'basil' is derived from *basileus*, the Greek word for 'king', and *basilikon*, meaning 'royal'. This derivation has led to speculation that it might have been thought of as the 'king of herbs' or used in royal medicines, probably as a digestive aid. The herbalist Parkinson considered that its smell was 'fit for a king's house', but also linked it with a superstition that connected basil with scorpions, saying that 'being gently handled it gave a pleasant smell, but being hardly rung and bruised would breed scorpions. It is also observed that scorpions doe much rest and abide under these pots and vessels wherein basil is planted' (Grieve 1992, p.87). Culpeper even supported the notion that smelling basil would breed a scorpion in the brain – perhaps not as strange as it sounds when the prevalent belief dictated that smells carried diseases, and some said that the name was derived from *basilisk*, a mythical, lizard-like creature that could kill with a glance...

Looking back in time, several varieties of basil have important and symbolic associations. Grieve (1992) tells us that in Persia, Malaysia and Egypt basil was scattered on graves and resting places, but that in ancient Greece it represented misfortune. Both the Greeks and Romans also believed that if the plant was badly treated it would flourish, going as far as shouting abuse at the seeds at planting time. It was also observed that basil would not flourish near rue, which was thought to be an 'enemy to poison'; now we can explain this as allelopathy. Despite this slightly sinister reputation, basil also acquired a reputation for promoting bonds between humans; in Moldavia there is a tradition that a young man will love a maiden if he accepts her offering of a sprig of basil, and in Italy it was regarded as a token of love. This theme is explored in Keats' writings, when he tells Boccaccio's tale of 'Isabella, or the Pot of Basil'. This story was part of the *Decameron*, a mediaeval allegory set in Italy at the time of the Black Death. Keats' adaptation tells the story of Isabella, whose family was planning her marriage to 'some high noble and his olive trees', but she falls in love with Lorenzo, who works for her brothers. When the brothers learn of this, they murder Lorenzo. However, his ghost speaks to Isabella in a dream, so she exhumes his body, and his head is planted in a pot of basil. Isabella tends this pot, as she pines away. As well as the representation of love, this also associates basil with final resting places.

Basil was grown in English herb gardens for culinary and medicinal use; it was used to treat nervous and digestive disorders and for its pleasing scent. Basil was added to sweeten washing waters, and it was included in nosegays; it was also a popular strewing herb.

Basil essential oil has a herbal top note, a sweet anisic herbal middle note, and a faint, warm dryout, but this depends on the variety and source. European basil, dominated by the light, woody floral linalool is typical, but the Comoran or 'exotic' basil contains a higher proportion of the phenolic ether called estragole, which has a sweet, herbaceous and anisic odour. The linalool or European basil is preferred in aromatherapy, because the estragole type has been associated with toxicity; it can only be used with caution but has useful antispasmodic and analgesic properties. The main uses of basil are as a stimulating, cephalic oil, useful for stress, and stress-related muscular pains and digestive problems.

Tulsi

Ocimum sanctum is native to Indo-China. It is often called holy basil, *tulasi* or *tulsi*. It has an aromatic, herbaceous, sweet, clove-like scent, partly due to the presence of eugenol and estragole, depending on the variety. Some varieties have a characteristic cassis (blackcurrant bud) note, due to the presence of a trace constituent (Kaiser 2006). There is also a lemon-scented (citral) variety. In India, tulsi is well loved and venerated; Hindu literature contains many legends about this plant. Tulsi is found in every market; it is planted in gardens and kept in homes, not only to sweeten the air, but also for spiritual protection. Tulsi is sacred to some Hindu deities such as Krishna and Vishnu, and also Lakshmi, the wife of Vishnu, and it is often planted near temples and courtyards to purify the air and invite divine presence. Many species of basil, including sweet and holy basil, are also used for their smoke. This practice takes place in countries such as Tanzania, Kenya, Uganda, West and South Africa, and one of the main uses is to drive away insects, especially mosquitoes, and to keep evil spirits at bay (Pennacchio *et al.* 2010).

The fresh, herbaceous, penetrating basil note can be found in fougère fragrances (Williams 2000), as in the top notes of *Azzaro pour Homme* (Azzaro), and Yves Saint Laurent's *Jazz* (Glöss 1995), and also in balsamic complexes (Jouhar 1991). In the original *Oscar de la Renta*, a basil and ylang ylang accord formed a bridge between the fresh citrus top notes and the sweet floral heart (Calkin and Jellinek 1994).

Hyssop

Hyssopus officinalis of the Lamiaceae family is commonly known as hyssop. The name comes from the ancient Greek *azob*, meaning 'holy herb'. Although it is no longer widely used, it was of significance in ancient times. Dioscorides tells us that it was used for cleaning sacred places; and hyssop is, for some, irrevocably associated with cleansing and purification. In the Bible it was the herb of David, who said, 'purge me with hyssop and I shall be clean; wash me, and I shall be whiter than snow.' As a purification herb, it was used for cleansing those with leprosy and their homes, and later it was used in the consecration of Westminster Abbey. In mediaeval times hyssop was a strewing herb and used in nosegays, and the fresh herb and its infusion and oil became a common household remedy.

The herb is highly aromatic, and its flowering tops were traditionally used in infusions for various ills, but particularly for the respiratory system (Gordon 1980; Grieve 1992). Hyssop flowers are very attractive to butterflies and bees, and hyssop honey was very highly regarded, so it was often grown in herb gardens and flower borders. Its essential oil has a strong, sweet, camphoraceous, warm, spicy odour (Williams 2000).

Hyssop essential oil, despite its good expectorant and mucolytic properties, is not widely used in aromatherapy because of numerous contraindications – the oil is moderately toxic, and has the potential to cause convulsions due to the presence of the ketones pinocamphone and *iso*-pinocamphone. Hyssop is one of the principal botanicals in Green Chartreuse liqueur. It is said that in 1605 a manuscript containing the recipe for an 'elixir of life' was given to Henri IV of France. This had been devised by monks with the intention of producing a medicinal liqueur, based on 130 botanicals and flowers in an alcoholic base. It was named 'Green Chartreuse' because of the chlorophyll extracted from the botanicals (Tonutti and Liddle 2010).

Lavender

Of all of the herbs in the Lamiaceae, lavender is probably the most popular, especially with regard to its scent. In fact, there are several species in the genus

Lavandula that have played a significant role in wellbeing, and these are the true lavender (*L. angustifolia*, *L. officinalis* or *L. vera*), French lavender (*L. stoechas*), spike lavender (*L. spica*), and the hybrid lavandin (*L.* x *intermedia*). The lavenders are aromatic, evergreen, woody shrubs, native to the Mediterranean coast, but they are now cultivated all over Europe, especially in France and Spain, and in other parts of the world such as Tasmania, for their essential oil.

Lavender gets its name from the Latin *lavare*, meaning 'to wash'. This comes from ancient Rome, when bathing water was scented with lavender. Like hyssop, lavender has acquired an association with cleansing, but perhaps on a more material plane. Like cardamom, lavender was also dedicated to Hecate, and her sorceress daughters Medea and Circe and, like many of the aromatic herbs, it was used to avert 'the evil eye' (Gordon 1980).

It was the fragrance of lavender that influenced its early uses. St Hildegard (1098–1179 CE) was a German writer, philosopher, mystic and Benedictine Abbess. Her holistic stance on healing, inspired by the natural world, has endured through her writings. She wrote *Physica* ('Natural Sciences') and *Causae et Curae* ('Causes and Cures'), and in this work she praised lavender above all other herbs. In in a chapter entitled '*De Lavendula*' she made specific reference to its scent, and this could be seen as indicative of its early popularity. According to Gordon (1980), in 1579 William Langham published *The Garden of Health*, where we can see that many uses were ascribed to the scent of lavender, such as comforting and clearing the head and sight, comforting the heart, reducing giddiness, and adding it to wine to temper its effects. Dried lavender was used to stuff cushions, apparently enjoyed by Charles VI of France, and during the Stuart period[1] in England lavender was being used with other flowers and herbs as ingredients for scenting bathwater; Parkinson (1567–1650) noted that lavender was used to perfume linen, clothing, gloves and shoes, and that the dried flowers brought comfort and could 'dry up the nature of a cold brain', and Gerard (1545–1611) suggested that it helped migraine, faintness and the 'panting and passion of the heart' (Gordon 1980, p.102). As might be expected, lavender was also a good strewing herb, used in houses and churches to prevent the plague. By the end of the fourteenth century lavender was being cultivated in the south of France for the nascent perfume industry, and lavender water was being used in *Hungary Water*, and also on its own in *Lavender Water*. In the eighteenth century it was being grown in Mitcham in England to produce essential oil for the House of Yardley's *English Lavender Water* – one of the few essential oil crops that can be grown successfully in Britain. However, the main area for growing aromatic crops for essential oils was the south of France. The First World War had a deleterious effect on the essential oil industry. The chemist and perfumer René-Maurice Gattefossé of the respected Gattefossé family had resurrected and reorganised the ailing essential oil crop growing and essential oil production industry in the south

---

1   The Stuart period (1603–1714) refers to the reign of the Scottish Stuarts, beginning with James I of England or VI of Scotland.

of France (Gattefossé 1992), and he was responsible for the modern approach to using essential oils for therapeutic purposes. Gattefossé called this *aromathérapie*. Lavender essential oil was one of the first to be investigated in this respect, and in 1991 Buchbauer *et al.* published the paper 'Aromatherapy: Evidence for sedative effects of the essential oil of lavender after inhalation.' Although aromatherapy was already becoming popular in the UK and English-speaking countries, this was a welcome piece of research that helped to substantiate the use of lavender as a sedative, relaxing scent. In aromatherapy true lavender is regarded as the most versatile essential oil, in terms of its therapeutic actions, and one can't help thinking that St Hildegard wouldn't be surprised!

There are significant differences in the different species and varieties of lavender. The true lavenders hybridise easily (they can interbreed within the genus), and this has given rise to many subspecies or varieties, such as *delphinensis*.

True lavender

True lavender essential oils have a herbal, slightly 'fruity', slightly floral, woody odour. The lavender from France, sold as '40/42' is typical. The '40/42' refers to its ester (linalyl acetate) content. Linalyl acetate can be present at anywhere between 36 per cent and 53 per cent (Price and Price 2007). High altitude French lavender, sold as '50/52' is also available, and in this a distinctive fruity 'pear drops' ester note is present. Linalyl acetate, along with *l*-linalool, may contribute to lavender's sedative effect on mice and humans (Buchbauer *et al.* 1991, 1993). Lavender absolute is bright green in colour and has an odour that is very similar to the plant, although more intense – sweet and herbaceous, with a green floral character and hay-like undertones.

True lavender essential oil is perhaps best known for its sedative, calming and mood-enhancing effects, evidenced in several studies on humans (Ludvigson and Rottman 1989; Diego *et al.* 1998; Moss *et al.* 2003; Lehrner *et al.* 2005). An animal study (Shen *et al.* 2005a) explored the effects of inhalation of lavender essential oil and isolated linalool on lipolysis (breakdown of fats), heat production and appetite. The results suggested that lavender, by virtue of its relaxing, stress-reducing action, also could also result in decreased lipolysis, increased appetite and thus weight gain. Price and Price (2007) noted that lavender is analgesic, anti-inflammatory, antispasmodic and cicatrising – key properties that determine lavender's broad spectrum of applications. However, Baumann (2007) did point out that lavender might just have a 'dark side', because a study (Prashar, Locke and Evans 2004) indicated that it might be toxic to endothelial cells and fibroblasts (found in the skin), and so, despite its undoubted therapeutic properties, lavender might not be the best choice in phytocosmeceuticals designed to combat skin aging.

Spike lavender

Spike lavender is obtained from *L. latifolia*, which is also known as *L. spica*, and it has a subspecies named *fragrans*. This essential oil has a very different aroma – it is lavender-like, but more camphoraceous, and lacks the soft, fruity notes of true lavender. This reflects its chemistry; although it contains linalool, it has almost equal amounts of 1,8-cineole, and camphor as a minor constituent. So, as its aroma might suggest, it is a much more stimulating oil, and useful for clearing the head, respiratory congestion and muscular aches and pains.

French lavender

L. stoechas yields an essential oil known in the trade as 'French lavender'. This is a smaller shrub than true lavender, and its flowers have a different form too – they are small, violet, and terminate in a tuft of brightly coloured leaflets. It gets its species name from the islands where it was abundant in ancient times, known to the Romans as the Stoechades, and now called the Hyères, a group of four islands off the coast of Hyère in the Var region of southeast France. For this reason, Grieve (1992) suggests that this was the lavender of classical times. In Spain and Portugal it was used for strewing the floors of churches and homes on festive occasions, and to make fires on St John's Day, when evil spirits were around. According to old Scandinavian and Slavic folk lore, this was the night when witches and demons were allowed to roam the earth. St John the Baptist's feast day was at midsummer, coinciding with the summer solstice and older pagan celebrations. Typically, the fires would be lit on hills at dusk, and allowed to burn until midnight.

L. stoechas was also an ingredient of the 'four thieves' vinegar' of the Middle Ages. (This concoction has its roots in Marseilles or Toulouse, where four thieves were robbing plague victims, without succumbing to the disease. They were caught, and revealed their secret recipe, which contained lavender, thyme, rosemary and garlic in vinegar.)

Apart from this, lavender had its own folk medicine uses, such as for healing wounds and as an expectorant and antispasmodic. The essential oil is more camphoraceous than that of true lavender, and it also contains an irritant ketone named fenchone; this limits its use in aromatherapy. *L. stoechas* is used in Unani Tibb medicine for brain disorders such as epilepsy; Zaidia *et al.* (2009) conducted an animal study which indicated that *L. stoechas* essential oil has anti-convulsant activity, which they attributed to its linalool, pinene and linalyl acetate content.

Lavandula x *intermedia*

The hybrid *Lavandula* x *intermedia* is a cross between true lavender and spike lavender; it yields an essential oil called lavandin. Its essential oil has a scent that is less 'fruity/pear drops' than high altitude true lavender, but not as penetrating and camphoraceous as spike lavender. Depending on the source, the essential oil contains moderate amounts of the dominant constituents of its 'parents' – *l*-linalool, linalyl acetate, camphor and 1,8-cineole. Like spike lavender, it is a useful mucolytic and expectorant and has analgesic potential, and it is more stimulating than true lavender. It is used to fragrance low-cost products and detergents.

Turin and Sanchez (2009) maintain that the best lavender fragrance is Caldey Island's *Lavender*, with Turin suggesting that 'lavender is summer wind made smell, and the best lavender compositions are, in my opinion, the ones from which other elements are absent, and only endlessly blue daylight air remains' (p.350). It would appear that the monks of Caldey Island in South Wales and the freelance perfumer Hugo Collumbien have achieved just this.

Lavender will also be found in colognes, lavender waters, fougères, chypres, ambers and floral perfumes (Jouhar 1991), including in the top notes of *Jazz* (Yves Saint Laurent) and in an accord with anise in the top note of Calvin Klein's *Calvin*; in the fresh, dry, herbaceous top note of Azzaro's *Azzaro pour Homme* and in the top note of the Houbigant's classic *Fougère Royale* (Glöss 1995).

Mint

Mentha is the mint genus, and within this there are many species and subspecies because, like lavender, the mints can easily hybridise. The best known species are spearmint (*M. viridis*) and peppermint (*M.* x *piperita*); we will also explore *M. pulegium*, which is commonly known as pennyroyal. The genus was given its name by Theophrastus, with reference to the Greek myth of *Minthe*. Minthe lived by the River Cocytus, which flowed into the River Acheron. She was a water nymph who was in love with Hades (or Pluto), the god of the Underworld. Persephone, Hades' consort, who had herself been abducted and forced to spend the winter months in the Underworld, found Hades and Minthe in a compromising position by the banks of the Acheron. In a jealous rage she transformed Minthe into a small, inconspicuous plant, so that no one would notice her and she would be trodden upon. Hades offered her comfort by giving her a distinctive scent.

In the light of this myth, it is poignant that mint was used from early times as a strewing herb, which would release its fragrance when crushed underfoot. Mint was also used as a culinary herb, and in traditional medicine the mints were digestive aids and used to alleviate pains. The mints all have fresh, penetrating odours, but no tenacity, and imperceptible dryouts. Many of them are important culinary herbs, and their main commercial use is in the flavour industry, or for the isolation of natural menthol, with only small amounts being used in fragrance.

Spearmint

Spearmint was, and remains, the most popular of the mints for culinary and flavouring purposes. It is native to the Mediterranean, and so was used by the Greeks and Romans, and is mentioned in ancient scriptures. The ancient Greeks, like the Arabs, would perfume the entire body, using specific scents on different body parts; and spearmint was used to fragrance the arms. It was also used in bathing water. In ancient Rome its flavour was greatly appreciated. Pliny the Elder said that 'the smell of mint does stir up the mind and the taste to a greedy desire of meat' (Grieve 1992, p.533). From this we can see that it had cephalic actions and was an appetite stimulant – and it is used in aromatherapy today for these same reasons. Spearmint was also used to scour food serving boards before their presentation to honoured guests. This was inspired by tale in Ovid's *Metamorphoses* of Philemon and Baucis, a couple who were noble, generous and kind, despite living their lives in poverty. Jupiter (the Roman equivalent of Zeus) did not believe that any mortals could be so good, and was considering punishing mankind. So he donned a disguise as a poor man, and with Mercury (Hermes to the ancient Greeks) paid a visit to their neighbourhood. As they expected, all the inhabitants turned them away – except for Philemon and Baucis, who made them very welcome, sharing what little they had. The wine pitcher never became empty, and the couple realised that they were in the presence of gods. As a reward, Jupiter granted them their desire – to live together as temple priests until they died together. At their death they were transformed into intertwined trees: she was transformed into the linden and he into the oak. This story suggested that everyone should be treated well, because you never knew when you would find yourself in the presence of a god – hence the use of spearmint at the table when entertaining guests. It was woven into garlands to be worn at feasts, and it decorated dining tables. It was also used to flavour wines and sauces, and it was believed that spearmint could prevent milk from turning sour. Spearmint was also valued as currency; the Pharisees (a social movement among Jews between 140 and 37 BCE) used mint, anise and cumin to pay tithes.

The Romans introduced spearmint to Britain, where it thrived in the damp climate, and it was certainly cultivated in the cloistered gardens in the ninth century. The early herbalists such as Turner (his *Herball* was published in 1568), Gerard and Parkinson all held spearmint in high esteem, making particular comment that its fragrance played a role in wellbeing. Grieve quotes Gerard: 'the smell rejoiceth the heart of a man, for which they used to strew it in chambers and places of recreation, pleasure and repose, where feasts and banquets are made' (1992, p.533). This mirrors ancient practices, exploiting the herb's refreshing scent and ability to stimulate the appetite and aid digestion. Later, Culpeper reinforced its cephalic effects, saying that the smell of spearmint was 'comfortable for the head and memory', whilst adding to its medicinal attributes. He suggested that it should form part of a tonic for 'delicate and consumptive young women'; his suggested treatment also incorporated a daily breakfast of a new laid egg, beaten with a large tablespoon of rum, a little shredded spearmint and a cup of new milk, to be consumed in the field with the milk-maid, with the added benefit of the morning air (Gordon 1980). Spearmint also acquired a reputation for being an effective breath freshener, and today it is the most popular flavour for chewing gum. Grieve (1992) makes reference to the observation that mice dislike the smell of spearmint, so it was used as a deterrent of mice. She also relates that mice love henbane (a toxic herb that was used medicinally, as an entheogen, in ritual, and as an apotropaic) and suggests planting spearmint between rows of cultivated henbane to reduce losses.

Spearmint essential oil has a sweet, warm, herbal and minty top note, a sweet, typically minty body, and no dryout (Williams 2000). Its main chemical constituent is *l*-carvone. Carvone is a ketone that has two 'chiral forms' – two molecules that are mirror images of each other. The *d*-carvone molecule has the odour of caraway, while the *l*-carvone molecule smells minty. Carvone is not toxic (Tisserand and Balacs 1995), and so, for children, spearmint is often thought to be a better option than peppermint (Lawless 1992).

In perfumery spearmint is used in soap perfumery for minty notes (Williams 2000), and can be used to impart 'lift and greenness' (Morris 1984). For example, in *Paul Smith London for Men* (Paul Smith) mint forms an accord with violet leaf, and in Davidoff's *Cool Water* it plays a part in the fresh, green, spicy top note. Spearmint specifically (rather than 'mint') is mentioned as a minor player in the herbaceous, fresh green top note of Chanel's *Egoïste Platinum* (Glöss 1995). Turin discusses the use of mint as a top note in Cartier's *Roadster*. Mint is a difficult scent to work with, because of its association with toothpaste, and the menthol note is cooling and fleeting. In *Roadster*, the top notes have an 'arresting freshness'. Shiso mint is an Asian mint, and this used in Heeley's *Menthe Fraîche* (Turin and Sanchez 2009, p.470), and paired with pandanus in Aftelier's *Shiso* (see also pandanus on page 318).

Peppermint

Peppermint is a hybrid species – a cross between spearmint and watermint (*M. aquatica*). It was cultivated in ancient Egypt and in Iceland in the thirteenth century – it is mentioned in their pharmacopoeias (Grieve 1992), but did not really gain popularity in western Europe until the eighteenth century. Peppermint is closely associated with England, especially Mitcham in Surrey, which was renowned for peppermint cultivation for essential oil.

Its essential oil varies in odour according to its source, but typically it has a strong, fresh, minty, green odour. Menthol is the main constituent, along with menthone – a ketone associated with effects on mucosal secretions and wound healing (Bowles 2003). The menthol content is responsible for the cooling effect when peppermint is applied to the skin.

In aromatherapy, peppermint has a long list of indications, but it is probably used most as an expectorant/mucolytic, for itching, nerve pain (especially migraine, neuralgia and sciatica) and digestive dysfunctions such as nausea, colic and irritable bowel syndrome (IBS). Research has substantiated some of these applications. For example, Gobel *et al.* (1995) conducted a double-blind, placebo-controlled study to investigate the effects of peppermint and eucalyptus essential oils on headache mechanisms. It was shown that a 10 per cent preparation of peppermint applied to the forehead and temples had a marked analgesic effect in relation to headache. Davies, Harding and Baranowski (2002) reported a case study of a patient suffering from intractable pain, thought to be due to an 'irritable nociceptor' pathophysiology. Peppermint essential oil (applied neat) was a very successful and quick-acting treatment for this type of neuropathic pain. Regarding its effects on IBS, a double-blind, placebo-controlled study (Cappello *et al.* 2007) demonstrated that peppermint oil, in enteric coated capsules, reduced the symptoms by 50 per cent in 75 per cent of the test group, compared with 38 per cent of the placebo group. In aromatherapy, peppermint oil is contraindicated for babies and young children as it can cause reflex apnoea, or laryngospasm (Tester-Dalderup 1980, cited in Price and Price 2007). Caution is also suggested with high doses, as this could cause sleep disturbance and skin irritation.

Peppermint oil is also used as a source to extract menthol; however, the field or 'corn' mint, *M. arvensis*, is more commonly cultivated for this purpose, as it has a much higher concentration of menthol – up to 95 per cent. This species is native to and grown in Japan, especially Hokkaido, Okayama and Hiroshima. Two varieties are known – Akamaru and Aomaru. The cornmint is collected in September, tied in bundles and hung up to dry for three weeks. The dried herb is then steam-distilled, and the crude distillate is put in metal containers at freezing temperatures. This causes the menthol to crystallise. Solid crystals of menthol also form on the surface of the distillate. The odour of menthol is very pungent, refreshing and typically peppermint-like. In Japan, it has acquired a cultural status similar to camphor.

Watermint

M. aquatica, watermint, one of the 'parents' of peppermint, deserves a brief mention. This is a very common species, generally thriving in wet habitats. Pliny mentions a 'wild mint' known to the Romans as *menastrum*, a name used for watermint in the fourteenth century. It had medicinal applications, but was not nearly as widely used as spearmint or indeed peppermint. It has a scent very similar to pennyroyal (Grieve 1992).

Pennyroyal

Pennyroyal, or *M. pulegium*, has a fresh, minty-herbaceous odour that is stronger and harsher that that of the other mints (Morris 1984). The Romans called it *pulegium* because it would repel fleas. It is the smallest of the mints and, like watermint, it thrives in damp ground. The herb was widely used, not for culinary purposes, on account of its pungent and disagreeable flavour, but to treat a wide variety of ills; Pliny listed 25 pennyroyal remedies (Gordon 1980), including those for purifying the blood, for flatulence, indigestion, colic, the common cold, delayed menstruation and gout (Lawless 1992). However, pennyroyal essential oil is toxic; it contains 55–95 per cent of a ketone called *d*-pulegone, and so it is not used in aromatherapy (Tisserand and Balacs 1995), and its flavour use is limited in some countries and banned in others (Morris 1984).

Díaz-Maroto *et al.* (2007) investigated the composition and olfactory profile of pennyroyal essential oil. They reported that pulegone itself had an intense mint, balsamic and pungent odour; while its isomer, *iso*-pulegone and piperitol, both with intense minty notes, also contributed to the characteristic pennyroyal aroma. They also suggested that the presence of 1,8-cineole added balsamic and eucalyptus-like notes, and small amounts of limonene, along with the aldehydes octanal and nonanal, added lemon notes. The spicy, thyme-like facet was due to carvacrol, a phenol, and its isomer, thymol. Their comments on the herbaceous element are interesting; they suggest that this might be due to the specific herb, and in the case of pennyroyal it might be due to hexanal and iso-pulegol. Fruity notes were contributed by β-damascenone, methyl-2-methylbutanoate and ethyl-3-methylbutanoate. The methodology of this study could have wider applications, and the analysis of pennyroyal has certainly revealed the importance of the individual constituents' contribution to the odour profile, but also the fact that it is their combinations that give a plant its aromatic signature. As we will see when investigating olfactory art (see Appendix D), the same applies to fragrance construction.

Origanum species

There are many species of *Origanum* that are strongly aromatic and have culinary and medicinal uses. They are native to the Mediterranean region, Asia and North Africa. There is often confusion over marjoram *O. majorana* and oregano *O. vulgare* because of the various species that are known by these names, and we even find 'marjoram' and 'oregano' herbs in the *Thymus* genus. For example, 'Spanish oregano' is in fact a species of thyme – *T. capitatus*. Genuine *Origanum* species include *O. vulgare* or common oregano, which has many varieties such as the subspecies *O. glandulosum* (the African variety), *O. virens* (of Morocco) and *O. heracleoticum* (of Greece, also known as winter marjoram). To complicate matters further, cultivated species go under names such as *O. onites* (pot marjoram); *O. majorana* was known in earlier times as knotted marjoram.

Sweet marjoram

What we now call sweet marjoram (*O. majorana*), was known to the ancient Egyptians, Greeks and Romans. According to the Greeks, marjoram was created by Aphrodite, and they called it 'joy of the mountains'. It was an ingredient in a tenacious perfume named after the ancient Roman word for marjoram – *Amaracinum*. Later Theophrastus wrote about *Amaracinum*, commenting that it was made from sweet marjoram roots, and stained pink with the flowers. The Romans clearly enjoyed the scent of sweet marjoram; it appears in several formulae for perfumes and unguents, and both the Greeks and Romans used marjoram to 'crown' young married couples, perhaps because of the connection with Aphrodite. In ancient Rome both marjoram and oregano (*O. vulgare*) were used as culinary herbs – especially in meat sauces.

Later, in mediaeval Europe, marjoram was a strewing herb, and used to polish furniture.[2] The fresh herb was to be found in nosegays and posies, and the dried herb in potpourri and in pillows to encourage sleep, and also to scent the winding sheets for the deceased. It was said that if marjoram grew over a grave, the deceased person was content. Marjoram was used in mediaeval cooking too, especially in

---

2   Some herbs, such as sweet marjoram and lemon balm, would simply be bunched and rubbed over wooden furniture, where their oils would impregnate the wood and leave a fresh scent.

bastings and 'dredgings' for joints of roasted meat. Before the advent of hops, marjoram was used in brewing to give bitter flavour to beer and ale (Gordon 1980); the dried herb and its extracts were used to flavour various foods, especially soups and sauces, including *shashlik* sauces ('*shashlik*' or '*shashlyk*' means skewered meat, a type of *shish kebab*, a popular dish in Eastern Europe, India, Mongolia, Morocco, Pakistan and Israel), and also liqueurs, vermouths and bitters (Baranauskiene, Venskutonis and Demyttenaere 2005).

Gordon suggests that oregano was the type used medicinally. However, Grieve (1992) states that their uses are similar.

Most commercially available essential oil is from the dried, flowering sweet marjoram; this has a warm herbal, camphoraceous, spicy scent that varies according to origins, which are usually France, Tunisia and Morocco (Lawless 1992; Williams 2000). Jouhar (1991) suggests that it is also tenacious, and reminiscent of nutmeg and mint. Myrcene, *para*-cymene, terpinen-4-ol and α-terpineol are typical components, some of which have analgesic properties (Bowles 2003), and this is one of the main uses of sweet marjoram in aromatherapy; it is also used to relax and promote sleep, along with lavender. Nutmeg and mint are also regarded as pain relieving, and so can complement sweet marjoram in this respect, as well as in odour. Although the scent of marjoram was favoured in ancient times, it is less popular in contemporary perfumery. It is used occasionally in herbal-spicy fragrances (Jouhar 1991; Williams 2000).

Oregano

Common oregano (*O. vulgare*), according to Lawless (1992), was the 'true' oregano of the herb garden, with an ancient reputation as a medicine for digestive complaints, respiratory problems and throat inflammation. Its essential oil has a camphoraceous, herbal top note, and a herbal, phenolic, woody middle and dryout (Williams 2000). The phenolic note gives a clue as to its chemistry, which is very different from that of sweet marjoram. It is dominated by carvacrol and thymol – strongly antiseptic phenols – with the capacity to irritate the skin. Lawless states that oregano oil is a dermal toxin, and for this reason it is contraindicated in aromatherapy, although it is found occasionally as a minor ingredient in fragrances such as in the dry, floral spicy heart of Yves Saint Laurent's *Jazz* and in the original *Silvestre* (Victor), playing a role in the spicy, resinous middle notes (Glöss 1995).

Rosemary

Rosmarinus officinalis is a strongly aromatic perennial shrubby herb with small, tough, linear evergreen leaves, and small pale blue flowers, native to the Mediterranean coast. The genus name translates as 'dew of the sea' (from *ros* meaning 'dew' and *mare* meaning 'the sea'), because the plant is often seen glittering with dew near the seashore.

Since ancient times, rosemary has been associated with improving the memory. In Greek mythology the Muses were the nine daughters of Zeus and Mnemosyne (her name means 'memory'). Their role was to act as inspiration and prompters of the memory for poets, writers, artists and musicians; and they are sometimes depicted holding sprigs of rosemary. Minerva, the Roman goddess of knowledge, wisdom and crafting was also associated with rosemary. According Spanish folk lore, when the Virgin Mary was fleeing from Herod's soldiers, she took shelter under a rosemary bush, hanging her blue cloak over it. When she removed the cloak, the white flowers had turned blue; and this gives another perspective on the derivation of its name – the 'Rose of Mary'. In Spain and Italy rosemary was thought to protect against witchcraft; in Sicily it was believed that young fairies took the form of little snakes and lay amongst its branches. In time, influenced by myths and folk legends, rosemary became a symbol of fidelity, and was entwined in scented bridal wreaths, while branches of rosemary, entwined with silk ribbons, were given to wedding guests. It also came to symbolise remembrance, and sprigs would be carried by mourners at funerals and cast on the coffin once it had been lowered into the grave (Gordon 1980; Grieve 1992).

Rosemary also had an impressive array of other properties. An eleventh-century Anglo-Saxon herbal mentions its use as a culinary and medicinal herb; it was one of the earliest herbs to be cultivated in monastery gardens; it was a bee-plant, a strewing herb, an insect repellent (it made insects and moths less 'merrie') and prevented bad dreams. Gerard advocated the wearing of a garland of rosemary around the neck to guard against the 'stuffing of the head and a cold braine' (Gordon 1980, p.147), while Culpeper suggested that it could be smoked in a pipe to help with respiratory problems, and that an ointment made from the leaves would alleviate 'cold benumbed joints'. Rosemary was also used in early colognes, along with lavender, and in cosmetic preparations to preserve beauty. Gordon (1980) suggests that the virtues of rosemary were perfectly summed up by William Langham in his 1579 work, *The Garden of Health*: 'Seethe much Rosemary, and bathe therein to make thee lusty, lively, joyfull, likeing, and youngly' (p.147).

Is there any foundation for the association of rosemary with memory, and its early therapeutic uses based on that? Contemporary research would suggest that there is. Studies have revealed that rosemary promotes alertness, although the effect is short-lived; that it can improve speed and accuracy in math tasks, and that its profile is similar to the effects of oxygen administration and the acute administration of ginseng (Diego *et al.* 1998; Moss *et al.* 2003).

In 2011 Dobetsberger and Buchbauer published a review of the effects of essential oils on the nervous system. They suggested that claims that oils which are often described as stimulating and activating and as enhancing cognitive functions, vigour and alertness – especially rosemary, peppermint, eucalyptus and jasmine – were supported by recent research. Additionally, the studies cited in that paper supported the established aromatherapeutic uses of these oils in conjunction with transdermal absorption and massage. Dobetsberger and Buchbauer's (2011) review of current research into essential oils and their actions on the nervous system mentioned that self-administered abdominal massage with rosemary oil can increase attentiveness, alertness, liveliness and joyfulness, while increasing breathing rate and blood pressure. It is quite striking how these words echo Langham's early observations about the effects of rosemary. Its pain-relieving property has also been demonstrated in several studies (Takakai *et al.* 2008).

In the Lamiaceae family there is potential for hybridisation between members of the same genus, as we have already seen in the cases of lavender, mint and marjoram; rosemary is no exception. There are several cultivated varieties, which give rise to essential oils with differing chemistry – these are called chemotypes. The ones that have applications in aromatic medicine and aromatherapy are CT 1,8-cineole (Tunisia), CT verbenone (France) and CT camphor (Spain). A 'typical' rosemary essential oil has strong, fresh, herbal, resinous top notes, and a herbal, woody, balsamic middle note with a dry herbal dryout (Williams 2000). Depending on the chemotype, it is dominated by 1,8-cineole or camphor (the verbenone type is rare), and this will affect the cineolic and camphoraceous aspect of the aroma. The other dominant constituent is α-pinene (Bowles 2003).

In perfumery, rosemary is often paired with lavender in colognes; it was included in Farina's first cologne. Caron's *Pour un Homme* has a classic accord of lavender, rosemary, bergamot and lemon providing the top notes, over a lavender heart and a vanillic, sweet, powdery base (Glöss 1995). Morris (1984) suggests that rosemary 'provides healthy, sportive and clean notes', but because it is distinctive, sharp and penetrating, and also inextricably associated with Italian and French cooking, its use requires skill.

Sage species and clary sage

In the *Tabula Salerni*,[3] there is a proverb: *Cur moritur cui Salvia crescit in horto?* This translates as 'Why should he die who has sage in his garden?' and refers to a species of sage known as *Salvia fruticosa* (Gali-Muhtasib, Hilan and Khater 2000). This Roman saying reflects the belief that sage conferred immortality. *Salvia*, the name of the genus, is from the Latin *salvere*, which means 'to be saved', and in past times the plant was referred to as 'sage the saviour', alluding to its healing properties. In the ancient Salerno school of medicine it was said that '*Salvia salvatrix, natura concilatrix*' – 'Salvia is a cure with a calming effect' (Valnet 1982, p.180). It is said that Louis XIV of France trusted sage more than his physician, and drank a cup of sage infusion every morning.

There are many *Salvia* species with both medicinal and culinary traditions of use. In folk medicine, they have been used to treat many ills, and especially for helping maintain and restore health, protect against infection, relieve pain, aid digestion and

---

3   The *Tabula Salerni* was a wax tablet of the Schola Medica Salernitana – the world's first medical school at Salerno in Campanula, Italy. It was founded on the site of a ninth-century monastery dispensary, and was hugely influential between the tenth and thirteenth centuries.

treat menstrual problems and infertility. Gali-Muhtasib *et al.* (2000) cite numerous modern studies that have elucidated *Salvia* species' therapeutic and medicinal potentials as antimicrobial agents, as spasmolytics and hypotensives, antioxidants and anti-inflammatories, for prolonging sleep, and treating Alzheimer's disease. Cabo *et al.* (1987) suggested that there were three broad types of sage, based on their dominant constituents: Group I consists of species characterised by α- and β-thujone; Group II by linalool and linalyl acetate; and Group III by 1,8-cineole and camphor (Gali-Muhtasib *et al.* 2000).

Sage is hardy, and has been cultivated in many countries for hundreds of years.

Most species have been of value in human health and wellbeing. However, as we will discover, one particular species, *S. divinorum*, has distinctive psychotropic effects, and *S. sclarea*, or clary sage, although it has the potential to cause mischief, has, overall, had a very positive impact on human wellbeing. We will begin by looking at the common sage and its history.

Common sage

Salvia officinalis is the common sage, native to the northern Mediterranean; it grows wild along the coast from Spain up to the eastern Adriatic, and on the mountains of Croatia.

To explore what lies behind its reputation for healing mind, body and spirit, we need to look at what the early herbalists wrote. Dioscorides maintained that sage was good for the liver and to make blood; it was a diuretic, and of use in consumption, for headaches due to cold rheumatic humours, joint pains, coughs, serpent bites and the plague. He also mentioned its ability to 'help the memory, warming and quickening the senses' (Grieve 1992, p.704). Gerard noted that it was 'singularly good for the head and the brain', that it stimulated the senses and the memory. On the physical level, sage strengthened the sinews, cured palsy and trembling, and was effective against serpent bites. It is still widely used in herbal medicine. In Italian folk medicine, sage is eaten to maintain good health – and it has a very long tradition of culinary use. Early recipes included traditional stuffing for duck, geese and pork, also sage and onion sauce and sage cheese. It is still widely used in Mediterranean and British cooking.

Sage essential oil, sometimes referred to as 'Dalmatian sage' on account of its original geographical origins, is derived from the leaves, and has a strong, sweet, herbal, camphoraceous odour (Williams 2000). The essential oil is dominated by α-thujone, β-thujone and camphor, so it belongs in Group I. These constituents are neurotoxic ketones, which requires that in aromatherapy it is used only very sparingly, if at all. Tisserand and Balacs (1995) state, 'the usual thujone content is sufficiently high to warrant its exclusion from aromatherapy.' Abuse of Group I and III *Salvia* species can lead to hypoglycaemia, epileptic reactions, loss of balance, tachycardia, muscle cramps and breathing difficulties – all toxic reactions due mainly to the thujones and camphor.

Salvia libanotica

The East Mediterranean sage, *Salvia libanotica*, is a popular plant remedy used in the Middle East to treat colds and abdominal pain. It has a very long history of use, since as early as 1400 BCE, and some of its common names are sage apple, *khokh barri* and *na'ama*. It was probably introduced to the region by the Greek colonists in the sixth century BCE, and is widely used in Lebanon, Syria, Palestine, Crete, Cyprus, Turkey, Greece, the south of Italy and Sicily. This species was formerly known as *S. triloba* because of its leaves, which have the appearance of three lobes, and it is sometimes still called Greek or Cretan sage. Nowadays it is estimated that most of the imported sage in the United States is *S. libanotica* rather than *S. officinalis*. In Lebanon both oil and water extracts are used internally, and externally to heal fractures, and it is widely thought that if it does not bring benefit, neither will it cause any harm. In Lebanon, Syria and Jordan, herbal practitioners regard it as a panacea, but its notable uses include treating headaches, sore throats and abdominal pains, and treating depression, as a tranquiliser and sedative. *Salvia libanotica*'s essential oil is characteristically camphor-like, and bitter, and it is dominated by 1,8-cineole and camphor (Gali-Muhtasib *et al.* 2000), rather than thujone, so it belongs in Group III.

Spanish sage

In 2003 Perry *et al.* conducted a pilot study to investigate whether Spanish sage (*Salvia lavandulaefolia*), could be used for dementia therapy. This was an open-label study, which involved giving oral doses to patients with Alzheimer's disease, and as such was not free from practice effects or expectations. However, overall there was a reduction in neuropsychiatric symptoms and an improvement in attention, and it was concluded that *S. lavandulaefolia* has pharmacological actions relevant to dementia therapy, and does not carry side effects – a recognised problem with conventional treatments. The potential ability of *Salvia lavandulaefolia* to improve cognition and protect against cognitive decline was investigated by Kennedy *et al.* (2010). The essential oil is dominated by camphor and 1,8-cineole, placing it in Group III, but some oils also contain significant amounts of limonene and pinene (Lawless 1992). The study by Kennedy *et al.* followed a preliminary *in vitro* investigation, and was a double-blind, placebo-controlled, balanced cross-over study that examined the cognitive/mood effects of a single oral dose of the extract in the essential oil. It was demonstrated that the extract improved both mood and cognitive performance in healthy young adults, and that it could be a potential treatment for dementia and the elderly; so this study certainly substantiates the use of sage to enhance cognitive ability.

Sardinian sage

The Sardinian sage (*Salvia desoleana*) was the subject of a study to explore its antifungal activity. Sokoviç *et al.* (2009) investigated this species indigenous to Sardinia, where it is used in folk medicine to treat menstrual, central nervous system and digestive disorders, much like the traditional uses of other sage species. Recognising the importance of finding medicinal compounds in therapeutic herbs, they focused on its antifungal potential because of the increasing number of fungal infections (especially in immunocompromised individuals) and the difficulty in treating these. First, they established that the main constituents were linalyl acetate, α-terpinyl acetate, linalool and 1,8-cineole; this places the Sardinian sage in Group II, and with lower toxicity than the other species discussed thus far. They observed a correlation between the chemical structure of the essential oil constituents and the antifungal activity – it certainly appeared that the chemical structure of the constituents affected the potency of each compound. However, what the study revealed was that the complete essential oil of *S. desoleana* was more effective than any of its individual components against all of the fungal pathogens tested; indeed, it had strong antifungal activity. This was explained by the synergistic activity of all of the components in the oil.

Salvia divinorum

In Mexico there are over 270 species of sage. According to Hanson (2010), one of these is the comparatively rare *Salvia divinorum*, found in the Oaxaca region of Mexico. It is known to the Mazatec people as *hojas* (leaves) or *hojas de la Pastora*, or *ska de la Maria Pastora*. It is possible that this is the species known to the Aztecs as *pipiltzintzintlithis*. Its fresh leaves are chewed, or made into an infusion and swallowed, or the dried leaves are smoked by shamans to induce hallucinations and trance during ritual and healing ceremonies (Hanson 2010). It is also used to treat a semi-magical condition called *panzón de barrego*, or swollen belly, believed to be caused by a curse from an evil sorcerer (Prisinzano 2005). The Mazatec consider that it is important to use only leaves that are free of insect damage. The effects are short-lived, lasting for up to an hour. Since the mid-1990s it has also been used as a recreational drug, and as such has been abused; it is now illegal in 13 nations, and 15 states within the USA.

Salvinorum A is a powerful hallucinogen; as little as 200μg to 1mg is enough to provoke a response. Roth *et al.* (2002) demonstrated that it binds to the κ-opioid (kappa-opioid) receptor in the brain, and this discovery stimulated further investigation. (The drugs known as opioids, which have a morphine-like action on the central nervous system, are mediated by four receptor families, designated μ, κ, σ and δ. These receptor families are distinguished by the drugs which bind to them and the responses those drugs produce.) Salvinorum A is different from other opioids in that it does not contain nitrogen, and its carbon skeleton and functional groups are different; broadly speaking, it is a diterpenoid with a neoclerodane carbon skeleton; and *S. divinorum* is the only botanical source of a hallucinogenic neoclerodane (Hanson 2010). Other classic hallucinogens such as LSD, psilocybin, dimethyltryptamine (DMT) and mescaline are active at the 5-HT_{2A} serotonin receptor, but salvinorum A shows no activity at this site (Roth *et al.* 2002, cited in Johnson *et al.* 2011).

Typically, recreational users smoke the dried leaves, or leaf extracts with enhanced salvinorum A concentration, or use tinctures for buccal administration; occasionally it is used via volatilisation. Its use is widespread; in 2006 it was estimated that at least 1.8 million people age 12 or older had used the drug in the USA, and most users reported that its effects are short-lived and are followed by positive effects such as increased insight and improved mood (Baggott *et al.* 2010, cited in Johnson *et al.* 2011). However, adverse effects have been reported, such as neurologic, cardiovascular and gastrointestinal effects. In a few cases, extended psychotic-type reactions have been experienced – but these were concurrent with the use of other drugs, and possible schizophrenic dispositions. Johnson *et al.* (2011) conducted a double-blind, placebo-controlled study of salvinorum A in four psychologically and physically healthy hallucinogen-using adults. The subjects inhaled volatilised salvinorum A, in increasing doses, randomly interspersed with placebo doses, in comfortable and supportive surroundings. It was found that the participants experienced changes in spatial orientation, and unusual and sometimes recurring effects such as revisiting childhood memories, cartoon-like imagery, and contact with entities. The experiences happened quickly after administration and lasted no longer than 20 minutes; there were no significant increases in heart rate or blood pressure, and there were no tremors. Johnson *et al.* concluded that inhaled salvinorum A was 'physiologically safe and psychologically well tolerated across the range of doses tested' (p.152) and that it 'occasioned a unique profile of subjective effects having similarities to classical hallucinogens, including mystical-type effects' (p.154). The case of *S. divinorum* reflects what Saniotis (2010) highlights as the western penchant for 'pathologising drugs', even those that have been used by 'indigenous and traditional peoples' foraging and usage habits of psychotropic and mood-altering substances' (Sullivan and Hagen 2002, cited in Saniotis 2010, p.480).

Clary sage

Clary sage, *Salvia sclarea*, and its close relatives *S. verbenaca* (wild English clary) and *S. praetensis* have an impressive and colourful past. Its name comes from its earlier folk name, 'clear eye'. If its seeds are put in water they form mucilage, which can be placed under the eyelids where it envelops any small irritating particles. The old herbalists called it *Oculus Christi*, meaning 'Christ's Eye'; however, Culpeper considered this blasphemous. Early culinary uses were clary leaf fritters; the leaves were dipped in a batter and fried, then served with meat. Clary wines were also popular, and allegedly had narcotic properties; the powdered seeds were added to wine to 'provoke lust' (Gordon 1980). Grieve (1992) explains that the wine merchants of Germany first used clary in wine – as an adulterant. It was infused with elderflowers and added to Rhenish wine to make it resemble muscatel, so that in Germany clary sage became known as *muskateller Salbei*, or 'muscatel sage'. In Britain it was also used as a substitute for hops in brewing ale and beer. This practice resulted in beer with intoxicating qualities, consumption of which was followed by a severe headache. Grieve quotes Lobel:

Some brewers of Ale and Beere doe put it into their drinke to make it more heady, fit to please drunkards, who thereby, according to their several dispositions, become either dead drunke, or foolish drunke, or madde drunke. (p.706)

Besides its potential to enhance the inebriating qualities of ale, clary sage also had some notable therapeutic properties. Clary infusion (and when added to beer) was used to treat 'women's diseases and ailments', and also digestive disorders and colic.

After World War I, the Gattefossé family was responsible for establishing clary sage as an essential oil crop in the South of France.

Clary sage essential oil has very distinctive odour. Williams (2000) describes it as having a sweet, herbal top note, a warm, herbal, tobacco-like middle with a warm, balsamic dryout. The dominant constituents are very similar to those of lavender – linalool and linalyl acetate. Therefore clary belongs in Group II. However, clary is complex, with over 250 constituents identified. It also contains an unusual constituent – sclareol, a diterpene alcohol. This is a comparatively large molecule, and molecules of this size are not common in essential oils, as they are often too big, and insufficiently volatile, to distil over into the essential oil. Sclareol is present at up to 7 per cent (Price and Price 2007). Its molecular structure resembles oestradiol, and it has been suggested that this is responsible for its 'oestrogenic' effects, although there is no evidence for this (Bowles 2003). Its scent is also able to bring about a state of euphoria, or high spirits. In 2010 Seol *et al.* conducted an animal study to examine the antidepressant effects of several essential oils, and demonstrated that of all the oils tested, clary sage, at a 5 per cent concentration, had the strongest antistressor effect, probably by modulating dopamine activities. They suggest that clary sage could be developed as a therapeutic medication for depression. This is another example of modern research throwing light on traditional uses of aromatics, and shows how we might in future harness clary's euphoric nature safely, effectively, and without a hangover!

Clary sage absolute is used in perfumery as a fixative and for imparting distinctive sweet, light, herbal, woody notes and warmth to fragrances. It can be used in a wide range of fragrance types, from chypre and fougère to orientals (Lawless 2009). Jouhar (1991) comments that clary absolute is subtle and long-lasting, and that the scent of the concrete resembles ambergris. Clary sage is dominant in the fresh, herbaceous top note of Hermès' *Equipage*, a spicy oriental with smoky, woody accords (Glöss 1995). Clary sage forms an accord with geranium, rose, carnation, anise and orris in the middle note of *Tuscany per Uomo Forte* (Aramis), and again with carnation and geranium in Rabanne's *Paco Rabanne pour Homme* (Glöss 1995); Turin and Sanchez (2009) discuss this citrus, woody fragrance, commenting that the 1973 version was the first of the aromatic fougères, a trend that developed and includes *Azzaro pour Homme* (Azzaro), *Rive Gauche pour Homme* (Yves Saint Laurent), *Yohji Homme* (a discontinued liquorice fougère by Yohji Yamamoto), *Or Black* (Pascal Morabito) and *Drakkar Noir* (Laroche).

Thyme

Thyme belongs to the genus *Thymus*, a large genus of over 100 species and varieties, in the Lamiaceae family. These include the common thyme (*T. vulgaris*), wild thyme (*T. serpyllum*), Moroccan thyme (*T. saturoides*) and Spanish thyme (*T. zygis*); we also have *T. capitatus*, known as Spanish oreganum, and *T. mastichina*, or Spanish marjoram (Soulier 1995). Thyme is a tough perennial herb, with tiny, dark green leaves. It is thought that what we now know as common or garden thyme is derived from the wild thyme that is native to the mountainous regions of Spain and the Mediterranean.

Early civilisations used thyme not so much as a culinary herb but for its scent and smoke – the genus name is derived from the Greek word *thymon* or *thuein*, which meant 'to make a burnt offering'. The Latin for thyme was *thymum*, and the old French word was *thym*. Its fragrance would certainly suggest that it was used as incense in early times. Evidence of this can be found in Virgil's *Georgics*, where it was used as an antiseptic fumigant, and Pliny the Elder suggested that burning thyme 'puts to flight all venomous creatures' (Grieve 1992, p.809). On the other hand, it is possible that the name comes from the Greek *thumus* (or *thymus*), a word that meant 'courage'. In those days thyme was considered to inspire invigoration. Thyme was a sacred herb of the Druids, who used it to lift the spirits and dispel negativity. The expression 'to smell of thyme' was a compliment, and thyme became a symbol of bravery and energy; mediaeval knights would wear an emblem of a bee and a sprig of thyme. In 1931, when *The Modern Herbal* was first published, Grieve (1992) noted that in the south of France wild thyme was a symbol of extreme Republicanism, and that tufts were sent with the summons to Republican meetings. It is also said that before going into battle, the Highland Scots would drink a beverage made from thyme to confer courage; wild thyme is the emblem of the Drummond clan. The wild thyme appears in other Scottish traditions. The folk ballad 'Wild Mountain Thyme' (Francis McPeake) is essentially a love song, containing the line 'wild mountain thyme grows among the Scottish heather' – perhaps an indirect reference to the custom for young women to wear a sprig of thyme, mint and lavender to attract a suitor. In folklore the thyme plant was the fairies' playground, and often a patch of thyme would be left undisturbed for their use. In Shakespeare's *A Midsummer Night's Dream* Oberon, the king of the fairies, says, 'I know a bank whereon the wild thyme grows,' referring to the bed of thyme on which the fairy queen Titania slept. The fairy association with thyme was notable; thyme was the main ingredient in a seventeenth-century recipe for a magic brew to help people to see fairies.

Bees are attracted to thyme, and it has long been noted that thyme honey is exceptional. In ancient times Mount Hymettus near Athens was covered in wild thyme, and the honey from this region was said to be the sweetest, so thyme became associated with sweetness too. Pliny commented that if thyme was blooming and abundant, the honey would be good (Gordon 1980; Grieve 1992).

Evidence of the use of *Thymus* species as a fumigant and incense can be found all over the globe. *Satar farsi* (*T. linearis*) is used in Nepal, *livantis* (the wild thyme of Cyprus, *T. integer*) is burned as a disinfectant, the garden thyme of Ethiopia (*T. schiperi*) is used as a condiment, and its infusion and smoke are used to treat gonorrhoea, cough and liver disease. The smoke of wild thyme (*T. serpyllum*) was used by the inhabitants of the Ubage Valley in the Alps de Haute-Provence in France as an antiseptic and to treat foot-and-mouth disease (Pennacchio *et al.* 2010). However, it is not just the smoke that has antiseptic qualities; through this and other practices, such as using thyme as a strewing herb, thyme became useful in the context of traditional herbal medicine too. Here we see many uses; infusions were used for excessive menstruation, aches and pains, while oil of thyme was used for sore throats and breathing disorders. Gerard recommended thyme for curing sciatica and headaches, and also for leprosy and 'falling sickness'. Culpeper said:

> It is a noble strengthener of the lungs, as notable a one that grows, nor is there a better remedy growing for whooping cough. It purgeth the body of phlegm and is an excellent remedy for shortness of breath. It is so harmless that you need not fear the use of it. (Grieve 1992, p.182)

Although thyme was not originally an important culinary herb, this did change, and it became widely used in the cuisines of all of the regions where it grew, especially as a preserver of meat.

According to Martí *et al.* (2007), in eastern Spain *Thymus piperella* is used mainly for flavouring stuffing, sauces, pickles, stews and soups, and to conserve and soften olives. It is also used in a distilled alcoholic beverage named *herbero*; this is known in the south of Valencia and north of Alicante, where it is well regarded as a digestive aid. In their investigation of its essential oil, Martí *et al.* found it to be non-toxic, and to have antispasmodic properties; this would help explain its use in the treatment of gastrointestinal disorders, such as diarrhoea. It also has antimicrobial activity; hence its use in preserving olives (and this also suggests that it would be of value in treating the intestinal infections that cause diarrhoea). So this species is not just of value as a culinary herb; but as such it may well be contributing to health in other ways.

Thyme has been cultivated as a decorative plant, and many cultivated varieties ('cultivars') are available. It is also grown for its essential oil, but, as might be expected, thyme oils vary widely in chemical composition and scent. In 1725 Neuiuiann, a German apothecary, isolated thymol from thyme essential oil. Thymol is a powerful antiseptic.

Common thyme essential oil is distilled from the fresh or partially dried leaves and flowering tops of the herb (Lawless 1992). The first distillate is red in colour and cloudy in appearance, and this is called 'red thyme oil'. It can be filtered and redistilled to produce 'white thyme oil'. Both have a sharp, warm, spicy herbal odour;

but white thyme has a sweeter top note. The linalool and geraniol chemotypes have softer, gentler, sweeter aromas, albeit with thyme's distinctive herbal signature.

In aromatic medicine and contemporary aromatherapy, several *T. vulgaris* chemotypes are available, including CT thymol, carvacrol, linalool and geraniol, named after their dominant constituents. From a safety point of view, oils with a high content of the phenols thymol and carvacrol are dermal irritants and strong mucous membrane irritants (Tisserand and Balacs 1995) and must be used with caution. This includes evaporation and inhalation, because of their capacity to irritate the mucous membranes of the respiratory tract.

Thyme is considered to be stimulating oil, useful for muscular aches and pains, respiratory congestion, coughs, debility and fatigue. It is also one of the best antibacterial essential oils.

Thyme absolute is also available, and this has a warm, herbal, woody aroma. In perfumery it can impart 'Mediterranean sunshine and body' (Lawless 2009, p.78).

Most of the typically herbaceous fragrances are in the Lamiaceae, but a few of importance are in the Asteraceae – *Artemisia* species and Roman chamomile.

Artemisia species

There are several notable aromatic *Artemisia* species: mugwort, wormwood, southernwood and tarragon. The genus is named after Artemis, the Greek goddess of the hunt (her Roman equivalent is Diana); she is often portrayed as carrying a bow and arrows. She was the daughter of Zeus and Leto, and, like her brother Apollo, she could send plagues and sudden death to mortals, but she was also the protector of young children and animals. Artemis is also associated with chastity and childbirth. Grieve (1992) elaborates on the name, quoting from the early work by Apuleius, the *Herbarium*:

> Of these worts that we name Artemisia, it is said that Diana did find them and delivered their powers and leechdom to Chiron the Centaur, who first from these worts set forth a leechdom, and he named these worts from the name of Diana, Artemis, that is Artemisias. (p.858)

Chiron represents the 'wounded healer'. Most of the aromatic *Artemisia* species are shrouded in superstition, and make fascinating study. Some of their more colourful associations are highlighted below, because these often give an insight into the underlying nature of the plants and their scents. The artemisias are known as bitter herbs. Bitters stimulate the taste receptors at the back of the tongue, and this has a priming effect on the digestive system. In folk and traditional medicine, bitters were used as tonics and to stimulate digestion and thus promote good health; the practice of adding bitter herbs to alcoholic beverages to be taken before meals gave rise to the drinks known as *aperitifs*.

Some *Artemisia* oils are used occasionally in perfumery, and quite often there are references to '*armoise*', the French word for artemisia, which is used to describe the oil of *A. vulgaris*. The common mugwort yields a bright green oil with a cineole-like odour (Jouhar 1991), which Lawless (1992) describes as colourless or pale yellow with a powerful, camphoraceous, bitter-sweet, herbaceous odour (p.134). The artemisia note is present in masculine chypre/leathery fragrances and Caron's *Yatagan*, a woody oriental launched in 1976, which also has wormwood in its top note; in Guerlain's *Derby*, released in 1985; and in the top note of *Aramis* (Aramis), which was composed by Bernard Chant (best known for *Cabochard*) (Grès 1959). Ralph Lauren's *Polo* is characterised by its patchouli/mossy/woody accord, but artemisia is paired with juniper berry in its herbaceous green top note. Serge Lutens' *Douce-Amère* opens with an absinthe theme, and tarragon is in the floral fougère masculine fragrance *Xeryus* (Givenchy) – a typical, somewhat 'loud' fragrance of the mid 1980s (Glöss 1995; Turin and Sanchez 2009).

Mugwort

Taking our cue from Apuleius, we will look first at mugwort. In fact there are two species that go by this common name – *Artemisia vulgaris* is the common mugwort, and *A. arborescens* is the great mugwort. It is sometimes known as armoise or wild wormwood. Mugwort is a common plant in many parts of Britain, and it closely resembles wormwood; the distinguishing feature is that its leaves are fluffy and white on the undersides only, and the leaf segments are pointed, not blunt as in wormwood. Before the use of hops, the flowering tops of mugwort would be dried and boiled with malt liquor, and this would be added to beer – so the common name is derived from 'mug', the drinking vessel. However, Grieve (1992) suggested that its name could also have been derived from the word *moughte*, a moth or maggot, because it was used as a moth repellent.

During the Middle Ages mugwort was known as *Cingulum Sancti Johannis*, reflecting the belief that St John the Baptist wore a girdle of mugwort when he was in the wilderness. This gave rise to many superstitions. Mugwort would protect the traveller from fatigue, sunstroke, wild animals and evil spirits, and it was worn on St John's Eve for protection from the evil that wandered the earth on that night. For this reason, in Germany and Holland, it is called St John's plant, and is gathered especially on his feast day. It has been used as a culinary herb – in parts of Europe it was used to flavour roast goose. In folk medicine its leaves and roots are used as a stimulant and nerve tonic; it was valued for palsy and hysteria, and 'quaking of the sinews'. It was also used to reduce fever, but its main use was as an emmenagogue, to bring on menstruation – reflecting Artemis' associations with both chastity and childbirth.

The common mugwort and its close relatives, *A. moxa* and *A. sinensis* (which are dominated by a constituent known as borneol), are used in an ancient form of acupuncture called *moxibustion*. For this the fluffy tissue on the underside of the leaves is dried and compressed, and formed into sticks; when lit and left to smoulder, the heat and smoke are held over meridians and specific points. This practice originated in the Ming Dynasty of China (1368–1644 BCE). Mugwort smoke was used for numbness and paralysis, eliminating worms, for treating skin problems such as acne, sores, toothache, dysentery, and for prolapse of the anus (Pennacchio *et al.* 2010).

Mugwort essential oils can be obtained from the leaves and flowering tops of both types, but they contain large amounts of thujone, a toxic ketone, and so they are not used in aromatherapy (Tisserand and Balacs 1995).

Wormwood

Wormwood, *Artemisia absinthium*, is a perennial herb with silver grey-green leaves covered on both sides with fine, white, silky hairs. It too is native to Europe, and has been widely cultivated. Ancient cultures believed that it was a powerful remedy that would counteract hemlock and toadstool poisoning, as well as 'the biting of the sea dragon'. Grieve (1992) suggests that it is one of the bitterest herbs known, second only to rue. In the Bible, King Solomon warns his son about a seductress: 'The lips of a strange woman drop as a honeycomb...but her end is as bitter as wormwood' (Gordon 1980, p.194). It was used in brewing instead of hops, and also figured in old love spells and charms. Grieve (1992) gives instructions for an old love charm that had to be prepared on St Luke's Day, consisting of marigold flowers, a sprig of marjoram, thyme and wormwood. These had to be dried before a fire, powdered, sifted and then simmered over a low fire along with virgin honey and vinegar. This was then used to anoint the individual before retiring, while repeating three times the lines 'St Luke, St Luke, be kind to me, in dreams let me my true love see' (p.859).

Medicinally, as its name suggests, the main use of wormwood was as a vermifuge – to help expel intestinal worms; but, like mugwort, it also had a role in preventing fleas, moths and insects. Bunches of wormwood were hung in homes for this purpose. It was observed that other medicinal herbs would not grow in the vicinity of wormwood, and now we know that this is an example of allelopathy. Wormwood was also recognised as an antiseptic – in 1760 a rumour that the plague had broken out in St Thomas's Hospital in London caused the price of wormwood to soar by 40 per cent. Other uses included appetite stimulation, insomnia, scurvy and, according to Culpeper, 'the hypochondriacle disorders of sedentary men'. Wormwood liniments were used for sprains and strains (Gordon 1980; Grieve 1992).

Wormwood has been added to alcoholic beverages for centuries. It was steeped in wine, which was taken before and after alcohol consumption to lessen its effects. The dark green oil of wormwood was used to make *purl*, an infusion made with ale or beer; this was favoured by seasoned drinkers as a morning tipple. In Scotland, whisky distillers used its seeds. Certain botanicals are important in the class of alcoholic beverages known as vermouths, and these are angelica, cinnamon, clove, coriander, dittany of Crete, marjoram, wormwood, mugwort and summer savory – all medicinal plants. In Europe, the legal definition of vermouth makes it obligatory for it to contain an aromatic *Artemisia* species – *A. absinthium* and *A. pontica* are the main species used. Because these are bitters they can, by reflex action, increase gastric secretions and stimulate the appetite; as a result of this, vermouths are considered to be aperitifs and are often consumed neat, or with water, or in cocktails. The cocktail ingredient 'Angostura bitters' contains *Galipea cusparia* extract to give a very high level of bitterness, and the beverage known as 'Campari' of Turin in Italy is probably the most bitter product on the market (Tonutti and Liddle 2010).

The most infamous aperitif of all time is probably absinthe. It was wormwood, which was included for its beneficial digestive effects, that was largely responsible for its reputation and downfall, resulting in a complete ban on its production in the early part of the twentieth century, until its subsequent reformulation and reintroduction much later in the century.

Absinthe was a pale green aperitif, with a very high alcohol content and an aniseed flavour; like pastis, it becomes cloudy when water is added. It was made with several botanicals including aniseed and wormwood. It had a strong and bitter flavour, and its consumption acquired paraphernalia such as special pierced spoons. These were designed to hold lumps of sugar over the absinthe glass, over which the water was poured. Absinthe reached its height of popularity with the artists, writers and actors, including Henri Toulouse Lautrec and Vincent van Gogh, who frequented Parisian cafés in the late nineteenth century. It was popularly called *la fée verte*, 'the green fairy', and the cafés introduced the concept of *l'heure verte* – 'the green hour'. Some of its drinkers believed that it heightened artistic awareness and aided sexual prowess, so its popularity grew, despite the adverse psychotropic effects of excessive consumption. Chronic abuse resulted in a syndrome named 'absinthism', which encompassed depression, psychosis and madness. The most dramatic example is that of van Gogh (1853–1890), who cut off his ear during a psychotic episode at Arles. (However, this was not due solely to absinthe. Based on his descriptions of his illness, he possibly suffered from temporal lobe epilepsy and manic depression, and so his severe mood swings would have been aggravated by absinthe, brandy, nicotine and turpentine; see Morrant 1993, cited in Tonutti and Liddle 2010.) In the early part of the twentieth century absinthe was banned because of its deleterious effects on individuals and society.

Originally the neurotoxic effects of absinthe were blamed on α- and β-thujones – the main constituents of wormwood essential oil. In 1993 Turner suggested that the thujone molecule shares some structural similarities with tetrahydrocannabinol (THC), found in cannabis, giving it the potential to cause psychotropic effects. Later Balacs (1998/1999) commented on a report in the *New England Journal of Medicine* concerning a case of wormwood poisoning. He suggested that α-thujone in the essential oil could interact with the same receptors in the brain as δ-9-tetrahydrocannabinol. However, a more recent investigation of three samples of absinthe – authentic pre-1915, post-ban 1915–1988 and modern commercial absinthe – suggested that 'absinthism' was due to the excessive use of alcohol, rather than its thujone content, which in this case was reported as β-thujone (Lachenmeier 2008, cited in Dobetsberger and Buchbauer 2011). Tonutti and Liddle (2010) note that the current version of absinthe, advertised as being 'of premium quality,' is made by distillation, has an alcoholic strength of at least 45 per cent volume, and must not contain artificial colours. The thujone content is limited by European and other regulations, as is the case with all vermouths.

Although it may seem that wormwood is the *bête noire* of the aromatic world, recent research has suggested that it might have a therapeutic role. Lachenmeier (2010) reported that studies have revealed potential medical uses for wormwood – including the treatment of Crohn's disease – and that it might even have neuroprotective effects that could be harnessed in the treatment of strokes. It is emphasised, however, that a thorough risk–benefit analysis is conducted, should the therapeutic dose exceed the current threshold dose set by the European Medicines Agency.

Southernwood

A. abrotanum is the botanical name for southernwood; it is now a familiar garden shrub, but it originally came from southern Europe (indigenous to Spain and Italy). Gordon explains that its name is a contraction of 'southern wormwood'. The species name is of unknown origin. It is an attractive plant, with finely divided, feathery, silver green leaves, and it is strongly aromatic. The ancient Greeks and Romans considered that it had magical properties and protected men against impotence, which led to the practice of placing sprigs of southernwood under the mattress. This reputation remained with southernwood, and inspired some of its folk names such as 'lad's love' and 'maid's ruin', and it was included in love potions, and country bouquets given as gifts but with the ulterior motive of seduction. Southernwood was also called the 'old man of southern Europe'.

It was used medicinally to expel intestinal worms, encourage menstruation and prevent the plague and 'gaol fever'. Parkinson suggested that, if burned, its ashes mixed with oil and rubbed into the face would encourage the growth of a beard in young men; it did not cure baldness, but along with rosemary made a good hair tonic. Its scent was thought to be invigorating, and it was used as a strewing herb. However, it seems that its folk traditions were perhaps more prominent than its medicinal uses.

Southernwood is a good flea and moth deterrent, and was used amongst clothing and linens for this purpose – giving rise to its French name *garderobe*. It was grown in chicken runs, where it was thought to promote good health and prevent mite infestation, as well as discouraging the habit of 'feather picking', which can lead to cannibalistic behaviour. It was also burned as incense – to keep trouble away and to repel snakes. Bees do not like southernwood, so small branches and sprigs were hung at windows and doors to discourage their entry. Perhaps the most charming use, however, was in the May Day custom of gathering dew. Maids would carry little southernwood and lavender brooms, and silver spoons to collect the dew, which was thought to clear and beautify the skin.

Today southernwood is not used in herbalism, except in Germany, where southernwood poultices are used on wounds and to draw out splinters – another traditional use.

Southernwood has a sharp, penetrating, pungent scent; the old varieties have a lemony character, and the more recent, cultivated variety has a more camphoraceous smell. Southernwood is bitter, but less so than wormwood; this quality is due to a sesquiterpene lactone of the 'absinthin' type. An essential oil can be produced, and there are two chemotypes – thujone and 1,8-cineole. The sesquiterpenes davanol, davanone and hydroxydavanone are also characteristic of both chemotypes (Gordon 1980; Grieve 1992; Katzer 2013).

Tarragon

Tarragon, *A. dracunculus*, is a perennial herb native to the south of Europe, and also parts of Asia and Siberia. In Britain it was first cultivated in Tudor gardens. The herb has long, narrow, green leaves, and its roots are coiled like little snakes. The species name *dracunculus* means 'little dragon', perhaps because of the appearance of the roots. Tarragon (*herbe au dragon*) is known as a culinary herb, perhaps best known in French cuisine, where it is present in some classic sauces such as *sauce tartare* and *sauce béarnaise*, and in tarragon vinegar, which was sometimes used to make mustard. Tarragon was said to temper the coolness of other herbs, and it was not included in soups because of its strong, pungent taste.

'Dragon herbs' were believed to cure the bites and stings of venomous beasts and mad dogs. Gerard maintained that if flaxseed was inserted into a radish root, or a sea onion, and planted, tarragon would grow.

There is little information regarding its early medicinal uses, although the leaves were 'heating and drying' and useful for the flux, menstrual problems and digestive problems, and its root was used to cure toothache (Lawless 1992), and John Evelyn said, ''Tis highly cordial and friend to the head, heart and liver' (Grieve 1992, p.792). Lawless (1992) comments that the maharajahs of India enjoyed tarragon tisane, and in Persia it was used to stimulate the appetite.

Its essential oil contains large amounts of estragole (also known as methyl chavicol), leading Tisserand and Balacs (1995) to advise that it should not be used in aromatherapy. However, Schnaubelt (1995) suggests that is it one of the best antispasmodic essential oils and can be used with caution for pain, spasm, and as a respiratory decongestant – which is one of its uses in herbal medicine. Tarragon oil, sometimes called '*estragon*', has a sweet, anisic, spicy-green odour that some have likened to basil – the dried herb loses this character.

Chamomile

According to Grieve (1992), because chamomile had been used by so many cultures, over such a long time, and because no plant was better known to 'country folk', the old herbals agreed that ''tis but lost time and labour to describe it' (p.185). For the sake of those who may be unfamiliar with chamomile, suffice it to say that *Anthemis nobilis* (sometimes called *Chaemamelum nobile*) is a strongly aromatic, low-growing, creeping perennial of the Asteraceae family; it has a grey-green, downy appearance, finely dissected, feathery leaves and small, white, daisy-like flowers. It was known to the ancient Egyptians, who valued it for its healing qualities, the ancient Greeks who observed its apple-like scent and called it *kamai* (ground) *melon* (apple) – hence the alternative genus name – and the Spaniards, who called it *manzanilla* (a little apple), the name also given to a light sherry flavoured with chamomile.

Chamomile is associated very much with England – despite its common name, 'Roman' chamomile. Here, it was one of the most popular strewing herbs because its strong, pleasant scent was released when it was walked upon. Chamomile lawns were popular long before grass was introduced for this purpose, and it would seem that the plant thrives when being compressed; the seats in 'herbares' (arbours) were also covered with chamomile. There was a saying, 'Like a chamomile bed – the more it is trodden, the more it will spread.'

Chamomile was said to symbolise 'patience in adversity'. It is also known as a 'companion plant', and the 'plant's physician' because it is protective of the health of other plants, even helping to prevent the damping off of seedlings in greenhouses. It is a gentle, non-toxic plant, unlike many of the others we have encountered in this family, but, just like southernwood, it seems that it is disliked by bees. There are single and double-flowered forms, and both were used as a tisane to relieve nausea and diarrhoea, and medicinally it was used as a tonic, digestive aid, painkiller and antispasmodic, and for its soothing and sedative effects. It is remains a useful remedy in contemporary herbal medicine (Gordon 1980; Grieve 1992).

Roman chamomile essential oil has a distinctive pale blue colour and a strong, fruity, apple-like herbaceous odour. The scent is intense and diffusive; it has a strong, fruity herbal top, a herbal, fruity, tea-like body and a warm, herbal dryout (Williams 2000). According to Bowles (2003) the essential oil is dominated by non-terpenoid esters such as isobutyl angelate. She cites Pénoël and Franchomme (1990), who state that such esters are especially oriented towards the head and the psyche, with cephalic and psychotropic characteristics.

In aromatherapy Roman chamomile is widely used as an anti-inflammatory, antispasmodic, calming essential oil (Price and Price 2007). Moss *et al.* (2006) demonstrated that the scent of Roman chamomile had a calming, sedating effect and reduced subjective alertness. However, as could be expected, these effects were influenced by induced expectancy. It is used occasionally in perfumery, but in small amounts and mainly in chypre type fragrances (Williams 2000). Calkin and Jellinek (1994), discussing the complex green note in *Fidji* (Guy Laroche 1966), also comment on the relationship between green notes and fruity notes. They suggest that trace amounts of the lower fruity esters can modify the harshness of some green materials; and so essential oils of Roman chamomile, and also basil and tarragon, have a useful modifying effect on powerful green scents, such as galbanum.

Green scents

In the natural aromatic palette, the most obviously 'green' odours are those of galbanum and violet leaf; however, we find an interesting combination of green, fruity and herbaceous types in tagetes, another member of the 'daisy' family, and also in blackcurrant bud.

Galbanum

The exclusively Old World genus *Ferula* of the Umbelliferae family contains around 130 species, growing throughout the Mediterranean to Central Asia; in Iran there are around 30 species, including *F. galbaniflua* (Dehghan *et al.* 2007). Galbanum is a large perennial herb which contains resin ducts. These exude a milky juice – a natural oleoresin as opposed to a pathological secretion – usually at the 'joints' of mature plants. Incisions are made at the base of the stem or at the root, so that the resin will collect there and solidify. Levant galbanum is soft, but Persian galbanum is more solid and hard. According to Grieve (1992), the best 'tears' of galbanum are pale on the outside, about the size of a hazelnut, and when broken open are composed of numerous clear, white tears. The type that is more common, and preferred because of its yield, however, is an agglutinated mass that contains red and white tears. This has a waxy consistency when warmed. Galbanum was widely used by the ancient cultures as incense; the Egyptians used it in embalming and in cosmetics (Lawless 1992).

Several *Ferula* species have been used in traditional medicine, notably as sedatives and for the treatment of digestive disorders, rheumatism and arthritis, headache and toothache (Dehghan *et al.* 2007). In Yemen *F. asafoetida* is known as *haltîda*, and the smoke from the burning resin is passed over the vagina after childbirth to help it contract. In the African American community of Detroit *F. foetida* is known as 'devil's dung' because of its foul smell (and taste), and its smoke is used to alleviate colic in children. *F. communis* is known as the 'giant fennel' (but is not a true fennel) in Bivona in Sicily, where parts of the plant are smoked to expel mucus (Pennacchio *et al.* 2010). So it is apparent that a wide range of therapeutic applications is attributed to *Ferula* species, and that some smell less than pleasant. (However, *F. galbaniflua* has an interesting scent.)

Lawless suggests that galbanum was used in a similar way to asafoetida, namely for treating wounds, inflammations and skin problems, as well as digestive and respiratory disorders. Grieve (1992) mentioned that galbanum was used as a stimulant, expectorant and antispasmodic – making it particularly useful for chronic bronchitis – and also in pill form for treating hysteria. In contemporary aromatherapy galbanum essential oil is indicated in circumstances that reflect its traditional uses – for skin problems, as an analgesic for the musculoskeletal system, and for respiratory complaints.

Galbanum essential oil has a very powerful, fresh, green odour, reminiscent of green bell peppers, or fresh peas in their pods, with maybe a slightly musty character at odds with the freshness. Williams (2000) describes it as having an intensely green, pine-like top note, a green, woody body, and a woody, balsamic dryout. This distinctive green note is partly due to the presence of trace amounts of a nitrogen-containing pyrazine, 2-methoxy-3-I-butylpyrazine (Gimelli 2001) and also undecatriene-3-one, which is also found in yuzu, an oriental citrus fruit (Omori, Nakahara and Umano 2011; see page 342). Galbanum essential oil is dominated by monoterpenes, including the pinenes, which account for the piney characteristics, and limonene.

In perfumery 'galbanol', a deterpenated product, is sometimes used; this does not have such noticeable piney notes. Galbanum resinoid is also employed as a fixative, and as a base note in green fragrances. (Although it is also green in nature, it is earthier.) Both Jouhar (1991) and Lawless (2009) comment that is used in the basis of opopanax perfumes, including those of old Arabic perfumery. Sanchez (in Turin and Sanchez 2009) discusses the nature of galbanum in modern perfumery; she considers it to be radically different from the other green odour types because it has a chalky and bittersweet character, 'reminiscent sometimes of dark chocolate and sometimes of old wood' (p.80). She also comments on its role in some classic fragrances: as a 'March wind' in Balmain's original 1945 *Vent Vert*; as 'the cold shoulder of an ice queen' in Chanel's *No.19*; and to impart a dry and powdery character to Lauder's *Alliage*, the first 'sports fragrance'. Earlier, in 1994, Calkin and Jellinek also wrote about galbanum in *Vent Vert*; originally, it had been combined with geranium in the top note, with both at unusually high levels, and they considered that 'sadly, the extreme character of this beautiful perfume has now been modified so as to appeal to a wider market' (p.134). The 1991 reformulation that Calkin and Jellinek are referring to was carried out because the original contained more than 1100 components; this was reduced to around 30. Turin analyses the demise of the original version, composed by Germaine Cellier, with its galbanum accord on the top, a long-lasting rose and jasmine heart, and a fresh, powdery drydown, and suggests that the second version was less 'symphonic', but it still had charm. However, another reformulation was undertaken in 1999, possibly to cut costs, and resulted in a much diminished, 'linear' fragrance with no relation to the original (Turin and Sanchez 2009).

Another galbanum-containing casualty of reformulation is *Cabochard* (Grès). When launched in 1953, this was a classic leathery chypre, whose top notes, provided by galbanum, armoise and basil, formed interesting relationships with the floral notes in the middle, especially with hyacinth which complemented the galbanum, and also with the leathery base (Calkin and Jellinek 1994).

One notable galbanum-containing fragrance that has survived more or less intact – the green floral *Chanel No.19* – was composed for Gabrielle Chanel (who at the time was in her eighties), by Henri Robert, and launched in 1971 (Turin and Sanchez 2009). Its top note is dominated by galbanum, supported by bergamot, lemon and ylang ylang; and any harshness from galbanum is tempered by amyl acetate (Calkin and Jellinek 1994), a fruity ester – a technique we have already mentioned in relation to *Fidji* on page 259.

Violet leaf

Viola odorata is the sweet violet – a small, delicate perennial that has heart-shaped, downy leaves and large, scented, deep blue or violet flowers. It has a creeping rhizome, and propagates by producing runners. It is native to Europe and parts of Asia, but has been widely cultivated for many years. There are over 200 species in the Violaceae family, such as the scented Parma violet (*V. alba*), the unscented dog violet (*V. canina*), the pansy or heartsease (*V. tricolor*) and *V. canadensis*, which is prolific in North America. The Parma violet will only flourish in a Mediterranean climate.

The name 'violet' is derived from the Greek *ione*. In Greek mythology Zeus was very fond of Io, but his consort Hera was very prone to jealousy. Fearing her wrath concerning the affair, and his concerns for Io's safety, he transformed Io into a white heifer, and to sustain her he caused sweet-scented violets to grow from the earth. Io's name lives on in the violet-scented molecules called 'ionones'. Grieve (1992) mentions Homer and Virgil, who wrote that the Athenians used violets 'to moderate anger, to procure sleep and to comfort and strengthen the heart' (p.835). She also mentions Pliny, who used a liniment of violet for gout and spleen disorders, and maintained that garlands or headdresses of violets could alleviate the effects of wine and prevent headache and dizziness. Paestum, near Salerno in Italy, is possibly best known for its three well-preserved temples, but it was (and still is), notable for its roses and violets. In ancient times these were valued in perfumery as well as medicine, and also for making wine. In the tenth century Apuleius' *Herbarium* mentions that *V. purpureum* was recommended for 'new wounds and eke for old', while Macer's *Herbal* (1552) suggested that violets were effective against 'wicked serpents'. Culpeper said that sweet violet was 'a fine, pleasing plant…of a mild nature, and in no way hurtful' (Potterton 1983, p.196). The leaves contain glucosides, and have had many therapeutic uses over the years, particularly in association with throat and mouth disorders.

Violet leaf concrete and essential oil are produced in the South of France; the absolute has 'an intense, rather unattractive, green and peppery odour' (Jouhar 1991). Like most absolutes, it is chemically very complex; the component that is responsible for the distinctive odour is 2-trans-6-cis-nonadien-1-al (International School of Aromatherapy 1993). In aromatherapy it is used in skin care, and for stress and insomnia and headaches – much like the ancients! However, recent research has revealed that violet leaf absolute may be of use in phytocosmeceuticals for sun-damaged skin and in anti-aging products (Baylac and Racine 2004).

In perfumery the green note is difficult to work with, because of the sheer intensity of naturals such as violet leaf and galbanum. However, violet leaf is used in trace amounts, for example, in typical rose bases (Calkin and Jellinek 1994). Lawless (2009) suggests that it can 'bring ylang absolute down to earth' (p.81), compliments osmanthus and mimosa, and combines well with orris concrete and lavender absolute. According to Morris (1984), its sharp, leafy scent 'adds an unusual vibrato to floral and chypre perfumes' (p.244). The green scent of violet leaf is used in *Eau de Cartier* (Cartier), *Verte Violette* (L'Artisan Parfumeur), *La Violette* (Annick Goutal) and *The Unicorn Spell* (LesNez).

Tagetes

Several species of *Tagetes*, which belongs to the Asteraceae family, have traditional therapeutic and ritual uses. *T. lucida* is known as the sweet marigold, and the ancient Aztec of Mexico used its smoke to dull the senses of prisoners prior to execution. It was also used in religious ceremonies. The Huichol of Mexico mixed its flowers with tobacco, for a hallucinogenic smoke, often accompanied by a maize beer – this was said to induce clearer visions. In parts of Africa, especially Zimbabwe, the smoke of *T. minuta* was used to repel mosquitoes, relieve dizziness and headaches, and for mental illnesses (Pennacchio *et al.* 2010).

T. minuta is known as the Mexican marigold, or sometimes the wild marigold or khaki bush. An essential oil is distilled from the bright orange, daisy-like flowers and flowering tops of this annual herb. The fresh oil is a liquid, which thickens and becomes sticky with age and exposure to the air. The top notes are green and herbal, giving way to a fruity, apple-like, green body, and then a fruity herbal dryout (Williams 2000). The main constituent of this essential oil is a ketone called tagetone, but it also contains furanocoumarins, and these cause phototoxicity. For this reason tagetes oil is not often used in aromatherapy, and its levels are restricted in perfumery.

Williams (2000) commented that it is used to impart apple notes in fragrances. Glöss (1995) lists it as a minor ingredient in some of the floral green fragrances, for example in the fresh, fruity top note of *L'eau d'Issey* (Myake); in the fruity green top note of *Calyx* (Prescriptives); and the fresh, green, fruity top note of *Eau de Givenchy* (Givenchy). Tagetes is also found in ambery oriental fragrances such as *Roma* (Biagiotti), contributing to its fruity green top note. Calkin and Jellinek (1994) discuss the structure of *Obsession* (Calvin Klein), another ambery oriental. Here tagetes is found in the fruity-green and herbal aspects of the top notes, where it brings an apple-like nuance.

Blackcurrant bud

The blackcurrant, *Ribes nigrum*, is native to the British Isles, but is widely distributed. It is cultivated for its berries which are used in jams and jellies and as flavours for icecream, yoghurts and alcoholic drinks. In the Burgundy region of France the bushes are pruned in winter, and an alcoholic tincture is made from the cuttings with dormant buds. When mature, this is used to enhance the flavour of blackcurrant juice. Apart from producing small, dark purple-black berries, blackcurrant is notable for the strong aroma of its leaves and flower buds. Grieve (1992) notes that in Siberia a drink is made of the young leaves which make 'common spirits' resemble brandy. Their infusion resembles green tea, and has cleansing and diuretic properties, while blackcurrant juice and blackcurrant jams and jellies are a folk remedy for sore, inflamed throats. Grieve also comments that goats enjoy the leaves, and bears like the berries.

Solvent extraction of the flower buds yields a concrete and an absolute (Jouhar 1991). The absolute is used in the flavour industry for its intense flavour, and in perfumery. It is a dark green paste with a characteristic strong, diffusive, penetrating odour, and it can be steam-distilled to yield an essential oil which has a similar scent.

In the perfumery industry blackcurrant bud is known as *Bourgeons de cassissier*, or *cassis bourgeons*. It is often described as green, fruity, minty, and even 'catty' (Lawless 2009). This is mainly due to its sesquiterpene constituents and the presence of trace amounts of sulphur compounds, specifically a thiole named 4-methoxy-2-methylbutan-2-thiol. The 'catty' element, for some, is reminiscent of male cat's urine, or the sexually related odour of the male cat. Calkin and Jellinek (1994) discussed the importance of such 'animal' smells in perfumery, and suggest that they may have an unconscious erotic effect.

In perfumery the fruity green notes in blackcurrant bud can be used to modify intense green odours, such as that of galbanum. We have already discussed the case of *Chanel No.19*, where the green notes are tempered by the addition of a fruity ester. Calkin and Jellinek (1994) highlight Jacomo's 1979 fragrance, *Silences*, where blackcurrant bud is used with galbanum to produce 'a perfume of outstanding individuality and beauty'. Guerlain's *Chamade*, composed by Jean Paul Guerlain and launched in 1969, was the first fragrance to use blackcurrant bud in this way. Its top note contains a green note, galbanum and blackcurrant bud accord, with hyacinth to complement the galbanum, and bergamot to reinforce the fruity aspects. *Chamade* is an aldehydic floral, but constructed in a typical Guerlain style, where the fragrance evolves and changes over time. Turin describes how it took him ages to connect the drydown on passers-by with its floral green top note, saying that 'Chamade is perhaps the last fragrance ever to keep its audience waiting so long while props were moved around behind a heavy curtain' (Turin and Sanchez 2009, p.167). Other fragrances that include blackcurrant bud are Van Cleef and Arpel's *First*, composed by Jean-Claude Ellena and launched in 1976, a floral with an animalic nature; and Annick Goutal's *Eau de Charlotte*, launched in 1982, with blackcurrant, mimosa and cacao.

Camphoraceous and cineolic scents

The words 'camphoraceous and cineolic' immediately conjure up an olfactory image of strident, medicinal proportions – perhaps with healthy connotations, but possibly not 'pretty'. However, some of these aromatics have made an enormous contribution to health and wellbeing, and some even have very attractive scents. We will begin by looking at bay laurel and myrtle, before progressing to the eucalypts and paperbarks.

Bay laurel

The bay laurel, *Laurus nobilis*, is a species within a small genus in the Lauraceae family. It is an evergreen tree with a smooth, reddish or olive green bark, sometimes multi-stemmed, and can reach 10–15 metres in height when mature. It has scented wood which is used in marqueterie, aromatic, dark green, glossy leaves, and black berries. The bay laurel is native to the Mediterranean, but will grow in colder climates, although not as vigorously. Bay laurel has already been mentioned in the context of the Elysian Fields of Homer's *Aeneid* (see page 40), and in our exploration of the Delphic Oracle, where it was sacred to Apollo and used by the Pythia in her preparations for prophesy.

The myth behind bay laurel perhaps tells us more about the nature of Apollo than the tree, but it does give some insight as to what the laurel came to signify. Daphne was a nymph, and a daughter of Gaia, the earth goddess. She was pursued by Apollo, who had killed her bridegroom; some versions of the myth also say that his heart had been pierced by one of Cupid's arrows, and so he couldn't help but fall in love with Daphne. She fled from him and, when caught, she asked the gods for help and they changed her into a laurel tree. Apollo then crowned himself with a circle of laurel leaves, and made the tree sacred to his divinity. The bay was therefore used to make garlands, and many depictions of great men of the time are portrayed wearing bay crowns. However, allegedly, Julius Caesar preferred to be crowned with Alexandrian laurel (*Ruscus racemosus*) which has broader leaves, and thus covered more of his bald head (Weiss 1997). A sprig of bay would be carried by soldiers to symbolise victory in battle.

By the Middle Ages a wreath of bay leaves and their berries also signified academic distinction, hence, for example, the English title of 'Poet Laureate'. The title of 'Bachelor' given to university graduates is derived from the Latin *baccalaureus* (berries and laurel). Because, in earlier times, university graduates were forbidden to marry (because it was believed that the duties of a husband and father would detract from their academic work), we still occasionally use the word 'bachelor' to denote an unmarried man. The name of the current continental European academic qualification is the '*baccalaureate*', again directly derived from the Latin (Gordon 1980; Grieve 1992; Weiss 1997).

Bay leaves were used to prevent contagion (according to Theophrastus, they would be held in the mouth as an antiseptic), and also to prevent intoxication. During an outbreak of the plague the Emperor Claudius and his court moved to Laurentium, which was famed for its bay trees, and close to where Pliny the Younger built his holiday villa.

The bay laurel tree was said to confer the gift of prophesy, probably because of the Pythia, and a withering and dying bay laurel tree was taken to be an omen of disaster. In 1629 all the trees at the University of Padua died, and this was said to foreshadow the great plague. In the same year Parkinson published *Paradisius Terrestris*, where he emphasised the importance of the bay tree for God and man, from the cradle to the grave. This heralded the popularity of the bay in Britain, where Culpeper noted that it resisted witchcraft and the many ills it could bring, and it was much used as a strewing herb by the 'wealthier folk'.

Grieve (1992) states that the leaves, berries and oil all have excitant and narcotic properties, and that they can reduce fever. She suggests that large doses, taken internally, can induce vomiting, and that external use is preferable, especially for sprains, strains, bruises and earache. In traditional Iranian medicine, bay laurel leaves are used topically to relieve rheumatic pain. In 2003 an animal study conducted by Sayyah *et al.* (2003) demonstrated that the leaf oil had pain-relieving and anti-inflammatory properties that were comparable with conventional analgesic and non-steroidal anti-inflammatory medications. They also noted that it has mild sedative properties.

Bay leaves are widely used in cooking; they have a sweet, warm, herbal, spicy flavour, and they are an important part of the classic French *bouquet garni*, a combination of a bay leaf, parsley stalks and thyme. Their earliest use was probably in the decoration of the boar's head served at feasts, complete with a lemon or apple stuffed into its mouth, and sprigs of rosemary in its ears…

In bay leaves the warm herbal note is possibly due to (Z)-3-hexenal. Bay laurel essential oil has an odour reminiscent of the leaves, but stronger; according to Williams (2000), it has a fresh, spicy top, a spicy, clove-like, sweet body and a spicy, balsamic dryout. Weiss (1997) also notes its aromatic, camphoraceous/cineolic notes, conferred by the high 1,8-cineole content. He notes that bay laurel is a major ingredient in a Syrian olive oil soap, Aleppo's *sabun bi ghar*, which has been exported for over 500 years. The berries yield an oil too – this is strongly aromatic, and used in combination with the leaf oil, cloves, cinnamon and pimento to make 'bay rum' – a hair tonic and fragrance. However, laurel leaf oil is a potential sensitiser and mucous membrane irritant (Tisserand and Balacs 1995), and according to Lawless (2009), its use is voluntarily restricted by some fragrance houses. Bay laurel leaf absolute is preferred; this has a fresh, warm, green, slightly spicy aroma, and lacks the strong camphoraceous character of the essential oil. Laurel leaf is present in the fresh, spicy herbaceous top notes of Dior's *Jules*, an aromatic fougère; the original version of Rochas' *Monsieur Rochas*, which is a fresh fougère; and in the middle note of Guerlain's oriental spicy *Héritage* (Glöss 1995).

Myrtle

Myrtus communis is a beautiful, fragrant evergreen shrub or tree; the young branches and twigs have a reddish colour, and the aromatic leaves are dark, glossy green. It produces scented, small white or pink flowers and red-blue or violet berries. It grows in Mediterranean regions and North Africa (Weiss 1997). Just as the bay laurel was sacred to Apollo, myrtle was sacred to Aphrodite – the sought-after and promiscuous goddess of desire. She rose, naked, from the foam of the sea – her name means 'foam-born' – and, riding a scallop shell, eventually settled at Paphos in Cyprus. Grasses and flowers sprang up under her feet as she walked, and when she flew she was accompanied by doves and sparrows. The origin of her association with myrtle is not very clear; however, there was certainly a strong connection, because many images and statues of Aphrodite, and her Roman equivalent Venus, portray her with myrtle at her feet. Myrtle was planted in the gardens around the Temples of Aphrodite and Venus.

The theme of myrtle being sacred to gods or important in worship, or appearing in prophesies, recurs across time and cultures. Myrtle was sacred to Shamash, the Babylonian sun god; its wood was used to make booths in the original Feast of Tabernacles, and in the Book of Isaiah in the Old Testament there is the promise of things to come – 'instead of the briar shall come up the myrtle tree' (Isaiah 55:13, King James Version, cited in Morris 1984). To the ancient Persians it was a holy plant, and in ancient Egypt women wore its blossoms together with pomegranate and lotus at festive occasions, while to the Jews it symbolised love and peace (Weiss 1997). Morris (1984) describes the 'Court of the Myrtles' at the Alhambra, and also the gardens of Baghdad, Damascus, Granada, Cordoba and Isfahan, where Myrtle is a well-loved aromatic plant whose crisp, pine-like perfume diffuses in the heat and fills the air. The entire plant is appreciated for it scent and beauty; and even in modern times its symbolism persists, as we can see in the tradition of using myrtle in bridal bouquets. Because of its old associations with Aphrodite and Venus, it was the custom in many Eastern European countries to hold myrtle over a bride's head. Queen Victoria was given a myrtle bouquet by Prince Albert's grandmother, and from this cuttings were taken and planted. From then until the present day, myrtle has featured in the bouquets of English royal brides, including Diana Princess of Wales and, more recently, Kate Middleton, now the Duchess of Cambridge, in 2011.

Myrtle also had medicinal and cosmetic uses. In ancient Egypt it was burnt as a fumigant. Dioscorides prescribed an infusion of myrtle leaves in wine for lung and bladder infections, and it was used when 'drying and binding' actions were required (Lawless 1992). In Europe a sixteenth-century skin care lotion called 'angel's water' was based on myrtle leaves and flowers. According to Bazzali *et al.* (2012), myrtle is known as a medicinal plant for its anti-hyperglycaemic, antiseptic and anti-inflammatory activities, and in folk medicine it is used in the treatment of urinary and respiratory diseases, including bronchitis and sinusitis, and also otitis, diarrhoea and haemorrhoids. It is also an antioxidant. In North Africa, where myrtle is prolific, an extract is made to treat coughs and chest complaints (Weiss 1997), and in southern Italy the leaves and branches are burned in traditional bread ovens to impart their fragrance to the bread (Pennacchio *et al.* 2010). The myrtle is late blooming, and so also important for bees and honey in the latter part of the season.

Myrtle leaf essential oil has a pleasant, fresh, camphoraceous, floral-herbaceous odour, with resinous undertones (Weiss 1997). However, there is a degree of variability in its chemical constituents, depending on its geographical source. A few major components are partially responsible for its odour; these are 1,8-cineole, α-pinene, myrtenyl acetate, limonene and linalool. Other monoterpene acetates such as linalyl acetate, bornyl acetate, terpinyl acetate and geranyl acetate also contribute to the characteristic fragrance. Additionally, four $C_8–C_{10}$ esters were identified by Bazzali *et al.* (2012), and these too contribute significantly to the fruity top note of myrtle essential oil. In particular, 1,8-cineole is associated with expectorant action – and so in aromatherapy myrtle essential oil is used for bronchitis, catarrh, and chronic coughs. It also has applications for skin care, colds and influenza (Lawless 1992). Schnaubelt (1999) suggests that it can be used with cypress in cases of pleurisy. However, the main commercial applications of the oil are in flavouring and also in alcoholic drinks. The berry oil is also used in bitters and liqueurs (Weiss 1997).

In perfumery some of its isolates or their synthetic equivalents are used. *Myrtenal* is powerful, sweet and herbaceous and used to impart a natural dry hay odour; *myrtenol* is warm, woody, herbaceous with a mild camphoraceous note, and used in spruce, lavender, citrus and bay type colognes; *myrtenyl acetate* is refreshing, sweet and herbaceous and can impart a fruity note. Myrtle itself is used to give a spicy-herbaceous element to fragrances, and also in leather accords (Jouhar 1991).

Medicinal and diffusive

Several of the aromatics explored so far have had a cineolic element, so now we will look at some that are indeed typified by this – the eucalyptus and paperbark trees that, like myrtle and clove, belong to the Myrtaceae family.

The Myrtaceae family is very large, comprising nearly 3000 species of evergreen trees and shrubs. Within the *Eucalyptus* genus there are around 700 species, and within the *Leptospermum* genus there are around 200, mostly native to Australia (Weiss 1997). *Eucalyptus* species, also known as gum trees, mallees and ironbarks, are very adaptable, and are found growing in a wide range of environments, some very different from Australia, although freezing ground is usually fatal. *Leptospermum* species, often called 'paperbarks', thrive in swampy terrain, and apart from Australia are found in Asia, Southeast Asia and the Pacific region.

Eucalyptus

The leaves of many *Eucalyptus* species have numerous oil glands located near the central veins, and so have very strong odours, which are especially noticeable if bruised, or after rain. In China eucalypts are known as 'the foreign stinking tree'. The volatile oil seems to have an allelopathic effect, because competitive species will not grow in their vicinity. Weiss (1997) cites Morikawa *et al.* (1995), who found that *Eucalyptus* leaves are able to absorb the nitrogen dioxide emitted in automobile exhaust gas, and suggested that plantations in cities might help reduce air pollution. Eucalypts are also associated with Australia's native marsupials, koalas: the leaves of some species are their main diet. In Australia *Eucalyptus* leaves and their oil are familiar household remedies for bronchial problems, and also for skin problems and wounds (Lawless 1992). The leaves of some species were smoked for general sickness, colds, influenza and fevers, and sometimes added to tobacco to enhance its flavour. The smoking of gum tree leaves to relieve asthma and bronchitis was prescribed by Australia's colonial doctors, but this practice was short-lived (Pennacchio *et al.* 2010).

Within the eucalypts there are three main groups, based on the chemical composition of their essential oils. The first group, and the one we most are familiar with, comprises the 'medicinal' oils, or '*eucapharma*' oils, that contain significant amounts of 1,8-cineole. There is also a group of so-called 'industrial' oils that are dominated by piperitone and phellandrene. The third group comprises the '*perfumery*' oils that are dominated by citronellal (Weiss 1997). Please refer to Table 9.1 for a summary of the common species discussed here, and their typical odours.

In the eucapharma oils, the oxide known as 1,8-cineole is present in some species at levels of up to 90 per cent. In 1996 Buchbauer reported that this constituent can increase cerebral blood flow; this explains why the typical eucalyptus smell can give a feeling of alertness. However, it can also have direct effects of the tissues of the respiratory tract, stimulating the cilia that have a 'sweeping' action and the goblet cells that produce mucus. This is why 1,8-cineole-rich oils are useful expectorants and mucolytics, as are menthone and carvone rich oils such as peppermint and spearmint. Typical of this eucapharma type are the Tasmanian (or southern) blue gum (*E. globulus*), the blue-leaved mallee (*E. polybractea*) and the green mallee (*E. viridis*), which frequently co-exist, and the gully-gum or Smith's gum (*E. smithii*). The so-called 'gum trees' got their name because of the dark coloured exudate from their bark, which was used in medicine and tanning leather. The 'mallee' type is distinctive; multiple stems arise from a common stock (botanically, this is a large lignotuber). The crude oils from the eucapharma group have an unpleasant odour that can irritate the respiratory tract. This is due to the presence of lower aliphatic aldehydes, which are removed by rectification (re-distillation and the fractions containing these components are removed).

The eucapharma oils are used in household products such as disinfectants, and in the flavouring of toothpaste, mouthwash and cough drops. As the name suggests, they are also found in pharmaceutical preparations such as pastilles, lozenges and syrups for coughs and colds. *Eucalyptus globulus* oil BP is a rectified product that has satisfied the stringent standards set by the British Pharmacopoeia, and has a 1,8-cineole content of 80–85 per cent. Cineole is easily isolated from these oils; it congeals at 1°C and can be frozen from the oil. A resinoid absolute can be derived from the leaves, and it has a very different odour from the typically cineolic distilled oil. Weiss (1997) describes it as 'a natural green odour with connotations of blackcurrant, together with those of fenugreek oil, lovage, and other persistent balsamic woody odours' (p.286), but he does not give any indication of its potential uses in perfumery.

The 'industrial' oils are obtained from the broad-leaved peppermint (*E. dives*) and the narrow-leaved or black peppermint (*E. radiata*). In these species, the leaves emit a strong peppermint smell if crushed. There are several distinct varieties within *E. dives*: one is rich in piperitone, which can be isolated and used as a raw material for the production of synthetic menthol and thymol, while another contains, like *E. radiata*, high levels of phellandrene, which is used in disinfectants and antiseptics. There is also a cineole-rich type that yields a eucapharma type of oil (Weiss 1997).

The third group is comprised of the 'non-cineole' oils, and includes the lemon-scented gum (*E. citriodora*) and lemon-scented ironbark (*E. staigeriana*); these will be discussed in Chapter 11, as they have lemon-like odours.

Table 9.1 Typical odours of some *Eucalyptus* species

Compiled and adapted from Weiss (1997).

Botanical and common names	Typical odour of essential oil
E. citriodora (lemon-scented gum)	Strong, fresh, rosy citronella.
E. dives (broad-leaved peppermint)	Fresh, camphoraceous, minty.
E. globulus (Tasmanian blue gum)	Refreshing, slightly camphoraceous, typical eucalyptus (cineolic).
E. polybractea (blue-leaved mallee)	Sweet-camphoraceous, cineolic.
E. radiata (narrow-leaved peppermint)	Powerful, peppery-camphoraceous.
E. smithii (gully-gum)	Fresh, cineolic.
E. viridis (green mallee)	Fresh, cineolic.
E. macarthurii (woolly-butt)	Fresh, sweet and rosy.
E. staigeriana (lemon-scented ironbark)	Sweet, fresh, fruity-lemon, verbena-like.

The cineolic eucalypts are widely used in aromatherapy; their main indications are for coughs, infections and sinusitis, muscular aches and pains, migraine, fatigue and general debility. Their odours are not suitable for fine perfumes, except for one species, *E. macarthurii*, or the woolly-butt tree, which yields one of the few *Eucalyptus* oils used exclusively in perfumery. The rectified oil contains around 85 per cent geranyl acetate, an ester with a sweet, floral, rosy and fruity odour, and geraniol, an alcohol that is also sweet and rose-like. This has potential applications in aromatherapy.

Paperbarks

Members of the genus *Melaleuca* are known as paperbark trees, because the bark resembles paper and can be peeled off in strips. The name *Melaleuca* is derived from the Greek word *melos*, which means 'dark' or 'black', and *leukos*, meaning white. The very first species within this genus was *M. leucadendron* (or the broad-leaved paperbark). It had a black-and-white appearance, because the papery bark on the higher branches was white, while the lower parts had usually been blackened by a forest fire. The trees are evergreen, with sparse foliage, and they also flower profusely, producing nectar and pollen; their honey is said to have health-promoting properties. *Melaleuca* species were used by indigenous peoples to relieve colds and headaches, simply by crushing the leaves and inhaling the volatile oil. The smoke from burning leaves was inhaled for various therapeutic purposes. The people of the Northern Territory smoked cajeput leaves for nasal and bronchial congestion, and the young leaves of the broad-leaved paperbark for colds, pain, fever, and malaise (Pennacchio *et al.* 2010). The name 'tea tree' was first used by Captain Cooke in 1777, when he instructed his men to drink a brew made from *Melaleuca* or *Leptospermum* leaves to prevent scurvy. The European settlers adopted the habit of inhaling crushed leaves and making infusions (Weiss 1997).

The species of commercial importance are *Melaleuca alternifolia* (the narrow-leaved paperbark or tea tree), *M. cajuputi* (cajuput) and *M. quinquenervia* (niaouli). The dominant constituents of their oils are terpinen-4-ol as well as 1,8-cineole. Terpinen-4-ol has a mild, peppery odour (Williams 2000). Tea tree oil has a very distinctive odour: spicy and aromatic, Weiss (1997) suggests that it has elements of cardamom, nutmeg and sweet marjoram. Terpinen-4-ol is usually present at up to 45 per cent, and 1,8-cineole at 3–17 per cent. Numerous studies have investigated its therapeutic properties. It is without doubt a useful antiseptic, with broad spectrum actions, and can be found in an array of personal care products – for acne, gingivitis, halitosis, toenail infections, *tinea pedis*, oral candidiasis and dandruff. It also has anti-inflammatory action. It is less known, however, that oral ingestion of the oil carries a risk of toxicity, especially for children, and that the oil deteriorates if not stored correctly. Degradation products in deteriorated oil have the potential to cause skin irritation (Faiyazuddin *et al.* 2009). It is also a dermal toxin in cats and dogs, so tea-tree oil should perhaps be avoided in pet care (Bischoff and Guale 1998).

Cajuput essential oil is extracted from *M. cajuputi*, which grows wild in Malaysia, Indonesia and Australia. Frequently this species is confused with *M. leucadendron* (Weiss 1997). The rectified essential oil has a pleasant but strong, camphoraceous, sweet odour (Williams 2000). 1,8-cineole dominates the oil at around 40 per cent. Its main uses are medicinal; Weiss suggest that in India, Malaysia, Indonesia and other Southeast Asian countries it is a panacea, widely and effectively used to treat intestinal worms, and also as an insect repellent. However, its use has been, to an extent, superseded by eucalyptus oils. In aromatherapy it is used as an antimicrobial, expectorant and analgesic.

Niaouli oil is obtained from *M. quinquenervia*, the leaves of the 'five-veined paperbark' which is native to Indonesia, New Caledonia and southern Papua New Guinea. The oil can be variable in chemical composition and odour, but typically can have 1,8-cineole at around 40 per cent and a sesquiterpene alcohol named viridiflorol at 18 per cent (Bowles 2003). Niaouli has a strong, sweet and camphoraceous/cineolic odour. In France it is more popular than *Eucalyptus*, and is called MVQ (*Melaleuca quinquenervia viridiflora*) oil. According to Schnaubelt (1999) it is important in French aromatic medicine, and one study indicated that niaouli oil had greater antibacterial action than eucalyptus, tea tree and others when used in massage practice (Donoyama and Ichiman 2006).

There is one paperbark species which is quite different in terms of chemistry, and thus aroma and potential applications, and that is *M. ericifolia*, the swamp paperbark, the source of rosalina oil. It is native to Australia and is found in coastal regions. The essential oil is obtained from the leaves and has a soft, pine-like, earthy aroma. There are two types: oils from the north give rise to the Type 1 essential oil, which is linalool-rich and cineole-poor; Type 2 oils come from the far south and are cineole-rich and linalool-poor (Brophy and Doran 2004). It is said to have properties similar to tea tree, and it is now being used in contemporary aromatherapy practice.

Most of the eucalypts and the paperbarks, then, yield scents that have a very positive impact on our wellbeing, ranging from hygienic applications and pharmaceutical preparations to inducing alertness. For many, their aromas are closely associated with the comfort that they bring to those suffering from colds and bronchial congestion. Many emit camphoraceous and cineolic odours that permeate the air and their environment.

Agrestic scents

The word 'agrestic' is used to describe odours that are associated with the outdoors and the countryside, so we will finish this chapter by exploring some of the aromatic plants that evoke this.

Many aromatic plant species have odours that can be classed as agrestic, but this category, like the herbaceous one, encompasses a range of odour types and characteristics.

In the deep, rich, earthy, woody group we will explore oakmoss, vetiver and spikenard, and also coffee, tobacco and the pungent cannabis. Hay is warm and mellow, and the meadows and hedgerows are host to some beautiful aromas. Birch tar is phenolic and can be used to evoke a smoky aroma. The smell of seaweed can remind us of the seashore; the 'marine' effect is difficult to achieve with naturals, but there are some synthetics and extracts that can be used to give this character. This chapter will conclude with patchouli, which really eludes categorisation. Patchouli manages to be deep, rich and dark, but with herbaceous, light top notes.

Rich, earthy, woody scents

Oakmoss and tree moss

These are not true plants, and are therefore unusual sources of aromatic materials. The full story of oakmoss as a fragrance spans centuries. Oakmoss and tree moss are lichens that grow on the bark of trees, particularly oaks and conifers. Lichen is a symbiotic organism, an association of an alga and a fungus growing together as one, and dependent upon one another for survival, although the fungal partner is dominant. Lichen produces a flattened structure called a *thallus* – this can be seen draping and trailing over the lower branches and twigs, and covering the bark of deciduous trees, particularly oaks. It has a moss-like appearance, hence the misnomer. *Evernia prunastri* is the most common species that yields oakmoss for perfumery. Two other species are extracted in China; these are *E. mesomorpha* and *Cetrariastrum nepalensis* (Joulain and Tabacchi 2009). Tree moss is obtained from lichens that grow on conifers – spruce, fir and pine. Their piney, coniferous, resinous odours can be detected in the lichen and its aromatic extract too. Other tree moss species include *Evernia furfuraceae* and *Usnea barbata*, the latter giving its name to usnic acid, a component with antibiotic properties. These antibiotic properties were exploited by the ancient Egyptians in the mummification process, where oakmoss, myrrh and pine resin were used to pack the cavities of the eviscerated body to help prevent putrefaction of the flesh.

Oakmoss

The oakmoss of ancient Egypt was *Pseudevernia furfuraceae*, which was imported from Greece. In sixteenth-century Europe oakmoss, this time *Evernia prunastri*, was a popular scent. In Elizabethan England it was used, along with orris root (the rhizome of the iris) and rose petals, to prepare a powder for perfuming the wigs that were fashionable at the time (Morris 1984). The scent of oakmoss is persistent and long-lasting, so along with its antiseptic properties it would certainly have helped mask any unpleasant odours.

Nowadays oakmoss is extracted using solvent extraction to produce the fragrant absolute; in reality this is a soluble resinoid (Joulain and Tabacchi 2009). It has a smooth, enveloping, rich, earthy, woody, resinous, warmly sweet, honey-like scent, with hay-like notes. Oakmoss is known as an excellent fixative and is important in the chypre type of fragrance. In the early 1900s, the perfumer François Coty became interested in this long forgotten fragrance, and, using his knowledge of the plant aromatics of Cyprus at the time of the Crusades, he created *Le Chypre*, which was launched with great success in 1917. Since then the chypre style has endured and developed, and the importance of oakmoss in perfumery cannot be overestimated. Three ingredients – oakmoss, labdanum and bergamot – form the structure of a chypre fragrance. Turin and Sanchez (2009) suggest that this accord gives two fundamental qualities – balance and abstraction – and it is a resinous quality that links the trio. A classic chypre perfume has a base of oakmoss, labdanum, sandalwood and musk, although patchouli and clary sage are often included. The heart is floral, often with rose and jasmine, and the top notes are provided by bergamot and other citrus oils. Jacque Guerlain's version of chypre, *Mitsouko*, was launched in 1919; he included iris and a fruity peach note based on undecalactone ('aldehyde C_{14}'). Despite more recent reformulation to satisfy European regulations that restrict the use of oakmoss, *Mitsouko* remains one of the best examples of the chypre style (Turin and Sanchez 2009). The genre evolved, and we now have chypre/fruity examples (like *Mitsouko*), chypre/floral, chypre/floral-animalic, chypre/fresh and chypre/green variants. The latter two are less overtly feminine or gender-specific, and masculine chypre types can be leathery, woody, fresh and citrus (Glöss 1995); see Appendix A.

Oakmoss absolute, despite its long tradition of use in perfumery, its unique and irreplaceable odour and fixative nature, now has severely restricted use, and a complete ban may be imminent. This is because it has the potential to cause sensitisation and cross-reactivity when applied to the skin. However, the situation is not quite as transparent as it may first seem. Joulain and Tabacchi (2009) discuss observations and events that have led to the current safety stance regarding oakmoss, and highlight several concerns. These include unfounded and misleading published reports, and a degree of uncertainty in relation to the conclusions drawn following some toxicological tests. Since the first observations of allergic contact dermatitis (ACD) in loggers in 1948, and the first skin-sensitising testing that took place in the late 1970s, fragrance manufacturers have made many efforts to identify the oakmoss allergens and produce extracts that are free of the offending components (such as atranorin, chloroatronin and haematomates). Several methods for the removal of these have now been patented, and all extracts with reduced levels gave good results when tested. Joulain and Tabacchi do comment that the problem is very complex, and highlight the real need for further bias-free experiments on both the analytical and toxicological aspects to establish the effects of the sensitisers, especially as it now seems that the regulation of chloranatronol and atronol in oakmoss absolute-containing products 'appears to be more important than that of the oakmoss absolute itself' (p.59).

Vetiver

Vetiveria zizanoides is a member of the Poaceae family of grasses, and is native to India. Its stems and leaves are erect, and develop from a branched and spongy rhizome. The roots emerge from the rhizome; they range in colour from yellow-white to reddish-brown or even black, depending on the soil, and form a fibrous mat. In African and Caribbean countries vetiver is cultivated for soil conservation; its extensive root mass can help prevent erosion by binding loose soil, and it is not the aerial, unscented grassy part that is of interest, but its fine mesh of fragrant, wiry roots. These can be used to make fans and screens (*tatties*), while the leaves are used to weave mats and as thatch. The rhizomes are hung in houses, sometimes dampened and placed in front of electric fans, where they release a cooling scent, or sewn into sachets to perfume drawers – so vetiver is really one of the original home fragrances.

Vetiver thrives in the tropics, especially in Java, where it is called *akar wangi*; this translates as 'fragrant root'. In Java, local rulers and dignitaries enjoy being cooled by large ceremonial fans woven from vetiver, and when the French *Compagnie des Indes Orientales* introduced vetiver to their colonies in Haiti and Louisiana in the eighteenth century, the 'Creole belles' began to use the vetiver fan (Morris 1984; Lawless 1992; Weiss 1997).

In its native India, vetiver has been used for a very long time indeed; it is mentioned in the ancient Hindu text, the *Atharvaveda*. In Sanskrit literature vetiver is called *reshira* or *sugandhimula*, later becoming known as *khas khas*, which in turn became *khus khus* in Europe (Weiss 1997). In Ayurvedic medicine vetiver is classed as a bitter, sweet and very cooling remedy. In the hot season, bundles of the roots are soaked in drinking water to stay cool, and to prevent Pitta (one of the three *doshas*; see Glossary) 'flare-up'. The incense and essential oil are used to cool the mind and improve concentration (Svoboda 2003). In addition to this, a decoction of the rhizomes is used to dissolve kidney stones, and a drink made from fresh rhizomes is regarded as a stimulant and a tonic, although Weiss (1997) does mention that it tastes unpleasant.

Vetiver oil is produced by steam distillation from the roots and rhizome. Turin describes the dried roots as smelling 'dry, dusty, austere, yet fresh' (p.547) and comments that no 'bottled' vetiver comes close to this (Turin and Sanchez 2009). The oil is produced commercially in China, and some oil comes from Central America, the Caribbean and Brazil. Oil from wild plants is known as '*khus*' in India. However, the best-quality essential oil frequently comes from Réunion; the Indian is good, but seldom available. Java oil is more readily available, but it is does not, according to Lawless (2009) have the depth and smoothness of the Réunion type. It is a dark brown to dark amber, viscous liquid, with a strong, sweet, rich, woody and earthy aroma (Weiss 1997; Williams 2000). Morris (1984) suggests that it is somewhat like the smell of a sliced raw potato. The odour is influenced by α- and β-vetivone and khusimone. It contains mainly sesquiterpenoids, the major component being vetiverol.

In aromatherapy vetiver is used in skincare, for arthritis, muscular pain, rheumatism, sprains and stiffness; and for the nervous system, encompassing debility, depression, insomnia and nervous tension (Lawless 1992). Schnaubelt (1999) and Price and Price (2007) suggest that it is an anti-infectious agent, a circulatory and glandular tonic, and an immunostimulant. In India and Sri Lanka vetiver is known as 'the oil of tranquillity', and this view has been adopted by aromatherapy practitioners. Vetiver attar is made by condensing the distillate into sandalwood oil. Vetiver concrete is also available, and this is thought to give a more accurate representation of the scent of the volatile oil in the rhizomes, so, as might be expected, it is preferred in perfumery work, blending and compounding. An oleoresin is produced if the concrete is further extracted, and a stable, rich-smelling extract can be obtained by molecular distillation (Weiss 1997). It is widely used – for its fixative qualities as well as its odour, especially with rose and opopanax, but also with patchouli, as a basis for oriental perfumes (Jouhar 1991).

Vetiver and vetiveryl acetate, which has a sandalwood-like quality, together form a woody accord that has been much used in perfumery – for example, in Paco Rabanne's *Calandre* (1966), a green, floral, mossy aldehydic with a metallic character (Calkin and Jellinek 1994). There are several fragrances that feature vetiver. *Habanita* (Molinard 1924) is an ambery oriental with a fruity top, a sweet floral heart and a sweet, balsamic, leathery base (Glöss 1995); Turin suggests that it has a vetiver and vanilla accord. Others include Annick Goutal's 'salty' interpretation named *Vetiver*, Etro's smoky, woody, 'liquorice and earth' *Vetiver*, Givenchy's *Vetyver* and Guerlain's *Vetiver pour Elle*, a floral (jasmine) version (Turin and Sanchez 2009).

Spikenard

Spikenard, *Nardostachys jatamansi*, is a herb of the Valerianaceae family that also includes *Valeriana officinalis*, the root of which has been used to aid sleep for thousands of years. It is native to India, China and Japan; it thrives at 3000–5000 metres in the Himalayan regions of India. Spikenard has pungent, aromatic rhizomes, and it too has been used since early times, when it was known as 'the root of nard', or sometimes locally as 'muskroot'. In India it was widely used as incense; and in the Sikkim Himalayas of India its smoke was used to drive away evil spirits. In the Manang District of Nepal it was highly esteemed, because it did not grow near human habitations and therefore was not 'contaminated'. In Ayurvedic medicine the roots were sun-dried and then soaked in ghee (clarified butter) before being smoked for the relief of asthma (Pennacchio *et al.* 2010). Spikenard is also used to balance all three *doshas*, and promote awareness and strength of mind. Morris (1984) comments that, to this day, Indian women perfume their hair with spikenard, as suggested in the tantric *Rite of the Five Essentials*.

India exported spikenard to the West, whereupon it became known to the Greeks and Romans. Dioscorides considered spikenard to be a warming and drying herb; he called it *gangitis*, 'product of the Ganges', and suggested that it was used to treat epilepsy, hysteria and convulsions, and that it could restore colour to grey hair. However, it was best known as a perfume; the ancient Romans used it in several formulations, such as *Foliatum* and *Natron*, both of which also were used to encourage hair growth, and *Regalium*, the 'Royal Unguent'. In the New Testament, John 12:3, it is recorded that Mary Magdalene anointed the feet of Jesus with a 'pound' of precious spikenard ointment. She was rebuked by those who witnessed this act, but not by Jesus. The Magdalene later became the patron saint of French perfumery; from mediaeval times onwards she was the patroness of the perfumery guild (Morris 1984).

Spikenard rhizomes yield an essential oil which has a pungent, earthy, valerian-like odour. Williams (2000) describes the top note as sweet, woody and spicy, the body as heavy, animalic, woody and spicy, and the dryout as woody and spicy. According to Lawless (1992), its principal constituents are bornyl acetate, *iso*-bornyl valerianate, borneol, patchouli alcohol, terpinyl valerianate, α-terpineol, eugenol and pinenes. These constituents would suggest that in aromatherapy it has uses for the respiratory system, skin care, insomnia, stress and tension. Dobetsberger and Buchbauer's 2011 review of essential oils and the central nervous system cited research which demonstrated that the inhalation of smoke of two Japanese incense ingredients – agarwood and spikenard oils – had sedative effects, and that their main constituents also produced such effects, even when administered in lower concentrations than those found in the oils.

Spikenard oil is not commonly used in modern perfumery, and its impact on wellbeing is historical rather than contemporary. It is the inspiration behind L'Artisan Parfumeur's *L'eau de Jatamansi*, which has a fresh, woody citrus top, with soft rose and a backdrop of spikenard and incense, and a dryout of a woody-balsamic benzoin (Turin and Sanchez 2009).

Coffee

Coffea arabica is the botanical name for coffee. Its name comes from Caffa, a province in Abyssinia. It was introduced to Arabia early in the fifteenth century, and then the Dutch introduced it to Batavia. In 1714 Louis XIV of France was presented with a plant, and it was this plant that reached Brazil and was the parent of all the coffee produced there. *C. arabica* is a tree that can reach ten metres in height, but in practice it is kept shorter so that the 'beans' can be harvested. It is an evergreen with very large, green, shiny leaves; dense clusters of white flowers are produced at the base of the leaves. These are followed by small red, fleshy, cherry-like, two-seeded berries. These seeds are the familiar coffee 'beans'. Once the beans are removed, they are roasted, and this process develops the volatile oil and acid which is integral to the aroma and flavour of coffee (Grieve 1992).

When coffee reached the western world, along with tobacco, cocoa and tea, it was originally viewed as an 'exotic novelty'. It arrived in Constantinople in the sixteenth century, and the first coffee shop opened in London in 1652 (Grieve 1992). In the West there were few native stimulants and euphoriants, and so these new 'soft drugs' offered respectable alternatives to alcohol. However, in the eighteenth century, some physicians and religious leaders took the view that new, fashionable habits such as tea and coffee drinking were 'enervating and unhealthy' (Jay 2010).

Coffee is a stimulant which can produce sleeplessness. Early medicinal uses were to counteract narcotic poisoning – in acute cases it was injected into the rectum. It was also used to help prevent the coma that follows a snake bite, to alleviate inebriation and as a diuretic. In Malaysia the leaves were infused – these contain more caffeine, its nitrogen-containing alkaloid, than the berries.

Coffee absolute has an aroma very similar to roasted coffee beans – deep, rich, warm and earthy (Lawless 2009). Although many people enjoy coffee as a beverage, it often seems that it is the aroma of freshly roasted and ground coffee beans that brings the most obvious reactions of pleasure. Coffee features in a few contemporary fragrances, such as Kenzo's *Flower le Parfum*, which Sanchez describes as a 'coffee vanilla', *Eau du Navigateur* (L'Artisan Parfumeur) which has roasted coffee and leather notes, and Jo Malone's *Black Vetyver Café Cologne*, which has a 'roasted caramelic top note accord' (Turin and Sanchez 2009).

Tobacco

We have already explored the importance of tobacco in ritualistic and shamanic practices, and its secular uses too. Smoking tobacco is an acquired habit – many will remember the first puff of a cigarette – and the anticipated glamour, or fitting in with the peer group, falling away as the dizziness hits... Here, we will not be considering the physiological effects of tobacco, but the tabac note in perfumery. This is the sweet, pungent, hay-like and slightly green smell of pipe tobacco, which, like the smell of coffee beans, can evoke feelings of pleasure.

Tobacco absolute is obtained by solvent extraction of semi-dried *Nicotiana tabacum*. Lawless (2009) described this as 'rich, warm, amber, with greenish hue and also deep, dark and mysterious' (p.81). He also commented that synthetic versions cannot approach the depth provided by the absolute. Tobacco concrete, absolute and resinoid are made in France, usually by the Grasse manufacturers, for use in the fragrance industry; Jouhar (1991) describes these as having the warm, intense odour of tobacco, and he too suggests that the absolute is essential to obtain genuine tobacco notes. Williams (1995), on the other hand, held the opinion that natural tobacco absolute prepared from cured tobacco leaves has a strong and unpleasant smell, and that only upon dilution does it allow its warm and mellow notes and compounding potential to be discovered. He suggested that harmonising notes included oakmoss, tonka bean or coumarin, vanilla or vanillin, and that these accords could be linked to heavy floral notes such as tuberose or honeysuckle, or guaiacwood or sandalwood. Although Jouhar (1991) noted that tobacco absolute was suited to 'masculine' fragrances (and Williams (1995) agreed), he also highlighted the use of a dominant tobacco note in a feminine fragrance – Caron's *Tabac Blond*, launched in 1919. This had rose-like, floral top notes, while the main theme was floral, tobacco and oriental. This was followed in 1966 by *Vacarme* (De Rauche), which had citrus, floral aldehydic top notes and a tobacco, woody, ambered, musky theme.

This book is not intended as a critique of fragrances, although respected critical reviews have been consulted. However, in the case of *Tabac Blond*, it is necessary to explain what happened to this first feminine tabac fragrance. Turin and Sanchez (2009) point out that the original *Tabac Blond* was a tribute to women who smoked. At the time of its launch, these women were very 'modern', and it was clearly intended to attract unconventional women; Stamelman (2006) quotes a Chanel advertisement of the time which stated, 'well-bred ladies will find [its scent] improper' (p.234). Turin and Sanchez maintain that the original was 'a terrific, edgy, weird, leather chypre' (2009, p.515). It has since undergone a few reformulations which made it sweeter, but recently the tabac element has become considerably diminished, leaving behind a 'cheap green chypre'.

There are still a few worthy examples of the tabac genre. *Tabac* (La Via del Profumo) is true to type, smelling like tobacco without being overly sweet, and *Tabacco* (Profumo di Firenze) gives the sense of a lit pipe, associating tobacco with incense and smoke.

Cannabis

Cannabis sativa is a large herb that belongs to the Cannabaceae family. It is native to India and the Middle East. The buds are picked and steeped in milk to make *bhang*, which traditionally is used to make a drink, or a sweetmeat called *majun*, and the little shoots are known as *ganga*, which is smoked like tobacco. A resin exudes from the leaves, flowering tops and stems. This is known as *churrus* or *charas*, and the traditional way of harvesting it was for leather-clad men to rush through the bushes, and then the resin would be scraped off their leather garments. However, in Nepal, the plant is squeezed between the hands, and in Arab countries it is rubbed carefully between carpets to harvest the resin. The resin is the product known as *hashish*. It is thought that the word 'assassin' is derived from this, because of the 'wild, fanatical courage' bestowed by its use (Grieve 1992).

Cannabis has been smoked across the globe for centuries. Its first use was probably as incense. It is thought that the ancient Assyrians used a cannabis fumigation to dispel the sorrow of grief (Manniche 1999). Indian yogis in Kathmandu smoked cannabis in preparation for meditation. Its hallucinogenic properties were also exploited by many peoples in India, Pakistan, Africa and Brazil, and the smoke also had medicinal uses – for example, to relieve the pain of childbirth, induce abortion, and alleviate asthma and coughs. The smoke was also regarded as a useful insect repellent (Pennacchio *et al.* 2010).

Dioscorides was certainly aware of cannabis, and it was mentioned in some early Renaissance herbals, although in these it was not noted for its psychoactive properties. However, tales of delirious hashish-eaters are recorded in the *Arabian Nights*. Jay (2010) discusses some early instances where cannabis was taken for its psychoactive effects. First was the case of Thomas Bowrey, a sea captain, who in 1689, on a voyage to Bengal, tried *bhang* – cannabis buds steeped in milk – but his description of its effects was not published. Later, in 1800, Napoleon's soldiers encountered hashish when they occupied Egypt.

The first detailed account of hashish use provided by a western observer was written in 1836. Jacques-Joseph Moreau de Tours was a Parisian psychiatrist who accompanied a patient to Egypt for a 'rest cure'. He was interested in the comparatively low level of insanity in the Arab world, and noticed that the main difference was that alcohol was not used, but hashish use was widespread. He returned to Paris with *dawamesc*, the bitter green hashish resin mixed with sugar and spices. His first dose of three grams before dinner produced helpless fits of laughter over the oysters, and hallucinations concerning a bowl of candied fruit. This experience led to self-experimentation and then experimentation with fellow doctors, writers and artists, in an attempt to understand insanity. The doses taken at the time are described as being fairly extravagant. As hashish use became popular with the Parisian bohemian counterculture, the *Club des Haschischins* was established at the Hôtel Pimodan; this was frequented by Honoré de Balzac, Gérard de Nerval, Alexander Dumas, Gustave Flaubert and Charles Baudelaire – all of whom referenced their experiences in their literary works. Jay (2010) focuses on

Baudelaire's observation that hashish intoxication has three distinct stages: 'the nervous thrill and giddy cheer of its onset, the overpowering sensory cavalcade of its peak and the oceanic calm tinged with melancholy in its wake' (pp.89–90). However, Baudelaire also wrote of the 'terrible cost' and how the 'soul-sickness of the morning after reveals the true nature of the forbidden game into which hashish lures the user by gratifying his natural depravity' (p.90).

By 1890 cocaine, opium and cannabis were all available in pharmacies. Cannabis was sold for insomnia, migraine and muscle spasm. Jay (2010) tells us that Queen Victoria's physician, John Russell Reynolds, wrote about cannabis in *The Lancet* in 1890, describing it as 'one of the most valuable medicines we possess'. It is highly likely that he prescribed it for the monarch for stomach cramps and childbirth. Later, in 1931, Grieve (1992) described the therapeutic and medicinal uses, noting that the principal use was for easing pain and inducing sleep. She also commented that its action was 'almost entirely on the higher nerve centres' and that it could produce 'an exhilarating intoxication', and in eastern countries was known as 'leaf of delusion', 'increaser of pleasure', and 'cementer of friendship'. However, she considered that the nature of its effects was dependent on nationality and individual temperament.

The psychotropic effects of cannabis are elicited by constituents known as tetrahydrocannabinols. In 2007 it was estimated that in the USA 28 per cent of persons aged between 18 and 25 had used *C. sativa* (USDHHS 2007, cited in Anderson *et al.* 2010). Smoking marijuana elicits acute subjective effects such as euphoria, depersonalisation, altered time sense, lethargy and drowsiness (Hollister 1986, cited in Anderson *et al.* 2010). Typically, these effects commence within minutes and can last for hours. Anderson *et al.* (2010) found that the acute effects can vary according to gender, and although there did not seem to be sex differences in marijuana's effects on cognition, the female participants in their study requested to discontinue the smoking session more often than the men, likely leading to an underestimation of differences.

C. sativa yields an essential oil from its flower buds and flowers, and it also yields a fixed oil from its seeds which has skin healing properties, and is used in massage practice as well as in phytocosmeceuticals. The essential oil has a characteristic 'cannabis' odour, which varies according to its composition and is related to many factors, such as the time of harvesting, the maturity of the flowers and ripeness of the seed. Depending on these factors, the oil can be dominated by monoterpenes or sesquiterpenes. Caryophyllene oxide is a minor constituent, but has a significant impact on the odour, and this is one of the components that sniffer dogs are trained to detect. The THC (tetrahydrocannabinol) component is non-volatile, therefore does not come over in the distillation process into the essential oil (Mediavilla and Steinemann, date unknown). It is thought that cannabis essential oil has analgesic and anti-inflammatory potential. For example, Tubaro *et al.* (2010) investigated the anti-inflammatory activity of isolated cannabinoids and cannabivarins from the flowers of non-psychotropic plants, confirming their anti-inflammatory activity but raising more questions about the cannabinoid receptors.

When pure cannabis resin is burning, it emits a pungent, spicy, almost incense-like, rich, sweet odour. The essential oil obtained from the leaves, flowering tops and entire herb is quite different. It is described by one essential oil trader as strong, earthy and harsh, with middle notes that are earthy green, fading to earthy and peppery and faintly sweet, with the pungent first impression dominating throughout (Michael 2013). Michael suggests, because of his personal experience, that cannabis oil should not be used by aromatherapists. In order to give an accurate description of the odour he 'inhaled' the oil for ten minutes. He reported that his head felt heavy, his ability to process thoughts slowed, he felt sleepy; and that absinthe and valerian oils had produced similar sensations on previous occasions. Several points emerge from this anecdotal report. First, these are psychotropic effects, and the psychoactive component in cannabis is not present in the oil. So is this a result of either pharmacological effects from volatile constituents, or via another mechanism such as hedonic valence or placebo effects? Grieve (1992) wrote that 'it is regarded as dangerous to sleep in a field of hemp owing to the aroma of the plants' (p.397), which certainly suggest that the volatiles as well as the cannabinoids could produce psychotropic effects. Second, Michael (2013) mentions that he has encountered this type of reaction with valerian (a soporific) and absinthe oils. Without doubt, other individuals will have had similar experiences with these oils, and perhaps this phenomenon warrants further study. Third, inhaling any essential oil for ten minutes does constitute quite a large dose; after all, over 2000 years ago, Dioscorides did note that whether a drug was a medicine or a poison was really a question of dosage.

Michael (2013) suggested that although the oil might not be suited to aromatherapy, it might be of interest to artisan perfumers. Given its odour profile, it is not the most likely candidate for fine fragrances; however, Turin and Sanchez (2009) reviewed a fragrance with a cannabis theme – Parfumerie Générale's *L'Eau Guerrière*. The first impression was of woody, camphoraceous, spicy and citrus notes, but after five minutes 'a note strongly reminiscent of cannabis resin' emerged.

Meadows and hedgerows

Here we will explore the archetypal agrestic scent of hayfields – sweet, warm, mellow and rustic. When individuals are asked what smells of the natural world bring them pleasure, a common response is the meadow, or new-mown hay.

Foin

The typical scent of new-mown hay is provided by two grasses – sweet alyssum (*Alyssum compactum*), which has a strong, sweet, honey- and pollen-like scent, and sweet-scented vernal grass (*Anthoxanthum odoratum*), which is widespread in pastures and hayfields in the southeast of the USA. It is also known as vanilla grass, holy grass and buffalo grass. It also has a distinct, sweet smell reminiscent of hay and vanilla, in part provided by coumarin and benzoic acid. Its essential oil is called flouve (from the alternative French name *Flouve odoronte*), which is sweet and hay-like, and reminiscent of mimosa. An absolute can be obtained; this is known as foin absolute. New-mown hay or *foin coupé* perfume was popular at the turn of the twentieth century. An important part of the hay-like odour is coumarin – a component of dried grass and clover, and also tonka bean. It was coumarin from tonka bean that was originally used in *foin coupé* perfumes, but this was replaced by the much cheaper and easier-to-use synthetic coumarin. According to Jouhar (1991), the *foin coupé* type of fragrance can be reproduced by combining synthetic coumarin with deterpenated bergamot and lavender, and then synthetic methyl salicylate (which has a wintergreen odour), clary sage and oakmoss. It is possible that foin absolute was used, along with oakmoss, to give a natural, mossy character in the base notes of Guy Laroche's *Fidji*, a green floral fragrance (Calkin and Jellinek 1994).

Hay

Hay absolute is used occasionally in perfumery. It is obtained by solvent extraction of dried alpine sweetgrass, *Hierochloe alpina*. This species is related to *H. odorata*, the sweetgrass that is used by the Native Americans in smudging ceremonies. Lawless (2009) commented that it was very seldom used in mainstream perfumes, because the synthetic coumarin is considerably cheaper. However, it has a beautiful scent – warm, sweet, rich, green and hay-like – and he suggested that it is 'perhaps a contender for a happy smell'. Sanchez suggests that hay absolute 'is a fantastically complicated smell, like the best pipe tobacco on earth, smoky and plummy with an angular, bitter vegetal pungency' (Turin and Sanchez 2009, p.172). It is used to good effect in Serge Lutens' *Chergui* – a tobacco oriental, with a heart of hay and iris. Hay is also present in *Fleur de Narcisse* (L'Artisan Parfumeur), *Vie de Chateau* (Parfum Nicolai) and *Fumerie Turque* (Serge Lutens).

Meadowsweet

It is worth mentioning *Filipendula ulmaria* at this juncture. This is meadowsweet, a plant that prefers to grow in damp ground, on the banks of streams, in meadows and hedgerows. From June to September it produces tall plumes with clusters of creamy flowers which have a fluffy appearance, with a heady, sweet, honey–floral odour; some say it is reminiscent of almonds, but this comes from its leaves. The impact of meadowsweet on wellbeing can be seen in its folk uses. It was one of the three herbs that were sacred to the Druids, and it featured in the Lammastide festival – a harvest festival held on 1 August. Meadowsweet was mentioned in Chaucer's 'The Knight's Tale', as a flower that was used in making mead and honey-wine. It is still used in herb beers. Later, both Gerard and Culpeper suggested that it could be infused in wine to acquire a 'merry heart'. Gerard also maintained that it was the best of the strewing herbs, 'for the smell thereof makes the heart merrie and joyful and delighteth the senses' (Grieve 1992, p.524). Meadowsweet was important in the development of aspirin; in 1839 salicylic acid was isolated from the flower buds. However, this could cause gastric discomfort, and so acetylsalicylic acid was developed and named aspirin, from acetyl and 'spirin', derived from the old name of the genus, *Spirae*. It is still used in herbal medicine for problems in the gastrointestinal tract. An essential oil can be obtained, and this contains salicylic aldehyde, phenylethanol, benzyl alcohol, and methyl salicylate (Mills and Bone 2000); Jouhar (1991) also mentions heliotropin and vanillin in connection with its scent.

Sweet clover

Sweet clover is another fragrant plant, a perennial herb that flourishes in meadows and pastures. *Melilotus officinalis* has a sweet scent similar to new mown hay or woodruff, due to the presence of coumarin. Sweet clover is a bee plant, whose name comes from *mel* (honey) and *lotus*: 'honey lotus'. Its dried flowers were used to perfume snuff and pipe tobacco, as well as to flavour tisanes and herbal medicines, and also cheeses such as Gruyère and the Swiss Schabzieger. According to Grieve (1992), the *Fairfax Still-room Book* of 1651 mentioned that clover was used in a bathwater recipe to counteract melancholy. It has a long tradition as a herbal medicine, mainly as a digestive, and it is used in modern phytotherapy to counteract swelling and oedema, as an anti-inflammatory, and to enhance immune function.

Like meadowsweet, sweet clover was important in the development of an important drug. 'Sweet clover disease' was a bleeding disorder in cattle that had eaten spoiled *Melilotus* hay. This contains dicoumarol, formed from coumarin by bacterial degradation. It is an anticoagulant, and its discovery led to the development of drugs such as warfarin.

The perfumes of meadowsweet and sweet clover are inextricably linked with the uplifting scent of meadows, and the best way to appreciate this is to smell them where they are growing, or to gather the blossoms and use them to scent the home. The scent of clover intensifies as it dries out, and so the dried flowers can be used as an all-natural potpourri.

May blossom

May blossom is a scent associated with the hedgerows that surround fields and pastures. This is the blossom of hawthorn, *Crataegus oxycantha* of the Rosaceae family, the common hedge tree of Europe. Its blossoms have snowy-white petals and bright pink stamens, and they have a heady, intoxicating, sweet, rich scent. In Celtic folklore the hawthorn is very much associated with the Fae; the Faery Queen is sometimes depicted beside a hawthorn tree. It was important in pre-Christian worship, where hawthorn trees were planted in circles; the site of Westminster Abbey was once called 'Thorney Island', because of a sacred stand of hawthorns. May blossom was used in garlands during May Day celebrations, but it was never brought into homes, as it was believed that this would bring illness and death. It has been noted that the initial odour of corporeal decomposition is sweet, and perhaps not unlike that of hawthorn blossom, and perhaps this is why the superstition arose.

In traditional herbal medicine the leaves, flowers and berries of the tree were used. The berries were used to treat heart problems, and the flowers and berries were used for sore throats and as a diuretic. More recently, clinical trials have indicated the efficacy of the flowers and leaves in the treatment of congestive heart disease due to ischaemia or hypertension, and also for the treatment of acne; it is thought to have anti-inflammatory activity, and may increase elasticity and hydration (Mills and Bone 2000).

In perfumery anisic aldehyde is used to recall hawthorn, whose natural scent is described by Jouhar (1991) as 'exquisite'. Hawthorn is not often mentioned as featuring in contemporary fragrances; however, Kenzo's aquatic floral *Flower* (launched in 2000) has hawthorn with rose, cassie and violet in its top note. It was also used in Guerlain's sweet floral fragrance *Après l'Ondée*, which was launched in 1905. According to Turin and Sanchez (2009), this fragrance displays the first 'serious' use of heliotropin, which has an odour reminiscent of cherry pie or almonds: very sweet, floral-narcotic and slightly spicy. *Après l'Ondée* is therefore characterised by this, and no doubt the sweet heady notes of hawthorn, but the effect is tempered by orris root and violet, anise and herbs.

Birch tar and cade oils

Another common response to the question about favourite smells in the natural world is the smoky smell of burning raspberry canes, or wood smoke. Birch tar oil and cade oil are sometimes used to achieve this effect in perfumery. Birch tar is produced by the destructive distillation of the bark of *Betula alba* and other birch species, followed by rectification. It has a persistent, intense, smoky, phenolic odour, with oily back-notes. Cade oil is similarly produced, by the destructive distillation of *Juniperus oxycedrus* wood, followed by rectification, resulting in a product with an intense, smoky, phenolic odour. Rectified birch tar was added to Guerlain's *Jicky* to impart the smoky note which was present in the impure vanillin used in the original formula (Turin and Sanchez 2009). Smoky notes in fougère and leather fragrances can be given by minute amounts of birch tar or cade (Williams 1995c).

The leather note can be composed of naturals, in addition to birch tar and cade (smoky), styrax, cassie (for a deep, intense leather effect), castoreum (animalic), and labdanum (for a leathery, smoky, ambery note) can all be used. Some perfumers also include myrtle, black tea, patchouli, or tobacco in leather accords. A synthetic that contributes to the leather note is isobutyl quinolone, which is itself earthy and root-like; and this combines well with vetiver and oakmoss. Sometimes traces of aldehydes C_{10} (waxy, orange peel), C_{11} (waxy and rosy) and C_{12} (smooth and violet-like) are included to give a smooth effect. A classic leather base is *Cuir de Russie* (Calkin and Jellinek 1994).

The 1924 fragrance *Cuir de Russie* (Chanel) was composed by Ernest Beaux, and it is said that the inspiration for it was a leather jewellery pouch. Essentially this was a jasmine floral with aldehydes, rose, ylang ylang and iris over a leather base. The use of birch tar is now restricted, but Turin comments that the reformulated fragrance has not suffered.

Other notable leather fragrances are Lutens' *Sarrasins*, which has an indolic jasmine paired with fruity leather, and *Knize Ten* (Knize). This was launched in 1924, and was composed by François Coty and Vincent Roubert; it is an ambery leather, and highly rated (Turin and Sanchez 2009). Glöss (1995) describes it as a leathery chypre, with a fresh citrus (bergamot and lemon) top, a dry, floral, woody middle featuring geranium and cedarwood, and a leathery base with musk, moss, amber, castoreum and vanilla.

Seaweed and the marine note

It is really very difficult to describe the smell of the sea, let alone define what constitutes it. For many years there was a popular notion that we smelt ozone – a molecule consisting of three oxygen atoms – that was responsible for the clean and bracing air at the seaside. Ozone has a faint chlorine-like smell; we can detect it in the air after a thunderstorm or heavy rainfall; some liken it to the smell around a photocopier. However, we now know that ozone has very little to do with the smell of sea air. Instead we need to consider what is in the natural environment that contributes to the smell, or sensation. It could be sand, salt, sea creatures, or algae, plankton, ocean bacteria, seaweed and their metabolites, in a myriad of combinations.

One of the main contenders is actually a gas – dimethyl sulphide, or DMS. This is produced by ocean-dwelling bacteria that colonise dying plankton and seaweeds, and in the natural environment it has a fishy, tangy smell. When the plankton or seaweed starts to decay, dimethylsulphoniopropionate (DMSP) is formed – this is a secondary metabolite in marine organisms such as algae. Just as in some terrestrial plants, these secondary metabolites are not part of essential growth and development processes, but are produced for other biological reasons. The DMSP is then converted by the bacteria into DMS, which is released into the seawater before escaping into the atmosphere. If plankton is under attack by one of any number of types of larger marine organisms, the released DMS attracts crustaceans and seabirds which will prey on the plankton predator, thus saving the plankton. So, DMS could also be a type of pheromone that acts as an SOS signal, but by declaring 'Lunch is here – come and get it'! DMS attracts seabirds – it may be a homing scent, or an aid to finding food. It is also involved in cloud formation, and therefore has a very important role in the ecosystem. We have a low olfactory threshold for DMS. It is often described as cabbage-like, and indeed it is released by several vegetables when they are cooked, before being oxidised in the atmosphere. It is also found in black truffles.

A study conducted by Silva, Rocha and Coimbra in 2010 revealed much about the smell of sea salt, finding a natural compound that is also important in the scent of some flowers. Marine salt is a product made in saltpans, through evaporation of seawater by wind, heat and sunlight. Although sea salt is an inorganic product, it does contain some volatile and semi-volatile components which arise from algae and bacteria, and perhaps environmental pollution. These compounds include alcohols, phenols, aldehydes, ketones, esters, other terpenoids and norisoprenoids, which are molecules formed by the degradation of carotenoids in plants, algae, fungi and bacteria. These are considered to be biomarkers of the marine environment, and, if measured, can give a 'fingerprint' of the marine salt. However, people who work in saltpans in regions such as Aveiro in Portugal and Guérande in France have reported smelling a violet-like odour on occasions. One of the carotenoids, β-carotene, can be degraded to β-ionone, a violet-scented compound that is present in many familiar natural products such as fruits, wines and the volatile oils of many flowers (see Chapter 10). It has a very low odour threshold, and we have already seen that its synthesis revolutionised the perfume industry. A recent study indicated that β-ionone might have health benefits, including chemopreventative and antitumour properties (Liu *et al.* 2008, cited in Silva *et al.* 2010). It is present at trace levels in marine salt from Aveiro and Guérande, but it has not been found in saltpans in the Algarve, south of Portugal, possibly because of the drier environment and Mediterranean influence.

So 'extracting' the smell of the sea is more or less impossible, but nevertheless there is a demand for natural and synthetic sea smells in perfumery and environmental fragrances. Perfumes have 'fantasy' marine themes – because most of us would not really want to smell of DMS, ozone or crustaceans... In this case, realism is not wanted, just a recreation of the sensation. There are a few fragrances that are evocative of salty, briny sea air, including i Profumi di Firenzi's *Brezza di Mare*, Profumum's *Acqua di Sel*, Montale's *Sandflowers* and The Different Company's *Sel de Vetiver*, which is claimed to smell like salt drying on the skin after bathing in the ocean.

There is an ever-expanding array of aromachemicals that deliver aspects of the marine smell – Algol, Ambrate, Aquanol, Calone (more for a freshwater effect), Decave, Florazon and 'maritime ozone' are just a few examples. A tincture that can be made of sand, seaweeds and shells will give a 'seashore' element to natural fragrances, and there are absolutes obtained from a few species of seaweed. These include *Fucus vesiculosus* absolute, which has a salty, briny, almost savoury green/marine odour, with no tangy/fishy notes. In low concentration it can impart a salty, oceanic note that adds interest to green/fresh fragrances. It is used to good effect in *Trade Wind* (Essentially Me), to give the sense of being on an exotic island. Sometimes juniper berry, oakmoss and vetiver can complement seaweed absolute; their 'natural' odours can give a sense of the outdoors. *Fucus* absolutes may also have a role to play in aromatherapy and phytocosmetology – they have anti-inflammatory activity, and could be used to protect the skin from UV damage (Baylac and Racine 2004).

Seaweed and the odours of the seaside emphasise the relationship of the sense of smell with our other senses, and indeed the role of odours in the ecosystem. The creative chef Heston Blumenthal embraces the multisensory aspects of gastronomy. He based the concept of sound paired with food on a study that had shown that oysters were rated as more intense and pleasant if consumed with the congruent sounds of the sea, than the incongruent sounds of a farmyard (Spence 2008). Blumenthal then created a dish named 'The Sound of the Sea', which combines our visual sense (the plate resembles a tideline, with flotsam and jetsam, beached greenery and foam) with a soundscape of the seaside and a breeze scented with 'sea odour'.

Patchouli

This section on 'agrestic' scents closes with patchouli. Its odour is quite unique in the world of plant aromatics, and perhaps 'patchouli' should be a distinct odour type. Patchouli, *Pogostemon cablin*, belongs to the large Lamiaceae family. In Southeast Asia, and especially India, there are around 40 different species, and several of these are cultivated for their oil – *P. comosum*, *P. hortensis*, *P. heyneanus* and *P. plectranthoides* – although oils from these species are not of the same quality as that of *P. cablin*. Its original home is unknown, and its regional names are similar; in Indonesia it is called *nilam wangi*, in Java it is *dilem wangi*, in Atjeh it is *nilam*, in Batak it is *singalon* and in Malaysia it has two names, *dhalum wangi* or *tilam wangi*. In ancient China patchouli was known as *guang huo hsiang*, which translates as 'Guangdong bean-leaf aromatic'. Its Sanskrit name is *tamala-pattra*, and in ancient Greece the imported herb was called *malabathron* (Holmes 1997). The genus name comes from the Tamil word *paccilai*, which means 'green leaf' (Morris 1984; Weiss 1997), or the South Indian Tamil word *paccixai* (Holmes 1997).

Patchouli is an aromatic, large, bushy tropical herb; its mid-green leaves are large and are covered in little hairs. When these are bruised they emit a characteristic scent, fresh, aromatic, reminiscent of herbs such as lavender and of beeswax polish. Patchouli has been used for its scent for thousands of years, beginning in Asia and the Far East. The herb was used in India and China by Buddhist monks to make a purifying bath, and it was also used as an ingredient in the water used to bathe images of the Buddha (Holmes 1997). In China patchouli was used to make a perfumed ink for writing on scrolls. Its leaves were dried, pulverised and used as incense, and its oil was used as perfume. The scent was known to be an insect repellent. The dried leaves, which turn a less attractive yellow-brown, were used to perfume fabrics and repel moths. The Arabs used it for carpets, and the Indians sprinkled the dried herb in layers to perfume and preserve woven shawls and jackets (Weiss 1997). It was the practice of packing fine shawls from Kashmir with coarsely ground, dried patchouli that was responsible for its popularity in Europe. In the early nineteenth century, during the time of Napoleon, trade between East and West grew rapidly, and carpets and fine 'cashmere' shawls, permeated with the aroma of patchouli, arrived in Europe. The scent was exotic, mysterious and sensual, and became loved by many – from the Empress Josephine, who wore the shawls over her gowns, to the painters and poets of the Romantic period.

In its native lands patchouli had also a medicinal tradition of use. The herb is used in Chinese medicine and in Ayurvedic and Greek traditions too. Holmes (1997) explores its physiological functions and indications, which include gastrointestinal deficiency, pain, insomnia, anxiety, varicose veins and haemorrhoids, scar tissue and numerous skin disorders.

Patchouli essential oil smells quite different from the fresh herb, and the fresh herb is not distilled because of the very low yield. In order for the cells to rupture and release the volatile oil, the herb has to be carefully dried first, and then lightly fermented to develop the aroma and increase the yield. Often harvesting is selective – only removing stems with three to five pairs of mature leaves. This allows rapid regrowth. Stems with leaves are dried for between two and five days, and special care needs to be taken to avoid the development of mould. The leaves are then stripped and placed in woven baskets, in small batches of 15kg, to allow the fermentation. Over-fermentation results in a mouldy note in the oil, so this must be avoided too. The process is controlled by 'nose'; experienced growers know when the leaves are ready. However, if the leaves are to be exported, they are dried and kept free of moisture (Weiss 1997).

The oil has a very distinctive odour; it is usually described as a base note, rich, sweet, herbaceous and aromatic, and with considerable persistence. It is also unusual in that it improves with age; Lawless (2009) wrote that it becomes 'more fruity, rounded and elusive'. Holmes (1997) gives a detailed description which gives a good sense of the aroma: 'sweet-rooty-musky, mossy, sweet-woody, with a weak, spicy top note and sometimes a hint of a green-floral, wine-like note (like that of Roman chamomile)' (p.18). Williams (2000) describes the top note as sweet, earthy, spicy, balsamic and rich, the body as powerful, spicy, woody, balsamic, earthy and rich, and the dryout as spicy, earthy, balsamic and rich. Calkin and Jellinek (1994) suggest that good quality patchouli oil has a character that is 'partly reminiscent of bitter chocolate and pepper' (p.129). Lawless (2009) suggests that 'the best patchouli should have an ethereal-floral character to its top note that is almost wine-like' (p.84). These various descriptions, although all representative of patchouli's scent, also give a sense of the various impressions it can give when interacting with individuals. Calkin and Jellinek (1994) also briefly discuss quality. If the oil has been distilled locally, in old-fashioned equipment, it can pick up a lot of iron. This can have a disastrous effect on the stability of a perfume compound. Williams (1995c) explains that iron, sometimes found in non-rectified patchouli oils, reacts with phenols such as eugenol, *iso*-eugenol, and all salicylates (aromatic esters) to give intense purple colours. The chemistry of patchouli oil is very complex, with around 60 constituents identified (Weiss 1997). The dominant constituents are the sesquiterpene alcohols – especially patchoulol (40%) according to Bowles (2003), and sesquiterpenes at up to 50 per cent, including α- and β-bulnesene (Price and Price 2007).

The oil is used as a food flavour – in sweets, baked goods, and some meats and sausages. The tar content of tobacco and cigarettes has been reduced by many manufacturers, and this has affected the flavour of the products, so patchouli oil is added to compensate for the changed flavour. The scent of patchouli has captivated generations. Holmes (1997) suggests that the fragrance of patchouli can affect the pituitary gland; endorphins are released which cause the sensations of wellbeing, emotional and sensual warmth, and this is very useful for those who are 'out of touch with their body and senses' (p.21). Holmes also makes the pertinent comment that:

> patchouli is perhaps the most overused social scent of recent decades, reminding us of the psychedelic 1970s – or the sinking 70s – with its legacy of drug abuse, the Vietnam War and social turmoil (despite that decade's enormous social change for the positive). (p.18)

Because of this, individuals who enjoyed patchouli in the early 1970s will still revel in its aroma, but those who dislike it will possibly retain negative associations with its use. For example, patchouli is very useful for masking other odours, such as the smell of marihuana.

Patchouli is also one of the most important raw materials of perfumery. Calkin and Jellinek (1994) devote an entire section to the 'patchouli floral perfumes', such as *Diorella* (Dior) and *Aromatics Elixir* (Clinique). The link between these superficially disparate fragrances is the relationship of patchouli with a synthetic – Hedione, or methyldihydrojasmonate, which occurs in jasmine absolute. This aromachemical is used to provide jasmine or magnolia-like effects, but rather than a rich, creamy character, it has fresh, citrus and green notes. Calkin and Jellinek argue that although *Diorella* and *Aromatics Elixir* are sometimes classed as chypres, their dominant floral notes and comparative lack of musk and animalic notes should place them in a separate category. Edmund Roudnitska was the first perfumer to use Hedione in 1966, in Dior's *Eau Sauvage*. This was a fragrance intended to be worn by both men and women, and is a fresh citrus fragrance with herbs such as thyme, basil and artemisia, but also jasmine, patchouli, Helional (which is sweet and hay-like, with an ozone note and a 'watery character'), eugenol, methyl ionone, woods and coumarin. *Diorella* (1972) is considered to be the direct descendant of *Eau Sauvage*; a feminine fragrance that epitomised bohemian chic. It too has a citrus top, and the heart is dominated by a jasmine note that is composed of Hedione, *cis*-jasmone and aromatic esters, and indole with a fruity aldehyde (C_{14}). Calkin and Jellinek (1994) note that Helional and eugenol form an accord with Hedione; this carries the character into the heart of the fragrance, in combination with a lot of patchouli (6%). Interestingly, when trying to define the Roudnitska 'signature', Turin and Sanchez (2009) asked each other an abstract question, regarding what course of a meal *Diorella* would be, and they concurred: 'Vietnamese beef salad' (p.206). This 'salty' or 'salami-like' note is due to the cresolic[4] aspect of lily (p.371). *Aromatics Elixir* was composed by Bernard Chant, and launched in the same year as *Diorella*. It is based on an herbaceous-patchouli-floral accord, but lacks *Diorella's* citrus top note; it has more emphasis on rose, and contained another important synthetic – hydroxycitronellal – which also formed an accord with patchouli. *Angel* (Thierry Mugler) is described as a 'fruity patchouli'; and although it is notable for its sweet candyfloss character provided by ethylmaltol, it has a Hedione and Helional accord in its top note – demonstrating yet again the close relationship of these aromachemicals with patchouli. Other fragrances that feature patchouli are *Tuscany per Uomo* (Aramis), a fougère with floral and resinous notes, and *Eau de Rochas* (Rochas), a cologne with a rich, woody, patchouli character (Turin and Sanchez 2009).

---

4   The cresolic note is given by a phenol, *para*-cresol, and its derivatives. It is tar-like and animalic; also important in narcissus fragrance.

CHAPTER 10

Flowers

Flowers and their scents have been used since antiquity for personal adornment and fragrance as well as medicines. Through the ages and across the globe, they have also acquired a tradition of rich symbolic and esoteric meanings. For example, in Tzotzil, a Mayan language, the flower is associated with song, and is a symbol of the spirit world. Flowers represent spiritual power and its manifestation in the body, specifically the heart, blood and eyes; they are also associated with fire, and are used to differentiate gender (Hill 1992).

In Europe in the nineteenth century, following the Napoleonic wars, there was increasing interest in new botanicals, an influx of exotic blooms into Europe, and the 'language of flowers' emerged. Goody (1993) analyses the phenomenon from its introduction by Lady Mary Wortley Montagu in 1718, who highlighted its oriental origins, to Goethe's 1819 poems on 'Secret Writing' about talismans and flowers, and Mme Charlotte de Latour's controversial *Langage des Fleurs*, which was largely based on an earlier anonymous work, but reprinted many times and translated into English, and which influenced later developments. Further controversy lay ahead; Christians believed that the meaning of flowers came from God, not pagans and their mythology, and later on Mme Charlotte de Latour was heavily criticised for her misunderstanding of old languages and resulting misinterpretation and oversimplification. Despite this, the language of flowers acquired religious, scientific and occult traditions, and even spawned a new study – botanology, the science of the mystical language of flowers.

There can be no doubt that for thousands of years flowers have appealed to our visual, tactile and olfactory senses, captivated us with their beauty, and seduced us with their scent. Tisserand (1985) describes how in ancient Greece the physician Marestheus recorded his observations of the effects of flower scents, noting that rose and hyacinth and flowers with fruity or spicy fragrances were refreshing, and would invigorate the tired mind, while the lily and narcissus were more 'oppressive' and could cause stupor if they were inhaled excessively (p.27). Tzvi (2011) discusses the views of Philo, in 2 Corinthians 2:14–17, when asked if nature, by producing flowers, was a temptation to sensuality. Philo was adamant that flowers were made to promote health rather than pleasure, but he did make the significant point that 'they are beneficial in themselves by their scents, impregnating all with their fragrance' (p.547). Much later, in 2008, Weber and Heuberger published the results of their research at the Fragrant Garden at the University of Natural Resources and Life Sciences in Vienna. They demonstrated that natural odours from blooming plants increased calmness, alertness and mood, and that the scents of flowering plants have beneficial effects on humans. These effects have also been observed with *shinrin-yoku* in Japan (see page 199). At the risk of being at odds with Philo and those who take the view that flowers are best used as medicines, we shall focus here on the aesthetics of floral scents and their influence on the psyche.

In this chapter we will explore some of the most important floral scents, beginning with the so-called *indolic* fragrances from flowers such as jasmine, gardenia, white champaca, orange blossom and tuberose. We will also discuss the *rose and the rosy-scented* botanicals geranium and immortelle. There is a myriad of variations in the floral scent theme, so we will also look at *violet* florals: orris root and violet flower and boronia; *green* florals such as hyacinth and narcissus, genet and broom, mimosa, cassie and linden blossom; *fruity* florals such as osmanthus, the *spicy* florals carnation and cassie, and heady *exotic* florals such as frangipani, ylang ylang and lotus. There are also some scented flowers that do not yield either essential oils or absolutes, such as *cottage garden* favourites the carnation, peony and lilac, lily and lily of the valley, so we will also mention these and look at how their aromas can be 'replicated' for perfumery. It really is impossible to cover all of the beautiful floral botanicals, and it is hoped that the ones included here are representation enough.

Indolic flower scents

Indole is a cyclic imine – a nitrogen-containing molecule – and is a trace constituent in the volatile oil of some white flowers. It is very important in their aroma, but in higher concentration it is highly unpleasant; Morris (1984) suggests that it can be perceived as the odour of putrefaction. Williams (2000) describes indole itself as smelling of mothballs, but faecal at 10 per cent and jasmine-like in trace amounts. It is added, sparingly, to heavy floral perfumes such as jasmine, lilac and gardenia. Williams (1995d) says that it has been likened to 'putting the sunshine in'. Indole also reacts with hydroxycitronellal to form a *Schiff base*, which has a very pleasant odour, without the disadvantage of adding indole itself, which can cause the products to turn pink within a few days!

Jasmine

There are many species of *Jasminum*, an evergreen climbing shrub that produces small, white, star-shaped, highly fragrant flowers, whose scent becomes more intense at night. In India there are at least 43 species. Jasmine originated in Kashmir, at the border of India and Iran. In Hindi it is known as *chameli. Jasminum officinale* from Persia was called *yasmin*, an Arabic word meaning 'fragrant'; while *J. sambac* from India was named after the Sanskrit *mallika*. Since ancient times, fragrant jasmine flowers have been used in garlands, as hair decorations, in worship and ritual, strewn at feasts, and used to scent bathwater. Its flowers were, and still are, used to scent and flavour teas in China. In India jasmine was used to scent ointments, body oils, hair dressings and perfumes, and the ancient Greeks and Romans used imported jasmine pomade. Weiss (1997) relates an anecdote about the Roman, Lucius Plotius, who while hiding from his political enemies was betrayed by the strong smell of his favourite jasmine fragrance! It also had medicinal uses – jasmine oil is considered to be an aphrodisiac, but is also a muscle relaxant and used to facilitate childbirth.

Three species are cultivated for their volatile oil: *J. auriculatum*, *J. grandiflorum* and *J. sambac*. These species are tropical/subtropical plants, and do not tolerate severe frosts. During the European Renaissance *J. officinale* was cultivated first in Italy and then in France for its use in fragrances. Budding *J. grandiflorum* cultivars onto the hardier rootstock of *J. officinale* (also known as 'poet's jasmine') resulted in plants that were more frost and disease resistant. By the end of the seventeenth century, Grasse was a major grower and processor of *J. grandiflorum*, and this peaked in 1920. Jasmine production moved to the then French colonies in Algeria and Morocco. Small amounts of jasmine are still produced in Grasse, Italy and Spain, but since the 1970s Egypt has been a major producer (Weiss 1997).

J. auriculatum is cultivated and processed in southern India, as is *J. grandiflorum*; however, the most common species in India is *J. sambac*, where it is known as 'Moonlight of the Grove'. Jasmine flowers are harvested manually, usually by young women or children; a highly skilled picker can collect three kilograms in six hours. Picking is usually carried out between dawn and 9.30–10.00am, and only half-opened and fresh, fully opened white flowers are selected – not buds or flowers that have started to turn yellow. Picking encourages further flowering; even if it rains the flowers are picked, despite the fact that they have no value. The harvested flowers must be processed very quickly because any delay reduces the yield and quality. Processing is either by solvent extraction for a concrete or by alcohol extraction of the concrete for an absolute. In times gone by, the flowers would be extracted by enfleurage.

In India, several other products are made with jasmine flowers. Attar of jasmine is made by hydro-distilling the flowers into sandalwood oil; it is estimated that 500kg of flowers are required to produce just one kilo of the attar. *Chameli ka tel* is a traditional perfumed oil made by extracting the flowers with hot sesame or groundnut oil. *Sira* is jasmine-scented sesame oil, made by spreading alternate layers of flowers and sesame seeds. The spent flowers are removed and replaced every 12 hours until the sesame seeds are impregnated with the fragrance of jasmine, then they are crushed and pressed (Weiss 1997). This product was, perhaps, the inspiration for the name of Patou's *Sira des Indes*, but not the fragrance itself, which has a fruity banana and pear element, and a champaca heart.

Jasmine absolute is a dark orange/brown liquid. It has over 100 constituents, but is dominated by aromatic esters such as benzyl acetate, methyl jasmonate and methyl anthranilate, and benzyl benzoate. Monoterpenoid alcohols such as linalool are present, as are the aromatic alcohols such as benzyl alcohol and the sesquiterpenol farnesol. The celery-like ketone *cis*-jasmone is found, and there are trace amounts of indole. The aroma varies according to its source, but is typically floral, fruity, heavy, and animalic with a waxy, spicy dryout (Williams 2000). Weiss (1997) quotes Arctander, who is generally considered to be the leading authority on natural fragrance description: 'An intense floral, warm, rich, highly diffusive odour, with a peculiar waxy-herbaceous, oily-fruity and tea-like undertone' (p.357).

There are subtle but distinct differences between the French *J. grandiflorum/ officinalis* absolute and the Indian *J. sambac*, which is, according to Lawless (2009), 'sweet, fresh, light white floral and lily-like, with a delicate, ethereal soft, green backnote' (p.72). A subjective description of the different nuances is that the *grandiflorum* is more 'restrained', and the *sambac* is more 'raunchy'.

Jasmine is often included in anti-aging phytocosmeceuticals; and this is supported by a study that demonstrated that it has free radical scavenging properties and may protect against UV-B induced skin damage (Baylac and Racine 2003).

In aromatherapy jasmine's main uses are for counteracting depression, stress and lack of confidence (Lawless 1992; Holmes 1998). In 2007 Hirsch *et al.* demonstrated that the aroma of jasmine could dramatically improve bowling scores. They suggested that it might do this by regulating mood, enhancing alertness and reducing anxiety, whilst improving self-confidence and hand–eye co-ordination. They concluded that a similar effect could be expected in other activities that involve hand–eye co-ordination and precision, so the results of this study have much wider relevance than to bowling alone. Hongratanaworakit (2010) conducted a placebo-controlled study to investigate the effects of abdominal massage with *J. sambac* oil. He showed that this not only had a physiologically stimulating effect, but also brought an increase in subjective behavioural arousal. So, this supports the use of jasmine in aromatherapy for its stimulating, activating effects.

Although jasmine's alleged aphrodisiac effects have not been proven, Holmes (1998) suggested that the euphoric nature of its scent might be mediated by two types of chemical opioid peptide neurotransmitters – the encephalins and endorphins. He explains that in Greek *euphoria* means 'wellbeing', and that jasmine fragrance might trigger the release of encephalins. Similarly, endorphins are related to feelings of wellbeing and possibly sexual desire, and so his hypothesis can help explain this aspect of jasmine's effects on the psyche.

The fragrance of jasmine is exhilarating and delightful. Classen *et al.* (1994) illustrate this by referring to a south Indian folktale of a king whose laugh would spontaneously spread the fragrance of jasmine for miles around. The perfumer Jean Carles described jasmine absolute as 'being to perfumery what butter is to *haute cuisine*: the effect of margarine is never quite the same' (Calkin and Jellinek 1994, p.93). As well as suggesting that jasmine absolute is one of the most important raw materials of perfumery, Jean Carles is also saying that small amounts of natural jasmine can make a huge improvement to a fragrance constructed with otherwise synthetic jasmine notes. Jasmine is often at the heart of a floral bouquet accord, usually with rose; this can be seen in numerous fragrances such as Yves Saint Laurent's *Rive Gauche* and Patou's *Sublime*, both aldehydic florals, and in Carven's

Ma Griffe, a chypre floral (Glöss 1995), which was composed by Jean Carles after he lost his sense of smell (Turin and Sanchez 2009). It is therefore quite difficult to single out fragrances that unequivocally represent the jasmine note in perfumery. *Joy* (Patou) was launched in 1935, with claims to being the most expensive perfume in the world. Its top notes are light, fresh and floral, and the main theme is floral and green, but with a jasmine accent (Williams 1995a). Jasmine is also common in the middle notes of chypre fragrances, such as Dior's *Miss Dior*, and it is the dominant floral in *Diorella* (Glöss 1995). A more recent jasmine/white flowers fragrance is Annick Goutal's *Songes*, and there are a few jasmine soliflores on the market too – Creed's *Jasmal* is a green jasmine, as is Keiko Mecheri's *Jasmine* (Turin and Sanchez 2009).

Gardenia

Gardenia jasminoides is a bush with dark green leaves and beautiful, heavily scented white flowers. Its botanical name suggests similarities to jasmine, and one of its common names is 'Cape jasmine'. The plant is native to the Far East, India and China, where the flowers are used to scent tea. Morris (1984) suggests that it is not possible to extract the scent from gardenia by 'any extractive process known', and Calkin and Jellinek (1994) simply refer to gardenia notes but do not list it as a 'natural'. An absolute can be produced; this has a sweet, rich, floral, jasmine-like odour, but it is seldom available (Lawless 1992). However, Jouhar (1991) suggests that gardenia yields an essential oil with an odour reminiscent of jasmine; it was dominated by benzyl acetate, but also contained linalool, linalyl acetate, and terpineol and methyl anthranilate, with traces of benzoic acid. Jouhar suggests that the characteristic odour is due to the presence of an aromatic ester, styrallyl acetate. Williams (1995d) concurs, noting that this occurs in gardenia absolute, and itself has a harsh, powerful, green, gardenia-like note. Calkin and Jellinek (1994) do mention the use of styrallyl acetate to impart a gardenia note in perfumes such as the floral bouquet heart of the original *L'air du Temps* (Nina Ricci). The gardenia note is also included in the top note of Dior's chypre *Miss Dior* and in Carven's *Ma Griffe*.

It is interesting that most of the fragrances with the word 'gardenia' in their name do not seem to live up to the promise. Turin and Sanchez (2009) comment that 'most gardenias fail to replicate the flower' (p.281). The first gardenia fragrance was Chanel's *Gardénia*, composed by Ernest Beaux and launched in 1925. Vosnaki (2011) explains that it was not originally intended to be a soliflore, but was chosen because of its resemblance to Coco Chanel's favourite but unscented flower, the camellia. Gardenia perfumes were very popular in the 1930s, and promoted as being reminiscent of the romantic gardens in the south of France, but fashions changed, and it disappeared in the 1950s. Over 60 years later, Chanel reintroduced a gardenia eau de toilette – *Les Exclusifs Gardénia*. The original version was in fact based on narcissus, but in an accord with styrallyl acetate and jasmine absolute. However, the contemporary version, composed by Jacques Polge, has obviously had to comply with the changed regulations, and is described as 'comparatively much thinner, stretched to its limit' (Vosnaki 2011). It is based on a white floral accord, and although it is said to have notes of gardenia, these are not detectable. It has a light, soft, vanilla base, which makes it an entirely different fragrance.

Tiaré is the name given to the flower of *Gardenia tahitensis*. This species is native to Polynesia, where the scented flowers are used in floral garlands known as *leis*, and worn by women as hair decorations; if a flower is worn over the left ear, it means that she is in a relationship, and over the right it signifies otherwise.[1] A beautifully scented product known as *Monoi Tiare Tahiti* is made by macerating the blooms in coconut oil; this is used in skin care. Ormond Jayne's *Tiaré*, Chantecaille's *Tiaré* and LesNez's *Manoumalia* are three examples of fragrances that feature this flower. According to Turin and Sanchez (2009), Sandrine Videault composed *Manoumalia* with reference to the natural flower, possibly inspired by her teacher, Edmond Roudnitska, who did the same with lily of the valley when composing *Diorissimo*.

Champaca

There are many species of *Michelia* in the large family Magnoliaceae. *M. champaca* and *M. alba* are two species that are valued for their scented blooms. They are tall, evergreen trees that can reach 30 metres in height, and native to the temperate Himalayan region, but are widely distributed throughout India (especially in the Eastern Ghats bordering Orissa and Andhra Pradesh), South China, Indonesia, the Philippines and some of the Pacific Islands.

In India, the flowers are produced once during the monsoon and again in the spring, when the powerfully scented golden-yellow (*M. champaca*) or white (*M. alba*) blooms cover the trees, and their fragrance permeates the air, especially at night. They are highly valued for their scent, which continues to be produced and released after picking, and they are used as decoration and at worship in temples. In traditional customs, women wear the flowers in the hair or behind the ears, where they open and release their scent. Champaca flowers are also used in garlands and for floating in water to scent rooms. There is limited local production of an essential oil by distillation, and champaca attar is also made. A commercial absolute is also available. Over 250 constituents have been reported, some of the major ones being linalool, methyl benzoate, benzyl acetate, *cis*-linalool oxide pyranoid, phenyl acetonitrile, 2-phenethyl alcohol, dihydro-β-ionone, α-ionone, β-ionone, dihydro-β-ionol, methylanthranilate, indole, methylpalmitate, ionone oximes and methyl linoleate (Rout, Naik and Rao 2006).

Jouhar (1991) describes champaca absolute as penetrating, warm, smooth and rich, with a neroli-like floral note accompanied by spicy, tea-like undertones. Lawless (2009) suggests that it has a powerful, sweet, heady, velvety, floral scent, with notes

---

1   The artist Paul Gauguin wrote that the Tahitians exude a 'mingled perfume'. Drobnick quotes Gauguin: 'A mingled perfume, half animal, half vegetable emanated from them; the perfume of their blood and the gardenias – *Tiaré* – which they all wore in their hair. "*Téiné merahi noa noa* (now very fragrant)", they said' (Gauguin 1957, cited in Drobnick 2012, p.12).

of lily, hay and orange blossom. The absolute is scarce, and it is not widely used in aromatherapy, although it might well have a relaxing or euphoric effect, rather like jasmine or orange blossom. Champaca is rarely used as the dominant floral in perfumery; more frequently it is used to enhance jasmine accords. However, it does feature in a few fragrances; we have already mentioned Patou's *Sira des Indes*, and it is also found in *Champaca* (Ormonde Jayne), which is a green floral (Turin and Sanchez 2009).

Orange blossom

The bitter orange tree, *Citrus aurantium* subspecies *amara*, yields four important aromatics – three essential oils and one absolute. These are *bitter orange oil* from the peel of its fruit, *petitgrain oil* from the leaves and twigs, and its blossoms yield *neroli bigarade* oil and *orange blossom absolute*. A so-called 'neroli' oil can also be obtained from the flowers of the sweet orange (neroli Portugal) and from lemon flowers (neroli citronier).

The bitter orange tree is native to Southeast Asia, and was introduced by traders to the Middle East and then to Europe. It is well established in the Mediterranean – especially Spain, which is associated with Seville oranges. The tree bears highly scented white flowers. In early times these were used to scent baths, especially in Asia. Neroli first become popular as a fragrance in the sixteenth century. The scent was named after a town called Neroli, near Rome, whose princess used the scent and thus made it popular. Other writers suggest that it was named after the Italian Duchess of Nerola, who scented her kid gloves with the fragrance. Over the years its use became widespread in Europe; it was enjoyed by the aristocracy and used extensively by prostitutes, acquiring a reputation as an aphrodisiac. However, white flowers also symbolise purity and chastity, so paradoxically orange blossoms were also used in bridal wreaths and bouquets, eventually superseding the rose in this role (Lawless 1994).

For essential oil and absolute production, flowers are harvested manually, when they have just opened but are not yet in full bloom. This should be done as early in the morning as possible to give the best quality oil. If unopened buds or wilted flowers are included, the product will have a grassy odour, while small leaves and their stalks will give an 'off-note'. Normally the flowers are spread in thin layers and stored overnight before processing. The yield is very low; one kilogram of blossoms gives just one gram of oil, so neroli is a very expensive product. However, there is also a valuable distillation by-product – orange flower water, which is used in flavouring and skin care. The fresh oil is clear and pale yellow, but it becomes darker with age. It must be stored in well-sealed vessels and in darkness; sometimes it is stored under a blanket of nitrogen to prevent oxidation. When fresh, the oil has a strong, orange-floral odour; it is diffusive but not persistent (Weiss). Neroli has a strong, light, floral, citrus top note, a floral, green, bitter body and no perceptible dryout (Williams 2000). Neroli bigarade essential oil is dominated by *l*-linalool, *d*-limonene, and β-pinene (Bowles 2003).

In aromatherapy neroli is used to alleviate muscular aches and pains, especially the stress-related variety, and for skin problems such as sensitivity and acne, and it is best known for its uplifting, anxiety-relieving and calming actions that are of value in both aiding sleep and counteracting fatigue. Weiss (1997) notes that neroli bigarade is a weak antiseptic, but has strong bactericidal action on *Staphylococcus aureus*, and that in traditional medicine it was believed to induce a semi-trance state when inhaled warm. This emphasises the difference between sniffing to detect and appreciate an odour, and inhaling a larger quantity of the vapour. Perhaps the main potential benefit of engaging with the scent of neroli is the dissipation of anxiety, and so the pleasure of being in the moment.

In perfumery neroli is an important ingredient in classic eaux de cologne (Chanel's version is a good example) and as a top note in many fragrances. It is often combined with bergamot, orange and ylang ylang (Calkin and Jellinek 1994). Turin and Sanchez (2009) mention a few neroli themed fragrances. These include *Néroli* (Annick Goutal), a classic green, citrus fragrance, and Creed's *Néroli Sauvage*, which is a fresh, green, woody neroli fragrance.

Neroli's solvent-extracted counterpart, orange blossom absolute, plays a role in the middle notes of perfumes. This is a dark orange-brown viscous liquid with a very different odour, and, when diluted, it is virtually identical to the blossoms. Williams (2000) describes it as having a strong, fresh, floral top, a rich, floral, animalic body and a rich, floral dryout. Aftel (2008) describes its fragrance as 'cool, elegant and intense…with suave strength and understated sexuality'. Chemically, it is also dominated by linalool, linalyl acetate, nerolidol and farnesol; the latter two are sesquiterpene alcohols that have been associated with anticancer effects (Bowles 2003). It also contains the rosy-scented phenylethanol and methyl anthranilate, a nitrogen-containing ester also found in mandarin oil (Weiss 1997) and important in the formation of Schiff bases, and also indole (Williams 1995c). *Sung* (Sung), in its original incarnation, was a green, fresh floral with orange blossom dominating the floral heart, but now it would seem that faecal notes are prominent. Orange blossom supported narcissus and jasmine in Caron's classic *Narcisse Noir*; however, this is now only available as an eau de toilette and has lost much of its impact. It also features in Jo Malone's *Orange Blossom Cologne* (Glöss 1995; Turin and Sanchez 2009).

Tuberose

Polyanthes tuberosa is a tropical perennial that emerges from a tuberous root in the spring. The name 'tuberose' reflects this, and the genus name comes from the Greek *polyanthes*, which means 'many-flowered'. Its leaves are long and slender and it bears heavily scented, waxy white, lily-like flowers, which open from the bottom to the top of a spike. There is a double-flowered variety that is used as a cut flower, but the single-flowered type has a stronger scent.

Tuberose is native to Central America, where the Aztecs knew it as *omixochitl*, meaning 'bone flower', with reference to the white colour of the flowers. Originally the tubers were exported from Mexico to the Philippines and then the East Indies. Tuberose reached Spain in 1594, and then France and Italy. It is now cultivated in France, India, Morocco and Egypt. Across the world, it is one of the most important flowers in garlands. In Hawaii it is used in garlands called *leis*, and in India it is culturally very important and used in wedding ceremonies and traditional rituals, in garlands and decorations. Here, all of its names refer to its fragrance: the Bengali name is *rajoni-ghanda* ('scent of the world'); in South India it is *sugandaraja* ('king of fragrance'). In China it is called *wan xiang yu* ('flower as precious as jade and becoming fragrant at night') or *yue xia xiang* ('fragrance under the moon'). Not only is it a night-blooming plant, it also continues to produce and emit its scent after it has been picked, so its volatile oil is extracted by solvent extraction or occasionally by enfleurage (Morris 1984; Lawless 1992).

The absolute is a soft, dark brown paste with a heavy, honey-like, sweet-caramel, floral aroma. Lawless (2009) suggests that it is sweet, heavy, floral and balsamic, with a slightly green, honey back note, and Morris (1984) comments that although it is intensely sweet, it has a 'curious camphor-like note'. Could this be the mothballs aspect of indole? Like most absolutes, tuberose is very complex, containing alcohols (nerol, farnesol, geraniol, and benzyl alcohol), aromatic esters (methyl benzoate, methyl anthranilate, benzyl benzoate, and methyl salicylate), eugenol and tuberone, a ketone (Jouhar 1991), and traces of indole. The scent of tuberose is said to have 'narcotic' properties. This term is widely used to denote a heavy, sleep-inducing scent, and over-use of such aromatics may indeed have a stupefying effect.

In aromatherapy, tuberose is used mainly for its fragrance, and to promote relaxation and sleep (Lind 1998). It is certainly one of the most expensive naturals, but this has not prevented it from being a prominent fragrance ingredient, and indeed a dominant floral in the 1970s and 1980s. Probably the first prominent, and now iconic, tuberose fragrance is *Fracas* (Robert Piguet), composed by Germaine Cellier and launched in 1948. Later, tuberose was prominent in many powerful, heavy, sweet fragrances such as *Giorgio* (Giorgio Beverly Hills), *Chloé* (Lagerfeld) and *Poison* (Dior). Turin and Sanchez (2009) discuss some of the more recent tuberose fragrances, including those that allow some of its more disturbing attributes to shine through. For example, both Luten's *Tubérose Criminelle* and Goutal's *Tubérose* display its facets of camphor, rubber and rotting meat. Kilian's *Beyond Love* is described as the 'best tuberose soliflore', composed by Calice Becker, who used fresh tuberose as an olfactory reference, and the best-quality absolute with traces of magnolia and iris to compose a scent as close to the flower as possible. However, Ropion took a more classical approach when composing Frédéric Malle's *Carnal Flower*, which has a 'euphorically beautiful, perfectly judged floral accord' (Turin and Sanchez 2009, p.162) of tuberose and jasmine.

Rose and rosy-scented botanicals

The rose

Roses belong to the genus *Rosa* in the large and diverse family Rosaceae. Weiss (1997) gives a comprehensive history of this genus, some species of which have captivated man since time immemorial. It is thought that the rose is native to the northern hemisphere, and all roses of the southern hemisphere have been introduced and cultivated. Rose fossils were found in Oligocene Period rocks from Oregon and Montana, and these are estimated to be around 35 million years old. Further on along the time-line, we find that roses were known to the Mesopotamians, from a cuneiform tablet that appears to refer to the rose and rosewater. We have already mentioned the importance of roses to the early Persian societies, and even to this day, to modern Sufis, the rose flower symbolises perfection, and its thorns the obstacles one must overcome to reach perfection. According to several accounts, when the Islamic prophet Mohammed was taken to heaven, some of his sweat fell down to earth where it was transformed into the rose. It is said that whoever smells the scent of a rose smells Mohammed. The rose can be a cultural 'mirror'.

The 'Blue Bird' fresco at Knossos in Crete depicts a light pink, five-petalled rose; this is over 3500 years old. Later, Herodotus (490–420 BCE) wrote that the exiled King Midas brought a 60-petalled, highly scented rose to Greece. Later still, Theophrastus indicated that roses were being classified into types. In his *Enquiry into Plants* he mentions both the dog rose (*kynosbaton*) and the cultivated rose (*rhodon*). Homer's *Iliad* of the ninth century BCE describes how the body of Hector, slain by Achilles, was anointed with rose oil before burial, so here we are beginning to see the value of the rose in the western world. We also know that the Roman writers Ovid and Virgil cultivated roses, so it is no surprise that Pliny the Elder made comments about how to improve roses, when to prune them and how to encourage flowering; he also described a 'hundred-petalled rose', which later acquired significance in perfumery. However, Pliny also described the medicinal importance of the flowers, listing 32 rose-based, perfumed remedies. In ancient Rome the rose and its scent reached a peak of popularity. The rose gardens at Paestum were established to satisfy the huge demand. There is no doubt that the fragrance of rose had a lot to do with this; however, by this time the rose was imbued with powerful symbolism – love, beauty, purity and passion – all explained by myth.

According to the Greek poet Anacreon, and myth, when the 'foam-born' Aphrodite emerged from the sea and came to land, white roses appeared where the foam dripped off her body, representing her purity and innocence. However, her reputation for purity soon changed, as she became the goddess of desire, and had many lovers. Adonis, the god of beauty and desire, was one of her favourites, and when he was wounded by a wild boar (possibly sent by Ares, the god of war – another 'favourite') and by dying in her arms, his blood fell onto a white rose, turning it crimson, and so the red rose came to signify desire and passion. Adonis' life, death and rebirth became the focus of a later cult, recorded by the Greek poetess Sappho around 600 BCE. She called the rose the 'queen of flowers'. Eros was the Greek god of love and desire, and the son of Aphrodite. Eventually, after a 'difficult' courtship, he married Psyche, who represented the 'soul of mankind', and this union was blessed by Zeus, who made everything 'glow with roses', and rose flowers were scattered over the land. The Romans adopted some of the myths, embellished them, and created their own too. They chose to believe that the rose was created by Flora, their goddess of spring and flowers. When one of her nymphs died, she asked the gods to transform her into a flower, and so Apollo (who had no Roman individual counterpart, and was their sun god too) gave her life, Bacchus (the Roman equivalent of Dionysus) gave her nectar, Pomona gave her fruit (the rosehip), and Flora gave her a crown of petals. Cupid was the Roman equivalent of Eros, and son of Venus (Aphrodite). When he was stung by bees who were visiting rose flowers, in revenge he shot his arrows at the roses. Where his arrows missed, thorns emerged. So when we read of the Roman customs of crowning bridal couples with garlands of roses, and decorating their statues of Venus, Cupid and Bacchus with the blossoms, we can begin to understand the significance that lay beneath these practices. We can see how important the rose was to the ancients, and throughout history its symbolism endured.

The rose also represented secrecy. This, too, has ancient origins, reaching back as far as ancient Egypt, where the rose was sacred to Horus. The Greeks translated his name as Harpocrates, and being represented as a naked youth with a finger-to-mouth gesture, he became the Greek god of silence. Aphrodite presented her son Eros with a rose, and he gave it to Harpocrates to ensure that his mother's indiscretions were kept secret. So the paintings of roses on Roman banquet-room ceilings signified that everything said under the influence of wine, *sub vino*, should remain *sub rosa*, that is, be kept in confidence. By the Middle Ages roses appeared on the ceilings of council chambers, and later they were carved on Christian confessionals, to signify secrecy.

The Jacobites were followers of a political movement in Great Britain and Ireland who aimed to restore the Stuart King James II of England and VII of Scotland, to the throne; he had been deposed in 1688 and replaced by his daughter Mary II, who ruled with William III (of Orange). The Stuarts were in exile, and the Jacobites believed that parliamentary interference with the succession of the monarchy was illegal; they resisted the Act of Union in 1707. A series of Jacobite rebellions ('risings') between 1688 and 1746 meant that the supporters had to plan their activities in secrecy, and so several gestures and symbols were used to signify support for the cause. One of the earliest Jacobite symbols was the white rose, which represented the exiled King James, with white rosebuds for his heirs Charles and Henry. The 'white cockade' evolved from this – this emblems of a rose made from white ribbon.

Weiss (1997) tells us that the first modern book on roses was *A Collection of Roses* written by Mary Lawrence in 1799, and that the most famous illustrations were in *Les Roses* by Pierre Joseph Redouté, published in three volumes between 1817 and

1824. These include the roses in the Empress Josephine's collection. Few botanicals have such a rich historical tradition, elements of which persist until the present day.

We also need to consider the botanical evolution of the rose from its early forms to the 150 species we know today, and its many more named subspecies (cultivars). *Rosa gallica* is the 'ancestor' of modern roses, and is probably the oldest type still in cultivation. It was known in 1600 BCE and is native to Europe, Turkey and Iraq; it is related to *R. phoenicia* and *R. damascena*. *R. canina* is the European dog rose, and when bred with *R. damascena* gave rise to *R. alba*, the white rose eventually adopted as the Jacobite emblem. When this was crossed with *R. damascena*, the result was *R. centifolia* – the 'hundred-petalled rose' that Pliny wrote about. The wild rose of China, *R. chinensis*, was crossed with *R. gallica* around 600 BCE and the result was the 'bourbon rose', the ancestor of the 'tea rose', the 'hybrid perpetual rose' and our modern 'hybrid tea roses'. Today, roses are placed in three groups. The canina group is native to Europe, western Asia and North Africa, and in it there are the albas, dog roses and sweet briars. *R. centifolia*, which is a complex hybrid, is also included in this group. (It is more commonly known as the cabbage or Provence rose, and characteristically has rich pink, very fragrant flowers that resemble a cabbage in shape.) The Gallicanae group relates to *R. gallica* as described above, and now includes cabbage types, damask roses, moss roses and Portland roses. Finally, the ancestors of the Chinensis group are two Chinese wild species – *R. chinensis* and *R. gigantea* – whose descendants include tea roses, noisettes, bourbons, hybrid perpetuals and hybrid climbing tea roses (Weiss 1997).

As these types are defined by their shapes and colours, they are also characterised by their scents. So, for example, Gallica roses are crimson, deep pink or mauve, sometimes with stripes or splashes of colour, and have an intense, spicy, 'old rose' perfume. Damasks are white to dark pink, and their perfume has a fruity characteristic.

Not all roses are scented; only 30 per cent of more than 3000 hybrid tea roses have strong scents (Helgeson 2011). Other modern hybrid tea roses display a wide variety of fragrance characteristics. For example, the cultivar 'Lady Hillington' has fresh, woody, powdery, fruity, green, violet-like and sweet notes; 'Diorama' (named after the couturier and the fragrance) has a tea-like, geraniol-like and violet-like note; and 'Grand Mogul' has a fruity, green and powdery note. Joichi *et al.* (2005) studied the scents of these typical tea-scented modern roses. The fresh scent of modern hybrid tea roses is mainly due to a constituent in the volatile oil called 1,3-dimethoxy-5-methylbenzene (DMMB); this has a fresh, earthy and phenolic spicy note, which is also found in their Chinese ancestor, *R. gigantea*. Joichi *et al.* also found the violet-like and earthy dihydro-β-ionol, the fresh leafy green *cis*-3-hexenyl acetate and, inherited from the European ancestry, the rosy-scented alcohols such as geraniol, citronellol, nerol and linalool. However, they identified another unique constituent, 1,3,5-trimethoxybenzene (TMB), which has a phenolic, spicy, earthy and animalic note, and suggested that this came from *R. chinensis* ancestors.

Calkin (1999) made a study of the diversity of old rose fragrance. He comments that the essential oil of *R. damascena* 'Kazanlik', the variety most widely cultivated for the production of rose otto, has over 400 constituents. Around 85 per cent of the oil consists of just four materials; another 10 per cent is represented by ten more constituents, while the remaining 5 per cent contains several hundred constituents. (This pattern can be seen in other scented species including jasmine and narcissus.) In gallica, damask, centifolia and alba roses, the major components are the 'rose alcohols', namely phenylethyl alcohol (or phenylethanol, which has a soft, petal-like, rosy character), citronellol (warm and vibrant rosy), geraniol (sharper rosy) and nerol (harsher and fresh rosy), occurring in varying proportions depending on species and variety. However, it is the hundreds of other minor and trace constituents that define the beautiful scent of the blooms.

In contrast, one of the ancestors of the tea roses, *R. gigantea*, has two major ingredients. One is dimethoxy toluene, which is present at 50 per cent and has a 'tarry and humid' element, and the other is dihydro-β-ionol, present at 10 per cent with an earthy, violet-like smell. This is also found in *R. chinensis*. The perfumes of their descendants, the hybrid musks and Banksias, have a violet character; the scent of a related constituent, dihydro-β-ionone, is more raspberry-like, and can be smelled in many modern hybrids. Other rose perfume characteristics include the exotic and spicy, verbena, and anise. This odour type is usually due to 4-vinyl anisole, and is present in many English roses that are commonly described as myrrh-scented. The Bourbon rose with its characteristic scent originated in the Réunion islands and was a hybrid of the autumn damask 'Quatre Saisons' and *R. chinensis* 'Old Blush'. The Bourbon rose became the staple of the French perfume industry; it flowers continuously and has a vibrant, rich fruity character. *R. moschata* is the ancestor of the noisette, and is known as the musk rose; it has a pungent, diffusive and clove-like scent, carried in the stamens. Calkin (1999) comments that it is unfortunate that this feature is absent in many modern roses: for example, a hybrid of the musk rose and *R. chinensis*, 'Blush Noisette', has an intense, green characteristic due to hexenals also present in its parents, and a sweet element contributed by phenylethyl acetate, which is present in small amounts in the musk rose. It is described as 'clove-scented', but this is only apparent when its stamens reach maturity. This difference between the scents carried in the petals and stamens has been used in fragrance composition. For example, 'Roseraie de l'hay' has a 'sumptuous' rugosa scent in its petals, while its stamens have a fresh, cucumber-like scent; this combination is also used by perfumers. Similarly, *R. gallica* petals have a typical old rose fragrance, which fades as the flowers mature and the light musky scent of the stamens comes to the fore.

Three species are important in the modern fragrance industry. These are *R. damascena*, *R. centifolia* and *R. gallica* (sometimes known as the 'apothecary rose'). These, and their hybrids, are extracted to produce essential oils, concretes and absolutes. Bulgarian rose oil is considered to be the 'standard' and the most desirable, but Turkish rose otto (here the essential oil is distilled from *R. damascena*) is also available and widely used. Rose oil from Morocco (where the essential oil is distilled from *R. damascena*), rose oil from France (where the essential oil is distilled from *R. centifolia*), rose oil from Egypt (distilled from *R. gallica* var. *aegyptiaca*) and rose oil from China (from *R. rugosa* and others) are also widely available. Absolutes include rose absolute 'centifolia', *rose de mai* absolute, which is produced in France and Morocco, and rose absolute 'damascena' from Bulgaria.

Chemically, the essential oil and absolutes are different. Rose essential oil is characterised by the presence of monoterpenes and their alcohols – geraniol and citronellol and small amounts of phenylethanol. The essential oil is colourless to pale yellow, with a deep, sweet, warm, rich, tenacious odour; the Moroccan (*R. centifolia*) oil has a less spicy note than the oils from Bulgaria or Turkey (Weiss 1997). Williams describes a typical Bulgarian rose otto as having a waxy, spicy, floral top, a warm, rich, floral, spicy body, and a warm, floral, spicy dryout. Rose absolutes have much greater amounts of phenylethanol than the essential oils – usually around 60 per cent (Tisserand and Balacs 1995), along with geraniol, citronellol, nerol and farnesol (Jouhar 1991). Absolutes are much darker in colour – orange-yellow to orange-brown, and have a much sweeter, richer odour. They have a floral, waxy, spicy top note, a sweet, rich, floral, spicy body and a warm, floral dryout (Williams 2000).

The aroma is thought to be antidepressant and an aphrodisiac. Hongratanaworakit (2009) demonstrated that transdermal absorption of rose can produce a state of relaxation, and supported its use in aromatherapy for the alleviation of stress, depression and anxiety, irritability and mood swings. Natural and synthetic rose is also of enormous importance in perfumery; it is present in the majority of fine fragrances and dominates several, and the following examples illustrate just some of the many ways that rose is represented in perfumery. *Rive Gauche* (Yves Saint Laurent 1971) remains a classic rose fragrance, and although it has been reformulated, Turin and Sanchez describe it as their 'reference' rose. *Tea Rose* (Perfumer's Workshop 1972) was perhaps the first 'niche' fragrance; it is a fresh, green rose soliflore. *Nahéma* (Guerlain 1979) is a vibrant rose fragrance, allegedly made with synthetics and no natural rose at all. In 1994 *Tocade* was launched by Rochas; this time the rose is showcased with vanilla in an oriental, ambery context. By contrast, *Homage* (Amouage) places rose in one of its ancient roles – in an attar-like fragrance where Ta'if rose is paired with Cambodian oud and Omani silver frankincense (Turin and Sanchez 2009).

Geranium

The common name 'geranium' is a little misleading, because here we are looking at *Pelargonium* species of the Geraniaceae family – aromatic, hairy, perennial shrubs that thrive best in warm temperate climates; there are around 250 species and many varieties. The glands that produce the volatile oil are numerous and located over the surface of the soft, hairy leaves, and the yield is good; around 700g of essential oil are obtained from 250kg of fresh leaves.

The *Pelargonium* genus was first named in South Africa, when *P. cucullatum* was collected from Table Mountain in 1672. *P. graveolens* was introduced to Britain in the early 1700s, and botanists at Kew Gardens studied the genus and produced many hybrids from the ornamental *P.* x *hortorum* and the rosy-scented type *P. graveolens* x *P. radula*.

Pelargonium was cultivated for essential oil for the first time in the early nineteenth century around Grasse in France. The main area of cultivation then moved to Réunion, where 'Bourbon' or rose geranium is produced (*P. capitatum* x *P. radens*), and now oils are produced in Algeria, Morocco and Egypt (Weiss 1997), and also India (with plants that originated in Réunion) and China (*P. roseum*, a hybrid of *P. capitatum* and *P. radens*).

The aroma of the oil will vary according to its geographical origin. Generally, the main constituents are citronellol, geraniol, linalool and *iso*-menthone, and it is their relative proportions that influence the odour of the oil. Geranium oil from Grasse has a fine, rose-like scent; however, it is the oil from Réunion that sets the standard for perfumery. This may have a fresh, mint-like note due to the *iso*-menthone, and also rosy, sweet and fruity notes. The Moroccan oil is dark to mid-yellow with a sweet, rosy and herbaceous aroma; Egyptian oil is yellowish-green with an aroma similar to that from Morocco. Oil from China is more variable in quality because of the differences in distillation methods and also the number of variants under cultivation. Generally, Chinese oil is a darker olive green with a harsher odour than Réunion, but more lemony and rosy, sweet and herbaceous; it is not considered a substitute for the others in perfumery (Weiss 1997).

In traditional medicine, geranium oil is an insecticide, nematicide and antifungal (Weiss 1997). It has many applications in contemporary aromatherapy too, such as for skin care, poor circulation, premenstrual syndrome, tension, anxiety and stress-related problems. Research has revealed that geranium can suppress inflammation and may be of use in the management of rheumatoid arthritis (Maruyama *et al.* 2006) and can relieve pain, even in cases of severe and disabling postherpetic neuralgia (Greenway *et al.* 2003). It has also been demonstrated that the scent of geranium can reduce anxiety (Morris *et al.* 1995).

Like rose, geranium is widely used in perfumery. Although many masculine fragrances contain rose, geranium is also used to impart its green, rosy notes, appearing less frequently in feminine fragrances. For example, in the chypre leathery *Knize Ten* (Knize) it forms an accord with cedarwood in the middle note, and in *Gucci pour Homme* (Gucci) geranium is used with carnation and patchouli. In the fougère, woody-ambery category, geranium, clary sage and carnation are used in the middle note of *Paco Rabanne pour Homme* (Rabanne). An example of geranium in a supporting role can be found in the dry, floral heart of Davidoff's fresh fougère, *Cool Water* (Glöss 1995). Geranium is rarely found in a leading role; however, Frédéric Malle's *Geranium pour Monsieur* (2009), composed by Dominique Ropion, pairs geranium with mint absolute and anise, over a warm, spicy base.

Immortelle

'Immortelle' is the French for 'everlasting', and here refers to *Helichrysum angustifolium* (or *H. italicum*), *H. orientale* (the essential oil) and *H. stoechas* (the absolute); however, over 400 species have been identified. *H. italicum* is a bushy, woody, aromatic herb of the Asteraceae ('daisy') family. Its brightly coloured flowers dry out and become papery as the plant matures, but remain colourful, so are often used in 'everlasting' flower arrangements. It is native to the Mediterranean region and North Africa, where, in traditional medicine, decoctions were used for asthma, bronchitis and whooping cough, and also for migraine, headaches and skin problems (Lawless 1992). Paolini *et al.* (2006) noted that within *H. italicum* there were three subspecies. These are *microphyllum* (Baleares, Sardinia and Corsica), *serotinum* (Iberian Peninsula) and *italicum* (Mediterranean basin).

Usually, the essential oil is obtained from the flowering tops of *H. italicum*. Its top note is rich, sweet and honey-like, the body is sweet, fruity and tea-like, and the dryout is warm and herbaceous. The essential oil contains an unusual group of constituents – italidiones – which are diketones. These are reputed to possess antibruising actions, and so in aromatherapy the oil is often used for superficial trauma to soft tissues. In 2007 Voinchet and Giraud-Robert investigated the therapeutic effects and potential clinical applications of *H. italicum* var. *serotinum* and a macerated oil of the musk rose (*Rosa rubiginosa*) following cosmetic and reconstructive surgery. The objectives of reducing inflammation, oedema and bruising were all achieved, and more than half of the participants were able to go home in five rather than the usual 12 days. The researchers attribute many of these effects to the italidiones, and commented that neryl acetate, a principal constituent, contributed to a pain-relieving effect. Post-operative scarring was also commented upon, and it was suggested that the musk rose oil helped to prevent scarring. Lawless (2009) suggested that in perfumery, immortelle deserved to be better known; however, Turin (Turin and Sanchez 2009) perhaps reveals why it is not more commonly used. He suggests that it has a 'difficult, burnt-sugar/fenugreek note', and that 'immortelle always sticks out'. He notes that Annick Goutal used immortelle very successfully in *Sables*: here, it sits on an amber base, and is a 'wonderfully original and satisfying fragrance' (p.482). He also comments on Dior's *Eau Noir*, composed by Francis Kurkdjian. In this interpretation of immortelle, it is paired with lavender to give the olfactory impression of 'sun-roasted garrigue, where both smells frequently co-exist' (p.235). Finally, the 'dusty spicy smell of immortelle' gives a seaside nuance in Parfums de Rosine's otherwise watery, fruity, rosy *Écume de Rose* (p.239) and is used, to great effect, in the interplay of freshness and dryness in Missoni's *Missoni Aqua*, composed by Maurice Roucel (p.383).

Violet floral scents: ionones and irones

Violet

We have already explored the intense green notes of violet leaf; however, in a few species, the violet flowers are highly scented. Grieve (1992) tells us that in ancient times the Britons used violets for cosmetic purposes, and the Celts steeped them in goats' milk to improve the complexion. Later on, the violet came to be associated with Napoleon Bonaparte. When he departed for Elba, his last message to his supporters was that he would return with violets, and so he was thereafter alluded to as *Caporal Violette*, and the violet became the emblem of the Imperial Napoleonic party. However, after he was exiled, his estranged consort Marie-Louise travelled to Parma and was charmed by the violets that were part of the local flora. She settled there, and encouraged their cultivation and the distillation of violet water at the San Giovanni Evangelista monastery. Not all violets are scented like the Parma violet, but it was observed that the unscented Toulouse violet does produce scent when grown in Grasse (Morris 1984). Violet flower absolute has a sweet, rich, floral scent, very similar to the fresh flowers, and Lawless (1992) suggests that in past times its scent was used to 'comfort and strengthen the heart' – and indeed one of the plant's folk names was 'heartsease'.

Extracting the scent from the flowers is possible, but a very costly exercise, as the yield is only 0.003 per cent. For this reason, violet scents are usually synthetic. An aromachemical known as ionone is used. This was first synthesised in 1893 by Tiemann and Kruger, as a by-product in the synthesis of irone. There are two isomeric forms – α-ionone and β-ionone – and a mixture of the two forms is known simply as 'ionone'. Because of its original synthesis, ionone was sometimes called 'irisone'; however, ionone itself can also be isolated from boronia and costus absolutes. It can be synthesised from citral and acetone. The ionones are an almost colourless liquid that is very prone to rapid deterioration, and so needs to be stored carefully in tightly closed containers, protected from light and at a cool, steady temperature. There are subtle differences in the odour between the two forms: α-ionone is floral, violet-like, woody and slightly fruity, while β-ionone is drier, woody-violet, slightly fruity and slightly oily, and reminiscent of cedarwood and raspberries. When diluted, ionone is reminiscent of orris, but when mixed with alcohol it is more like fresh violets. Both forms can cause olfactory fatigue; that is, if they are smelled over a short period of time, their odours can no longer be detected because the olfactory receptors become 'numb'. The α-isomer is more versatile and is used in violet fragrances such as *'violette de parme'* and other floral perfumes, although the β-isomer also finds applications in violet and jasmine fragrances, woody fragrances and also in fruity perfumes for lipsticks. There is also a series of methyl ionones; the most widely used is γ-methyl-ionone. This does not occur in nature, and is a colourless liquid with a soft, sweet, violet-like and woody scent. Gamma-methyl-ionone is used in violet and floral fragrances and also woody ones; it is considered to be an excellent blender which can contribute powdery characteristics (Jouhar 1991; Williams 1995d). There are very few violet soliflores on the market today; however, Penhaligon's *Violetta*, Annick Goutal's *La Violette* and Caron's *Violette Précieuse* are three good examples (Turin and Sanchez 2009). Guerlain's classic (1905) *Après l'Ondée* has a fresh, floral violet and bergamot top over a floral (carnation and ylang ylang) heart and a sweet powdery base, and Yves Saint Laurent's *Paris* (1985) has a heart dominated by a violet and rose accord (Glöss 1995).

Orris

Orris is an exquisite scent, but not one that can be experienced directly in nature. It is a waxy, white solid that is obtained by steam distillation of the powdered rhizomes of *Iris pallida, I. germanica* and *I. florentina*. In order to allow the fragrance to develop, the rhizome must be washed, peeled and then dried under controlled conditions for three years. This is therefore a very costly raw material in perfumery, so what are its origins? These species are 'flag' irises, decorative perennials with distinctive scented flowers and elongated, sword-shaped leaves that emerge from a creeping, fleshy rhizome known as orris root.

The iris is named after the goddess of the rainbow, reflecting the many lovely colours of flowers in this genus. The ancient Egyptians placed the three-petalled flower on the brow of the sphinx and on the sceptre of their kings, the petals representing faith, wisdom and valour. The Romans dedicated the iris to Juno, consort of Jupiter.

Orris root was known to Theophrastus, Pliny and Dioscorides. In ancient Greece and Rome it was valued for its medicinal properties; it was crushed and infused in wine for bronchitis, coughs and hoarseness, and also to treat headaches and diarrhoea. The ancient Greeks and Romans also used its juice in cosmetics and perfumes, although the fresh root is not scented (Grieve 1992; Lawless 1992). When fresh, the roots are acrid and pungent to taste, but this disappears in the dried roots, when they begin to develop a violet-like aroma.

In Tuscany, the orris root is called *giaggiolo*, and its planting and cultivation is taken very seriously. The plants take three years to mature, reaching over a metre in height, before the rhizomes are harvested, trimmed, peeled and dried. In fact, there are several different varieties in the orris root of commerce – however, 'Florentine' iris was well regarded. In England, in the time of Edward IV, his wardrobe accounts of 1480 indicate that powdered orris root was mixed with anise and used to perfume linen, and during the reign of Elizabeth I (1558–1603) it was known to 'cloth-workers and drapers', who used the roots to trim the materials to make 'swete clothe'. Also, in his *History of the Vegetable Kingdom* (1868), the physician, scientist and prolific writer Dr William Rhind noted that orris gave a 'peculiar flavour' to artificial brandies and that the root was used in Russia to flavour a honey and ginger beverage (Grieve 1992, p.437).

The orris of perfumery is a very costly, waxy, solid material, sometimes called 'butter'. It is not a concrete, although it has been called this because of its appearance. It is still sourced in Florence, but often processed in southern France and Morocco. It has a sweet, violet-like and woody scent with moderate tenacity; and has a muted, almost sad character in comparison with the lively and joyful nature of, for example, jasmine. Orris' notable constituents are irone, aldehydes C_9 and C_{10} and myristic acid. Irone (α-irone) is 6-methyl-α-ionone; it was first isolated from orris roots in 1893 by Tieman and Kruger, and has the soft, sweet, diffusive odour of orris and violets. The isolate and its synthetic equivalent are not stable, and must be stored in small volumes, sealed under nitrogen. On exposure to the air, it oxidises and spoils very quickly. Although within orris oil, it is protected by the myristic acid it should still be stored carefully, away from light and heat, and in a tightly sealed container. Aldehyde C_9 (nonanal) in dilution is sweet, rosy, fresh and waxy, and orange-like, and C_{10} (decanal) is powerful and waxy, and pleasant only in very high dilution. In recent years the synthesis of α-irone from α-pinene has become established, and so iris perfumes have become more commonplace. In the iconic *Iris Gris* (1947), composed by Vincent Roubert for Jacques Fath, the somewhat sombre orris was paired with a lactonic (milky) peach base (Persicol). More recently, Frédéric Malle's *Iris Poudre*, composed by Pierre Bourdon, used the same idea, resulting in a powdery, fruity iris. *Chanel No.19* (Chanel) is a green floral, with orris and rose in the heart; the top is green and the base woody, mossy and powdery (Glöss 1995); this fragrance can give a cool and aloof effect. In contrast, Annick Goutal's *Heure Exquise* also combines green (galbanum) and iris, but with a woody, animalic base, giving a much warmer, more intimate effect. In Guerlain's *Iris Ganache*, composed by Thierry Wasser, iris appears in a sweet violet, gourmand style of fragrance; Guerlain's *Insolence*, composed by Maurice Roucel is in a similar style, but using 'red fruits'. However, the iris fragrance that seems to be heading for cult status is Serge Lutens' *Iris Silver Mist*, again composed by Maurice Roucel. This is an ethereal, powdery, rooty interpretation of orris (Turin and Sanchez 2009).

Boronia

Boronia megastigma is the brown boronia, a bushy evergreen shrub belonging to the Rutaceae (citrus) family. It reaches around one metre in height, and has small, aromatic leaves and small, cup-shaped flowers. These are intensely fragrant, and are chocolate brown-red on the outside and yellow inside. Brown boronia flowers smell like freesia and osmanthus, and are valued in flower arrangements in its native Australia. There are around 95 species in the genus, all but one occurring in Australia.

Boronia concrete and absolute are produced in southwestern Australia and Tasmania. The absolute is a dark green, viscous liquid with a fresh, fruity, spicy, tea-like character and a rich floral undertone (Lawless 1992; Leffingwell 1999–2001). Morris (1984) describes its scent as rich in violet notes, with a fresh top note and a rich, warm body, while Lawless (2009) concurs, adding that it has lily and freesia notes against a soft green back note. Boronia is used as a food flavour – it imparts body and a natural character to raspberry, strawberry and peach flavours.

For some time it has been established that boronia contains β-ionone. It also contains other ionones and related constituents such as α-ionone, β-ionol, dihydro-β-ionone, dihydro-β-ionol and 3-hydroxy- (E)-β-ionone. However, linalool, linalyl acetate and a series of 8-hydroxylinalool esters, and methyl jasmonate and related compounds are also present, and these too will have an impact on the aroma (Leffingwell 1999–2001).

Boronia is not a prominent or well-known perfumery material. It was exhibited at the British Empire Exhibition in 1924, but is rarely available, and has gained iconic status in the natural perfumery profession (Lawless 2009); for example, Aftelier's *Lumière* is based on Tasmanian boronia with blue lotus and frankincense.

Green florals

Narcotic florals

Hyacinth and narcissus are linked in Greek mythology, because both are symbolic of the cycle of life, death and rebirth, or transition and transformation. In these myths we can see a similar theme to that of Adonis and the rose.

Hyacinth

Hyacinthus was a beautiful youth, and lover of Apollo, but Zephyrus, god of the west wind, was also fond of him. Apollo taught him many skills such as archery, music, divination and throwing the discus. Apollo threw the discus and, trying to impress, Hyacinthus ran to catch it; however, the jealous Zephyrus blew the discus off course, and it hit and killed the youth. Apollo transformed his blood into the hyacinth flower, rather than have him descend to Hades. Sometimes it is said that the letters '*ai, ai*' were traced on the flower, so that Apollo's cries of grief would always be heard. Some versions of the myth suggest that the iris was the flower that represented his transformation, while others versions suggest that Hyacinthus was taken to the Elysian Fields by Aphrodite, Artemis and Athena. His tomb was at the foot of Apollo's statue at Amylcae, southwest of Sparta, and in the Mycenaean era a cult grew around him. Every summer, in Sparta, the three-day festival of *Hyacinthia* was held; the first day was spent mourning his death, but the following two days celebrated his rebirth.

The hyacinth emerges from a round bulb; it has bright green, lance-shaped leaves, and spikes of very fragrant, bell-shaped flowers. Linnaeus first called the hyacinth the flower of grief and mourning. As the related, but largely unscented, wild bluebell of the British Isles did not appear to have anything written on it, the early botanists named it *Hyacinthus non-scripta* (Grieve 1992). Despite the fact that it does not have a scent, when in full flower, bluebell woods are very special places to be; they can impart the sense of being at the fringe of another world, and have inspired many fairy tales and even fragrances.

The hyacinth that is grown for its oil is *Hyacinthus orientalis*. This is sometimes called *jacinthe* oil, and is cultivated commercially in both Holland and France. The absolute is a dark greenish liquid that has a very powerful, sharp, green, leaf-like odour, only pleasant on dilution, and only resembling hyacinth on extreme dilution (Jouhar 1991). At the time of writing, hyacinth absolute is very scarce; however, synthetic hyacinth is easily obtained. There is a marked difference in the fragrance: the synthetic version lacks the deep green-earthy note, and sweet green-floral notes dominate. Hyacinth absolute has a complex composition. It contains phenylethanol, eugenol, methyl eugenol, benzoic acid, benzyl acetate, benzyl alcohol, cinnamic alcohol, cinnamyl acetate, benzaldehyde, cinnamic aldehyde, methyl- and ethyl-*ortho*-methoxybenzoate, methyl methyl anthranilate, dimethyl hydroquinone and *N*-heptanol. Its odour is said to be narcotic, uplifting, refreshing, invigorating, and it may enhance creativity. The scent was used in ancient Greece to refresh the mind (Lawless 1992), and in Islamic culture hyacinth is said to sustain the soul; indeed, Mohammed himself suggested that scent itself was 'bread for the soul'. In a study of the mood-altering and enhancing effects of fragrances, Warren and Warrenburg (1993) found that hyacinth fragrance evoked happiness, sensuality, relaxation and stimulation, while decreasing feelings of apathy, irritation, stress and depression.

Hyacinth features in many classic and well-regarded fragrances. Guerlain's *Chamade* has a hyacinth and galbanum accord, Annick Goutal's *Grand Amour* is a floral bouquet with a powdery hyacinth character, and Serge Luten's *Bas de Soie* pairs hyacinth with iris. A hyacinth and oakmoss accord can be found in 'vintage' Guy Laroche's floral green *Fidji* and Chanel's *Cristalle*, a citrus chypre (Glöss 1995; Turin and Sanchez 2009).

Narcissus

Narcissus was a very different character, and perhaps less likeable than Hyacinthus, but his myth has a similar theme. His name is derived from the Greek word for 'sleep' or 'numbness'. He was the son of a river god and a nymph, and became a hunter who was renowned for his beauty. He had many suitors, both male and female, including the mountain nymph Echo, who pined and dwindled to an echo after he rejected her. Nemesis, the goddess of anger, was either petitioned for help or angered by his attitude, and so caused him to love himself, since he would not love others. He saw his reflection in a pool, fell in love with it and couldn't leave. Some versions say that he wasted away and died, and others say that he committed suicide. Either way, his transformation and 'rebirth' was symbolised by the appearance of the narcissus where he lay. He did not have a cult following, but leaves us with the concept of narcissism, and the scent of his flower has narcotic effects, perhaps reflecting his characteristic state of emotional numbness.

The genus *Narcissus* contains *N. pseudo-narcissus* (daffodil), *N. jonquilla* (jonquil) and *N. poeticus* (narcissus), from which an essential oil (ex-enfleurage) and an absolute can be obtained. The plant is cultivated in the Mediterranean, Morocco and Egypt for its aromatic extracts. Apparently it is not named after the Narcissus of myth, but from the Greek *narkao*, 'I grow numb', because the plant has narcotic properties. Grieve (1992) quotes Pliny, who described it as *'narce narcissum dictum, non a fabuloso puero'* which translates as 'named Narcissus from Narce, not from the fabulous boy' (p.573). She goes on to elaborate, saying that Socrates called it the 'chaplet of the infernal gods' because of its effects; an extract of the bulbs, if applied to open wounds, caused staggering, numbness of the nervous system and paralysis of the heart. Ancient Greeks planted *Narcissus* species near tombs. The bulbs of *N. poeticus* are even more poisonous than the daffodil, and Grieve suggested that 'the scent of the flowers is deleterious, if they are present in any quantity in a closed room, producing in some persons headache and even vomiting' (p.573). Despite this, the scent is well liked, and narcissus absolute is used in perfumery. It has a tiny yield, but is produced in small quantities – for example, in the Lozère, in the Languedoc Roussillon region of France. It is a dark orange/olive green, viscous liquid with a heavy, sweet, herbaceous, hay-like, earthy, floral odour. It only smells like narcissus on extreme dilution. Like all absolutes, it is chemically very complex, containing phenylethanol, α-terpineol, *l*-linalool, methyl ionone, anisic aldehyde and benzyl acetate (Jouhar 1991). There are trace amounts of indole, and since it is a white flower, this may not be surprising. According to Lawless (1992), it has antispasmodic, aphrodisiac and narcotic actions, and can be used in aromatherapy for its fragrance alone.

Narcissus absolute is used in the all-natural fragrance *Narcissus Poeticus* (Annette Neuffer); this also contains galbanum and blackcurrant bud, a pairing already seen in *Chamade* (Guerlain), and has a smooth, sweet base of vanilla, sandalwood and tonka bean. Indeed, the drydown of *Chamade* is described by Turin as 'beautiful, a strange, moist, powdery yellow narcissus accord that had the oily feel of pollen rubbed between finger and thumb' (Turin and Sanchez 2009, p.167). *Escada* (Escada) is a fresh floral. The top notes combine hyacinth, galbanum and peach, the heart is based on an accord of narcissus, tuberose and jasmine, and the base is floral and powdery, with cedar and heliotrope. A fragrance that showcases the hay-like nature of narcissus is L'Artisan Parfumeur's *Fleur de Narcisse*, which has notes of narcissus, hay, hyacinth, blonde tobacco, iris and blackcurrant bud over a moss and leather base. The classic *Narcisse Noir* (Caron 1912) featured narcissus and jasmine, and also the related jonquil in its heart note (Glöss 1995), but according to Turin and Sanchez (2009), the reformulated version is a sweet, jasmine and orange blossom cologne.

Calkin and Jellinek (1994) analyse the construction of Guy Laroche's *Fidji*, launched in 1966. This fragrance had a light green, floral character, and they comment that its green note was very complex indeed, with no one specific note predominating. They suggest that this might have been achieved with the use of several compounds or bases, including a hyacinth and a narcissus, perhaps with natural narcissus and violet leaf.

Honey and hay-like florals

Genet and broom

Genet is the name given to the absolute derived from *Spartium junceum*, commonly known as the Spanish broom, which was known to the ancient Greeks and Romans. It is related to the common broom of temperate northern Europe, *Cytisus scoparius*. (The species name comes from the Latin *scopa*, meaning a 'besom' or 'broom'.) The shrub is called 'broom' because traditionally the branches and twigs were made into brooms, and in Madeira woven into baskets, while in Scotland and the north of England it was used for fencing and thatch, cords and coarse cloth.

Broom belongs to the Leguminosae family whose members bear their seeds in pods, and is grown as an ornamental. It is a large woody shrub with long, bright green, flexible stems, small, narrow green leaves and yellow, pea-like, scented flowers, borne in racemose inflorescences (i.e. the individual flowers are formed on individual stalks on the main axis, as, for example, in the lupin).

The broom has an interesting history. Apart from its considerable uses in making household materials, it became a heraldic emblem. In early days it was adopted as the symbol for Brittany in France. When Geoffrey of Anjou was heading into battle, he pulled a piece of broom from a steep bank and announced, 'This golden plant, rooted firmly amid rock, yet upholding what is ready to fall, shall be my cognizance. I will maintain it on the field, in the tourney and in the court of justice' (Grieve 1992, p.125). Then Fulke of Anjou used it as his emblem, as did his grandson Henry II of England (1133–1189), who claimed the province. Henry used its mediaeval name, *Planta genista*, thus giving his line the name 'Plantagenet'. After Henry's death the broom appeared on the seal of his son, Richard I (1157–1199), which was its first heraldic appearance in England. An alternative version of its early use in Brittany suggests that a prince of Anjou assassinated his brother, and, overcome with remorse, made a pilgrimage to the Holy Land. Each night of the journey, he scourged his flesh with a brush of 'genets', and adopted the broom as his emblem so that he would not forget his repentance. In 1234 Louis of France founded a special order, whose token, called the *Colle de Genêt*, was made of alternating symbols of the *fleur de lys* and the broom flower; the motto was 'Exaltat humiles', 'He exalteth the lowly'. The order was bestowed on Richard II of England; this was a great honour, and on his death his tomb in Westminster Abbey was decorated with a broom plant, with open, empty pods.

The broom also had its own specific folk traditions. For example, if the broom was covered in flowers, it signified times of plenty. At the Whitsuntide festival it was in full bloom, and used for decoration rather than domestic chores. An old Suffolk saying was 'If you sweep the house with blossomed broom in May, you are sure to sweep the head of the house away' (Grieve 1992, p.125). It was used as a substitute for rosemary in rustic wedding bouquets.

Broom plays an important part in the ecosystem. It can help prevent soil erosion, and it tolerates sea air and salt spray, colonising sand dunes after the mat-forming grasses. It provides shelter for game birds too. Buds of the common broom were eaten as a delicacy, and the flowers and flowering tops were made into a decoction or infusion which was used as a cathartic and diuretic. It contains an alkaloid called sparteine that is toxic in large doses and scoparin, a glucoside. The Spanish broom is considerably more toxic, and cases of poisoning were recorded when the two types were confused (Grieve 1992). The yellow flowers have also been smoked for their psychotropic effects (Pennacchio *et al.* 2010).

As in traditional medicine, in perfumery the two types should be differentiated. Common broom (*Cytisus scoparius*) absolute is sweet and honey-like, and is produced in the south of France and Morocco. Genet absolute, obtained from the yellow-golden flowers of Spanish broom, is a dark brown, very viscous liquid that has a tenacious, sweet, rosy floral odour with green, herbaceous and hay-like notes (Jouhar 1991). Broom has been used since the sixteenth century in perfumery (Lawless 2009) and occasionally in contemporary perfumery. For example, Dior's *Dune* contains broom in its top note, possibly inspired by the scent of the plant growing on sand dunes, and Lauder included it in the heart notes of *Wild Elixir*, along with gardenia, orris, jasmine, muguet and water lily notes.

Farnesol, sweet, delicate florals

Mimosa

Mimosa and cassie belong to the same genus – *Acacia*, which is, like broom, in the Leguminosae family. The wood and bark of many *Acacia* species are used for their smoke (refer to Table 3.1). The acacias are a group of evergreen trees and shrubs, and some can reach 30 metres in height. They are often the 'pioneer' trees that grow after forest fires. The floral emblem of Australia is *A. pycnantha*, sometimes called mimosa (a name also given to the flowers and the absolute of *Acacia dealbata*, a small tree that is native to Australia, but also grown in France, Italy and India). In its native Australia it is known as the 'silver' or 'blue wattle'; the early settlers used it to make wattle and daub huts, and the silver or blue description might refer to white lichen that can cover its bark, or perhaps its silvery, blue-grey leaves. Like broom, its flowers are born in racemose inflorescences; and each bright yellow flower is globe-shaped and composed of 13–42 tiny individual flowers. The flowering tips and shoots are cut and used in floral decorations; mimosa flowers are a traditional gift on International Women's Day on 8 March. In Grasse in France, *La Fête du Mimosa* is held every February to celebrate the golden flower that has come to represent the end of winter.

Mimosa flowers have a delicate scent, candyfloss- and honey-like, but balanced with a sharper green note. Mimosa flowers and twig ends yield an absolute that has a powerful green-floral odour; this is mainly produced in the south of France (Jouhar 1991). Lawless (1992) suggests that it has a slightly green woody-floral odour and recommends it for anxiety, stress, tension and over-sensitivity. One of its main constituents is farnesol, a sesquiterpene alcohol.

In perfumery it is often used in lilac and lily of the valley re-creations (Jouhar 1991). Fragrances that feature mimosa are L'Artisan Parfumeur's *Mimosa pour Moi*, Kenzo's *Fleurs d'Hiver/Winter Flower* and Annick Goutal's limited edition *Le Mimosa*. *Cinéma* (Yves Saint Laurent) is a quiet, powdery, sweet interpretation of mimosa, and Divine's *L'Infante* is a rich, complex and intense natural mimosa fragrance (Turin and Sanchez 2009).

Cassie

Cassie, *Acacia farnesiana*, is a thorny bush or small tree similar to mimosa, which is cultivated in southern France and Egypt. Native to tropical and semi-tropical regions, possibly the West Indies, it is named after the Villa Farnese in Italy, where it was introduced as an ornamental: Odardo Farnese and the cardinal Alessandro Farnese established one of the first private botanical gardens at Carparola in the sixteenth and seventeenth centuries. Sometimes it is called opopanax, but it bears no relation to *Commiphora*. In India attar of cassie is a popular perfume; in the West the yellow, fluffy flowers are solvent-extracted to yield cassie absolute. Lawless (1992) describes it as having a warm, floral-spicy scent with a rich balsamic undertone, and it is this balsamic warmth that distinguishes it from mimosa. The odour, described as 'exquisite' by Jouhar (1991), has spicy and floral notes; it finds applications in violet or jasmine and rose accords. It is also said to have a powdery floral, violet-like top note (International School of Aromatherapy 1993). Like all absolutes, it is chemically very complex, and contains benzyl alcohol, methyl salicylate, farnesol, geraniol and linalool (Jouhar 1991; Lawless 1992). Cassie is sometimes used in leather accords to impart intensity. *Une Fleur de Cassie*, composed by Dominique Ropion for Frédéric Malle, is considered to be one of the best examples; here cassie is included in a 'symphonic' floral (Turin and Sanchez 2009).

Linden blossom

Tilea vulgaris, the linden (or lime) tree is native to Europe. It is a tall, deciduous tree with bright green, heart-shaped leaves. It bears clusters of strongly scented yellow-white flowers, called linden or lime flowers. These flowers have a long herbal tradition. Linden tisane, made from the dried flowers and known as '*tilleul*', is widely used as a calming tea, and its other uses in herbalism are for indigestion, palpitations and nausea, migraine, hypertension and fevers. This is the tisane that, paired with a madeleine, evoked the first recorded 'Proustian' memory. Grieve (1992) notes that if the lime blossoms are old, a tea made from them will have a narcotic effect. Linden blossom honey is regarded as being one of the finest, and had medicinal as well as culinary uses. The linden tree also features in Greek mythology: Philemon and Baucis, who wanted to spend eternity together, in the end were transformed into intertwined trees; he became an oak, and she became the linden.

Linden blossom concrete and absolute may be obtained from the blossoms, and are used in perfumery. The absolute is a yellowish, semi-solid paste with a green-herbaceous aroma; it is dominated by farnesol, which links it with mimosa and cassie. In aromatherapy linden blossom absolute is indicated for cramps, indigestion and headaches (Lawless 1992).

Current linden fragrances include *Tilleul* (D'Orsay), *Eau de Noho* (Bond No.9) and *Eau du Ciel* (Annick Goutal), where the top note is a linden and rosewood accord, and its green character and relationship with the violet is exploited in the heart note of violet leaves, iris, neroli and orange blossom. Corfan (2010) commented on the aroma of a recently available linden blossom CO_2 extract that is much closer to the scent of the fresh linden flowers. He described it as having honey, aromatic, broom, hay, violet leaf and chamomile notes, with an animalic, civet-like drydown. It is expected (and hoped) that this will open up new possibilities for linden blossom in perfumery.

Exotic florals from the East

Aglaia

Aglaia species are members of the family Meliaceae, which is the 'mahogany' family of tropical and subtropical regions such as Southeast Asia, northern Australia and the Pacific. The name *aglaia* is derived from the Greek word which means 'to make more beautiful', and Aglaea is the name of one of the Three Kharites in Greek mythology. The Three Kharites (or Charites), were the daughters of Zeus and Eurynome or Dionysus and Aphrodite. Aglaea represented 'splendour' and Euphrosyne 'mirth', while Thalia represented 'good cheer'. There are many regional variations regarding the symbolism. They are perhaps better known by their Roman name of the Three Gratiae, or Graces, and the numerous sculptures and paintings of them.

Aglaia spectabilis is a medium-sized tree that produces numerous highly scented, small yellow flowers. In Papua New Guinea it is known as *waso-no*, which means 'good-smelling'. In their natural state, the flowers have a 'quite transparent, ionone-floral and aromatic-floral scent, accompanied by a watery-fruity note typical of watermelon' (Kaiser 2006, p.84). Kaiser gives their constituents as (*E*)-ocimene, linalool, methyl benzoate, (*Z,Z*)-nona-3,6-dienol, β-ionone and (*E,E*)-2,6-dimethyl-1,2-epoxyocta-3,5,7-triene – the last of which gives a highly diffusive, fresh floral note which, if synthesised, could present new opportunities in perfumery. A reconstruction of the aglaia scent based on Kaiser's analysis was the inspiration behind Hugo Boss's *Hugo Boss Woman* in 1998 (Schilling *et al.* 2010). However, aglaia absolute, obtained from the flowers of *A. odorata*, is also available. This species is commonly known as the Chinese Rice Tree, and is native to China, Cambodia, Taiwan, Thailand and Vietnam. It does not appear to have gained much use in mainstream perfumery, but it is well known to natural perfumers. It has a light and fresh floral scent with jasmine and lemon-like notes, and for this reason it is considered valuable for linking these two odour types in natural compositions. Anya McCoy's *Light* (Anya's Garden) has aglaia with genet in the middle note, a citrus (cédrat and yellow grapefruit) and juniper berry top, and an ambergris and frankincense resinoid base note.

Osmanthus

Sweet osmanthus, *Osmanthus fragrans*, is an evergreen shrub native to China and some parts of Japan. According to Kaiser (2006), it is known as *kweiha*, and is one of the ten traditional flowers of China, where it is regarded as a very beautiful fragrance. Osmanthus is a medium-sized woody shrub, and although it is regarded as an autumn flower, some varieties can bloom all year round, and these are named 'osmanthus four seasons'. The flowers can vary in colour according to type, from silvery white to reddish orange, but the ones with orange-yellow flowers are regarded as the best. Monks have cultivated it for centuries, and osmanthus groves can be found at Buddhist temples. When in flower, a diffusive, fruity-floral scent fills the air, and even when the flowers fall, covering the ground, the fragrance is emitted for many hours. In China the dried flowers are used to enhance the flavour of green and black teas.

The golden-orange flowers are used for the extraction of the very expensive osmanthus absolute. Kaiser (2006) suggests that this 'quintessential scent of China', contributes a 'unique balance between floral and fruity notes' (p.29). Osmanthus absolute is an amber or green viscous liquid which has a distinctive, complex odour; it is rich, sweet, honey-like and ethereal-floral, reminiscent of plums and raisins (Leffingwell 2000) and apricot (Warren and Warrenburg 1993). Constituents that are important in its odour are β-ionone, dihydro-β-ionone, γ-decalactone and related lactones, linalool, nerol and geraniol (Kaiser 2006). Warren and Warrenburg's study (1993) on the mood effects of fragrance found that the scent of osmanthus (a synthetic version) had stimulating and 'happy' qualities, and could prominently reduce apathy and depression. Since then osmanthus has become part of mainstream perfumery, with several well-known fragrances claiming to include an osmanthus note, such as *Escape* (Calvin Klein 1991, since reformulated) and *Sunflowers* (Arden 1993). Calkin and Jellinek discuss its role in Calvin Klein's powdery, sweet, rosy floral *Eternity* (1988), where a rich osmanthus complex, and possibly a natural absolute, is used to give a floral-fruity character to an otherwise synthetic, 'luxury toilet soap'-like heart. Lawless (2009) commented on his experience working with osmanthus in composing *Kuan Yin* (Essentially Me); it produced unexpected delicate notes of peach blossom. However, Turin and Sanchez (2006) discuss the challenges of osmanthus in perfumery; they suggest that it is actually a 'ready-made' fragrance, and that the perfumer's skill is in reviving it after the solvent extraction process. As an example, they follow the work of Jean-Claude Ellena in relation to osmanthus. In 2001 he composed *Osmanthus* for The Different Company, which captured its nature perfectly and combined it with peach and lemony top notes. Later, in 2005, he composed *Osmanthe Yunnan* for Hermès. This combined osmanthus with Yunnan smoked tea notes, freesia, orange and apricots, and Turin and Sanchez (2006) describe it as 'a perfume of pure happiness' (p.427). This sounds very like the effect that Warren and Warrenburg's research suggested.

Pandanus

Pandanus species of the Pandanaceae family are sometimes called 'screw pines'; they are palm-like trees and shrubs, ranging from one metre to 20 metres in height, and grow all over Southeast Asia. Typically, they produce 'prop roots' that help anchor them in the soil, and have a broad canopy of strap-shaped leaves and large, heavy, pineapple-like fruits that ripen from green to orange-red and are eaten by a wide range of creatures – bats, rats, crabs, elephants and monitor lizards. The strap-like leaves are cut into strips and used to weave baskets, mats and ropes. The leaves of *P. amyryllifolius* are used in Southeast Asian cuisine to flavour rice and curry dishes, and also desserts such as *pandan* cake. In India they are used to flavour ordinary long grain rice, as distinct from basmati rice; this is because the constituent that gives the aroma and flavour, 2-acetyl-1-pyrroline, occurs naturally in basmati rice. *P. odoratissimus* grows in India on coastal belts and river banks, and is found in thickets in tidal forests.

The scented 'flower' that is so important in Indian culture is not a true flower, it is a male spadix, enclosed in a long, fragrant bract. It is very large, and creamy white or yellow in colour. These flowers are used to make oils, perfumes and lotions. They are used in garlands and hair ornaments, but are not offered in worship. This is because they are said to have been cursed by the Lord Shiva.

Three scented products are made from the flowers, which must be harvested in early morning and processed quickly, as they lose their scent when the calyx is opened; extraction is by basic hydro-distillation. *Attar kewra* is obtained by distillation into sandalwood oil. This is used as a perfume, and also to flavour tobacco and make incense sticks. *Rooh kewra* is the pure essential oil; it is costly and valued as a perfume, but is also used in medicine as an antispasmodic and stimulant, as well as to treat headache and rheumatism. Finally, *kewra water* is a by-product of distillation and has culinary uses (Gupta 2013).

Kewra oil has a powerful, sweet, lilac, green and honey-like odour. Gupta (2013) states that the main constituent responsible for the aroma is phenyl ethyl methyl ether, although Jouhar (1991) mentions phenylethanol, benzyl alcohol and its esters benzyl acetate, benzyl benzoate and benzyl salicylate, linalool and geraniol, linalyl acetate, santalol, guaicol and an unusual constituent, ω-bromstyrene, which itself has a harsh, hyacinth-like odour.

Kewra is not widely used in western perfumery. However, two all-natural fragrances feature it. These are Anya's Garden *Fairchild* and Aftelier's *Shiso*. It is worth mentioning the notes in these fragrances, because they illustrate the construction of natural fragrances and also shows the creative use of materials to achieve specific effects. *Fairchild* was composed by Anya McCoy. Here, pandanus is used along with tropical flowers in the top note. The middle note is comprised of many of the aromatics discussed in this chapter – three jasmines (*grandiflorum, sambac* and *auriculatum*) white and gold champaca, and ylang ylang. The base note contains seaweed, ambergris, smoked sea shells and oakmoss; this would suggest that the intent was to recreate the ambience of a tropical beach. *Shiso*, composed by Mandy Aftel, sounds quite different, with more of a spicy, woody, Asian theme. Here the top note is provided by clove and pepper, the middle by pandanus with *shiso* (an Asian mint) and geranium, and the base is sandalwood, patchouli and oud.

Lotus

We have already explored the importance of the blue lotus of the Nile to the ancient Egyptians, and the sacred lotus of India has a similar significance to Buddhists and Hindus. There are many parallels in the symbolism between these related species, especially in relation to the diurnal pattern of the flowers opening and closing; both flowers were said to be the home of the sun god. The Indian type is *Nelumbo nucifera*, of the Nelumbonaceae family; it is a true lotus rather than a water lily. It was originally native to the lakes of Kashmir, but spread over the Indian subcontinent. Monks carried it all over Southeast Asia; its seeds can remain viable for over 1000 years. Like *Nymphaea stellata*, a water lily, it is an aquatic perennial, with blue, white or white-and-pink-tipped flowers. Buddhists adopted the lotus as a symbol of *dharma* because its roots are in the mud but it rises to the surface and the light, where it produces large, flat leaves and beautiful scented flowers. The flowers are diurnal; they close at night and open in the morning, before closing again in the late afternoon.

The symbolism surrounding the lotus is considerable – the Buddha is depicted as sitting on the flower, and the *Asvins*, the youthful twin gods of the dawn, wore a garland of blue lotuses. The pink lotus is very much associated with Kuan Yin, who represents the principle of compassion; in every Chinese Buddhist temple there is a shrine to her, and it is usually adorned with pink lotus blooms (Lawless 2009). Hindu deities are also portrayed holding the lotus, and it is used as incense in temples. The flowers symbolise immortality, resurrection, and transcendence too, as they emerge from dried-up pools following the monsoon. When the flowers open, they emit an exquisite scent. Kaiser (2006) notes that the poems written about the lotus exhibit a 'positive synaesthesia of appearance, cultural feelings and olfactory perception' (p.120). He mentions that, when experienced out of context, the scent is warm-herbaceous, sweet, aromatic and somewhat medicinal, largely due to its main constituent 1,4-dimethoxybenzene. There are several cultivars, and they all have similar scents; *Nelumbo lutea*, the yellow-flowering American lotus, has a more pronounced jasmine note.

Lotus absolute needs to mature in order to develop its fragrance. McMahon (2011b) describes pink lotus absolute as a deep pink, viscous liquid with a rich, sweet floral heart, fruity/leathery notes and a powdery, spicy dryout. White lotus is a dark brown, viscous liquid with a similar odour but an animalic, herbaceous dryout.

Many commercial fragrances list the lotus note, and in most of these it is probably difficult to discern. Jouhar (1991) noted that 'lotus' perfumes were mixtures of linalool and phenylethanol, with traces of patchouli and γ-undecalactone (peach aldehyde), fixed with amber and benzoin resinoid. However, *Royal Lotus* (Anya's Garden) is an all-natural fragrance with blue and pink lotus, and jasmine and orange blossom, and Essentially Me's *Kuan Yin* and *White Blooms* have pink lotus in supporting roles.

Tropical florals

Frangipani

According to Jouhar (1991), 'Frangipanni' was the name given to a jasmine-like perfume that was popular in the middle of the nineteenth century. It was not linked to a botanical species, but to the name of an ancient Roman family whose descendent invented a method of perfuming gloves. Frangipani is the tree whose botanical name is *Plumeria*, after the French botanist Charles Plumier. It is believed that *Plumeria* was native to tropical America or the Caribbean, and was then introduced to Australia. It is now present across tropical regions.

Plumerias are small trees with scented flowers; their fragrance is more intense at night, in order to attract their pollinators, the sphinx moths. They do not produce nectar, but the moths continue to transfer pollen from flower to flower in their quest for it. *Plumeria* is a deciduous tree with thick branches that contain a milky latex. Its leaves are arranged in a spiral at the ends of the swollen branches (Tohar *et al.* 2006). *Plumeria* has large, waxy, five-petalled flowers that are beautifully formed and can be found in many different colours: deep pink buds opening to light pink; or red tinged with apricot; pale pink with pale yellow centres; yellow with gold centres; deep pink with cream and yellow centres; creamy white with pale yellow deepening to gold centres, and pure, waxy white.

Like all highly scented and striking flowers, frangipani has acquired cultural traditions, but because of its spread in tropical regions, these are quite varied. The fragrant frangipani flowers are very beautiful, and have acquired a variety of meanings in various cultures, such as new life, creation, dedication and devotion. In Sri Lanka *Plumeria* is known as *araliya*, 'the temple tree', because it is planted near temples and shrines, and in India this is also the case (McMahon 2011c). In Bali the flowers are offered in temples. However, in some Southeast Asian cultures, they are believed to shelter ghosts and demons, and are often planted in graveyards; in Bangladesh they are associated with death and funerals, as are other white flowers. Despite association with a vampire, in Malaysia it is a popular garden plant, known locally as *kemboja*. A more positive theme can be found in Hawaii and the Pacific Islands; the Hawaiian culture regards the frangipani flower as a symbol of everything good. In Hawaii, Tahiti, Fiji, Samoa, Tonga and the Cook Islands the flowers are used in making *leis* (garlands), and, like the tiaré flowers, are worn by women as hair decorations that indicate their relationship status.

Plumeria species have several uses in traditional medicine. A decoction of the bark is used as a purgative, emmenagogue, diuretic, and to reduce fever, it is also said to cure various venereal diseases. *Plumeria* is also among the traditional plants that have been found to possess antitumoural and antimicrobial properties; it might also be effective against parasitic infestations. In Thailand an infusion of the flowers is applied to the skin after bathing, as a cosmetic (Tohar *et al.* 2006). In Ayurvedic medicine frangipani is used to calm fear and anxiety, and also to treat tremors and insomnia. In India incense sometimes contains *Plumeria* species, indicated by the word *champa*; perhaps *Nag Champa* is best known in the West, this combines frangipani with sandalwood and the water-absorbing resin of *Ailanthus malabarica*.

This is a Southeast Asian rainforest tree, whose resin contains small amounts of the psychoactive β-carboline, also found in tobacco. The scent of the flowers depends on the variety and the person describing the scent; Criley (2001) maintains that *Plumeria* flower fragrances can be weak, mild or strong, and that the strongly scented varieties can be described in terms of other fragrance types such as citrus, coconut, rose, cinnamon, carnation, jasmine, gardenia, fruity and woody. It is worth looking in more detail at the fragrance variations, which can (but only up to a point) be explained by chemistry. In two studies (Omato *et al.* 1991, 1992, cited in Criley 2001) analysis of the essential oils of two varieties – 'Common Yellow' and 'Irma Bryan' – showed significant differences in their constituents which could help explain the odour differences. Criley reported that 'Common Yellow' was dominated by phenylacetaldehyde which has a penetrating, pungent, green-floral, sweet hyacinth odour, and linalool, with *trans, trans*-farnesol, β-phenylethanol, geraniol and α-terpineol, and that two trace components, neral and geranial, contributed to its citrus notes. 'Irma Bryan' was dominated by β-phenylethanol, which has a sweet, rosy scent, and contained almost three times as much as did 'Common Yellow'. It too contained phenylacetaldehyde, but at a lower level, and other constituents such as methyl cinnamate, which is spicy and fruity.

A few years later Tohar *et al.* (2006) investigated the aroma and chemical composition of a further three *Plumerias*. The white-flowered *P. acuminata* had a sweet floral, fruity-fresh green and woody fragrance. It was rich in esters, notably benzyl salicylate, which has a mild, sweet, floral-balsamic odour, and neryl phenylacetate, which is fruity, rosy and apple-like. It also contained *trans*-nerolidol, found in all of the species examined (this has a mild, pleasant floral odour), linalool and geranial, which contributed to the citrus note of the oil. The reddish-orange flowers of *P. rubra* had a strong, sweet scent. It too was characterised by esters, notably phenyl ethyl benzoate, but also benzyl salicylate, which has a faint, sweet, floral odour and phenyl ethyl cinnamate, which has a rosy, honey-like scent. However, the presence of δ-terpineol, *trans*-nerolidol and farnesol were thought to enhance the scent of this variety. The red-flowered *P. rubra* had a sweet, tea rose-like scent, with spicy-herbaceous characteristics. Its main constituents were hexadecanoic acid, linoleic acid, tetradecanoic acid and dodecanoic acid, making it very different from the others analysed. In this case it was minor constituents that contributed to the odour; geranyl isobutyrate, geraniol, neryl formate and menthone could have given the tea rose character; linalool, farnesal, farnesol and *trans*-nerolidol could have given the sweetness, while the peppery, spicy herbaceous element may have come from terpinen-4-ol (mild lilac), caryophyllene (clove-like), methyl cinnamate (balsamic, fruity, strawberry-like) and methyl salicylate (sweet medicated and fruity). The studies have all had value, in that they have elucidated chemical 'markers' for the fragrances of different varieties of *Plumeria*, but they also show us that the fragrance of the flower (and indeed any flower) is far greater than the sum of its constituents, as we saw when discussing fragrance philosophies in Chapter 5.

So, if indeed there is such a thing, a 'typical' frangipani absolute has a rich, exotic, heady floral aroma, with sweet honey-like notes and fruity notes; the scent is said to bring comfort, impart inner peace and release tension (McMahon 2011c). Turin and Sanchez (2009) suggest that frangipani can be either jasmine-like or peach-like. Frangipani can be found in the heart notes, along with champaca, of the fruity floral *Sira des Indes* (Patou). Turin and Sanchez mention two frangipani fragrances: Chantecaille's light, woody floral *Frangipane* and Ormonde Jayne's *Frangipani Absolute*, a fresh and intense floral that smells somewhere between jasmine and peach. *Songes* (Annick Goutal) was composed by Isabelle Doyen in 2005; the creative brief was inspired by the scent of frangipani at dusk on the island of Mauritius. It opens with a jasmine accord which gives way to frangipani, tiaré, ylang ylang and vanilla.

Ylang ylang

Cananga odorata var. *genuina* is a tall tropical tree that can reach 35 metres in height; under cultivation it is pruned to about three metres. It is native to Southeast Asia, has naturalised in Burma, Malaysia, Indonesia, Papua New Guinea, the Pacific Islands and the Philippines, and has been introduced into many other tropical regions including the Caribbean and the Indian Ocean. It is said that ylang ylang was 'discovered' on the island of Ceram in the Indonesian archipelago by the Dutch Captain d'Etchevery in 1770.

The name 'ylang ylang' is a Tagalog[2] phrase that means 'flower of flowers' (Morris 1984); the words are derived from *ilong-ilang*, a Philippine phrase that describes how the flowers flutter in the breeze. The genus name, *Cananga*, is probably derived from the Malaysian *kenanga*. In Tamil ylang ylang is called *karumugai*, and in Sri Lanka it is known as *wanasapu*.

Ylang ylang has slightly aromatic thin, oblong leaves with a pointed apex, and numerous, yellow/green highly scented flowers.

The flowers have an intense floral, narcotic fragrance, and they are used for personal decoration and to scent fabrics, homes and clothing; in Indonesia it is a folk custom to perfume the bed linen of newly married couples with ylang ylang

---

2   Tagalog is an Austronesian language spoken in the Philippines. It means 'river dweller'.

flowers (Weiss 1997). Locally produced oils have been used in folk medicine for cosmetic and skin care purposes, but the commercial value of ylang ylang oil has been recognised for some time and commercial cultivation and oil production have been well established in Indonesia and Madagascar, and also Réunion, Comoro and the Philippines, for some time. Weiss (1997) suggests that the first distillation of the oil is credited to Albertus Schwenger, who operated a small mobile still in the Philippines in the mid-nineteenth century, and the first commercial operation was started by Steck, who ran a German apothecary, and his nephew Paul Sartorius; the oil was marketed as 'Ylang Ylang Oil Sartorius' and it gained an international reputation. Ylang ylang oil was one of the new scents exhibited at the Paris World Exhibition in 1878 (Morris 1984). Because of world wars, economic forces and inclement weather – the cultivated areas are subjected to damaging local cyclones – some regions fared better than others in terms of oil production. Most oil is now produced in Indonesia and Madagascar.

Morris (1984) notes that by 1893 ylang ylang oil had become one of the mainstays of French perfumery, the finer grades being preferred to oils from related species, or lesser grades which are known as cananga. The flowers must be harvested carefully to yield the best oil. Initially the flowers have little scent, and have green petals covered with fine white hair that disappears as they mature. Within two to three weeks the petals turn from pale green to yellow, and their scent becomes stronger. They are ready for harvest when two little reddish spots appear on the base of the petals. The flowers are harvested manually; Weiss (1997) comments that an experienced picker can collect 20kg per shift, but the flowers must be treated gently, because bruised or damaged ones will result in off-notes in the product. They must be distilled as soon as possible after picking to give a good yield; 2.0–2.5 per cent is expected. As delays are inevitable, the flowers are spread out in the shade to avoid fermentation before processing.

Fractional steam distillation of the flowers produces four or five grades of essential oil, and each fraction has a different chemical composition and odour. The grade known as 'extra' is preferred for its fragrance, but the absolute has an odour closer to that of the flowers. Ylang ylang extra has a sweet, persistent, floral odour with a 'creamy' top note. Williams (2000) describes it as having a strong, medicated, floral top note, a medicated, floral, fruity body and a medicated, floral spicy dryout. Its chemical composition is very variable; however, it will usually contain linalool, geranyl acetate, benzyl acetate and methyl salicylate (which is responsible for the slightly medicinal note), phenyl methyl ethers (15%), sesquiterpenes such as farnesene and caryophyllene, and phenols, including eugenol. The extra has higher levels of p-cresyl methyl ether, methyl benzoate, linalool, methyl acetate and geranyl acetate than the other grades (Weiss 1997).

Ylang ylang has long been considered an aphrodisiac – its scent is considered to be very relaxing yet highly euphoric – and so in aromatherapy its scent is used to relax and uplift, and to help the individual to connect with their senses and the physical realm. In 2004 Hongratanaworakit and Buchbauer conducted a study which demonstrated that ylang ylang had a 'harmonising' effect, where blood pressure and heart rate decreased whilst attentiveness and alertness were increased. In 2006 the same researchers investigated the effects of ylang ylang oil, this time via absorption through the skin. Again, it was demonstrated that there was a significant decrease of blood pressure and increase in skin temperature in the ylang ylang group compared with the placebo. The ylang ylang group also reported feeling more calm and relaxed than the control group.

Moss *et al.* (2006) investigated the cognitive effects of ylang ylang aroma, and demonstrated that ylang ylang could significantly increase calmness, but it decreased alertness and reaction times, and impaired memory and processing speed. So there is little doubt as to the relaxing effects of the fragrance of ylang ylang, and its use in aromatherapy massage.

In perfumery it plays a major role; its jasmine-like aspects blend well with rose, and it is often found as a modifier in synthetic lilac and violet accords (Jouhar 1991). Ylang ylang is very versatile. For example, it is in the green top notes of Chanel's *No.19*, along with galbanum, bergamot and lemon; in the heart of the classic chypre *Miss Dior* (Dior) along with fruity jasmine notes and rose; in the heart of Patou's fruity floral, *Sira des Indes*, along with frangipani and champaca; with vanilla in Maître Parfumeur et Gantier's *Fleurs des Comores*; and with rose in the sweet floral heart of Molinard's oriental ambery *Habanita* (Calkin and Jellinek 1994; Glöss 1995).

Cottage garden scents, restricted access only

The well-loved fragrances of 'cottage garden' flowers are perhaps most captivating when smelled *au naturel* – in some it is simply not possible to extract their aromas, and in others the yield is so low that commercial scale extraction is not feasible. Some of their scents, however, can be recreated by the skilful blending of synthetics and naturals. Calkin and Jellinek (1994) explained that most floral bases were constructed with the same eight materials, and that it was their relative proportions that determined the characteristic of the base. These ingredients were phenylethanol (mild honey, rose or hyacinth-like), hydroxycitronellal (delicate, mild, floral and linden blossom-like), benzyl acetate (floral, fruity and jasmine-like), phenylacetaldehyde (intense green and hyacinth-like), citronellol (fresh, sweet, light and rosy), hexyl cinnamic aldehyde, α-terpineol (sweet, floral and lilac-like) and indole (jasmine-like on dilution) – and depending on the ratios, a jasmine, lilac, muguet or hyacinth-like scent could be created. However, while new scent molecules are being synthesised, others, including many of the above that were previously available, are now restricted, and so there is a constant state of flux. Until fairly recently, if any product contained a fragrance, this could be simply labelled as 'parfum', but now in Europe, since March 2005, all cosmetic and detergent products have had to declare the presence of 26 materials (Cadby *et al.* 2011). The International Fragrance Research Association (IFRA) publishes details of all recommendations and restrictions on their website; the reader is encouraged to visit this for current information (see the websites in the 'Recommended Reading' section at the end of the book).

Carnation

There are only two plant species with a carnation scent, and these are *Dianthus caryophyllus*, the carnation, and *D. plumarius*, the pink – both of which enjoy a dry, sunny, Mediterranean climate. Its psychotherapeutic effects have not been explored in the literature, but several individuals who have had the opportunity to experience its scent in an aromatherapy context have expressed feelings of 'comfort' and 'joy' or of 'being carefree', and a few have commented that it evoked positive childhood memories of playing in a garden. It is possible to produce carnation essential oil, which has a rich, clove-like scent, and an absolute is occasionally available; it has a very powerful fragrance and is extremely costly to produce. The absolute is a green or brown, highly viscous liquid or paste, with sweet, herbaceous, honey-like, minty floral and spicy-clove notes. The main constituents of carnation oil are benzyl benzoate (sweet balsamic), eugenol (warm spicy clove-like), phenylethanol (mild rose or hyacinth-like), benzyl salicylate (mild balsamic floral) and methyl salicylate (fruity medicinal). Most 'carnation oil' on the market is synthetic. The carnation scent can be mimicked using eugenol with *iso*-eugenol, which has a light, flowery, carnation-like and spicy scent, and other spice bases. Other aromachemicals that are important in carnation accords are *iso*-amyl salicylate, a highly aromatic, clover-like aromachemical, and benzyl *iso*-eugenol, which is mild, balsamic and carnation-like. In Calkin and Jellinek (1994) carnation compounding notes include ylang ylang extra, perhaps modified with benzyl acetate; rose notes derived from geraniol modified with, for example, phenylethanol; geranium oil; floral modifiers such as Hedione (methyl dihydrojasmonate, which has a sweet, floral, jasmine-like odour); spicy notes from eugenol and *iso*-eugenol; honey notes from various phenylacetates and perhaps honey or beeswax absolute; cinnamon notes from cinnamic alcohol and its esters; balsamic floral notes from benzyl salicylate; sweet notes from vanillin and heliotropin; and some naturals to give variants on the carnation theme. The naturals might include spices such as clove bud or black pepper, earthy freshness from carrot seed, florals such as rose or iris, and woods such as the rosy guaiacwood or cedarwood. Rosy notes can even come from citronella oil.

There are severe limits imposed on eugenol and *iso*-eugenol, and so, although it may have seemed that carnation soliflores had simply gone out of fashion, the reality is that they are disappearing (Alavi 2012). However, the carnation note is present in many masculine fragrances, appearing more often than rose. In Paco Rabanne's *Paco Rabanne pour Homme*, carnation forms an accord with clary sage and geranium in the middle note; in Hermès' *Equipage*, Shulton's *Old Spice* and numerous others it is paired with cinnamon, and in Guerlain's *Habit Rouge* there is a carnation and patchouli accord. Armani's *Armani Eau pour Homme* features carnation with bay and jasmine in the middle note (Glöss 1995). Guy Laroche's *Fidji* had carnation and orris in the heart, and in Dolce & Gabbana's first feminine fragrance, the aldehydic floral *Dolce & Gabbana* (1992), a carnation note has an enormous impact, although it is not listed by Glöss as a major floral ingredient (1995).

Lilac

The lilac is a spring flowering shrub, probably originating in Iran and introduced to Spain in the sixteenth century. The lilac flower has a sweet, fresh, heady, honey-like, spicy, cinnamon-like, floral scent. The essential oil does not resemble the lilac in its scent, and is very difficult to produce. Although small amounts of the absolute have been prepared on a small, experimental scale, this does not have the odour of the fresh flower either. A lilac alcohol has been identified, and this has four isomers, making up some 70 per cent of the oil (Jouhar 1991; International School of Aromatherapy 1993). So the lilac fragrance is made by compounding synthetics and naturals to give an interpretation of the scent. Calkin and Jellinek's (1994) basic materials for a lilac base included phenylethanol; α-terpineol for its lilac-like scent; ylang ylang extra, perhaps modified by linalool or an aromatic ester such as methyl benzoate (fruity floral, blackcurrant, ylang ylang and tuberose-like on dilution); muguet notes from hydroxycitronellal; green notes from phenyl acetaldehyde; anise notes from anisaldehyde; sweet floral notes from heliotropin; floral-cinnamon notes from cinnamic alcohol, clove-like notes from *iso*-eugenol, and indole. Naturals might include cinnamon bark. Houbigant's *Quelques Fleurs* (1912) had a dominant lilac note, as did Caron's *Fleurs de Rocailles* (1993). However, hydroxycitronellal is now severely restricted by anti-allergen guidelines (Alavi 2012) and this has had an impact on the recreation of lilac bases. Lilac soliflores are non-existent, but the lilac note can be found supporting other florals. For example, Guerlain's *Nahéma* has a peach and floral top note over a rose heart, which is supported by ylang ylang, jasmine, lily of the valley and lilac. A similar theme can be found in the heart note of Balenciaga's *Le Dix*, composed by Francis Fabron in 1947, where the top note is aldehydic, but the rose heart is supported by lilac, lily of the valley, jasmine, orris and champaca.

Lily

The lily has been a favourite perfume for millennia; the ancient Egyptians would macerate the flowers of *Lilium candidum* in oils to extract their fragrance. However, it is not possible to extract the scent from any of the various species of *Lilium*, and so the lily note in perfumery is always composed of synthetics and naturals. Again, 'lily aldehyde' or hydroxycitronellal was the predominant constituent of lily bases, often with linalool, α-terpineol, and traces of jasmine (Jouhar 1991). The original *L'air du Temps* (Nina Ricci 1948) had a lily note, modified with the subtle character of benzyl salicylate. However, we have just noted that hydroxycitronellal has been restricted, and so has benzyl salicylate, and although the current version of this fragrance is still an 'amber lily', Turin and Sanchez (2009) remark that it has become diminished, and is now 'worn so thin that you can see its bones and nothing else' (p.77). Many modern perfumes have a lily note buried within floral bouquets, such as Lauder's *Beyond Paradise*, and in Yves Saint Laurent's *Paris* a lily note, along with lily of the valley, orris, jasmine, linden blossom and ylang ylang, supports the main theme of the violet and rose heart. There are very few lily soliflores, but Cynthia Rowley's *Flower* is an 'accurate' representation, as is Guerlain's *Aqua Allegoria Lilia Bella*, and Penhaligon's *Lily and Spice* combines the lily note with saffron. Roméa d'Améor's *Les Maîtresses de Louis XIV* was composed by Pierre Bourdon, and combines lily with lily of the valley (Turin and Sanchez 2009).

Lily of the valley

Lily of the valley is *Convallaria majalis*, also of the Liliaceae family. It is a small perennial, with small, bell-shaped, white or occasionally pink flowers. Its delicate beauty and fragrance have been appreciated for many years; the flowers have a delicate, green, rosy floral scent, but extraction of this is not possible. In a study in 1993, Warren and Warrenburg found that a synthetic recreation of lily of the valley fragrance (described as a 'living flower fragrance') increased both stimulation and relaxation, and lowered depression, apathy and irritation. The subjects in the study reported that its scent produced a heightened sense of calm, with an increase in awareness and energy; effects that appear to be similar to those of jasmine fragrance.

Lily of the valley probably originated in Asia, but now grows wild all over Europe. The species name, *majalis*, means 'that which belongs to May', named after Maia, the mother of the Greek god Hermes. According to legend, the origin of the thick carpets of lily of the valley in St Leonard's Forest in Sussex was St Leonard's long battle against a dragon in the woods near Horsham. He did not survive, but wherever his blood fell, lily of the valley sprang up to commemorate the struggle. Another gentler legend tells that in wooded glades, the scent of lily of the valley attracts the nightingale, and leads him to select his mate (Grieve 1992). In France, on May Day, it is still customary to give posies of the flower to friends and loved ones. This practice was instigated by Charles IX of France, who received lily of the valley as a lucky charm, and thereafter, each year would offer flower posies to the ladies of his court. The lily of the valley (*muguet*) came to be a symbol of springtime, and in France it is sold tax-free. The perfumer François Coty gave gifts of lily of the valley every year, with flowers picked from the grounds of his Chateau de Puy D'Artigny (Morris 1984). In 1936, shortly after he died, and as a tribute, Coty launched a lily of the valley fragrance called *Muguet des Bois*, composed by Henri Robert. This had a fresh, green, floral top note, a lily of the valley heart with lilac, rose and jasmine, and a sandalwood and musk base note (Glöss 1995).

The archetypal lily of the valley fragrance was Dior's *Diorissimo*, composed by Edmond Roudnitska in 1956. The original had a leafy green top note, a delicate but intense lily of the valley heart, supported by lilac, jasmine and rose, and a soft sandalwood and civet base (Glöss 1995). Turin and Sanchez (2009) relate a delightful 'legend' about how Roudnitska went about composing *Diorissimo*: he planted lily of the valley in his garden in Cabris, near Grasse, so that he would have a natural reference for its perfume. The most recent version of his classic fragrance is harsher, and more jasmine-like than previous versions.

The components of a muguet base were hydroxycitronellal (maybe with Lyral and Lilial), cyclamen aldehydes (these have a floral green, cucumber-melon-like odour), linalool, phenylethanol and citronellol for the rosy aspects, benzyl acetate as modifier, green notes from phenylacetic aldehyde, and floral cinnamate derivatives such as cinnamic aldehyde. When we consider the case of lily of the valley we see just how severely the ingredient restrictions have impacted on perfumery. Turin and Sanchez (2009) explain that the hydroxy aldehydes such as hydroxycitronellal and Lyral (which has a soft, delicate floral scent – lily, cyclamen, muguet) and other aromachemicals such as benzyl salicylate do not have particularly powerful odours. This meant that they were used in fairly large quantities in what were very popular fragrances, and unfortunately allergies were a consequence in some users. Turin and Sanchez describe the restriction on hydroxycitronellal as a 'huge loss' and say that it is no longer possible to create a good muguet fragrance. When the accords of earlier years are examined, such as the Mellis accord (see page 220), we can see the devastating effect of the restrictions, and the impact on what Calkin and Jellinek (1994) refer to as the 'floral salicylate perfumes' with their lilac, lily of the valley or carnation notes (eugenol, and *iso*-eugenol) enhanced by salicylates such as benzyl salicylate. This group of perfumes, although not usually included in genealogies, includes Nina Ricci's *L'air du Temps*, Guy Laroche's *Fidji*, Cacharel's *Anaïs Anaïs* and Yves Saint Laurent's *Paris*, and an examination of their recent reviews, especially if comparing 'vintage' with current versions, makes sad reading. However, the work of fragrance chemists such as Roman Kaiser might point to a happier future. For example, a compound called 2,3-dihydrofarnesol was isolated from a Ligurian lemon flower. Dihydrofarnesol is found in many other flower scents; it has a fresh, aldehydic odour, and is a 'particularly important' component of the scent of lily of the valley. Another compound, (Z)-4-hepten-2-yl salicylate, was discovered in the 'Indian Ashok Flower' and this has a white-floral, lily and salicylate odour (Schilling *et al.* 2010).

Honeysuckle

As might be expected, honeysuckle (*Lonicera periclymenum* and *L. caprifolium*) does not readily yield its scent either. It is a twining climber, and many varieties produce abundant, highly scented flowers. It is probable that it originated in Asia Minor, but it is now widely cultivated in many countries. An essential oil can be obtained, but only in tiny quantities, and it is unusual in that it does not appear to contain aldehydes, ketones or nitrogenous compounds. Its scent has been described as falling between jasmine and narcissus, and can be mimicked by building on lily of the valley bases with the alcohols found in jasmine and rose and their absolutes, along with traces of tuberose, mimosa and violet leaf (International School of Aromatherapy 1993). Before the increase in raw material restrictions, honeysuckle fragrances could be composed of 'rhodinol' (which is *l*-citronellol, a sweet, rosy-floral alcohol), benzyl acetate, linalool, methyl anthranilate (an orange blossom-like and fruity ester) and heliotropin (Jouhar 1991). Some fragrances do contain honeysuckle notes, but Turin and Sanchez (2009) comment that it is not possible to create a convincing honeysuckle soliflore, because it does not 'hold together' (p.173). Probably the best way to experience the delightful fragrance is to smell the flowers on a warm summer evening.

Peony

The common garden peony, *Paeonia officinalis*, bears flowers that have a delightful, subtle scent. The genus allegedly got its name from the Greek physician Paeos, who used the plant to treat gods and mortals wounded in the Trojan War. In ancient times the peony was thought to have divine origins; it was an emanation of the moon that would shine at night to protect shepherds and their flocks, and the crops. It would also drive away evil spirits and avert tempests. The root was used as an antispasmodic and to treat convulsions, and also lunacy (Grieve 1992), possibly because of its associations with the moon. Peonies such as the red-flowered *P. delavayi*, the yellow-flowered *P. lutea* and their hybrids also have beautiful perfumes. *P. lutea* has a fresh, soft, floral perfume, with as 'cassis-like fruitiness' (Kaiser 2006, p.207); important constituents in its odour are linalool, cinnamyl alcohol, β-ionone and a form of indole, and the cassis note is contributed by traces of 4-methyl-4-sulfanylpentan-2-one. The beautiful ornamental tree peony, *Paeonia* x *suffructicosa*, originated in China and was introduced to Japan, America and Europe. Their flowers are good antioxidants that may have a potential role in preventative medicine, and products such as peony pollen-yam yoghourt,[3] and nutritious peony wine, peony-scented tea and oil have been developed. Recently, the planting of the tree peony in China has been expanded because of this potential for health enhancement.

Given the limited studies to date, Li *et al.* (2012) made an analysis of the peony volatiles. Their study of 30 cultivated varieties allowed them to identify five fragrance patterns: woody (*cis*-ocimene), rose (*d*-citronellol), lily of the valley (linalool), phenolic (1,3,5-trimethoxybenzene, TMB, also found in Chinese roses) and one unidentified type, which was characterised by pentadecane, also found in Qimen black tea.

Jouhar (1991) mentions a peony ketone that can be isolated from *P. montana*; this has a pungent, warm, aromatic and slightly hay-like scent. Peonies do not readily yield essential oil or absolutes, so in mainstream perfumery the peony note is always synthetic. Perhaps of all the floral scents, the peony suffers from the worst interpretation and representation, at least in terms of the scent of the flower.

---

3   Peony pollen yam yoghourt is made with peony pollen (about 0.5%), yam (around 35%) and honey; it is valued as an antioxidant.

For example, Turin and Sanchez (2009) discuss the peony element in the oriental woody rose fragrance *Tuscany per Donna*. Here the peony is represented as a 'sharp, fluorescent pink, sulphurous grapefruit peony in the modern style' (p.530). They also mention Thierry Mugler's peony version of the successful gourmand fragrance *Angel*, named *Angel Pivoine*, and Floris' *Fleur*, which is a fruity peony. Peony might just be another case where it is perhaps best to connect directly with the flower to experience the beauty and pleasure of its scent.

CHAPTER 11

Citrus, Lemon-Scented Botanicals and Fruity Fragrances

Citrus comprises the smallest group of fragrance types, but it has an important place in wellbeing. The majority of us will already have experienced the uplifting effects of citrus scents; they can gently elevate our mood if we are feeling low, and calm us if we are agitated or frustrated. *Lemon-scented botanicals* include herbs such as lemon balm, fruits such as *Litsea cubeba*, grasses such as lemongrass, and some eucalypts, and so we will consider how their scents too have impacted on our wellbeing. Finally, fruity scents, although present in the natural world, are more difficult to isolate or extract, but they are important in fragrance, and so their synthetic versions will be mentioned.

Citrus

When we refer to a 'citrus' scent we mean the fresh, zesty, fruity scent of the peel of citrus fruits. Citrus trees all belong to the genus *Citrus*, which is placed in a sub-family called the Aurantioideae within the larger family, the Rutaceae. The genus is very variable in appearance, containing some large and some small trees, some bearing large fruits and others small fruits, in colours that vary from green through to yellow and orange. However, all the essential oil-yielding *Citrus* species are spiny, evergreen shrubs or small trees with fragrant white flowers and leaves, and edible fruits. The leaves are dotted with volatile oil glands, and 'petitgrain' *leaf oil* is produced in some species. Generally the flowers are highly scented, and some species yield *flower oils*, such as neroli and orange blossom. Citrus fruits and plants are termed *agrumes*, which means 'sour fruits'. The *fruit oils* are found in numerous volatile oil sacs in the outer skin or peel. The fruit is actually a special type of berry called a *hesperidium*, where a tough outer layer protects fluid-filled segments. The peel of the citrus fruit is known as the *flavedo*. The very outer layer is a thick cuticle, and under this is the exocarp. This contains chloroplasts, the photosynthetic cells that contain chlorophyll while the fruit is unripe, and are therefore green. As the fruits ripen, the green chlorophyll breaks down and xanthophyll and carotene pigments become dominant, and so the colour changes gradually from green to yellow-orange. The oil sacs within the flavedo are in fact volatile oil-producing glands. They can store the volatile oil, and as it accumulates the pressure within these specialised cells increases; this is known as turgor pressure. Under the flavedo, the *albedo* is found. This is a thick, spongy layer that surrounds the fleshy, juicy segments. It is often referred to as the pith, and it contains vitamin C, sugars, cellulose and pectins. Within the centre of the fruit there is a pithy axis around which the segments are packed, each surrounded by a thin membrane. The seeds (pips) are arranged around the central axis, embedded in the juice sacs (Weiss 1997).

The genus probably originated in Southeast Asia, with the main centre being northeast India, Burma, the Yunnan province of China and the Pacific Islands, although the exact origins are not known, lost in a maze of extensive hybridisation and cultivation. Only one type – the grapefruit – originated in the New World (Weiss 1997). The generic name *Citrus* referred to the type known now as the 'citron' (*Citrus medica*). It is derived from the Greek word *kedros*, which means 'cedar', possibly because the Hellenistic Jews used this very large fruit in place of the cedar cone at the Sukkot festival, or the Feast of the Tabernacles. Svoboda and Greenaway (2003) suggest that all species are derived from three species: *Citrus medica* (the citron), *C. maximum* (the pomelo, or shaddock in Barbados) and *C. reticulata* (the mandarin). Weiss (1997) notes that it is not possible to say when citrus was first domesticated, and no truly wild ancestors have been identified. It is possible that *C. aurantifolia*, the lime of India, is one of the ancestors too. The taxonomy (the classification and naming) of the genus is not always clear, again because of the hybridisation and numerous cultivars that now exist. To complicate matters, we now have many hybrids within species such as the 'tangor', a cross between the tangerine and the orange, and the 'rangpur', a cross between the mandarin and the lemon. Furthermore, genetic mutations have resulted in varieties such as the Washington navel orange, and the grapefruit cultivar known as 'Thompson pink' is a *periclinal chimera* – a mutation where one of the layers of the fruit will be of a different genetic type.

Although citrus fruits are eastern in origin, they probably spread west at the time of Alexander the Great, and are now consumed worldwide and grown wherever the climate allows. They are not generally frost-hardy. Citrus has been cultivated since at least 2100 BCE in tropical and subtropical regions of Southeast Asia (Natural History Museum, date unknown). We do know that the citron was grown in Greece in the first century and Italy in the second century CE. Its species name *C. medica* was given by Linnaeus, and comes from its ancient name the 'Median apple'. (Theophrastus in his *Enquiry into Plants* noted that it was an inedible 'apple' native to Media, which had been part of Persia.) Many citrus species have been widely used in cookery and confectionery, and many would also have been used in traditional folk medicine; for example, lemon infusion or diluted lemon juice was used as a febrifuge, to lower high temperatures and fevers, and also as a diuretic, and to manage cases of acute rheumatism. Lemon (like other citrus species) is a good astringent, and can be used as a gargle in cases of sore throat, or to counteract itching and combat haemorrhage. Famously, lemon juice was known to prevent scurvy, a disease caused by deficiency of vitamin C, and from the late sixteenth century both lemon and lime juice were carried on ships undertaking long voyages for this purpose (Grieve 1992). In the ancient system of Ayurvedic medicine, the lime is a panacea. It is sour, bitter, astringent and cooling, and it is claimed that there is no disease that this fruit does not have the potential to treat.

Apart from the bitter orange, whose juice is of little value, the citrus peel oils are usually a by-product of the juice and canned fruit industry. Citrus essential oils can be either cold-pressed or distilled. Most lemon and sweet orange oil is cold-pressed, where pressure is applied to the fruit, and the volatile oils and juice are drawn off at the same time, but into separate channels. If the essential oil is extracted prior to the juice, the fruits are first scarified (abraded) to rupture the oil cells, and then pressure is used to extract the volatile oil. Large volumes of water are required to prevent the oil being re-absorbed into the peel. The first stage of extraction results in a volatile oil, wax and water emulsion, which is then filtered; the sludge is removed and the filtrate is centrifuged to remove particulate matter. This is followed by de-waxing and clarification. Even after this processing, some waxes may remain, and can be seen as a slight haze in chilled, cold-pressed citrus oils. An earlier method of cold extraction was 'ecuelling', using an *écuelle à piquer* (lit. 'pricking bowl') where the whole fruits were either manually or mechanically rolled over sharp projections. This ruptured the oil cells in the peel, and the oil was released and collected. This method obviously involved minimal processing, and it is still used for small quantities of high-quality bitter orange or lime oil. Some oils, such as lime, are more commonly distilled than cold-pressed. After crushing to remove the juice, the fruit mass is left to separate into three layers: the middle layer is run off to produce the juice, while the pulpy and volatile, oil-rich top and bottom layers are distilled to yield the essential oil. The destinations of most citrus essential oils and their derivatives are the food and drink, condiment, perfumery, cosmetics, pharmaceutical and industrial fields. Seed oils are also produced, and these may have pharmaceutical applications due to their potential antimicrobial activity (Weiss 1997).

Sometimes citrus oils are subjected to further processing before reaching their destinations. Citrus oils can contain high proportions of terpenes, especially *d*-limonene. Terpenes can cause problems with solubility when the oils are being incorporated into products, and so some oils are deterpenated for the flavour and fragrance industry. Terpenes can be removed without adversely affecting the aroma, which in most cases is mainly due to aldehydes. So removing all or some of the terpenes can improve the odour, reduce water-solubility problems and improve stability. Deterpenated oils are called 'folded oils', they are more concentrated – for example, a ten-fold oil will contain only 10 per cent of the original terpene content;

the most common strengths are five-fold for lime, ten-fold for lemon and twenty-fold for sweet orange. The deterpenation process is accomplished by distillation, solvent or CO_2 extraction. Solvent extraction also removes any waxes that remain, and these products are also known as 'washed' citrus oils. The limonene and other terpenes that are removed have a commercial value too; their solvent properties mean that they can be used in detergents, resins and adhesives. One terpene in particular, d-limonene, has other uses too – for example, in the synthesis of synthetic spearmint flavour (Weiss 1997; Costa *et al.* 2010).

Cold-pressed citrus oils often contain furanocoumarins, which are constituents that are implicated in phototoxicity (Tisserand and Balacs 1995). Phototoxicity is a type of toxicity associated with the reaction of some chemicals with sunlight. If a photosensitising or phototoxic substance is applied to the skin, and then exposed to ultraviolet light or sunlight, skin damage and burning results. This is because some chemicals, such as the furanocoumarins that are found in some essential oils, are stored in the upper layer of the skin for up to 48 hours, where they can 'absorb' UV light before releasing it into the skin in one concentrated burst. In the case of bergamot oil, which contains a furanocoumarin known as 'bergapten' (5-methoxy psoralen), a condition called berloque dermatitis, permanent pigmentation resulting from sunburn, can result. In the 1960s and early 1970s bergamot was actually incorporated into some suntan lotions to accelerate the acquisition of a sun tan, but now all phototoxic oils are carefully controlled and restricted in the fragrance and cosmetic industry. Because furanocoumarins are not volatile compounds, if citrus oil is distilled, they do not appear, but sometimes, as in the case of bergamot oil, they can be removed so as to remove the risk of phototoxic reactions.

All of the commonly available citrus fruit oils are used in aromatherapy, but those that have been further processed after extraction are avoided, with the exception of 'furanocoumarin-free' (FCF) bergamot. Without exception, citrus scents are regarded as 'uplifting' and 'refreshing', and can be useful for those suffering from stress and depression. Depression is associated with an increase in sympathetic nervous activity and decreased parasympathetic nervous activity, and dysregulation of the psychoneuroimmunological balance. There is some research that supports the view that citrus oils can be used therapeutically in cases of mild depression. In 2001 Heuberger *et al.* showed that both d- and l-limonene increased systolic blood pressure, but only the d-form, the type that dominates citrus oils, caused subjective alertness and restlessness; the l-form had no effects on psychological parameters. Correlational analysis[1] of the results showed that changes in the autonomic nervous system (ANS) and self-evaluation were related to the subjective evaluation of the odours, and that both pharmacological and psychological mechanisms contribute to the effects. Hongratanaworakit and Buchbauer (2007a) investigated the effects of massage with kaffir lime peel oil on human autonomic and behavioural parameters.

---

1   This is a statistical technique used in sociological analysis. It measures the strength between variables; a value of +1.00 indicates a perfect positive correlation, 0.00 means that there is no relationship, while -1.00 is a perfect negative correlation.

It caused an increase in blood pressure and decrease in skin temperature compared with the placebo group; and the kaffir lime group rated themselves as more alert, cheerful and vigorous than the control. Based on this study, it would seem that kaffir lime peel oil has activating effects. In the same year the same researchers (Hongratanaworakit and Buchbauer 2007b) conducted a study that investigated the effects of transdermal absorption of sweet orange oil, but this time the participants were prevented from smelling the oil. They found that autonomic arousal was decreased, and feelings of cheerfulness and vigour were reported. This type of effect could be due to a quasi-pharmacological mechanism. Two years later a study conducted by Saiyudthong *et al.* (2009) investigated the effects of massage with lime essential oil. This demonstrated that systolic blood pressure was decreased after a single massage with lime, suggesting reduction of sympathetic activity and potentiation of the parasympathetic response. It was acknowledged that massage alone could produce these effects, but that the lime essential oil potentiated the parasympathetic response. This highlighted the paradox that while fragrance alone can increase alertness, if applied topically with massage it can have a relaxing, stress-relieving effect. So, this illustrates how the context in which a fragrance is experienced can affect the responses. Following previous studies on the antidepressive effects of inhaling citrus fragrances, Komori (2009) conducted a study on the effects of inhaling lemon and valerian essential oils on the ANS in healthy and depressed male subjects. This study showed that in the healthy subjects, lemon stimulated sympathetic nerve activity and the parasympathetic nervous system. However, the depressed subjects, who already had enhanced sympathetic activity, showed a decrease relative to enhanced parasympathetic activity, after inhalation of lemon. Valerian, which has a long tradition of use as a sedative, did not stimulate sympathetic activity in any of the test subjects in this study. Overall, the studies cited here not only support the aromatherapeutic use of citrus oils for alleviating stress and depression, they also support the quasi-pharmacological (see above) and hedonic valence (see page 34) theories that attempt to explain the effects of odour.

Although most citrus oil research has focused on their effects on the ANS and mood, they have other useful physiological actions; for example, Baylac and Racine's research (2003) has indicated that citrus peel oils may have anti-inflammatory activity. Citrus oils are also important in the food industry. They are thought to have health-promoting effects – for example, as dietary antioxidants. In 2009 Patil *et al.* conducted an *in vitro* study of lime essential oil to investigate its possible use in the prevention of colon cancer. The lime oil that they used contained *d*-limonene at 30.13 per cent and d-dihydrocarvone at 30.47 per cent, along with 'verbena', β-linalool, α-terpineol and *trans*-α-bergamotene. It was demonstrated that the lime oil was able to inhibit the proliferation of colon cancer cells, and that the likely mechanism was the induction of apoptosis (programmed cell death). This study certainly suggests that lime oil may have wider potential health benefits, and perhaps supports the way in which it is regarded in Ayurvedic medicine.

We will now take a brief look at some of the fragrant citrus oils, and a few that are less well known. Citrus oils are among the most volatile; they are top notes that evaporate readily, and disappear comparatively quickly. When typical citrus oil (lemon, for example) is put on a smelling strip, the immediate impact is given by its *d*-limonene, which accounts for around 70 per cent of the oil. This evaporates first, giving a fresh, sharp, citrus impression. Then the moderately volatile components, present in much smaller amounts, such as the aldehydes citral and nonanal, and esters such as geranyl acetate, start to evaporate, their odours mingling with that of *d*-limonene and the other terpenes such as β-pinene, and γ-terpinene. The aroma on the strip becomes stronger and more pronounced, sweeter and fruitier, less sharp. In a fairly short time this starts to fade, until all that is left is a faint, nondescript dryout. You do not need to wait long to reach the heart of a citrus note. This is why, in perfumery, citrus is always in the top notes of compositions, and why citrus-dominated fragrances such as the eaux de cologne have no tenacity.

Citron or cédrat

It is fitting to begin this exploration with one of the ancestral species – *C. medica*, the citron or French cédrat of perfumery. The fruit resembles a large lemon; but the resemblance ends when it is cut open. The pulp is dry, with very little juice, and it has a considerable albedo, or pith, which adheres to the segments. Its candied pith is eaten, and in the East the fruit is used to make jams and pickles.

It is thought that in Greek myth the 'golden apple' that Paris gave to Aphrodite (with serious consequences, eventually resulting in the Trojan War) was actually a citron. In Rome, where it was erroneously believed that quinces were citrus, the citron tree was called *Malus citreum*, later shortened to *citreum* (Natural History Museum, date unknown). Although the pulp is inedible, as Theophrastus noted, the citron did have therapeutic uses, and macerated in wine it was believed to counteract poisoning. Pliny the Elder was the first to call it 'citrus', also describing its attributes, including its powerful smell, which repelled insects, and that it was an antidote to poisoning. The citron is also mentioned in Islamic texts.

Cédrat essential oil is valued in perfumery because, like bitter orange, it has greater tenacity than many citrus oils, and although it has the characteristic sharp citrus odour, it also has intensity and depth. Citron can be found in Guerlain's fresh citrus *Eau de Fleurs de Cédrat*.

Bergamot

Bergamot oil is obtained from *C. aurantium* subsp. *bergamia*, and is the most important citrus oil from the fragrance perspective. Its botanical origins are unclear, and we do not know whether this valuable subspecies is a mutation or a hybrid. Bergamot essential oil production became established in Italy in the sixteenth century; bergamot is named after the town of Bergamo in the Lombardy region of Italy where it was used in local folk medicine to reduce fever and to treat intestinal worms. Even today the most significant producer is Italy, with oils from Reggio

Calabria in southern Italy being regarded as the best available. Small plantations are present in the Ivory Coast, Africa, and Argentina and Brazil.

Bergamot fruits are inedible, with an acidic and bitter taste. The peel is smooth and thin, and the fruits are small, spherical and yellow when ripe.

In Grasse, around 1745, there was a short-lived practice of incorporating bergamot rind into small papier-mâché boxes, but this custom died out after 1832.

The oil is widely used in perfumery, and to flavour Earl Grey tea, tobacco, and many foods (Lawless 1992; Weiss 1997; Costa *et al.* 2010).

Bergamot essential oil has a light olive green colour, the shade being determined by the stage in the season that the fruits are harvested. It fades with time, eventually becoming yellow to pale brown in colour. Bergamot does not have the typical citrus, zesty aroma of the other citrus peel oils. Aftel (2008) described the aroma as having 'an extremely rich, sweet lemon-orange scent that evolves into a more floral, freesia-like scent, ending in an herbaceous-balsamic dryout'. Tisserand (1985) suggested that it is 'sweet and citrusy, but has a warm, floral quality absent in lemon and orange, and reminiscent of lavender or neroli' (p.189). Williams described it in terms of its notes: the top is fresh, sharp and citrus, and the body is citrus, herbal and peppery. Lawless (2009) concurs with the peppery note, but also includes its floral aspect.

There is a great deal of variation in its composition, usually related to its geographical origins (Weiss 1997). According to Price and Price (2007), the major components are alcohols such as linalool, esters including linalyl acetate, and monoterpenes including *d*-limonene, α- and β–pinene and γ-terpinene. Between 4 per cent and 7 per cent of the oil is comprised of non-volatiles, including bergapten. The IFRA currently suggests a maximum of 0.4 per cent bergamot oil in the final 'leave-on' products for application to areas of skin. So, to achieve a completely safe level of bergapten, and thus remove the risk presented by bergamot oil, the bergapten has to be removed, or reduced to a level of 15 ppm in the final product. Bergamot essential oil is a good antiseptic and has many aromatherapeutic uses; for skin problems, itching, sore throat and tonsillitis, loss of appetite, urinary tract infections, colds, fevers and influenza, as well as for anxiety and stress (Lawless 1992).

Bergamot is an essential component of eau de cologne type fragrances. In Muelhen's *4711 Echt Kölnisch Wasser*, it is the dominant citrus in the fresh top note, with lemon, orange, petitgrain and neroli; the heart contains rosemary and rose. Farina Gegenüber's *Original Kölnisch Wasser* has the same ingredients in the top and heart, but also includes carnation. Roger and Gallet's *Jean Marie Farina* cologne is another variation on the same theme; it has a top note of bergamot with lemon, petitgrain, orange, mandarin and rosemary over a floral neroli and carnation heart.

Bergamot is extremely versatile, and appears in all the other fragrance categories too. Along with oakmoss and labdanum, bergamot is important in the chypre structure, and so it is found in most chypres, especially the fresh type. Dior's *Eau Sauvage* combines bergamot, lemon, basil, cumin and a fruit note in its citrus fresh top note. Miyake's *L'Eau d'Issey pour Homme* has a fresh, cool top note with bergamot, green notes, lemon, orange, tarragon, melon, aldehyde and pineapple. (We will return to these fruity elements at the end of this chapter.) The leathery chypre fragrance *Knize Ten* (Knize) has the classic cologne accord in the top note; and the woody chypre *Vetiver* (Guerlain) has bergamot, lemon, mandarin, neroli and coriander. The oriental spicy fragrances that feature bergamot include Guerlain's *Héritage*. In some of the feminine fragrances bergamot plays a less dominant role, but is included across the categories. It is most prominent in those with fresh citrus top notes, such as Chanel's *Cristalle*, and is included in the top note in most feminine chypre fragrances too.

Bitter orange, sweet orange, mandarin and tangerine

Bitter orange

C. aurantium subspecies *amara* is the botanical source of three oils – bitter orange peel, petitgrain and neroli. (We have already discussed neroli and orange blossom absolute, the indolic florals, in Chapter 10.) The name is derived from the Sanskrit *nagaranga*, the Hindu *naranja* and the Arabic *naranj*, the Latin *aurantium*, the Spanish *naranja*, the Italian *arancia*, and eventually the French *orange* (Natural History Museum, date unknown), and the first mention of the orange is in Arabic writings (Grieve 1992). The subspecies name *amara* means 'bitter'.

Bitter orange is also known as the sour or Seville orange, and originated in Indonesia. It was introduced to Spain by Muslims in the twelfth century, hence its name of Seville orange, and from there it was taken to the New World (Natural History Museum, date unknown).

The bitter orange fruit is spherical, medium to dark green, becoming more yellow as it ripens, and yields bitter orange oil. The fruits have a long history of culinary and medicinal uses. The main use for the whole fruit is for marmalade. The liqueur *Curaçao* is flavoured with the unripe fruits. Bitter orange is also used to flavour baked goods and soft drinks, and to aromatise drugs. Since the tree is native to Asia, its flowers and fruits are used in oriental medicine – mainly as remedies for the myriad disorders of the digestive system, as a cardiac tonic, and for anxiety.

The scent of bitter orange essential oil is fresh and delicate, with sweet floral elements, and a green note can be detected. It is more subtle and fresh than sweet orange, and has a more tenacious, floral undertone (Aftel 2008; Lawless 2009). The major components include terpenes at around 90 per cent, (particularly *d*-limonene), linalool, linalyl acetate and decanol. Deterre *et al.* (2011) made a study of the key aroma compounds in bitter orange essential oil and a macerate-distillate extract. These are summarised in Table 11.1. As a consequence of their findings, Deterre *et al.* (2011) suggest that maceration of bitter orange peel in an alcoholic solution, followed by a batch multi-stage distillation, makes it possible to eliminate some of the 'off' odours that can be present in the essential oil.

Table 11.1 Bitter orange aroma compounds

Compiled and adapted from Deterre *et al.* (2011).

Aroma compound – essential oil	Odour
α-pinene	Floral
Octanal	Green
Limonene	Citrus
Linalool	Floral
α-terpineol	Green?
Linalyl acetate	Floral
E,E- or *E,Z-* 2,4-decadieneal	Frying
dodecanal	Not determined
Caryophyllene	Green
Unknown compound	Plastic note
Aroma compound – heart cut of the macerate-distillate	**Odour**
Myrcene α-phellandrene Limonene	Citrus and mint
z-linalool oxide α-terpinolene Linalool Neral	Floral

Using the model of fragrance energetics (see Chapter 5), Holmes (1997) suggests that, because of its green citrus character, bitter orange can help counteract anger and frustration by imparting regulating, cooling, relaxing, clarifying sensations. Bitter orange oil is used in aromatherapy and artisan perfumery, but is not so prominent in mainstream perfumery. Its comparative tenacity is used to extend the grapefruit top note in Hermès' *Eau de Pamplemousse Rose* (Turin and Sanchez 2009).

It is worth mentioning petitgrain briefly at this point. It is not a citrus peel oil, but is obtained from the bitter orange tree's leaves and twigs. 'Petitgrain bigarade' has a floral, sweet, orange-citrus scent; Weiss (1997) notes that the product from Paraguay, 'petitgrain Paraguay', has a stronger, sweet, woody-floral aroma. The essential oil is dominated by linalyl acetate, but also contains monoterpenes and their alcohols. It is used in aromatherapy; Schnaubelt (1999) recommends this oil to balance the autonomic nervous system; Franchomme and Pénoël (1990) support this, in addition to citing its antispasmodic, anti-inflammatory, anti-infectious and antibacterial properties. In perfumery it is often found alongside bergamot in eaux de cologne.

Sweet orange

C. x *sinensis* is the sweet orange; as its name suggests, it is native to southwest China where it borders Burma. It was known as *C. aurantium* var. *dulce* (*dulce* meaning 'sweet'). It is a hybrid, probably a cross between *C. maxima* (pomelo) and *C. reticulata* (mandarin). The sweet orange is one of the best-known citrus fruits and is now widely cultivated for consumption and its juice. The familiar yellow-orange fruit is oval or ellipsoidal with a smooth peel. The cold-pressed oil, once known as 'oil of Portugal', is pale yellow-orange to dark orange, but the colour does vary according to the cultivar used and the country in which it is grown. The blood orange cultivar is highly rated by Aftel (2008). Typically, the aroma is fresh, fruity, and very similar to the peel when scarified. Its top note is sweet, light, fresh and citrus, the middle is citrus and aldehydic, and the dryout is faint and pithy (Williams 2000). The main constituents are monoterpenes, mainly limonene; the aldehydes octanal and decanal have a significant impact on the odour. Linalool, octyl and neryl acetates are also present (Weiss 1997).

Franchomme and Pénoël suggest that its aromatherapeutic uses are for dyspepsia, insomnia, anxiety, and as an air disinfectant. Sweet orange petitgrain oil is produced by distilling the leaves; monoterpenes are the main constituents of this type of petitgrain. Like bitter orange, sweet orange is used in colognes, but does not normally dominate; however, Hermès' *Eau des Merveilles* is described by Turin and Sanchez (2009) as a 'salty orange' fragrance. Orange also features with patchouli and lavender in LUSH's *Karma* solid perfume.

Mandarin and tangerine

Mandarin and tangerine are generally considered as one species, usually *C. reticulata*. 'Tangerine' is the name used in English-speaking countries and 'mandarin' elsewhere (Weiss 1997). The mandarin *C. reticulata* originated in China, and the tangerine may be a hybrid species, *C. x tangerina*. The Natural History Museum (date unknown) suggests that mandarins such as the cultivar 'Emperor' have yellow or pale orange fruits, and that tangerines have deep orange-red fruits. The 'clementine' originated in Algeria. Dugo *et al.* (2011) also highlight the confusion in the literature regarding the classification of the mandarin. They suggest that the correct denomination for mandarin of the Mediterranean basin is *C. deliciosa*. This area is the main producer of the oil, mainly in Avana and Tardivo di Ciaculli. Aftel (2008) asserts that the oil sold as tangerine is much preferable to mandarin for perfumery.

The fruit is a flattened sphere, with a peel that may vary from green in unripe fruits to yellow and deep orange-red, depending on the cultivar. The unripe green fruits yield the oil that is preferred in perfumery; this is light yellow in colour. When the fruits reach the final stage of maturity the skin is barely attached to the pulp, and the oil will be red or orange in colour, depending on how it has been extracted; so mandarin is sold as green, yellow or red. Obviously, the chemical composition of the oil will vary too.

Generally, the aroma is intense, sweet, and very occasionally not very pleasant – a fishy note may be present due to the presence of anthranilates, which are nitrogen-containing esters. According to Price and Price (2007), the major constituents are usually monoterpenes, dominated by limonene at 65 per cent or more; alcohols, including linalool; short chain fatty aldehydes at around 1 per cent; trace amounts of thymol, and sometimes anthranilates. Thymol and dimethyl anthranilate contribute to the aroma, even although they are present only in traces (Weiss 1997). Dugo *et al.* analysed Sicilian mandarin oil over the entire growing season, but weather and other factors were variables that could not be controlled. The composition of the volatile fraction of the oils agreed with previously published data, and Dugo *et al.* identified three new components in the non-volatile component – demethyl-nobiletin, *iso*-sinensetin and demethyl-tangeretin – and their findings may help identify quality parameters for mandarin essential oil. Mandarin petitgrain is produced by steam distillation of the leaves; its main constituents are citral and linalool.

In aromatherapy the uses of mandarin/tangerine are very similar to the ones already highlighted in citrus oils. The scent is regarded as calming, and thus useful for tension and insomnia. In perfumery green mandarin is included in citrus accords, and according to Lawless (2009) it can add sharpness to floral blends.

Japanese connections

These are lesser-known citrus scents which are either just finding their way into perfumery or aromatherapy, or have the potential to do so.

Tachibana

C. tachibana is a species related to mandarin, and much associated with Japan. Its fruit is used as a motif at New Year or coming-of-age celebrations, and it is cultivated at Japanese shrines. Its flower oil has massive potential; it has a floral, jasmine-like and orange flower-like scent, and its main constituents are linalool and γ-terpinene. The peel oil has a sweet, green, juicy odour, and is dominated by limonene and linalool (Ubukata *et al.* 2002, cited in Svoboda and Greenaway 2003).

Jabara

Omori *et al.* (2011) investigated a rare essential oil extracted from *C. jabara*. They describe jabara as a sour citrus, indigenous to Kitayama village, Wakayama, in Japan. It was certified as a new species in 1971, and is related to *yuzu* (see below). It is thought that jabara evolved through natural selection from the hybrids of other species in the region, such as yuzu, *kunenbo* and *kishu-mikan*. The fruit is juicy and mainly seedless; it is used as a seasoning, and in drinks, vinegar and jam.

It was the potential of jabara's juice to counteract the symptoms of Japanese cedar pollinosis (JCP) that highlighted its potential as a therapeutic and cosmetic ingredient. The pollen of the Japanese cedar (*Cryptomeria japonica*) is responsible for an allergic disease which is so prevalent that it is considered a public health problem in Japan. The symptoms are tear production, red eyes, sneezing and running nose. Jabara extract is already included in some phytocosmeceuticals as a soothing, anti-allergenic ingredient.

Jabara has a unique odour – and so the researchers analysed the aromatic compounds in the peel extract to try to identify some of the constituents responsible for this. The oil contains a relatively high proportion (around 47%) of myrcene, and this in itself is very unusual for citrus peel oil. Myrcene, which is thought to be the most important constituent in jabara's aroma, has, according to Williams (2000) a sweet, fresh, light, balsamic odour; however, Omori *et al.* describe this as 'metallic and resinous'. Limonene is also present (around 28%) imparting its fresh but weak citrus odour, as is γ-terpinene (around 15%) which has a terpeney, sweet, citrus scent with tropical and lime nuances (Brechbill 2007). Small amounts of β-phellandrene, and α- and β-pinene were detected; oxygenated compounds such as geraniol were present only at around 0.6 per cent. Omori *et al.* also identified some unusual constituents that played a major role in its odour – a group of undecatetraenes, which have potent green and fruity odours, and 7-methyl-1,6-octadien-3-one, which has a metallic and mushroom-like odour. Unfortunately they do not give an odour profile of the whole oil but, given the information, we can use our olfactory imagination.

Yuzu

Yuzu is a hybrid of *C. ichangensis* (the Ichang lemon or papeda) and the sour mandarin; it is named *C. x junos*. It originated in East Asia, grows wild in China and Tibet, and was introduced to Japan and Korea. Its fruit resembles a grapefruit, with a green or yellow uneven peel (Masayoshi 2010). In Japanese cuisine the peel is used as a garnish, and the juice as seasoning or in a citrus sauce called *ponzu*. It is also used in teas, vinegars and alcoholic drinks, and in Korean cuisine in marmalade-like syrups. It also has a strong, fragrant aroma; in Japan, on *Tōji*, the winter solstice, it is customary to bathe with yuzu oil or the cut fruit in bathwater. The yuzu bath is called *yuzuyu* or *yuzuburo*, and is a cleansing and fortifying ritual.

Yuzu essential oil is a floral citrus, in the manner of bergamot. Two constituents have recently been identified as important in its odour; undecatriene-3-one has been recently identified and 1,3,5,7-undecatetraene contributes to the green aspect (Omori *et al.* 2011).

Yuzu is being used to scent personal care products and in perfumery. Turin and Sanchez (2009) give two examples – one with a yuzu note but no actual yuzu, and the other in a citrus fantasy fragrance. The first is *Yuzu Ab Irato* (Parfumerie Générale), where the yuzu note is achieved with an accord of mint and pepper; it is more complex than cologne. The second is *Yuzu Fou* (Parfum d'Empire), which is described as a 'baroque fantasy of citrus'. Apart from yuzu, grapefruit, bitter orange,

orange blossom, sweet orange and verbena can also be detected, mixing sweet, sour and savoury elements.

Lemon and lime

Lemon

It is believed that the name 'lemon' (*C. limonum* or *C. limon*) is derived from the Sanskrit word *nimbuka*, which became *limum* or *limu* in Arabic, but either way, the tree probably reached Europe via Persia or Media (Grieve 1992). It probably originated in the Himalayas in north Burma and south China, and it is a comparatively recent introduction to India. The lemon is thought to be a hybrid of the citron and the pomelo. It was introduced to Haiti by Columbus on his second voyage in 1493, while the Arabs took the lemon to East and Central Africa, where 'rough' lemons naturalised along the Mazoe River in Zambia. Rough lemons are used as the woodstock for sweet oranges, lemons and mandarins.

The lemon is now widely used as a flavouring and garnish, in perfumes and cosmetics, and for citric acid and pectin production (Natural History Museum, date unknown).

The main producer of essential oil is Sicily. The fruit is ovoid, yellow when ripe, with a smooth or rough peel, depending on the variety. The cold-pressed oil is clear, a pale to greenish yellow that turns brown with age, and the odour is fresh, sweet and lemony (Weiss 1997). The principal monoterpene is *d*-limonene at approximately 70 per cent; however, citral has a major impact on the odour. The oil is phototoxic due to the presence of non-volatile furanocoumarins, and it may cause dermal irritation in some people (Lawless 1992).

Williams (2000) describes cold-pressed lemon as having a light, fresh, sharp citrus top and a strong citrus body, with very little dryout. Lemon is often found with bergamot in top notes, as, for example, in Lancôme's *Ô* (Glöss 1995); with citrus and moss in Annick Goutal's *Eau d'Hadrien* eau de parfum and eau de toilette; and in the unusual fougère *Eau de Réglise* (Caron), where it is in the top note with roasted coffee (Turin and Sanchez 2009).

Lime

The native East Indian lime, *C. aurantifolia*, is possibly one of the ancestral types. However, the lime that is more familiar to us is derived from the Indian citron, and is classed as *C. medica* var. *acida*. This variety probably originated in northern India, where it is still widely grown and used in traditional medicine. The lime was taken to the Americas by the Spanish and Portuguese in the early 1500s, and introduced to the Florida Keys (the reef islands off the southwest coast) around 1838, where it became naturalised and consequently known as 'Key lime' (Hodgson 1967). Its fruit is nearly spherical, small and greenish to light yellow in colour.

As already mentioned, distillation is the usual method of extraction for lime oil, although small amounts of expressed oil are available. Distilled oil is produced from both ripe and unripe fruits, while the more expensive expressed oil comes mainly from green, unripe fruits. The chemical composition of lime oil is variable, but distilled oils have less citral, β-pinene and γ-terpinene, and more *p*-cymene, terpinen-4-ol and α-terpineol than the expressed oil (Weiss 1997). Franchomme and Pénoël (1990) state that lime oil is sedative, anti-inflammatory, anticoagulant and antispasmodic, suggesting that it is indicated for anxiety and stress, and inflammatory and spasmodic problems of the digestive system. In perfumery lime oil has a more distinctive odour than some of the other oils, and is instantly recognisable. Jo Malone's *Lime Basil and Mandarin Cologne* is a good example, and Guerlain uses lime with linden blossom very successfully in *Eau de Cologne Impériale* (Turin and Sanchez 2009).

There are other species that are commonly known as lime. Sweet lime (*C. limetta*) is native to South and Southeast Asia, but also cultivated in the Mediterranean. Its Arabic name *limu shirin* is derived from the Persian words meaning 'lemon sweet'. It has a green, sweet juice; and sweet lime juice, or *mosambi*, is the most commonly available citrus juice in India, Pakistan and Bangladesh. Its essential oil is produced in small volumes in Sicily; it has a lemon-like scent (Weiss 1997).

The kaffir lime (*C. hystrix*) of Indonesia is used in traditional medicine, and as an insect repellent. The peel oil is dominated by *d*-limonene and β-pinene, and its relaxing properties have already been discussed. Kaffir lime leaves have a distinctive appearance; they are constricted in the middle and so resemble double leaves. These are widely used in Southeast Asian cuisine; they are an ingredient in Lao and Thai curry pastes. The leaf oil scent is characterised by *l*-citronellal, and it also contains citronellol, nerol and limonene. This isomeric form is interesting, because it is the *d*-isomer that is normally found in lemon-scented essential oils such as lemon balm and lemongrass.

The Australian finger lime (*C. australasica*) is one of three *Citrus* species native to Australia, along with *C. australis* (Australian round lime) and *C. glauca* (desert lime). *C. australasica* is unique in terms of shape, colour and aroma; it is finger-shaped, up to ten centimetres in length, can be green, red, purple, black or yellow in colour, and has a fresh, green odour. It is sometimes called 'lemon caviar' because, when cut open, the green-yellow vesicles burst out, like caviar. The fruits are eaten fresh, sometimes with seafood, and added to alcoholic drinks. Delort and Jaquier (2009) analysed finger lime essential oil, and besides *d*-limonene they found *iso*-menthone, which is not usually found in citrus oils, and citronellal, and identified six new terpenyl esters. They suggested that the limonene/*iso*-menthone/citronellal composition is unique in the citrus family.

C. medica var. *sarcodactylis*, although it is not described as a lime, is another unusual variant called 'Buddha's hand' or the 'fingered citron'. This originated in northeastern India or China, and has a thick peel and no flesh, and is often seedless. The pith is not bitter and can be candied, and the fruit can be sliced and used as a garnish. It has elongated, finger-shaped sections that take either a closed or an open hand form. The fruit is highly fragrant, and is used in China and Japan to scent rooms and clothing (Morris 1984); the closed hand form, which resembles the prayer position, is offered in Buddhist temples.

Pomelo and grapefruit

Pomelo

C. maxima, the pomelo, probably originated in China. This is one of the largest fruits, round or pear-shaped, and reaching 30 centimetres in diameter. The Natural History Museum (date unknown) suggests that it reached the Mediterranean as a curiosity around 1000 CE. It is believed that in the 1600s its seeds were taken from the East Indies to Barbados in the Caribbean by Captain Shaddock, hence its name 'shaddock' there. Its pith is bitter and is discarded, but the pink, red or yellow-white flesh is sweet and mild, and it is eaten as a dessert fruit, candied, made into marmalade or used in stir fry dishes. In China the leaves are used in ritual bathing to cleanse and repel evil.

Grapefruit

Until fairly recently, little distinction was made between the pomelo and the grapefruit, and commercial cultivation of the grapefruit did not commence until around 1880. The grapefruit is a hybrid of the pomelo and the sweet orange, and common cultivated varieties are 'Marsh', 'Thompson Pink Marsh' (which arose as a mutation) and two red-fleshed mutations, 'Ruby' and 'Web'.

The grapefruit is known as *C. paradisi*; the large, light yellow to orange-coloured fruit is eaten primarily as a 'breakfast' fruit, and is the source of a peel oil (Weiss 1997). Grapefruit essential oil is a relative newcomer to perfumery, having become available only at the beginning of the nineteenth century (Aftel 2008). It can be produced by steam distillation or cold expression of the peel. The cold-pressed oil is yellow to pale orange/yellow; the aroma is sweet and fresh, similar to the fruit itself, and deteriorates rapidly on exposure to the air (Weiss 1997).

The major constituent of the peel oil is *d*-limonene (approximately 84%); the grapefruit-scented nootkatone (an isomeric form of a ketone based on a terpenylcyclohexanol structure) and traces of a sulphur-containing compound give the oil its distinctive aroma (Williams 1996). Lawless (2009) suggests that the yellow type is preferable to the pink or red variants, as it contains slightly more nootkatone. Monoterpenes make up about 95 per cent of the oil (Weiss 1997). It does not appear to be strongly phototoxic; however, Tisserand and Balacs (1995) suggested that in aromatherapy the maximum concentration of grapefruit should be 4 per cent, due to the potential for phototoxicity.

Dietary grapefruit has acquired popular associations with weight loss. Harris (2006) cites Shen *et al.* (2005b) who demonstrated that the scent of grapefruit could affect autonomic nerve activity, increasing lipolysis and metabolism, thus reducing weight in rats. (Lavender, which was investigated in a similar manner, had the opposite effects.) In general terms, this can be interpreted as the fragrance of grapefruit having activating effects.

Williams (2000) gives the odour profile of grapefruit as a fresh, citrus top, an orange-like body and a pithy dryout. The grapefruit note, and the expensive and subdued nootkatone, is apparently quite difficult to work with. Guerlain's *Aqua Allegoria Pamplelune* is possibly the best example of a grapefruit fragrance, and in this it is used with a 'pink floral accord'. As in the case of *Eau de Pamplemousse Rose* (Hermès) (see page 339), the top note of grapefruit is vivid and realistic, but not sustained, and Jo Malone's *Grapefruit Cologne* is pleasant but 'unremarkable' (Turin and Sanchez 2009).

Lemon-scented botanicals

Lemon-scented species are characterised by a few constituents – notably the aldehydes citral (which is the name given to the naturally occurring isomers neral and geranial) and citronellal (usually the *d*-isomer), and also *d*-limonene.

The citral found in citrus oils has a slightly different odour from that of other lemon-scented botanicals; and this is probably related to the relative proportions of the isomers. Citral is not very stable, and can cause problems such as discoloration. It is used in the synthesis of ionones (Jouhar 1991). Citral is thought to have anti-inflammatory, sedative and antifungal properties (Franchomme and Pénoël 1990; Lis Balchin 1995). Lawless (1992) suggests that it may cause dermal irritation or sensitisation in susceptible individuals, and so, in aromatherapy, oils with a high citral content should be used with care. However, other components present in complete essential oils, such as monoterpenes like *d*-limonene, might reduce the potential for irritation.

Citral has a strong lemony odour, while citronellal has a powerful fresh, green lemon odour with faint rosy herbaceous undertones, and *d*-limonene has a weak lemon aroma. These constituents are widely distributed, occurring in herbs, grasses, fruits and leaves. Svoboda and Greenaway (2003) give a comprehensive list of lemon-scented plants: lemon-scented herbs include lemon-scented varieties of thyme (*Thymus* x *citriodorus*), creeping lemon thyme (*T. praecox*), basil (*Ocimum* x *citriodorum*), mint (*Mentha piperita* var. *citrata*), bergamot mint (*Monarda citriodora*), lemon catmint (*Nepeta cataria* 'Citriodora') and savory (*Satureja biflora*). The lemon-scented grasses are lemongrass and citronella, and the Myrtaceae family has lemon-scented myrtle, crimson bottle brush, lemon-scented gum and ironbark, and lemon tea tree. The small fruits of *Litsea cubeba* (may chang) are also noted for their lemon fragrance. A selection of lemon-scented botanicals is explored below.

Lemon balm

Melissa officinalis, lemon balm, or sometimes bee balm, is a popular bushy, perennial 'cottage garden' herb of the Lamiaceae family. Its leaves have a distinctive lemon scent and flavour. It was known to the ancient Greeks and Roman; Pliny and

Dioscorides suggested that it could close wounds and supress inflammation. The early herbalists knew it as 'balm' and it was highly regarded, especially for disorders of the nervous system. It was also a popular strewing herb. Lemon balm was an ingredient in 'Carmelite Water', which was enjoyed on a daily basis by Charles V of France, and John Evelyn was not alone in the opinion that 'balm is sovereign for the brain, strengthening the memory and powerfully chasing away melancholy', while balm steeped in wine 'comforts the heart and driveth away melancholy and sadness' (Grieve 1992, p.76). Here we have a pleasant, lemon-scented herb with a well-established reputation for aiding mental faculties and cheering the spirit; it is not surprising, therefore, that its essential oil has been the subject of studies investigating the management of dementia. Ballard *et al.* (2002) reported that *Melissa* essential oil could reduce agitation in severe dementia, and extend the time spent on constructive activities while reducing the time of social withdrawal. Following this study, Elliot *et al.* (2007) conducted a preliminary investigation to determine the bioactivity of the oil, especially in relation to its ability to bind with the key neurotransmitter receptors that are important in the mediation of agitation. They found that *Melissa* had a wide receptor-binding profile (greater than that of lavender), which could explain its calming and cognition-enhancing actions. They also suggested that the topical application or inhalation of *Melissa* could be a better way of delivering a treatment for agitation than intra-muscular injections or tablets.

The essential oil has, according to Williams (2000), a citrus, herbal top note, a herbal body and no dryout. In aromatherapy lemon balm is not widely used; it is has a low yield and is therefore expensive, and because of this it is often adulterated; it can be difficult to obtain the genuine, unadulterated oil. *Melissa* oil contains around 80 per cent citral, the naturally occurring mixture of the isomers geranial and neral, with a strong lemon odour. Citral is often cited as a potential skin irritant with sensitising (allergic reaction) potential. It also contains citronellal, but at a lower level; a high level is an indicator of adulteration (Sorensen 2000). Citronellal has a fresh, lemon-citrus, slightly floral-rosy aroma.

Lemon verbena

Despite the name, which can sometimes be confused with lemon balm, lemon verbena is botanically distinct. It is *Lippia citriodora* (sometimes *Aloysia triphylla*) of the Verbenacea family, a deciduous shrub with lemon-scented leaves, native to South America but now widely cultivated, especially in the south of France. The leaves, even when dried, retain their odour, and so lemon verbena (*verveine citronelle*) tisane is a popular beverage. It does have therapeutic actions, and can be used to reduce fever and aid the digestion (Grieve 1992).

Its essential oil has a fresh, fragrant, fruity citrus, sweet floral scent (Williams 2000), but is not used in aromatherapy and rarely in perfumery because of its skin-sensitising and phototoxic potential (Jouhar 1991). It contains 11–36 per cent geranial, 7–12 per cent neral and 4–23 per cent *d*-limonene (Svoboda and Greenaway 2003). Tisserand and Balacs (1995) discuss both the essential oil and the absolute. The oil has mild to moderate irritation capacity, strong sensitising potential and mild phototoxic potential due to photocitrals, and is not used in fragrances. However, the absolute can be, but in restricted amounts; it is not phototoxic and not irritant, but is a potential sensitiser. Turin and Sanchez (2009) discuss a citron and verbena accord in Guerlain's *Eau de Guerlain*, which has a coherent drydown and 'completely transcends the cologne genre' (p.225); they suggest that it is the best citrus fragrance available.

Lemongrass

The genus *Cymbopogon* (previously known as *Andropogon*) consists of 50–60 species of tropical, perennial, tufted grasses, some of which have extremely aromatic, lemon-scented foliage. These include *C. nardus* (Ceylon citronella), *C. winterianus* (Java citronella), *C. citratus* (West Indian lemongrass) and *C. flexuosus* (East Indian lemongrass) These oils all come from the Far East – India, Sri Lanka, Indonesia and Malaysia – and the oils are usually steam- or hydro-distilled (Weiss 1997).

West Indian lemongrass is only produced under cultivation. It is grown mainly in Argentina, Brazil, Guatemala, Honduras, Haiti and other Caribbean islands, Java, Vietnam, Malaysia, Sri Lanka, Madagascar and the Comoro islands, and also in the Philippines, China, India, Bangladesh, Burma, Thailand and Africa. East Indian lemongrass is grown in southern India, mainly in Kerala.

There are two varieties – the white-stemmed and the red-stemmed – and it is usually the latter that produces the 'typical' oil. Both varieties have long narrow leaves and they rarely flower. The young leaves contain the most oil. The leaves are harvested and, prior to distillation, allowed to wilt for two days, in order to give a higher yield and increased citral content. They are also finely chopped prior to extraction (Lawless 1992). Oils from both types contain around 80–85 per cent citral; it tends to be slightly higher in the East Indian type. They both contain geraniol, at about 3–5 per cent, perhaps slightly more in East Indian oils, which also have considerably more methyl heptanol. However, the West Indian type contains around 20 per cent myrcene, while the East Indian has only traces. This is the second time we have encountered high levels of this component in lemony-scented oil – it was also dominant in jabara (citrus) oil (see page 341). Myrcene is thought to have pain-relieving qualities, and lemongrass oil is often used in aromatherapy for this purpose. An animal study conducted by Seth *et al.* (1976) suggested that injected lemongrass oil had tranquillising and analgesic effects. More recently, Faiyazuddin *et al.* (2009) reviewed the antimicrobial activity of lemongrass, and recommended it for the treatment and control of acne.

Lemongrass essential oil has a strong, lemony herbal aroma, with a herbal, oily dryout (Williams 2000). Because of the instability problems inherent in citral, there are many other lemon-scented botanicals and aromachemicals that are preferred in fine perfumery. However, lemongrass is used for citrus effects in household and industrial products, and is a valuable source for the isolation of citral (Williams 1995c).

Citronella

Citronella oil is obtained from *C. nardus* and, rather than being dominated by citral, it is characterised by citronellal. *C. nardus* is grown mainly in Sri Lanka, and another species that produces an essential oil, *C. winterianus*, is grown throughout the Far East, and now also in Central and South America. The two types are generally known as Ceylon and Java types. The Ceylon type has a floral, woody, grassy and leafy scent, while the Java type is sweet, fresh and lemony. The difference lies mainly in their geraniol content, which is higher in the Ceylon type, contributing to the floral notes. Like lemongrass, citronella oil is an industrial oil, used in insect-repelling products, in household and industrial cleaning products, and for the isolation of geraniol, citronellol, citronellal and menthol synthesis (Weiss 1997).

Weiss (1997) also makes a very interesting comment: orang-utans produce a citronella-smelling exudate that appears to repel insects...so perhaps this slightly harsh, unrefined scent is important not just for human wellbeing.

Lemon scents in the Myrtaceae family

Lemon-scented eucalyptus

Eucalyptus citriodora is the lemon-scented eucalyptus or gum, a medium to tall eucalypt with leaves that emit a strong lemon aroma when crushed. To obtain good-quality oil, the leaves and twiglets must be distilled as soon as possible after harvesting; after 24 hours the yield may be diminished and the odour characteristics changed, especially in terms of its aldehydes (Weiss 1997). The oil has a strong, fresh rosy-citronella odour; the ISO (International Organization for Standardization) specification states that it should contain a minimum of 70 per cent citronellal (Weiss 1997). Citronellal may have calming and antifungal properties (Bowles 2003); Price and Price (1997) state that it has bacteriostatic properties which are due to a natural synergism between citronellal and citronellol, and that the oil is active against *Staphylococcus aureus*. They also claim that it has antifungal activity. Therefore, although it is not classed as a 'medicinal' essential oil, it may have considerable use in treating some infections, perhaps even methicillin-resistant *Staphylococcus aureus* (MRSA). Because of its high citronellal content, like citronella, it too is considered to be an industrial oil, with applications in insect-repelling products. It is used as a source of natural citronellal, which is used to make hydroxycitronellal – even now one of the most widely used materials in perfumery.

Lemon-scented ironbark

E. staigeriana is the lemon-scented ironbark, a medium-sized eucalypt with highly lemon-scented leaves. It has a pleasant, sweet, fresh, fruity-lemon, verbena-like scent, and in this case citral and citronellal are not important. The odour is conferred by geraniol, methyl geranate, geranyl acetate, *d*-limonene, β-phellandrene and neral (one of the citral isomers). The oil is produced in Guatemala and Brazil, and is used in perfumery, toiletries and flavouring, but there are some stability problems and so it is not used in soaps (Weiss 1997).

Lemon-scented tea tree

Leptospermum petersonii is the lemon-scented tea tree, a small shrub or tree that is often grown as an ornamental tree or in hedging. The crushed leaves have a powerful lemon aroma, and can be distilled to produce an essential oil which also has a lemony, pungent, diffusive odour. This is typically composed of citral and citronellal, but also eugenol, *iso*-pulegol and hydrocarbons. It is used for the isolation of citral, which is then used to produce ionone. Weiss (1997) comments that once included in a formula, it is difficult to remove and substitute with something else, because it is so distinctive. The terpeneless version also has reduced citral content, and has an intense, fresh scent; it is also more stable and is used in toiletries.

Lemon-scented myrtle

Backhousia citriodora is the lemon-scented myrtle, from the tropical and subtropical rainforests in Australia. Svoboda and Greenaway (2003) describe this as an attractive evergreen shrub or bushy tree, with lemon-scented leaves that turn from reddish-green to glossy green as they mature, and creamy white flowers. They note that the essential oil from its leaves contains very high levels of citral, and their analysis confirmed that neral was present at 37–42 per cent and geranial at 44–49 per cent. Lawless (2009) discusses *Myrtus citriodora*, also known as lemon myrtle. This oil usually comes from Spain, and is described as a warm Mediterranean herbal with a strong lemon character.

Litsea cubeba

Litsea is a fairly large genus in the Lauraceae family, and *Litsea cubeba* is a small tropical tree native to East Asia, notably China, where it is cultivated. Here it is called *may chang*, but it is also referred to as tropical verbena. It has fragrant flowers and leaves which, like the other botanicals discussed in this section, emit a lemon scent when crushed. Although the leaves and bark can yield an oil, it is the small, peppercorn-sized fruits, that are extracted to give an intense, lemony, fresh and fruity essential oil. This is sweeter than lemongrass but less tenacious, and the citral content is in the region of 85 per cent (Weiss 1997). Bowles (2003) suggests that its essential oil contains geranial (40%), neral (33.8%) and limonene (8.3%); according to Lawless (1992), it can be used in aromatherapy for its antiseptic and deodorant qualities, and as sedative that can combat tension and stress-related conditions. Litsea oil is also an important raw material for the isolation of citral and subsequent synthesis of ionones, but it is also used in citrus perfumes. Its intense, fresh, fruity lemon characteristics can contribute to the middle notes of fragrances, unlike the citrus oils.

Some fruity fragrances

We will conclude this chapter by looking at fruity scents other than lemon or citrus.

Fruity scents are almost universally liked and enjoyed, especially when in context, or perhaps in personal hygiene products such as shower gels or handwashes. Indeed, fine fragrances with a subtle fruity aspect are also widely appreciated; however, if the fruity note is too dominant, the composition will not usually be described as refined or sophisticated! The types of odours we will be discussing here are those of apples and pears, tropical fruits such as pineapples, bananas and mangos (and coconut), and drupes such as cherries and plums, peaches and apricots. The scents of soft fruits such as strawberries, raspberries and blackcurrants are also used in perfumery. These scents cannot be extracted for use in fragrances, but there are now many fragrance chemicals that can be combined to replicate the essence of their aromas, and some that are generally fruity but not specific. For example, nonyl acetate is fruity, floral and diffusive, and the ubiquitous linalyl acetate, found in many essential oils, has a fruity, bergamot- and pear-like odour. Novel aroma molecules are being developed all the time, so any list will go out of date very quickly, and those mentioned below are intended simply to give an idea of what is possible. Brechbill (2007) is a useful resource for those interested in this topic, and Turin (2006) gives an unsurpassed and readable perspective on aroma chemistry. Fragrances that feature some fruity notes are given as examples, using Turin and Sanchez (2009) for reference.

Apples and pears

Apple notes can be given by diethyl malonate, ethyl-2-methylbutyrate, hexadrenyl-iso-butyrate, 'Verdox' (Brechbill 2007) and *iso*-amyl-*iso*-valerate (ripe apples). Some fragrances have a fruity apple theme, such as Donna Karan's *Be Delicious*. The pear note can also be found in fruity fragrances. Some aroma compounds that can give this effect are *iso*-amyl acetate, which is also banana- and apple-like; hexyl acetate, which is like a fruity green pear; and phenyl acetate, which is floral green and pear-like. 'Anapear', methyl-(*Z*)-4,7-octadienoate, was first isolated from Indonesian passion fruit, and the (*E*)-isomer was synthesised to result in a pear-like, powerful, green, fruity and aldehydic compound (Schilling *et al.* 2010). Lauder's *Beautiful Sheer* is a pear-floral fragrance and Caron's *L'Anarchiste* is apple lavender, while Frédéric Malle's *Outrageous* has notes of crab apple and musk (Turin and Sanchez 2009).

Tropical fruits

Turin (2006) discusses fresh pineapple and banana, noting the cheesy aspect that they have because their smells are given by butyric esters: when eaten these release butyric acid into the nose, and this has a buttery, cheesy odour. Pineapple effects can be imparted by allyl cyclohexylpropionate, which itself is sweet, fruity and pineapple-like and can be used in traces to give fruity top notes; allyl caproate has a powerful pineapple scent, while allyl amyl glycolate is more green and can impart intensity. 'Pharaone' has a green, powerful and diffusive pineapple scent.

Turin and Sanchez (2009) comment that the only true pineapple fragrance was Patou's *Colony*, and that L'Artisan Parfumeur's *Ananas Fizz* is more like grapefruit than pineapple, although the name would suggest otherwise. A fruity pineapple and green banana effect can be imparted by ethyl caproate, while *iso*-amyl propionate can give a sweeter banana and pineapple note.

A banana effect can be given by *iso*-amyl caproate, while hexenyl acetate gives an unripe banana odour. Again, a dominant banana characteristic is not usually found in fine fragrances, but some, such as Patou's *Sira des Indes*, have a fruity top note that is suggestive of bananas and pears.

According to Burr (2007), the scent of green mango was the inspiration for Jean-Claude Ellena's composition for Hermès, *Le Jardin sur le Nil*; however, according to Turin and Sanchez (2009), this fragrance is 'woody fresh', and not reminiscent of green mango.

Coconut can also feature in fragranced products. Coconut 'aldehyde' is γ-nonalactone; this has a creamy, sweet, coconut odour, while octalactone is more intense, with a coumarin-like, spicy note. Monyette Paris' *Monyette Paris* is a coconut tuberose that utilises coconut lactones (Turin and Sanchez 2009).

Cherries, plums, peaches and apricots

The damascones can convey various impressions of dried fruits; α-damascone is intensely fruity and plum-like, rosy when diluted, and damascenone (trimethyl cyclohexdienyl butanone) is reminiscent of plums and raisins. A sharp plum and apple odour can be contributed by *N*-heptyl formate, and trimethyl cyclohexadienyl butenone has a fruity, plum and raisin character. 'Nectaryl' is reminiscent of peaches and apricots. Several aromachemicals can impart a peach note, including γ-undecalactone, peach lactone or 'aldehyde' and 'Persicol' (δ-undelactone, a lactonic peach base) that was used in Jacques Guerlain's fruity chypre milestone, *Mitsouko*. Many fragrances have subtle peach elements. For example, Guerlain's *Chant d'Arômes* is a floral with peach, as is their *Nuit d'Amour*. Boucheron's *Jaipur* was composed by Sophia Grojsman, and, according to Turin and Sanchez (2009), is reminiscent of apricot tart, with an apricot and plum accord and a woody, rosy heart. Guerlain's *La Petite Robe Noir* is a fruity gourmand fragrance that features 'black' notes, including that of black cherry; the 2013 edition features blackcurrant too.

Strawberries, raspberries, blackberries and blackcurrants

Strawberry ester, ethyl methyl phenyl glycidate, gives sweet, fruity, strawberry notes and is widely used in fragrances. Cyclopentadecanolide smells of blackberries and musk, and is used to enhance fragrance diffusion. Donna Karan's *DKNY Delicious Night* is a fruity chypre that features blackberry notes (Turin and Sanchez 2009). Raspberry ketone is *para*-hydroxy-benzyl acetone, and dihydro-β-ionone is reminiscent of raspberry, as is the floral fruity 'Berryflor'. Givenchy's *Hot Couture* has raspberry notes, as does Prescriptives' *Calyx*. Methyl benzoate is intensely fruity, floral and blackcurrant-like, and 'Datilat' has a complex odour, floral with aspects of blackcurrant, plums, roses, tobacco and honey. Cartier's *So Pretty* is a fragrance that Turin and Sanchez describe as a 'blackcurrant chypre' (p.505).

Watermelon and cucumber

Before concluding this brief foray into fruity fragrances and aromachemicals, the topic of melon–cucumber also needs to be addressed. This note became popular in fragrances in the 1990s with the introduction of 'Calone', and has persisted. Apart from Calone, 'Helional' (which has also a metallic element) and 'cyclamen aldehyde' can give this watery melon and cucumber effect. Issey Miyake's *L'Eau D'Issey* (1992) is typical; apparently the Japanese designer asked for a scent that smelled like water. This spawned a myriad of other aquatic, melon–cucumber fragrances such as Bulgari's *Aqua pour Homme Marine*, Rochas' *Aquawoman*, Kenzo's *Flower*, Armani's *Acqua di Giò*, and Profumum's *Acqua di Sale*. (Please see Appendix A.)

CHAPTER 12

Attars and the Role of Fragrance in Unani Tibb Medicine

JEANNIE FATIMEH GRAHAM

Attars are natural fragrance oils used as part of the holistic healing system of Unani Tibb eastern medicine. Although they can be used purely as scents, they also have the potential to heal on a physical, emotional, mental and spiritual level. Attars were first produced by Ibn Sina, known in the West as Avicenna. He was an eleventh-century Arabian alchemist and physician, and is considered to be the greatest individual physician who ever lived. It was Avicenna who, in a scientific way, subsequently developed the use of attars for healing. Prior to this, perfumes were comprised of viscous ointments, thick resins and gums.

Attars

Attar is an ancient Persian and Arabic word, which translates as 'essence' or 'sweet smell'. Attars are alcohol-free, natural fragrances; the addition of alcohol to these pure essences would destroy their very essence and render them unsuitable for traditional Unani Tibb healing purposes. Traditional attars are concentrated aromatic blends, extremely popular in the Indian subcontinent and the Middle East, where they are renowned for their arousing aroma, which is both sensual and spiritual.

The attar manufacturing process begins with the delivery of fresh flowers in jute sacks, which are then weighed, quality checked and then emptied out into large copper stills to which a similar amount of water has been added. (A minimum of 80–100kg of flowers per kilogram of base oil are required to produce one kilogram of attar.) The mouth of the filled still is then plastered with clay and a lid clamped tightly on it, making it totally airtight, except for a small hole in the lid through which a pipe of hollow bamboo wrapped either in coconut twine or a coarse cloth is pushed, to collect vapours into a second copper receiver. This receiver remains immersed in a shallow tank of water to help condense vapours. The coconut twine or cloth serves to absorb the heat from the bamboo pipe, preventing it from overheating from the vapours.

The still, containing the mixture of flowers and water, is heated from below by wood charcoal or even cow dung. Attendants skilfully monitor the stills to ensure that correct temperatures and speed of distillation are maintained for individual attars. They do this by adding or removing wood to and from the fire, and by regularly feeling the outside of the still and placing their ears to it, to listen intently for any variation in the sounds from within. A skilled attendant is able, just by feeling the rounded part of the receiver under water, to ascertain exactly when the correct quantity of vapours has condensed inside the receiver. Once that moment arrives, he then wraps a wet cloth around the body of the still, which temporarily halts the distillation process. The full receiver is replaced by an empty one, which in turn may be replaced by yet another. The process is repeated several times, with further batches of flowers being added each time and the water in the tank changed frequently to prevent overheating. The actual distillation process can take up to six hours.

The oil and water mixture can subsequently be separated, either by running off the condensed water vapour through a small capped outlet at the bottom of the receiver, or by pouring the mixture into an open trough. The base material is then poured into leather bottles to remove any sediment and excess moisture. The leather of the bottles is semi-permeable, allowing water to flow out, and the attar to remain. In attar distillation no separate condenser is used in the process, as the long-necked, round copper receiver also acts as a condenser. Copper is used for the stills because it is a good conductor of heat. The unique fragrance of the flowers is captured by the base oil in the receiver, which acquires their specific scent.

The receiver would traditionally contain a base of pure sandalwood oil, but, regrettably, it is not uncommon nowadays for sandalwood oil to be substituted with liquid paraffin, or, even worse, with DOP (dioctyl phthalate). Although attars are still extracted into a pure sandalwood base by some high-quality producers, the attar industry of today has been hit by an ethical and financial dilemma as a result of the rising cost and scarcity of pure-quality sandalwood oil. Many attar producers have been struggling financially, and their profits have declined from what was once a staggering 900 per cent of costs to currently a slim 10–20 per cent margin. This has inevitably resulted in higher retail costs and a decline in sales. In response to this fall in profits and rising costs, it is becoming more and more common for liquid paraffin to be used for the manufacture of cheaper attars. Unfortunately, whereas, as recently as six years ago, the ratio of attars based on sandalwood oil to those based on liquid paraffin or DOP was 80:20, that has now inverted to a disturbing ratio of 10:90. DOP is also recognised as a carcinogenic agent, not unbeknown to attar manufacturers; yet, driven by profit margins, they continue to use it. The result is that today, more than ever, it is vital to ascertain the quality of source and supplier when using attars, especially when using fragrant oils for spiritual and healing purposes. What is perhaps just as alarming is that the target market of attars has now altered considerably, with almost 90 per cent of attar production now being targeted at the tobacco industry to be used as flavouring. With this changing profile of the natural attar industry, many of the well-established manufacturers are now additionally beginning to produce synthetic perfumes (Behl 2008).

Effective healing and desired spiritual success can only be achieved using pure oils. This is especially true when using attars in the spiritual realm. For the practitioner of Unani Tibb therefore, ascertaining the source and quality of attars to be used is extremely important, and it is essential to use only attars with the purest of base ingredients, which have had no alcohol, chemicals or preservatives added during their processing, and have not been produced with child or forced labour, or caused any negative environmental effects. This is because when the attars are used for healing purposes, or especially spiritual advancement, it is of paramount importance that no negative energy is transmitted into the attars. There are many attars available worldwide that are labelled as 'attars', but do not meet this required standard, so extreme vigilance is required to select only the purest attars for use, taking into account the aforementioned criteria.

Attars are usually categorised according to the type of raw material used. There are 'floral attars' produced from a single species of flower – for example, rose, gardenia, honeysuckle, lavender, lilac and lily. Then there are 'herbal and spicy attars', which include henna, amber and musk, for example. Once single scented attars have been produced, it is also traditional practice for several natural attars to be selected and blended together to produce unique scents, particularly for use as perfumes. So although there is a vast range of individual oils of attar, which in addition to their healing purposes are also used in their own right as fragrances, such as sandalwood, patchouli and lavender, many attars are also combinations of oils, sometimes as many as 40, blended together according to centuries-old, secret family formulas. For healing and spiritual purposes, it is more common for single scents to be used, but there are a few notable exceptions, such as the magnificent *Jannat al Ferdows*, which translates as 'gateway to paradise'.

As attars are highly concentrated, it is more usual for them to be sold in small quantities. The shelf-life of an attar is permanent, with the scent of some attars increasing in strength and becoming more aromatic as they age. Traditionally, attars were sold in intricately decorated glass bottles, reflecting their high status, magnificence and exclusivity. Attars are even considered by some to be the most precious material possessions a person can own. There is an old tradition in the Middle East involving attars, where it is customary, as guests are leaving the home, for the hosts to offer them an attar as a leaving gift.

The Unani Tibb humoural system of medicine

In order to understand how attars are used as tools in healing, it is essential to have at least a basic comprehension of the Unani Tibb humoural system of medicine, and the way that healing is approached in this system. Unani Tibb medicine is based on the methods of medicine used and taught in ancient Greece, Arabia and Persia. 'Unan' is the Arabic and Persian word for the country Greece, and 'Unani' literally means 'from Greece'; 'Tibb' is an Arabic word meaning 'medicine' or 'nature' – a reference to classical Greek medicine. These methods themselves included aspects of Egyptian and Mesopotamian healing methods from even more ancient times. Unani Tibb traces its roots back to the classical Greek physicians Hippocrates (circa 460–370 BCE) and Galen (circa 129–217 CE) and the later renowned Arab physician Razi, known as Rhazes in the West (865–925 CE). But it was the Persian medical scholar Hakim Ibn Sina (980–1037 CE), known more commonly in English as Avicenna, who subsequently developed the teachings of his predecessors into a comprehensive healing system, enriching it with elements of the medical traditions of Persia, Arabia, India, China and classical Greece. His renowned medical encyclopaedia *The Canon of Medicine* was translated into Latin in the twelfth century, and set the standard for medicine worldwide. In this work Avicenna enriched Persian medicine with Greek, Islamic, Chinese and Ayurvedic medical teachings to establish what we now refer to as Unani Tibb medicine. The 'silk route', spanning the distance from China and linking Persia, Arabia and India, also played a vital role in helping to make possible the distribution of knowledge between these regions.

A belief central to Unani Tibb is that good health, a contented state of mind and balanced emotions represent the normal constitution for human beings. As a person can be knocked out of balance by emotional, psychological, social, environmental, dietary or spiritual factors, Tibb uses a holistic set of principles to diagnose and treat various conditions, based on each person's body type, personality and *mizaj*, or individual metabolic constitution. Each item of food we eat, or each medicine, herb or scent we use internally or externally, has its own *mizaj*. In addition, a medicine or food that has positive effects for one person may be detrimental to a person of a different *mizaj*. It is this factor that Unani Tibb takes first into account when treating patients, and appropriate herbal treatment and attars will subsequently be selected for each individual and guidance offered in the appropriate choice of foods and lifestyle, all suitable for that person's specific constitution. An important principle governing Unani Tibb medicine is that no treatment should ever impair the body's natural functions.

In his *Canon of Medicine* Avicenna defined Unani Tibb as: 'the science of which we learn the various states of body, in health and when not in health, and the means by which health is likely to be lost and, when lost, is likely to be restored' (Howell 1987, p.58–59). He promoted the concept that the chief function of a physician is to aid the body's natural forces when fighting a disease.

The healing system of Unani Tibb adheres to the humoural theory, which takes as its premise the presence of four humours in the body. The blood humour is referred to as *dam*, phlegm as *bulgham*, yellow bile as *safra* and black bile as *sauda*. Sickness and disease are seen as resulting from imbalances in these humours.

A physician of Unani Tibb is referred to as a *hakim; hakima* if female. He or she will diagnose a patient's condition in terms of a surplus or deficit of one or more of the four humours, and will then attempt to address and ultimately cure these symptoms by administering herbs or attars capable of re-establishing a harmonious relationship between the *bulgham, dam, safra* and *sauda* humours. In addition to herbal treatment, other techniques used to cleanse the body and restore humoural balance include *mushil* (purging), *taariq* (sweating), *hammam* (balneology), *hijama* (cupping) and *riyazat* (exercise).

Unani Tibb, as a tradition, heals using herbs, minerals, diet and attars in a way similar to how a western herbalist would, but before commencing any treatment, it is essential for a Tibb practitioner to assess the patient's *mizaj*, which can be very broadly understood as metabolic type or constitution, but relating to the basic primary elements. Once this is ascertained, the *hakim* will then suggest lifestyle and dietary changes and prescribe herbs, minerals and attars; the aim is to rebalance the patient physically, emotionally and spiritually. The herbs, minerals and attars have the ability to rebalance, because they too have their own *mizaj* and will be carefully selected to work on imbalances in one or more of the humours.

According to Unani Tibb there are four primary elements, referred to as *arkan*. These are simple individual substances that cannot be dissolved into simpler entities. Any matter found in nature is formed by a combination of these elements, with qualities varying depending on the specific nature of each constituting element. Each of these primary elements contains two of the properties of heat, dryness, cold or moisture.

One of the two properties is always active and one is passive – 'heat' and 'cold' being active, and 'moisture' and 'dryness' being passive. If we take *Fire* as an example, it contains the two properties: *hot* and *dry*. *Heat* is the active property here and *dryness* is the passive property. Two active properties cannot be found together in one element – for example, an element cannot be both hot and cold. *Earth* and *Water* are also 'heavy' elements: they are strong, negative, passive and female, *Fire* and *Air* are 'light' elements: they are weak, positive, active, and male.

Table 12.1 The four primary elements and their attributes

Active	Passive	Light/heavy	M/F	+
Fire (*nar*)	hot	dry	light	male
Air (*hawwa*)	hot	moist	light	male
Water (*Ma*)	cold	moist	heavy	female
Earth (*ardh*)	cold	dry	heavy	female

These four elements are the basic building blocks of all substances in nature, including the human body, animals and plants. The elements are used both to explain the origins of disease and to describe them diagnostically. Balanced health depends on a proper balance of these four elements. In addition, each element and its qualities can be related to seasons, time of day, organs of the body and types of disease. This system of corresponding attributes is extremely important in Unani Tibb medicine, resulting in a holistic system of diagnosis and treatment.

A person is born with a predominance of one element over the others, and this determines their temperament. Healing is then a matter of balancing these elements, or the humours resulting from these elements, through physical, emotional and spiritual channels. The ratio of these humours in relation to each other will change over a person's lifetime, although most people have one dominant humour. Furthermore, the humours change according to the seasons and the time of day. An important factor is that the effects of one humour can be offset or modified by those of another. No one is born with 25 per cent of each humour, and what counts as an optimal balance for one person will differ from what counts as an optimal balance for another. A person's temperament or *mizaj* is characterised by these humours and their subsequent effects, and careful study of them assists in the selection of appropriate remedies for each individual patient.

If we consider diseases and herbs with respect to the primary elements and their qualities, care can be taken to select the most beneficial remedies with the qualities appropriate to balance a patient's humours. If the attributes of the herb or drug being used to treat do not match those of the patient and the disease, treatment may end up not only being ineffective, but also producing side effects. With modern pharmaceutical medicine, side effects are common and there is usually no way of predicting which patient will react adversely. Similarly, when herbs are taken off-the-shelf, without due consideration for a patient's *mizaj*, treatment may also be ineffective.

The humours relate to each of the temperaments as follows.

- Blood humour (hot and moist) relates to sanguine temperament: *dum.*

- Phlegm humour (cold and moist) relates to phlegmatic temperament: *bulgham.*

- Yellow bile humour (hot and dry) relates to choleric temperament: *safra.*

- Black bile humour (cold and dry) relates to melancholic temperament: *sauda.*

It is also common for people to have combined temperaments, as in the combinations below:

- sanguine/phlegmatic
- sanguine/melancholic
- phlegmatic/sanguine
- phlegmatic/choleric

- choleric/phlegmatic
- choleric/melancholic
- melancholic/sanguine
- melancholic/choleric

The *sanguine temperament* is connected closely to the blood humour and the stimulation of the veins and arteries, which provide our bodily energy. Common qualities observed in sanguines are that they have a tend to have a ruddy appearance, or redden easily, with smooth, firm, moist and warm skin; are of a medium build; have a good appetite and digestion; have light yellow urine and firm brown faeces; have usually pleasant dreams and are generally of a happy disposition. A sanguine person will suffer more from imbalances during spring or summer, or if exposed to wind or heat. Typical signs of excess sanguine humour are usually related to the circulatory system.

The *phlegmatic temperament*, closely linked to the phlegm humour, relates to the expulsion of excess and unnecessary substances from the body. Phlegm plays a necessary role in the body during bouts of cold and flu, with copious amounts of it being expelled by the body through the nose in an attempt to clear out toxins and bacteria. The phlegm humour has a beneficial cooling and moistening effect on the heart, and strengthens the function of the lower brain and the emotions. Phlegm maintains proper fat metabolism and the balance of body fluids, electrolytes, and hormones via the circulation of lymph and moisture through the body. On the other hand, excess phlegm in the system can manifest as excessive sleepiness, dullness, slowness, heaviness, forgetfulness, runny nose, poor digestion, and pale and cold skin. Phlegmatic types tend to have pale, smooth, soft, cold and moist skin; a short stature, often with a flabby build; poor appetite; slow or weak digestion; thin and pale urine and pale and loose faeces; frequent dreams of water; and apathy. Phlegmatics often suffer from disorders of the central nervous system, such as multiple sclerosis, muscular dystrophy or cerebral palsy, and disorders in their fluid metabolism.

The *choleric temperament* is linked to the yellow bile humour, whose receptacle is the gallbladder. The yellow bile humour warms the body and increases both physical and mental activity. The choleric temperament is also closely associated with the nervous system. Cholerics tend to have yellow, rough, warm and dry skin; a short stature with a lean body build; a strong appetite; overactive digestion; and thick orange urine and dry, yellow faeces. Signs of choleric humour excess include excessive leanness of the body, hollow eyes, irrational anger, a yellow tinge to the skin, a bitterness in the throat, a stronger than average pulse, disturbed sleep, and frequent dreams of fire, lightning or fighting. Those of a choleric temperament may suffer from anxiety, agitation, nervous exhaustion, insomnia and strokes.

The *melancholic temperament* is linked to the black bile humour, which has the spleen as its receptacle. Melancholics tend to have brown, rough, dry and cold skin; a medium or slim body build; a large appetite; slow digestion; thick, pale urine and dry, black faeces; and to suffer from worry or grief. They may often drag their feet, acting as if their bodies were a burden to them, and also feel severe physical pain from the slightest of injuries. In *The Traditional Healer's Handbook* Hakim Chishti describes the black bile humour as 'consisting of a cool and thick earthly aspect which is prone to coagulation and a more fluid, vaporous substance' (Chishti 1991).

In normal quantities, this stimulates the memory and creates a practical and pragmatic personality. However, if the coldest part of the black bile humour is not eliminated properly, it can settle in tissues and form tumours. Signs of excess in the melancholic temperament include irrational fears, rough and swarthy skin, leanness, insomnia, nightmares, a weak pulse, a preference for solitude, thin clear urine and frequent sighing.

A practitioner of Unani Tibb will assess a person according to the above body types or combinations of types in great detail, and treatment will be designed to rebalance any excess of humour, using lifestyle changes, therapies, herbs and attars. Hakim Avicenna, who introduced us to the world of attars, invented the process of steam distillation, and was the first person ever to distil the oil of rose, also developed the use of attars for physical ailments using specific scientific formulas and designed an elaborate system whereby attars and flowers were also assigned the properties of hot and cold, moisture and dryness. This allowed treatment of physical conditions by considering the inherent imbalance and temperament of an individual and rebalancing with an attar of an appropriate temperament. Avicenna was also the first person to apply oils in a therapeutic sense to balance the emotions.

In planning treatment with herbs or attars, the practitioner will take into account the fact that plants and their derivatives are recognised not only as being 'hot' or 'cold', and 'dry' or 'moist', but as having a certain degree of potency of these qualities. So each herb or attar can be hot or cold and moist or dry in the first, second, third or fourth degree. When a herb or attar is sought out, depending on how far out of balance the patient has become, a herb or attar of a lesser or a higher degree of the opposite quality will be selected. The two qualities within the herb or attar may also differ – so, for example, a herb or attar may be used, that is hot in the second degree and dry in the first degree.

The practical use of attars in Unani Tibb medicine

Attars used as fragrance

Only a few drops of attar are required when using as a fragrance. The etiquette in receiving an attar is to offer your right hand palm down, so that the person offering the attar can apply it over the back of your hand. You should then rub the back of that hand onto your chin and cheeks and across the opposite wrist, rubbing both wrists together, and then across the front of your clothing. When applying directly on yourself, you should place one of the fingers of the left hand over the top of the attar bottle and tip the bottle to wet the finger. Then the tip of this finger should be rubbed well over the back of the right hand. Ideally, before continuing, you should lift the back of the right hand up and hold it a little way away from the nose, and then take a few deep breaths to breathe in the essence of the attar. You should then rub the back of the right hand over the back of the left hand, creating some friction and heat, which will release more oils. You can then rub the backs of both hands onto your neck, wrists and clothing.

Attars used as incense

According to Avicenna, this method of using attars has a particularly strong effect, especially on the heart. This mode of application releases the essence of the oil into the air and disperses it. It is also an effective means of administering the properties of the attar to children or others who may be less compliant in using them. Two to four drops of a selected attar should be dropped onto a piece of charcoal or placed in an oil burner, and used in a way similar to that for essential oils (Chishti 2003).

Attars used in massage

Attars are excellent for treating physical imbalances. They can be used with a carrier oil such as olive oil or sweet almond oil at a ratio of 2–4ml to 120ml base oil.

Attars used in bathing treatments

A few drops of attar can be added to a small amount of milk, and mixed to disperse the oil before adding to a bath full of warm water. The advantage of using attars in this way is that the essence of the attar is released, meaning that it can be inhaled over an extended period of time. It also enables the whole body to be treated. Caution should be taken to avoid excess.

Attars used as a fomentation

One to three drops of attar should be added to approximately two litres of warmed water in a container with a lid, and shaken vigorously. A further two litres of warmed water are then added to this liquid, and it is shaken again. A piece of cheesecloth should then be dipped into this warmed attar water and placed over the area to be treated (Chishti 2003).

Attars used in meditation

Attars are frequently used for spiritual practises and meditation. When used for this purpose, prior to ritual prayers, or before sufi *dhikr* or spiritual chanting circles, attars are offered to those who are gathered, who then apply them with the hope of opening their heart, receiving assistance on their spiritual journey, and reaching elevation to another level.

Therapeutic applications of attars

Attars can be applied in specific ways, to strengthen individual systems of the body (Chishti 2003):

- To strengthen the brain: frankincense and rose.

- To strengthen the heart: sandalwood, amber and rose.

- To strengthen the liver: amber.

- To strengthen the stomach: rose.

- To strengthen the nervous system: frankincense.

- To strengthen the female reproductive system: rose and sandalwood.

- To strengthen the male reproductive system: myrrh, musk, violet and amber.

As already discussed, Unani Tibb medicine assesses each person according to their particular temperament, which will include elements of heat or cold, moistness or dryness. Attars, too, are classified based on their effect on the human body, and will warm, cool, moisten or dry the body. If a person is suffering from an *excess of cold*, typical signs could include a weak digestion, lack of thirst, a tendency to phlegm and catarrh and a laxity of joints. Signs of *excess heat*, on the other hand, could include fatigue, excess thirst, a bitter taste in the mouth, a weak and rapid pulse, lack of energy, and inflammatory type conditions. *Excess moisture* in the body could result in symptoms similar to those of excess cold, as well as puffiness, a tendency to diarrhoea and upset stomach, excess sleep and excess saliva and nasal secretions. *Excess dryness*, on the other hand, may manifest as dry and rough skin, insomnia and wasting of weight. By way of an example, someone suffering from a cold/moist imbalance would be prescribed an attar that had hot/dry qualities. Depending on the degree of cold or moist imbalance, or which quality was dominant, an appropriate attar would be selected. But further care would still need to be taken to monitor the degree of each quality. For example, if a person of a cold and dry temperament required a heating attar, it would be inadvisable to prescribe one that also had drying qualities of a high degree, as this would increase the patient's dryness; but a heating attar with only one degree of dryness would be acceptable.

Examples of heating oils

- Amber hot 2° and dry 2°

- Frankincense hot 2° and dry 2°

- Lavender hot 1° and dry 2°

- Lilac hot 3° and dry 1°

- Lily of the valley hot 3° and dry 3°

- Musk hot 3° and dry 3°

- Patchouli hot 2° and dry 2°

Examples of cooling oils

- Jasmine cold 1° and moist 1°

- Myrrh cold 2° and dry 2°

- Rose cold 2° and dry 2°

- Sandalwood cold 2–3° and dry 2°

- Violet cold 1° and moist 1°

Specific points of application

In addition to considering the temperament of the disease and the attar, and matching these accordingly, specific points of application are also indicated for particular conditions. For heavy eyelids, itchy eyes or halitosis, attars are applied to the nape of the neck. For pain in the upper arms or throat, or to generally relax the solar plexus, the attar is rubbed gently between the shoulderblades. For any type of tremor of the head, or for a range of conditions of the head, face, teeth or ears, drops of attar are placed on the back of the neck. An attar can be applied under the chin to treat conditions of the teeth, throat and jaw, or to generally cleanse the head. Applied to the legs, attars assist in cleansing the blood and promoting menstrual flow. Placed over the ankle bone is specific for suppressed menses, sciatica and gout. The area behind the knee is the application location for ulcers of the leg and foot. The inner thighs are the areas used to treat inflammation of the upper thighs themselves, haemorrhoids, and conditions of the bladder and uterus; whereas the area of the front of the thighs is specific for inflammation of the testicles, or to treat leg ulcers. To treat conditions of the hip joints and sciatica, an attar can be applied to the outer thighs (Chishti 2003).

Specific methods of use

Methods of using attars can also be specific to the conditions presented. For headaches or migraine, for example, attars of violet or sandalwood would be used, either as an inhalation or as a foot massage. To treat a black eye, one drop of rose attar is diluted in 30ml of olive oil and rubbed over the injured area; and for an itchy nose one drop of rose is diluted in 7.5ml of either almond or olive oil and rubbed gently just inside the nose. If there is excessive sneezing, rose attar is diluted, again in olive oil, at a ratio of one drop to 15ml and rubbed on the outside of the nose, but also on the palms of the hands and soles of the feet. One drop of myrrh, sandalwood or rose attar diluted in 15ml of olive oil can be applied to the external ear to help cure earache. And to help those suffering from insomnia or general agitation, four drops of either rose or violet attar are added to 4ml almond oil and applied to the soles of the feet, the external ear and the back of the neck.

There is a very precise method of using attars for treating emotional and mental imbalances, including depression. One to two drops of an appropriate attar are placed on a piece of cottonwool the size of a small pea. This is then inserted under the ridge (inferior antihelix crus) of the right ear only, above the opening (not inside the ear). It is important to apply the attar to the right ear and not the left. The essence is absorbed via the cells in the skin and has an immediate effect on the mind and emotions. To achieve its optimum effect, there is also a precise method of using attar of amber, an extremely popular attar used by both men and women. (Attar of amber is produced from the fossilised sap of ancient *Pinus succinefera* conifers. It has a warm, rich, sweet, deep and sensual smell.) The specific method is to place a dot of the attar on the index finger of the right hand and rub this between the index finger and the thumb before applying it to the third eye, located between the eyebrows, and massaging it in gently. This will result in an immediate focus of the mind and increase in perception and mental alertness. Amber is known to have aphrodisiac properties; it is also used for treating asthma and rheumatism, and is believed to offer protection against negative energy (Chishti 2003).

Attars and the heart

In the medical system of Unani Tibb, the heart is considered the most important organ. Avicenna concurred with the prophetic tradition of the Prophet Muhammad in this regard:

> There is one organ in the body, which, if it is well, the whole body is well; and if it is ill, the whole body is ill. And this organ is the heart. (Chishti 1991, p.238)

Avicenna discusses many diseases of the heart – for example, embolism of cardiac arteries and inflammation – but for him, the heart possessed a much greater function than simply that of a muscular pump. He believed the heart to be a reservoir of divine potentialities and to be greatly affected by emotions such as pleasure, sorrow, joy, grief, revenge, anxiety and exhilaration. He considered blockages of the heart to be the result of disturbance of the breath or imbalances of rhythm, for example. Avicenna argued that the first purpose of treating any cardiovascular disease was to purify the blood, as he saw the blood as the means to refine the *pneuma* or vital force. This could be achieved by the use of minerals, herbs, diet, climate change or attars (Ibn Sina 1993). Avicenna was so convinced of the value of attars in treating heart conditions that he once remarked that 'all aromatic oils are cardiac drugs'. He considered that attars had a unique ability to restore harmony to the human body, as well as encouraging the emergence of divine potentialities. He stressed that:

> The vital power of the heart is attracted to aromas. In cardiac drugs great consideration is given to aromas, because the heart is the seat of the production of the vital force of the body. (Chishti 1991, p.238)

Of the 63 cardiac drugs mentioned by Ibn Sina, 40 were in fact attars. The heart is also the chief mechanism and tool used to develop and advance the soul (Chishti 1991).

The rose

Both the rose and attar of rose have a unique status. Rose is the most superior of all the floral scents and is referred to as the 'queen of scents'. The rose symbolises love, truth and beauty. Attar of rose, although elegant and feminine, is also frequently used by men in the Middle East, especially as part of religious ceremonies. There is a sufi spiritual legend which considers that the first thing ever to be created in the universe was the 'Soul of Prophecy', which was created from the Creator's own light (*nur*). One drop of perspiration of the Soul of Prophecy was subsequently taken to create the 'Soul of the Rose'. This tale serves to illustrate the spiritual significance of the rose, which is seen not only as representing love and beauty but also as a representation of perfection, containing the pure essence and light of the Creator (Chishti 2005). In fact, the rose is the very symbol of sufism, and it is also called the 'Mother of Scents' and the 'Queen of the Garden'. The allure, splendour, and sweet scent of the rose can only be found at the very end of a long, tough and very thorny stem. This, for the sufis, symbolises and parallels the mystic path to the Creator.

The rose is also considered to have the most refined essence of all flowers, and because of this it is traditionally used to absorb and convey the blessings of saints from their shrines. It is traditional practice for visitors to shrines to place rose petals on the tomb of the saint. The visitors return later and collect the petals they have left. The soul of the saint is considered to be a living thing, which means that the petals left at the tomb are perceived to have absorbed the essence of the saint, and this essence of rose is then used for healing purposes. In the same way, attar of rose is believed to absorb spiritual blessings and the blessings of angels, when used in prayer or meditation.

The scent of attar of rose helps create a serene, peaceful and tranquil atmosphere. It also conveys an inner strength, yet at the same time presents an outer softness. Rose works simultaneously on a physical, emotional and spiritual level. It is a purifying attar and the least toxic of all scents. It is excellent to use around children, who are often attracted to its scent, and is by far the most common attar used by the sufis. Astrologically, the ruling planet of this attar is Venus.

The sufi path

Attar essences can be collected from many plants, but for use in the spiritual arena the sufis and their followers have tended to use predominantly those which have been divinely recommended. These include, in addition to rose, amber, frankincense, jasmine, myrrh, violet, sandalwood, musk, henna, 'oud (see page 160) and *Jannat al Ferdows* – all of which are pure oils, except the last, which is a blend. There is a tradition which states that attar of jasmine can heal up to 70 different illnesses. Violet attar is also unique, in that it has the ability to be heating in the winter and cooling in the summer (Ispahany 1956).

The sufi mystics of Islam consider attars central to their journey. They believe that, just as human beings, in addition to having a physical body, also have an absolute essence, referred to as a soul, which will be extracted at death, so each flower and plant also has an essence in addition to its physical form. Because plants are viewed as having such an essence, the sufis consider that beautiful scents in the form of attars created from plants and flowers will have a profound effect on the human soul, which itself yearns for beauty. Just as important, the sufis believe that angels too are attracted to beautiful scents, and this is why followers of the sufi path apply attars or rosewater before their meditation and prayer sessions, hoping to attract angels to their gatherings. Attars are an integral part of sufi meditation circles, and it is common to see attars offered around prayer circles and applied before they begin, although many do this purely in emulation of the Prophet Muhammad, as he was renowned for having used attars, rather than from an awareness of any healing or spiritual properties of the attars themselves. The Prophet Muhammad was known to have had a special container in which he stored attars, and there are traditions passed down relating to him applying attars, especially attars of rose and musk, to his head and beard.

Spiritual use of attars

The highest-level use of attars is considered to be a spiritual one, rather than a physical one: that of adjusting and balancing the spiritual stations, and treating emotional and spiritual health. According to Unani Tibb medicine, when we treat a patient, we cannot overlook the emotional and spiritual dimension of that person, and these dimensions need to be treated alongside the physical body.

The soul is seen as eternal and indestructible. It is believed that the soul is placed in the body by the Creator at the moment of conception, and remains with us until death, at which time the spirit and soul separate. The sufis have developed specific spiritual practices to develop the soul and aid the seeker on their spiritual journey, and the application of attars to adjust and rebalance the soul are an integral part of this practice.

The sense of smell has long been linked to the spiritual realm, and the life story of Farid ud-Din Attar, one of the most respected sufi poets and sheikhs ever to have lived, serves as an excellent illumination of this. The works of Farid ud-Din Attar have been translated into many languages and read and studied worldwide, one of his most popular works being *Mantegh e Tir* (*The Conference of the Birds*).

Farid ud-Din Attar was born in Nishapur, northeastern Iran, sometime between 1120 and 1157, into a long line of *attaars*, or perfumers, hence his name. He grew up immersed in and surrounded by attars and their magnificent scents, and was gradually taught the knowledge that encompassed this field of study. It was typical in those days for medicines to be sold alongside attars, and this is how it was in Attar's family business; the attars on the shelves were considered as much a part of medical treatment as the herbs and medicines. Attars were part and parcel of the healing process and definitely more than just perfumes. As Farid ud-Din grew into a young man he started work in this family dispensary as a perfumer himself, blending and selling attars, as well as becoming skilled at practising medicine. The time he spent working in the dispensary with attars was to serve as the basis for discovery of his spirituality and the beginning of his ultimate spiritual journey. It is believed that he authored much of his poetry in his dispensary.

The story is told that one day a dervish called at Attar's dispensary in the hope of collecting alms for charity, but when he arrived, Farid ud-Din was so occupied going about his business, seeing to his patients and selling attars, that he completely ignored him. The dervish approached Farid ud-Din for alms a second time, but this time he spoke his thoughts out loud. He wondered how, when Attar was so busy accumulating wealth, he would manage to depart this world, since it would mean leaving behind all the material goods he had amassed. Attar simply replied: 'I will give up my ghost as you will.' No sooner had Farid ud-Din said this than the dervish lay down on the floor, closed his eyes, declared adamantly: 'There is no god, but God', and passed away. It was this event and encounter with the dervish that changed Attar's life forever and opened his eyes to his future spiritual path. Many of Attar's works focus on cutting ties with the material world (Friedlander 1992).

The sufi tradition developed the spiritual use of aromatherapy by relating different scents to the stations the soul passes through on its journey of return to the Creator, and to the various physical, mental and spiritual illnesses that reflect the soul's growth through its respective stages. The soul is seen as our link to the Infinite; attars have a vital role to play in this spiritual journey, and are used within each spiritual station to bring about balance (Chishti 2005). Over time, as we use attars, we gradually develop more awareness of the subtleties of our souls, which are part of the divine plan of existence. Sufis consider that we can either experience life from a purely physical point of view, or from that of our soul, which is one of a higher perspective. Each station of the soul is called a *maqam*, which translates as 'resting place'. At the more advanced stages, a sheikh or guide is essential to guide a follower through the phases. These *maqam* are enumerated and described slightly differently depending on the sufi order, but it is usual to refer to between five and seven major stages. Each spiritual station relates to different physical and spiritual ailments or diseases, and specific attars are recommended to use at each different stage when embarking on a spiritual journey of advancement.

The initial resting place is referred to as the *Maqam an-Nafs* or the 'Station of Egotism' and represents egotism and all the appetites of our physical life. This is the stage we are born into. As infants we have a pure desire for our needs to be satisfied. Adults in this stage also demand their desires to be fulfilled, but these are no longer for basic survival needs, but rather gluttony, wealth, fame, status or sex, for example, and the more these aspirations are fed, the stronger they actually become, as they can never be satisfied. In this initial stage, the station of *nafs* (egotism), the sort of physical ailments to be expected include obesity, gout, eye disease, hypoglycaemia, jaundice, cancer, heart attacks, alcoholism and drug abuse. Likely spiritual illnesses might include depression, fear, anxiety, self-doubt, sexual perversion and mental illness. Attars of rose and frankincense are recommended for both the physical and spiritual ailments in this 'station of egotism' and in addition, for this level, attar of musk is used for physical conditions and attar of violet for spiritual conditions. The Farsi word for the burning *nafs* is *atesh*, which means 'fire'. It is a perfect analogy, for just as with a small fire, which may burn slowly to begin with, the more we put into it and 'feed' it, the larger the blaze becomes. In the same way, the appetites of the human body grow more fiercely if they persist into adulthood and no effort has been made to control this ego of the physical body, which requires the setting of limits (Chishti 2005).

The next station is the *Maqam al-Qalb*, the 'Station of the Heart'. Once a seeker arrives at this *maqam*, a sequence of events will begin to occur. A move from one station to the next comes as a result of focus on self-development, discipline and appropriate guidance. Seekers will work on developing themselves, accept responsibility, work with regularity and try to instil courage, kindness and justice as personal qualities within themselves. As they leave the previous station, they will start to reduce the amount of food they eat and limit themselves to eating only *taher*, or pure food and drink. All these endeavours serve to enhance the condition of their soul. Once they have entered this stage and as they advance, the soul will begin to gain precedence over physical desires, and as a result excesses start to be driven from the physical body. This toxic elimination process may manifest in physical signs such as skin eruptions, fevers, kidney disease, headaches, sensitivity to toxins, diarrhoea, aches and pains and a general irritability. Emotional and spiritual elimination signs often include an exaggeration of self-importance, fear of failure, extreme anger, lack of concentration, and emotional excess (Chishti 2005).

Attars are the ideal medium for treating these conditions. They are also used as a preventative measure to keep such sicknesses from occurring in the first place when the seeker enters this stage. They help by retaining a steady balance and by quietening the soul. Amber, rose and musk are the attars that would be prescribed for the physical ailments of the station of the *qalb*. For spiritual and emotional imbalances, sandalwood and violet would be used. Attar of sandalwood, for example, is quietening to all of the senses. All appetites of the body, whether sexual appetite or appetite for food, lust for material things or fame or self-importance, will be soothed.

Once the station of the heart has been established, the seeker has the capacity to travel onwards, but the journey is now impossible without the assistance of a guide or teacher. This is because it is difficult to truly view ourselves. We can see a reflection of ourselves, but not our real self, and without a guide this can result in self-deception, so the seeker needs to be prepared to submit to a spiritual guide (Chishti 2005). For all of the more advanced stages from here on, a sheikh is essential to guide followers through them, and to instruct those on the path in the application of essential and intense spiritual practices specific to each stage. Those who attempt to develop on their own will be misled by their own *nafs* or ego.

In the spiritual station of *Maqam ar-Ruh*, the 'Station of Pure Spirit', the student on the path could begin to suffer from corrupted appetite, fatigue, muscular disease, auto-intoxication or psychosis. Attars of 'oud, henna, amber and musk are the appropriate scents to use here. Spiritually, the ailments encountered may include arrogance, pride, forgetfulness, self-deception and lack of concentration, for which attars of violet, rose and sandalwood are appropriate. The *Maqam as-Sirr* is a spiritual level known as the 'Station of Divine Secrets', where physical ailments such as feelings of suffocation and pain in the heart may be expected to occur, as well as spiritual conditions of over-sensitivity, false interpretations, irrationality, disconnection with reality, and even rejection of belief in the Creator. Attars of 'oud, sandalwood and henna are recommended for the spiritual ailments, and *Jannat al-Ferdows* for any physical diseases. Some seekers become so overwhelmed at this stage that they are unable to leave; they become divinely intoxicated. At the levels of *Maqam al-Qurb*, the 'Station of Nearness to the Creator' and *Maqam al-Wisal*, the 'Station of Union with the Creator', there tend to be no physical ailments, only spiritual conditions such as excessive ecstasy, incessant weeping, incoherence and total silence, for which attars of rose and amber are recommended (Chishti 2005).

Corresponding to each of these stations of the soul, and attuned to specific frequencies, are subtle spiritual energy points, termed *lata'if* (*latifa* in the singular). Each *latifa* can be activated by spiritual experiences and practices, and attars applied to them. These points are vital for balancing the body's energies, and their imbalance results in sickness. According to the spiritual Masters of the Naqshbandi-Haqqani Sufi Order, there are seven *lata'if* which are used in spiritual healing: *Nafsi, Qalb, 'Aql, Ruh, Sirr, Khafa* and *Akhfa*. The *Latifa al-Khafi*, which according to some is located in the middle of the forehead (between the eyes or in the third eye position), translates as 'mysterious' or 'latent'. This stage represents intuition and is closely related to the sense of smell (Mirahmadi 2005).

The journey of the soul through the different *maqamat* and the *lata'if* energy points illustrates the role spirituality plays with respect to various illnesses and why the spiritual aspect of our persona cannot be ignored when considering how best to tackle and treat illness and disease. For addressing all imbalances, especially spiritual ones, attars are our closest allies.

> The art of healing was dead, Galen revived it; it was scattered and dis-
> arrayed, Razi rearranged and realigned it; it was incomplete, Ibn Sina
> perfected it. (Ansari 1976)

As part of this 'perfection' of the art of healing, Avicenna developed the use of attars. These attars are indispensable to the Unani Tibb system of medicine, for physical and emotional healing and spiritual advancement, but they can also be used solely as aromatic scents. This form of aromatherapy, using attars to restore harmony, is, in essence, medicine for the soul. Whether attars are applied directly to the skin and subsequently absorbed via the cells of the skin, or are inhaled via the olfactory system, they can have an almost immediate effect; or they may require time to work with the body to heal. Attars can adjust emotions, states of mind and the spiritual side of a person, and many physical diseases will respond beneficially to their correction. But the spiritual aspect will always take precedence over the physical.

In Conclusion

CHAPTER 13

Cultivating the Olfactory Palate

How many of us educate our olfactory palates or meditate on scent? With all of the scented products available to us, and the sophisticated ways of perfuming our world, comparatively few of us take the time to actively develop our sense of smell. In this concluding chapter we will consider why we should, and how we can, develop our olfactory palate. We will begin with a comparison of those who have not cultivated their sense of smell with those who have, by looking at novices and experts. The Japanese art form of *koh-do*, the incense ceremony, will also be discussed, and we will look at ways of using its principles to engage with scents. Finally, we will explore the role of fragrance in meditative practice, altered states of consciousness and the noetic experience, which takes our appreciation of fragrance to an entirely new level.

Novices and experts

> To the unlearned nose, all odours are alike; but when tutored, either for pleasure or profit, no member of the body is more sensitive. (Piesse 1891, cited in Dalton 1996)

Dalton (1996) made some pertinent observations about skilled perfumers. She noted that individuals who have outstanding ability in other fields, such as athletics, art or music, have been the subject of intense interest: what led to their ability and expertise, how they trained, how they learned to optimise their talent. By contrast, perfumers who display creativity and artistry in the realm of scent have not been subjected to the same scrutiny; indeed, the individuals behind fragrances are rarely acknowledged. Dalton examined the sensory and cognitive aspects of perfumery by comparing 'novices' (nonperfumers) with 'experts' (perfumers), and identified three areas pertinent to developing expertise in odour perception. These are olfactory sensitivity, discrimination and memory.

Sensitivity

When we are born, we have a fully functional olfactory system. This serves us well; however, our culture does not demand that we actively nurture our sense of smell. Therefore most perfumers start out with a perfectly 'normal nose'. Dalton (1996) noted that some perfumers do have an exceptional degree of sensitivity, but then so do many non-perfumers. The difference is that perfumers have experience, which leads them to a higher level of olfactory acuity. Early research had indicated that novices can quickly attain increased olfactory sensitivity simply by repeated exposure to single odorants (Semb 1968, cited in Dalton 1996; Rabin and Cain 1986). In 1996 Dalton and Wysocki conducted a study which involved exposing novices to two odorants, *iso*-bornyl acetate and geraniol, in the context of weekly tests over a six-week period. The odour detection thresholds increased by an average of 256-fold over this period, showing that a dramatic improvement can be achieved simply by repeated exposure, and that the sensitivity differential between novice and perfumer can be very quickly reduced.

There are physiological and genetic factors that can be responsible for variation in the ability to detect and perceive odours. Olfactory sensitivity is diminished by the aging process, and some psychiatric disorders which feature depressive components can also affect olfactory perception. Lombion-Pouthier *et al.* (2006) investigated the effects of some psychiatric disorders on odour perception, and found that, compared with a control group of healthy subjects, depressive patients had poor sensitivity and poor detection abilities, and that they overrated pleasantness of odours; anorectic patients had high sensitivity but overrated odour intensity and underrated pleasantness; and those who had alcohol or drug addictions had impairments in the ability to identify odours. Since the olfactory pathways are directly connected with the limbic system, and mood disorders involve the brain structures that constitute the limbic system, these olfactory variances are probably physiological expressions of the diseases investigated.

Many individuals, including perfumers, also have olfactory 'blind spots'; these are possibly genetically determined. For example, Stansfield (2012) notes that around 50 per cent of adults cannot detect the odour of the hormone androsterone, found in human perspiration, even when it is presented at artificially high levels. Amongst those who can detect it, 15 per cent describe it as smelling like rubbing alcohol. Partial anosmias are not uncommon either; in this case the individual has difficulty in perceiving, or cannot perceive, certain odorants. Calkin and Jellinek (1994) suggest that even a few very skilful perfumers are not able to smell some perfumery materials, such as musks or woody odorants, in their pure form, although they can detect their effects within a composition. For example, Turin (2006) discusses the widely used (and now restricted) ester, benzyl salicylate, which has a very weak, sweet, floral-balsamic smell; some perfumers cannot detect it at all, but can immediately recognise its presence in a formula, where it has the ability to enhance the richness and depth of floral compositions. However, a perfumer's skills extend beyond olfactory sensitivity, and the next distinguishing factor between novice and expert is discriminatory ability.

Discrimination

Laska and Ringh (2010) identify two commonly agreed measures of olfactory sensitivity. One is the *detection threshold*, which they define as 'the lowest concentration at which an odorant can be detected or discriminated from a blank stimulus'. The other is the *recognition threshold* or 'the lowest concentration at which an odorant can be assigned a recognisable quality, or can be discriminated from another odorant' (p.806). The detection threshold is lower than the recognition threshold. However, Laska and Ringh took a different approach to establishing the gap between detection and recognition; they used a performance-based measure rather than verbal labelling, thus avoiding semantic ambiguity. Their 2010 study, which used a series of aliphatic aldehydes, found that at the group level, there was a factor of 100 times separating the ability of the best and the worst, but some individuals within the group could discriminate between aldehyde pairs presented at a factor of three above detection level. This shows a considerable variation in ability.

One of the biggest differences between novices and experts is the ability to discriminate between odorants in a mixture, as evidenced in another study conducted by Livermore and Laing (1996). When asked to identify some of the components of various mixtures which contained between two and six odorants, untrained participants performed very poorly in comparison with perfumers. Even with prior exposure to some of the components, they were only able to identify the components of a binary mixture 12 per cent of the time.

There is also the ability to verbally label odour perceptions. This, too, can be learned; further studies of longer-term adaptation to odours have revealed that repeated exposure to single odorants, in conjunction with standard odour descriptors and qualities, enhances the individual's ability to verbalise their sensory perceptions (Dalton and Wysocki 1996). Contemporary research has suggested exactly the same. Barkat *et al.* (2012) commented that the olfactory system needs to process complex stimuli all of the time since, in natural conditions, odours come from mixtures of odorants, so our olfactory receptors must interact with neural processing of the signals. However, because of the complexity of natural odours, competition may occur at the level of the receptors and there may be inhibitory interactions at the neural level. Their perspective suggests that the perception of a mixture is not as the sum of its components. There are two ways of looking at this. First, in, for example, a binary mixture, each component might be distinct and identifiable, and the processing can be described as dissociative, analytical or elemental. Second, the mixture might be perceived as a distinct entity, with a quality that neither of its components possesses; this perception is called associative, synthetic or configurable processing, and it may be weak or strong, depending on the constituents. Barkat *et al.* suggest that in humans, when just two components are involved, there is little evidence to support the latter, but with more than four components, new odour sensations can indeed be produced. This of course can be witnessed in perfumery. Burr (2007) relates an interview with the perfumer Jean-Claude Ellena, who is skilled at creating an olfactory impression with comparatively few ingredients. During this interview Ellena demonstrated that if *iso*-butyl phenylacetate (sweet, synthetic-chamomile-like) was combined with ethyl vanillin (gourmand vanilla), the combination smells like chocolate, which itself contains around 800 molecules; and the same ethyl vanillin, combined with cinnamon, orange and lime essences, can give a realistic impression of Coca Cola.

It is believed that binary mixtures can stimulate cortical neurons that are not stimulated by the individual odorants, and one of the difficulties inherent in investigating this is the human difficulty in conveying the perception of odour quality (Barkat *et al.* 2012). However, this too is something that needs to be learnt, and the only way to do it is to practise. By doing this, a cognitive aspect joins the sensory processing, and odour memory is developed.

Implicit and semantic olfactory memory

Dalton (1996) suggested that olfactory expertise appeared to be characterised by differences in the way odour memory is stored and organised, and in the way this information is evaluated and applied. Perfumers therefore need to train their cognitive processes, which give the associations between the sensory impact of an odour and the ability to recognise it, label it and then compose with it. This ability is described by Barkat *et al.* (2012) as requiring both a perceptual and a semantic knowledge of odours.

In 1999 Degel and Köster investigated the influence of odours on human performance and implicitly learned odour memories. (Their findings regarding lavender and jasmine were discussed in Chapter 2.) During the course of this study they demonstrated the existence of implicit odour memory. Odours are expected in some situations, such as kitchens and train lavatories, more than others; but if a subject is unknowingly exposed to an odour, they will later connect this odour to the place where they had prior experience of it – even if they remain unaware that there was an odour in the place where they were tested. The biggest surprise was that implicit memory only works in subjects who do not know the odour well enough to be able to name it. Degel and Köster ask: does the presence of a name in the verbal memory block the build-up of new episodic memories, or does it block retrieval of the odour from the implicit memory? They also suggest that, once an odour has entered the semantic memory, this takes over and inhibits episodic memory, to prevent subsequent interference. This could explain why proactive interference (the restriction of new learning by prior learning), is so strong in olfactory memory. This study also revealed another 'accidental' finding, which was at odds with conventional understanding: the non-identifiers had a better *implicit* olfactory memory than those who could identify the odours. Generally it is thought that knowing the correct name for an odour has a positive effect in odour recognition tests, and so this must be due to *semantic* memory, not implicit odour memory. Köster *et al.* (2002) conducted a further study on implicit odour memory, which suggested that both proactive and retroactive interference (the latter being the reduction of prior memory by new learning) do occur in the pre-semantic, episodic memory, where odours are linked to the context or environment in which they are first encountered, even without knowledge.

Valentin, Dacremont and Cayeux (2011) investigated whether sensory training could improve short-term olfactory memory as well as improve long-term semantic odour memory. The participants in this study were experts (perfumers and flavourists), trained panellists and novices. They were asked to study three sets, each with three, six and 12 odours, of both a) common and unusual perfumery and b) flavour raw materials, with encoding instructions. As expected, the experts had superior recognition performance, but the magnitude of the effect of expertise was modified by the type and number of odours. For example, in the case of common odours, the experts' performance was significantly better for the large set of 12. The effect of expertise was also significant for all three sets of uncommon odours. Valentin *et al.* concluded that experts develop a better olfactory short-term memory than novices, because of their training. They also suggested that odours are represented both perceptually and verbally in short-term working memory. So indeed the belief that in order to become an expert, motivation, perseverance and deliberate practice are required, appears to be sound.

Dalton (1996) suggested that experts also use a strategy known as 'chunking'. For example, we can memorise telephone numbers more easily if we break them into short sequences – and the same technique can work with odour memory. A perfumer can look at a list of ingredients, and rather than see a long list, will recognise accords that give specific effects.

Jean Carles recognised the huge reliance that perfumers place on cognitive skills when he said that the most important attribute in a perfumer is a good olfactory memory. Perfumers create fragrances from the memory of odours, so composition is a cognitive process. This is why Carles could still work as a perfumer after his sense of smell declined. The development of creative expertise is reckoned to take ten years of creative activity, over and above the preparation that leads to this stage – as evidenced in other disciplines, from chess to art and music (Dalton 1996).

Talking the talk and walking the walk

In Chapter 6 the concept of odour vocabulary was introduced. This is considered vital for the aroma-profiling of single aromachemicals, 'naturals' composed of perhaps hundreds of constituents, and perfume compositions; in other words, it allows for the description of single components and complex compositions using a common language. The ability to verbalise is also a clearly important distinction between novices and experts. It is also important if there is a desire to engage more fully with the olfactory sense and reap the benefits.

A rich language that needs to be learned in context

Odour descriptions are complex, and the way in which odour vocabulary is used by untrained individuals can be very variable. For example, Mensing and Beck (1988) and Donna (2009) commented that the 'fresh' dimension was often misinterpreted; this might be because, for example, some citrus fragrances or oils have a trigeminal component that is associated with energetic, 'fresh' or clean feelings; or perhaps their overuse in products related to energetic activities or cleaning has influenced interpretation (Porcherot *et al.* 2010).

It is also often said that untrained individuals have difficulty in describing odours because of a deficiency in their olfactory vocabulary. There is sometimes also the 'tip of the nose' moment: 'I do know this smell but I cannot find the words for it right now!'

Manetta *et al.* (2011) suggest that verbal representation of fragrances can be achieved through the use of metaphor and analogy, and that it also depends on the conditions under which individuals are asked to describe fragrances. In their 2011 study they investigated the olfactory lexicon, and they also varied the context, so that participants were asked to describe fragrances in a triadic task and a sorting task. They found that a high percentage of the frequently quoted words were common to both tasks, and that the descriptions of fragrance were 'numerous and rich'; they collected around 50,000 words. It is interesting that this methodology provided a context for odour description, a factor that is absent in many other studies.

The odour perception space

In 2009 Zarzo and Stanton examined the 'odour perception space' and the 'odour descriptor space' – the perceptual and sensory maps for odour description – with the intention of identifying their underlying dimensions and working towards the development of a 'standard' sensory map of perfumery odour descriptors. Following analysis of two databases of odorants using a statistical method known as principal components analysis (PCA), they looked at a wide range of schemes for classifying odours, including Jellinek's Odour Effects Diagram (1951), Harder's 'Discodor' (1979), Tisserand's mood cycle (1988), Thibaud's semantic odour profiles (1991), the Aftelier Natural Perfume Wheel (2006) and the Edwards Fragrance Wheel (2008). These were then compared with the PCA results. A high level of consistency was found, and modifications to these schemes were suggested to improve it further. It would seem that the correlations between Jellinek's and Edwards' schemes, when compared with the databases, were remarkable, and because the 'Fragrance Wheel' is so comprehensive and current, if modifications are made we might be closer to having a standard sensory map. However, debate continues over some details, such as reference materials for odours. For example, galbanum resinoid and patchouli were the materials most often selected for 'green' and 'earthy' respectively, but they have also been assigned to 'tart' (dry) and 'dusty' respectively. The metallic note is another area where there is discord. This has been associated with both geranium and bay, which was selected as the reference material, even although the metallic note is very minor in bay. So, because of our inability to quantify or qualify smells with unbiased instruments, and our reliance on our noses and words – which can be biased because of our humanity, our gender, our physiology, our culture and our experiences – these minor discrepancies will probably stay with us. However, Zarzo and Stanton indicated that there is a general consensus of opinion regarding fragrance classification and description, and they have made an enormous contribution to the odour descriptor space.

Cultivation of the sense of smell

The more we penetrate odours, the more they end up possessing us. They live within us, becoming an integral part of us, participating in a new function within us. (Roudnitska 1991, cited in Aftel 2008, p.44)

What is of interest here is how to cultivate the olfactory sense for pleasure and wellbeing. There are many ways in which we can approach this; simple daily awareness is a starting point. It is thought that by actively using the sense of smell, even when it is in decline due to advancing years, connections can be made between the receptors and neural circuits, and olfaction can be stimulated. Actively smelling materials that are pleasant, several times a day, is enough to stimulate the receptors (Byron 2013). In addition, we can adapt the novice perfumer's path, and systematically work with the odours of essential oils and absolutes – see Appendix D for a guide. With regular practice the ability to detect, discriminate and describe odours develops. The process of olfactory learning is inherently enjoyable and rewarding, and in itself can contribute to feelings of wellbeing. However, there are additional benefits, one of which is revealed by *koh-do*.

Koh-do

The Japanese art of *koh-do* can give us an indication not only of the pleasure of heightened olfactory awareness, but also of what is happening at the biological level. The historical origins of *koh-do*, a traditional art of incense appreciation, were introduced in Chapter 3 (see page 80). In the *koh-do* ceremony the participants 'listen' to *koh-boku* (incense). They discriminate and appreciate the differences in the fragrances of six kinds of incense, using a shared palette of descriptors. Japanese incense is traditionally based on agarwood; as we have seen, there will be variations in its quality and scent. There are six types – *kyara*; *sumatra* or *sumotara*; *sasora*;

rakoku; managa or *manaka;* and *manaban* – but the incense is not named either after these or for its appearance, but according to the images described by the symbolic characteristics inspired by the fragrances (Fujii *et al.* 2007). Morita (1992) noted the descriptions given by Ashikaga Yoshimasa in sixteenth-century Japan. *Kyara* he described as gentle and dignified, with a touch of bitterness, and compared the fragrance to an aristocrat in its elegance and gracefulness. In contrast, he described *sumotara* as sour at the beginning and the end, saying that it was sometimes easily mistaken for *kyara*, but that it had something distasteful and ill-bred about it, like a servant disguised as a noble person. From this we can get an idea of the elaborate use of analogy, and also the writer's ideas about social organisation!

Incense discrimination is not like discriminating between, for example, rose and jasmine absolutes; it is more like discriminating between different species of rose and their geographical origins – and this despite the fact that the intensity of the incense fragrance is very low compared to that of an absolute or essential oil.

Fujii *et al.* explain how incense is described using five symbolic axes: sweetness, bitterness, sourness, hotness and saltiness – words that normally describe taste sensations. Each of these axes has a combination of several characteristics specific to incense, and a quantitative element is also applied, so that the *koh-do* master (expert) who has mastered these axes can describe the sensation in terms of a five-dimensional symbolic space, having learned to 'form and manipulate abstract images from complex olfactory stimuli'.[1] In *koh-do* this knowledge is shared and compared. The reasoning process is one of the highest cognitive functions and takes place in in the prefrontal cortex (PFC) of the brain. Using near infrared spectroscopy, Fujii *et al.* (2007) examined the prefrontal activity of masters and beginners during an incense discrimination task. They found that with the masters, in the early listening phase, the first inhalation provided names and stimulus images to the left and right PFC. This is the phase where the first impression is formed. During the discrimination phase, the PFC shapes and sorts the stimulus images that have been pre-processed, and sends a query to the knowledge base by name or image. The response is then received, and the result compared with the image being generated by the incense stimulus. This final processing takes place by communication between the left PFC, which retrieves the name, and the right PFC, which is concerned with the shape of the image, until the best conclusion is reached. This is an example of abductive reasoning, where a conclusion is drawn from multiple premises. Beginners appeared to have more difficulty reasoning about the olfactory stimulus, and did not show dynamic, organised PFC patterns. This might be because they did not have a pre-learned *koh-boku* knowledge base, or perhaps because, although they could create

---

1   The five dimensions are arranged around the circumference of a circle. Depending on the strength of each characteristic, a dot can be made on a line between the characteristic and the centre of the circle. The position of the dot can be near the centre (weak presence) or near the circumference (strong). The shape that results from joining the dots will give a sort of 'starburst' effect, a pattern that represents the olfactory characteristics. This technique is also used in organoleptic analysis of foods and drinks.

internal images, they could not represent these images in the symbolic space. In other words, they had not learned to manipulate abstract concepts.

Kumikoh shows another way of appreciating incense, this time in a literary context. The 'composer' gives a title which reflects something inspirational, such as a sunset, an image given by a story, or a literary piece such as a *waka*, a Japanese poetic form. Then the 'master of the incense ceremony' will select a range of incenses, so that the sunset or the poem can be played out in the realm of fragrance. This way of appreciating fragrance can be practised by novices and experts, but *kumikoh* must be conducted by someone skilled in the management of incense burning and knowledgeable about the rules of etiquette too, and the participants must first be able to identify the characteristics of the six incense types. The records of *kumikoh* are maintained on sheets of rice paper using calligraphy, and sometimes participants will compose a poem. The correct identities and correspondences and the short story or poem are shared at the end, so that the participants can gauge their performance and progress (Morita 1992).

Fujii *et al.* (2007) showed that masters of *koh-do* had achieved the highest levels of cognitive processing that are possible. When the expert in perfumery is compared with the *koh-do* and *kumikoh* master, we can see many parallels, especially in terms of discrimination, olfactory memory and creativity. It is suggested, therefore, that an expert perfumer is also capable of the highest level of cognitive processing – abductive reasoning – and that taking steps to cultivate our olfactory palate will also improve our cognitive functioning.

Koh-do is a social activity, and fragrance appreciation is also something that can be shared, either in person, in books or online. Once the journey has started, a new world opens up on entering the world of fragrance literature. Discussion about scent will reflect its multisensorial aspects, and can also explore its significance beyond the senses.

Transcendence – fragrance beyond the sensorial realm

In 1982 Arthur Deikman noted that meditation was 'the best known technique of mystical science'. Very broadly speaking, there are two types of meditation – concentration and mindfulness. The *concentration* technique is derived from yoga, where the focus might be an object such as a candle flame, or sound and words, as with a mantra. *Mindfulness* (or insight) meditation is a Buddhist practice, and, in contrast, aims to allow unbroken, detached attentiveness to any thoughts and sensations that may arise – whatever enters our consciousness. It is a much more dynamic process. However, both types of meditation ultimately allow us to detach ourselves from the transient realm of the mind and the emotions. Then we can leave behind any analytical thoughts, or problem-solving activity, or the need for emotional and sensory stimulus, and enter a mode of awareness and allowing, or receptivity. The ultimate goal of meditative practice, as practised in yoga and Buddhism, is to reach a state of pure awareness that is known as *Nirvana*, enlightenment or truth.

Although fragrance is often used to accompany meditative practices, it can also be the focus of meditation. Lawless (2010a) compared the experience of smelling with 'awareness and enquiry' with the 'just sitting' method of meditation. He explained that this method is a practice of body awareness; it is known as *shikantaza* and is attributed to the Zen master Dogen. In order to still the mind, awareness is deliberately shifted to the body, which is always present, unlike our thoughts, and, with practice, mind and body become harmonised.

Reflective awareness, meditative trance and transcendence

When we fully engage with a fragrance, we first enter a state of *reflective awareness*. This is inherent within cognitive processes and allows an individual to maintain a degree of ordered thinking. But what happens when a trance state is entered?

Trance is an altered state of consciousness. In Chapter 2 Wolinski's concepts of trance states and therapeutic trance were introduced. Glicksohn and Berkovich Ohana (2011) note that there are many different concepts of trance, and different routes to entering a trance state, such as *hypnosis*, or *concentrative* or *mindfulness* meditation. Rapaport (1951, 1967, cited in Glicksohn and Berkovich Ohana 2011) had suggested that reflective awareness plays an important role in both cognition and consciousness, and Glicksohn and Berkovich Ohana explain that, in a trance state, reflective awareness is restricted or even absent. For example, if a trance state is reached by hypnosis, reflective awareness is absent.

Concentrative meditation is different. If there is intense focus on an object, the background is less important and can fade from awareness; this means that the object becomes de-contextualised. This is called the 'figure–ground' distinction (Glicksohn 1998). Focusing on a perceptual experience is at the heart of many meditative practices, and scent meditation would fall into this category. As the meditation progresses, detachment from language and thought follows, reflective awareness becomes restricted, and 'trance logic', a different, perhaps more primitive type of thinking, emerges. The individual is no longer bound by reasoning, distinctions between cause and effect may vanish, and opposites can co-exist (Ludwig 1967, cited in Glicksohn and Berkovich Ohana 2011). A meditator might experience 'vivid imagery, inward absorbed attention, positive affect, decreased self-awareness, and increased alterations in the state of consciousness and varied aspects of the subjective experience' – all suggesting a high level of trait absorption (Pekala, Wenger and Levine 1985, cited in Glicksohn and Berkovich Ohana 2011, p.54).

In concentrative meditation, it is recognised that a series of states of consciousness emerges from the trance state. Practitioners of this method can progress to the practice of *mindfulness* meditation. There are distinctions between the two methods. In mindfulness meditation, the figure-ground balance is dynamic, and rather than restricted reflective awareness, there are multiple layers of reflective awareness.

Unlike concentrative meditation, there are no defined stages in terms of states of consciousness, and 'after many years of practice, there is a sudden and dramatic reorganisation of cognition' (Glicksohn and Berkovich Ohana 2011, p.54). Advanced practitioners can be aware of spontaneous changes in consciousness, transcendent experiences, showing reflective awareness during the meditation.

Glicksohn and Berkovich Ohana (2011) investigated the incidence of transcendence during meditation amongst a group of experienced meditators. Using electroencephalograms (EEG), they were able to demonstrate a particular pattern of cortical activity in the brain that accompanied the transition from trance to transcendence. This was characterised by the balance of alpha–theta activity along the anterior posterior axis. They suggest that there is a shift from absence of reflective awareness in trance, to multiplicity of reflective awareness in transcendence.

Meditation can also induce synaesthesia (Glicksohn and Berkovich Ohana 2011); this word is derived from the Greek *syn* (union) and *aesthesis* (sensation). From the biological perspective, synaesthesia is a neurological condition where two or more of the senses are interconnected in the mind (Stansfield 2012). For example, sounds or words or smells can be perceived also as colours, and smells can be perceptually linked with colours, sounds and words. Odour has many established cross-modal associations, and if scent is used as the perceptual experience, perhaps there will be much greater opportunity for synaesthetic experiences. Fragrance has accompanied meditative practices for millennia; is this perhaps because of scent's inherent ability to induce synaesthesia? Scent with meditation, or concentrative meditation with scent, might just promote more vivid and spontaneous imagery, sounds, music and tactile sensations than mediation without scent. It is possible that in some spiritual practices, scent-induced synaesthesia manifests as fragrant visions or presences. It is also possible that scent and meditation can facilitate a 'bifurcation of being', a metaphysical state where we exist simultaneously in two spaces at once – such as in shamanic trance, or entering a fully immersive virtual-reality environment…where the possibilities are endless (Morie 2008).

Noetic insight

Hewitt (2011) explains that 'noetic insight involves direct access to knowledge beyond that which is available through the five senses or through reason' (p.177). Typically, the 'feeling of knowing' can manifest as sudden insight, sudden creativity, the 'eureka effect'[2] or the 'Aha!' moment, and there is a usually a strong element of sensing the interconnectedness of all things. It is embedded in the unconscious mind, and the stronger the association with the conscious mind, the more 'right' it

---

2   'Eureka!' was the exclamation uttered by ancient Greek mathematician and engineer Archimedes (287–212 BCE) when he had a sudden insight about the displacement of bath water; it is said that he leapt out of the bath and ran naked through the streets, such was his desire to share his discovery. The 'eureka effect' is therefore the sudden and unexpected resolution to a question.

feels. Noetic insights can be experienced in altered states of consciousness, such as in meditation, shamanism and the use of hallucinogens.

It is thought that psychedelic drugs such as LSD alter the functioning of neurotransmitters and reduce activity in the prefrontal cortex where higher cognitive functions occur, whilst stimulating the limbic system. This may produce altered states of consciousness (ASCs), but these will be experienced and interpreted within their cultural context. 'Typical' effects include changes in sensory perception, changes in temporal perception, changes in body image, vivid images, heightened awareness of colour, abrupt mood changes, enhanced memory, ego dissolution, a sense that telepathic communication is possible, empathy, concern with philosophical, cosmological and religious questions, and an apprehension of the world being experienced (Masters and Houston 1966, cited in Hewitt 2011, p.180). There are also frequent 'Aha!' moments and epiphanies; the psychedelic experience is filled with mystical or religious meaning for 35–50 per cent of users.

However, with the exception of the flash-insights of those considered to be geniuses, intuition was until very recently regarded with great suspicion by both the scientific and mainstream religious communities, because the phenomenon could not be measured or verified. Hewitt points out that since the 1970s this has changed; knowledge of neurotransmitters and the advent of the EEG, along with magnetoencephalography (MEG), neuroelectric and neuromagnetic source imaging and positron emission topography (PET), have elucidated the working of the brain and produced a revolution in the cognitive sciences. She tells us that some, such as geneticist Dean Harmer, have proposed that a specific form of the VMAT2 gene (the 'God gene') predisposes an individual to spiritual experiences, while others, such as Michael Persinger, demonstrated that magnetic fields delivered via a 'God helmet' can induce perception of a 'presence'. Those cases of epilepsy where altered sensory perceptions precede a seizure and synaesthesia also include elements of noetic insight.

Synaesthesia is not noted as a dysfunction but, like psychedelic experiences, it is linked to biochemical and neural processes. It may even be linked to the evolution of human consciousness, including the development of language and metaphor. Hewitt (2011) cites Hunt (2005), who suggested that synaesthesia may be linked to the human capacity to use symbols. Hewitt suggests that synaesthesia might be 'a core element of noetic experiences' linking 'core sensory experiences and cross-modal perceptions with a sense of knowing' (pp.190–191), and that a biopsychosociological model offers the best way of understanding noetic insight.

This, then, must include the contribution that quantum physics can make. Radin (2006, cited in Hewitt 2011) posed the question: can one mind influence another? Certain particles can exist simultaneously in many states, there is a non-local connection between them, and only when they are observed or measured do they become real. So if there is a quantum 'fabric' or 'matrix' in which all elements, including human consciousness, are connected, then these 'entangled minds' (Radin 2006, cited in Hewitt 2011) may be related to our noetic experiences. Hewitt likens this to a 'cultural psyche', which is reminiscent of Jung's notion of the 'collective unconsciousness'. She suggests that this 'feeling of knowing' may be a sensory ability.

It is clear that the olfactory sense, with its rich cross-modal associations, is entangled in ASCs and the noetic experience. Moeran (2009) notes the observations of Douglas (1975) who suggested that smells were 'matter out of place' and therefore formless and able to cross boundaries, and also Turner (1969) who wrote that smells were 'neither here nor there…betwixt and between' (p.440). Scents have long been linked with the sacred, the divine, transition and transcendence. This can be seen in the hymns of the theologian known as St Ephrem the Syrian (306–373 CE), which abound with eloquent olfactory metaphors, and indeed imply that scent itself is the means to spiritual experience. For example, Harvey (1998) quotes lines from Ephrem's 'Hymns on Paradise', where paradise is described as 'that treasure of perfumes' and 'that storehouse of scents' (p.122). She suggests that, to Ephrem, the fragrance of Paradise was life-giving: '…for its scent gives nourishment to all at all times, and whoever inhales it is overjoyed and forgets his earthly bread; this is the table of the Kingdom' (p.122). Ephrem frequently referred to 'The Fragrance of Life', a non-cognitive yet revelatory knowledge of divine being, and the revelation occurs 'from within and without: as the divine is mingled with the senses, the senses can perceive the divine in the world they experience' (Harvey 1998, p.110).

Final thoughts

The exploration of the world of plant aromatics, and indeed perfumery, can open up a new internal landscape – there are just so many scents to discover and experience. Fragrance belongs to a vibrant invisible dimension that will impact on how we feel, think and behave. It can be a messenger and a guide. We have looked at fragrance from many different perspectives, from its earliest uses to the present day, from the biological to the quantum, and this has shown us the extent and depth of its influence on individuals and societies; fragrance and wellbeing are inextricably linked.

According to Morita (1992), a sixteenth-century Zen priest suggested that incense holds ten 'virtues'. These virtues could also attributed to fragrance, and they are presented below.

- It brings communication with the transcendent.

- It purifies the mind and body.

- It removes uncleanliness.

- It keeps one alert.

- It can be a companion in the midst of solitude.

- In the midst of busy affairs, it brings a moment of peace.

- When it is plentiful, one never tires of it.

- When there is little, still one is satisfied.

- Age does not change its efficacy.

- Used every day, it does no harm.

(Morita 1992, p.104)

Examples of each of these virtues can be found throughout this exploration of plant aromatics and the psyche. In Chapter 2 (on page 42) we asked if we could define wellbeing as a state of being where we are 'calm but alert, perhaps feeling a sense of wonder, or being engaged in a creative activity, or observing and immersing the self in beauty and connecting with the natural world, centred in awareness rather than mental activity, and, most importantly, being completely and utterly in the moment'. It is now very clear that, if this is accepted as a reasonable definition, then fragrance can certainly help us experience a state of wellbeing. This can be enjoyed by simply taking the time to actively use our sense of smell, with awareness and respect, and always remembering to pause, reflect and appreciate the beautiful scents that surround us in the natural world.

Fragrance helps us be in 'the moment', and experience the health of 'the ordinary mind'; it can be part of our *dharma*. So, even if we take only small steps to cultivate our appreciation of fragrance, our lives will surely be enriched.

Glossary

ABSOLUTE: a highly concentrated aromatic extract of the concrete (see below); obtained by alcoholic extraction.

ACCORD: in perfumery, a combination of aromatics that combine to give a particular fragrance effect.

ACETYLCHOLINE: a molecule which is released at the neuromuscular junction and causes contraction, but it has a wider role as a stimulant of the autonomic nervous system, as a vasodilator and cardiac depressant.

AGRESTIC: an odour that is reminiscent of the countryside.

ALCHEMY: the protoscience that preceded chemistry. Different cultures adopted different goals and approaches, but these were always highly symbolic – for example, the search for the 'philosopher's stone' in the endeavour to turn base metal into precious metal (e.g. lead into gold); or the extraction of the life force (quintessence, or fifth element) from plant material by distillation.

ALIPHATIC: a carbon chain structure. A lower aliphatic aldehyde molecule (for example) has a short carbon chain and an aldehyde functional group (a carbonyl group with a hydrogen atom bonded to the carbon atom of the group).

ALLELES: alternative forms of the same gene.

ALLELOPATHY: a type of competition between plants. Plants must compete with each other in the environment for resources such as light, nutrients, water and space. Many of the secondary metabolites, including some terpenes, can inhibit the growth of other species in the immediate vicinity.

AMBER: a perfume note that is powdery and reminiscent of vanilla.

AMYGDALA: a set of neurons in the medial temporal lobes of the brain where emotions are processed and memories are consolidated. It has a primary role in the formation and storage of memories that are triggered by emotional events, and sends signals via the hypothalamus to activate the sympathetic nervous system. It is also part of the limbic system, which is associated with pleasure, fear and aggressive behaviour.

ANIMALIC: an odour reminiscent of an animal source – musk, castoreum, civet. An example of a plant aromatic with an animalic odour is ambrette seed; this is often used as a botanical musk substitute.

ANTINOCICEPTIVE: reduces sensitivity to painful stimuli.

ANTIPRURITIC: relieves itching.

ANXIOLYTIC: anxiety-relieving.

APOPTOSIS: programmed cell death; a normal physiological process in maintaining homeostasis and tissue development in multicellular organisms.

APOTROPAIC: type of magic intended to ward off evil, to protect against misfortune by means, for example, of good luck charms, talismans, amulets, gargoyles on buildings, carved pumpkins on Hallowe'en, or even crossing the fingers.

AROMA-CHOLOGY: the study of the psychological effects of odours.

AROMATHERAPY: the therapeutic application of essential oils and aromatic plant extracts in a holistic context, to maintain or improve physical, emotional and mental wellbeing.

ATTAR: an ancient Persian and Arabic word, which translates as 'essence' or 'sweet smell'. Attars are alcohol-free, natural fragrances; traditional attars are concentrated aromatic blends, extremely popular in the Indian subcontinent and the Middle East, where they are renowned for their aroma, which is both sensual and spiritual.

BASE: a perfume base is a ready-made composition of perfume materials designed to give a specific effect. Perfume bases can be viewed as building blocks around which a fragrance can be constructed.

BASE NOTE: an odour that persists after the top and middle notes have evaporated; usually given by constituents with low volatility. Also known as the dryout note, or the drydown.

BEESWAX ABSOLUTE: a rich, warm, honey, and hay-like extract of honeycombed beeswax.

BEHEN OIL OR BEN OIL: a cold-pressed oil from the seeds of *Moringa* species – the tropical 'horse radish' or 'drumstick' tree. It has a high content of oleic acid, and is very stable. Theophrastus noted its 'receptiveness for taking in odours'.

BIOSYNTHESIS: the building up of more complex chemical compounds from simpler ones within a cell.

BODHISATTVA: a Sanskrit word meaning a level of spiritual achievement, or an heroic aspirant to enlightenment. In art it refers to a male or female figure with a peaceful, god-like appearance – for example, Maitreya (male) and Sarasvati (female).

BODY NOTE: also known as the middle note, this is the sensory impact of the moderately volatile constituents of an aromatic material or a perfume, with traces of the top notes and the emergence of the base notes becoming apparent; has intermediate lasting power.

CALYX: the cup-like structure, formed by the sepals, that encloses and protects a flower as it develops.

CAMBIUM: a plant tissue that lies between the bark and the wood. One of its main functions is the production of new cells.

CAMPHOR: natural camphor is referred to as *d*-camphor because it is optically active – it will bend a beam of polarised light to the right. (The *d*- stands for *dextro*-rotatory.) Synthetic camphor, or camphor derived from fractional distillation of petroleum, is a fraction of the cost, but it is not optically active. It can also be obtained from pinene, converted to camphene and then treated with acetic acid and nitrobenzene to form camphor.

CARPEL: the structure that bears and encloses the ovules in flowering plants. It is comprised of the ovary, style and stigma.

CASSIS: a term used to denote a blackcurrant fruit aroma or flavour.

CASTOREUM: the beaver has glands under its tail which secrete oil that waterproofs its coat to prevent waterlogging. Castoreum is the dried secretion of these glands; an absolute and tincture is used in perfumery. The tincture has a tenacious, leather-like, phenolic odour that is often used in leather and tabac masculine fragrances.

CEPHALIC: benefits the head and mind; stimulating to the thought processes.

CHARGE: the aromatic material introduced to the extraction vessel.

CHIRAL: a term used to denote that a molecule has two forms. Some isomers have the same molecular formula, but the orientation of the atoms is subtly different. In simple terms, the two forms could be described as 'handed', or are mirror images of each other. Chirality is important in how a molecule will smell, and in its potential biological activity.

CHOLINERGIC: stimulating the production of acetylcholine. This is a molecule which is released at the neuromuscular junction and causes contraction, but it has a wider role as a stimulant of the autonomic nervous system, as a vasodilator and cardiac depressant.

CHYPRE: François Coty created the first modern chypre fragrance in 1917. It is a perfume type containing a base accord of oakmoss, labdanum, sandalwood and musk (and often including patchouli and clary sage), and a floral heart (often rose and jasmine), with a bergamot top note.

CINEOLIC: a eucalyptus-like odour.

CICATRISANT (CICATRISING): promotes healing by formation of scar tissue.

CIS- AND TRANS-ISOMERISM: a type of geometrical isomerism; cis-isomers have groups of similar atoms on one side of a double bond, trans-isomers have the same groups of atoms on the opposite sides of a double bond. Examples are geraniol (cis-) and nerol (trans-).

CIVET: the glandular secretion of the civet, Viverra civetta and other Viverra species (small animals related to the weasel). In its raw form it has a pungent, repellent, faecal odour. A tincture is made from the secretion of the abdominal glands, for use in perfumery; this is sweet and reminiscent of animal fur, and used to impart lift to chypre and delicate floral perfumes. The main constituents are civettone and skatole.

CONCRETE: an aromatic solid or semi-solid extract containing essential oil, waxes and pigments, obtained by solvent extraction of aromatic plant material.

CONTINGENT NEGATIVE VARIATION (CNV): an electrical phenomenon in the human brain, manifesting as an upward shift in brain waves, as seen on the EEG, when the subject is expecting something to happen.

CORYLOPSIS: a Japanese shrub named Corylopsis spicata (related to witch hazel), which bears pendulous racemes of yellow, cowslip-scented flowers. Its scent can be mimicked by a combination of lily, ylang ylang and small amounts of patchouli.

CYCLAMEN ODOUR: from the flowers of an alpine plant of the primula family; a strong jasmine-like scent with a strong undertone of humus under trees in a forest, and elements of lily, violet and hyacinth.

DHARMA: a path or way of living that involves following a set of ideals and philosophies, especially those of the Buddha, and the cultivation of mindfulness and wisdom, which leads to enlightenment or nirvana.

DIFFUSIVE: a characteristic of some fragrance compounds, essential oils and absolutes, where the scent rapidly permeates the atmosphere.

DITTANY OF CRETE: a 'wound herb', also used for disorders of the head and for opening obstructions; valued by ancient cultures, but superseded by sweet marjoram and oregano.

DOSHAS: in Ayurvedic texts, the elements are combined into pairs, giving three *doshas* – *Vata* (Ether and Air), *Pitta* (Fire and Water) and *Kapha* (Water and Earth) (Frawley and Lad 1986). The *doshas* have behavioural, emotional, cognitive and physical/physiological correspondences. Each and every human being, as part of nature, has their own particular mix of the three *doshas* which gives rise to that individual's unique constitution, or *pakriti* (Svoboda 1984).

DROPSY: an old term meaning oedema, the accumulation of fluid in the tissues.

DRYOUT: the odour that remains when an aromatic material is in the very final stages of evaporation.

E- PREFIX: abbreviation of the German *entgegen*, 'opposed to', in relation to the *trans*-isomer.

EMMENAGOGUE: promotes menstruation.

ENFLEURAGE: the process of absorbing the fragrance from fresh flowers of a single species into a purified fatty medium over a period of time, to produce a pomade.

ENTHEOGEN: a psychoactive drug used in a religious, shamanic or spiritual context, for healing, transcendence, revelation, meditation. The word is derived from the ancient Greek *entheos* and *genestai* meaning 'that which causes one to be in god'.

ENZYME: a biochemical catalyst.

EPIPHYTE: a plant which does not have roots in the soil, but lives above the ground, supported by another plant or object. It obtains its nutrients from the air, rainwater and organic debris. Many orchids are epiphytes and the typical habitat is the canopies of tropical rain forests.

ESSENTIAL OIL: a volatile product, obtained by a physical process from a natural source of a single botanical species, which corresponds to that species in name and odour.

ETHNOGRAPHY: a method of enquiry in the exploration of specific human cultural phenomena.

EVAPORATION: the change in physical state from liquid to gas/vapour.

EXPRESSION: a mechanical process of scarification and compression for obtaining the volatile oil from the flavedo of citrus fruits.

EXTRACT: the soluble matter obtained from an aromatic plant by washing with a solvent that is then recovered by vacuum distillation. Extracts include concretes, absolutes and resinoids.

EXTRAIT: the French word for 'extract'. Originally, extrait perfumes were produced by alcoholic extraction of enfleurage pomade. Early extraits were of the floral type, such as rose, jasmine, tuberose, cassie, violet, jonquil, bitter orange blossom and mignonette. The term came to describe strong alcoholic solutions of perfume compound (or essence), and it is currently used to describe the strongest form of alcoholic perfume that is commercially available (between 5–20% of perfume compound in strong ethanol).

EXUDATE: a resinous substance produced by the cambium of some woody plants; aromatic exudates include benzoin, frankincense and myrrh.

FIXATIVE: a perfume ingredient that can prolong the lasting power of the main theme of a fragrance.

FOUGÈRE: literally 'fern', a perfume type, usually containing coumarin (a hay-scented aromachemical) and lavender oil; derived from the scented soap *Fougère Royale* (Houbigant 1882).

FRACTION: in perfumery, refers to a separately collected portion of the distillate. In the distillation process, portions will have different boiling points, and these can be collected in different receivers. This is known as fractional distillation.

GENUS (PLURAL GENERA): the taxonomic category between family and species.

GEOSMIN: an organic chemical – a bicyclic alcohol – responsible for the earthy taste and smell of beets; also the smell in the air after rain has fallen on dry ground.

GLANDS: (essential oil-producing) glandular cells, glandular hairs; a group of one or more cells whose main function is to secrete a plant's volatile oil – for example, glandular trichomes common in the Lamiaceae; vittae or resin canals in the Umbelliferae; secretory cells in flower petals, secretory cavities in the peel of citrus fruits.

GRAPE POMACE: also called grape marc, this is the leftover skins and seeds after pressing. It is used to produce pomace brandy, and beverages such as *grappa* or *zivania*.

GRIFFIN: a mythical creature, considered to be the 'king' of creatures. One of its roles was to guard treasures. In ancient Greece it had the body, tail and hindquarters of a lion, and the head, wings and front feet of an eagle.

HELIOTROPIN: an aromachemical that can be derived from naturals such as pepper oil, or by the oxidation of *iso*-safrole. It is a crystalline solid with a smell reminiscent of cherry pie or almonds; very sweet, floral-narcotic and slightly spicy. It is used in floral perfumes and is a popular modifier.

IMMUNOGLOBULINS: antibodies.

INDIAN ASHOK FLOWER: the fragrant flower of the rainforest tree *Saraca asoca*. It is sacred in the Indian subcontinent, being associated with the *Yakshi* – tree deities – and it is also related to fertility. Kamadeva, a Hindu god of love, is often portrayed holding an ashoka blossom.

IN VIVO **AND** *IN VITRO*: Latin terms used to describe experiments either within the living, or living tissue (*in vivo*), or outside living tissue in a testtube (*in vitro*, literally 'in glass').

ISOMER: one of two or more compounds where the molecular formula is identical but the atoms are arranged differently – for example, α- and β-pinenes are identical apart from the position of a double bond.

JIMSONWEED: the colloquial name for *Datura stramonium*; a corruption of the name of a small town, Jamestown, in Virginia.

KINNI-KINNICK OR KINNIKINNICK: a native Algonquin word for a wild tobacco-based smoking mixture. Sometimes the bearberry plant (*Arcostaphylos uva-ursi*) was smoked, and this too was referred to as kinni-kinnick.

KUNDALINI: the concept of a dormant force that lies coiled at the base of the spine. In yoga, if this is awakened, deep meditation, enlightenment and bliss may be attained.

LIGNOTUBER: a tuber that arises from adventitious roots (i.e. roots that arise from the base of the stem; can be seen in the form of 'suckers') and then becomes woody (lignified).

MAENAD: literally means 'raving one'. The Maenads were originally nymphs who cared for Dionysus, and as he came of age they worshipped him. Thereafter they travelled, usually alone, seeking tribute to Dionysus. If this was withheld, they became frenzied, developed talons, and went on a rampage of destruction; they would leave a trail of chaos, with inhabitants of villages in the grip of sexual frenzy and intoxication, and complete loss of sensibility.

MAY BLOSSOM: hawthorn, *Crataegus oxycantha*, of the Rosaceae family, a common hedge tree of Europe, whose blossoms have a sweet, heady scent. In perfumery, anisic aldehyde is used to recall this odour type.

MAY DAY: 1 May, the Celtic festival of Beltane, similar to the festival of Flora in ancient Roman times; a celebration of spring and fertility.

METOPION: a compounded perfume with therapeutic properties.

METRORRHAGIA: irregular uterine bleeding, particularly between menstrual periods.

MIGNONETTE: the flowers of *Reseda odorata*, indigenous to Egypt and the Mediterranean. The absolute has an odour reminiscent of violet leaves.

MOTOR ACTIVITY OR RESPONSES: responses to a stimulus that produces movement.

MUCOLYTIC: reduces the thickness of mucus in the respiratory tract.

MUSK: the abdominal glands of the male musk deer of the Himalayas, Tibet and North India contain a secretion that can be made into a tincture for use in perfumery – although most of the perfumery musks are now synthetic. The tincture has a radiant, sweet, fresh odour with fruity notes.

NATURAL KILLER CELL: a type of white blood cell that is critical in the immune response.

NMDA RECEPTOR: a glutamate receptor that is involved in synaptic plasticity and memory function; a mechanism for learning and memory. Synaptic plasticity is the ability to change the strength of the connection (synapse) between two neurons, according to the use or disuse of the transmission.

NORADRENALIN OR NOREPINEPHRINE: a hormone and neurotransmitter which has a wide range of effects, including the 'fight or flight' reaction to stressful situations.

OLEO-GUM RESIN: a plant exudate composed of water-soluble gum, resin and volatile oil.

OLEORESIN: a plant exudate consisting of resin and volatile oil.

OLFACTION: the sensory process of detecting smells.

OPTICAL ISOMERISM: where the molecule of one form is the mirror image of the other form – for example, *d*- and *l*-limonenes and *d*- and *l*-carvones. Also known as stereoisomerism.

PERCOLATION: an old method of extracting aromatic plants, based on the principles of diffusion and osmosis. It was similar to maceration, but a quicker process. The plant material was placed in a vertical container, and the solvent (water and alcohol) was added from the top. The solvent would sink to the bottom and was then slowly recycled back to the top. The process was repeated until the solvent had removed the aromatic part of the plant material.

PHENOLIC: pertaining to phenols – molecules characterised by the presence of a benzene ring (AKA aromatic ring) structure with one or more hydroxy groups bonded directly to this. In terms of odour description, phenolic denotes a medicated/disinfectant-like, often powerful odour, that relates to phenols such as thymol and carvacrol (in thyme oil), and is often related to or the tarry/smoky odour type.

PHENYLETHANOL: 2-phenylethyl alcohol, the main commercial alcohol apart from ethyl alcohol, and the most used fragrance in the perfumes and cosmetics industry. It is a minor constituent in narcissus, hyacinth, geranium Bourbon, and Aleppo pine, rose and jasmine flowers; up to 60 per cent in rose absolute. It has a rose-like aroma.

PHYTOCOSMECEUTICAL: in the cosmetic industry, cosmeceuticals are multifunctional topical skin care products that are designed to influence the biological functions of the skin, offer protection, promote health and improve the appearance. A phytocosmeceutical contains plant-derived functional ingredients.

POMADE: a product of the enfleurage process – a fragrance-saturated fat.

PROPHYLACTIC: prevents disease or infection.

PSYCHONAUTICS: a methodology to describe and explain the subjective effects of altered states of consciousness, including meditation and the use of psychoactive drugs; distinct from recreational drug use because of the intent to explore traditional wisdom.

PSYCHOTROPIC: mood-altering.

RACEMIC MIX: a naturally occurring mix of two enantiomers (optical isomers) of a compound – for example, *d*- and *l*-linalool.

RACEMOSE INFLORESCENCE: an inflorescence is a flowering system consisting of more than one flower. A racemose inflorescence is where the individual flowers are formed on individual stalks on the main axis, as in, for example, lupins and broom. A *spike* is a racemose inflorescence on which the flowers are sessile (without stalks) and are borne on an elongated axis. This can be seen in *Lavandula* species.

RECTIFICATION: a process of re-distillation of an essential oil to eliminate unwanted constituents, or to standardise the product.

RESINOID: the product of solvent extraction of an oleo-gum resin or an oleoresin, which contains the odorous constituents.

SALTPETRE: a naturally occurring form (white crystalline) of sodium nitrite.

SAPONINS: bitter tasting glycosides (sugar compounds) formed from a sugar and a non-sugar molecule (an aglycone) in which the aglycone part is a steroidal alcohol. They are soluble in water, and produce foam. Many saponins are toxic to mammals and fish. The steroid hormone diosgen is obtained from saponins in yam (*Dioscorea*) species.

SATYRS: the male companions of Dionysus and associated with Silenus. They typified a free and carefree life, and had goat-like features (a tail, ears and phallus); similar to the Roman faun, portrayed as half man (upper) and half goat (lower).

SCARIFICATION: the process of scraping the surface of citrus fruits to allow mechanical expression of the volatile oil.

SCHIFF BASES: aromachemicals formed when aldehydes are reacted with methyl anthranilate (a nitrogen containing aromatic ester); also known as aldimines.

SECONDARY METABOLITE: in contrast to primary metabolites such as glucose, secondary metabolites are chemicals produced in the plant that are not involved in growth and development, but often in response to stress or injury. Examples of plant secondary metabolites include the terpenes and phenylpropanoids – common volatile oil constituents.

SEDATIVE: relaxing in effect, reducing activity, promoting sleep.

SEMANTICS: from the Greek word *semantikos* ('significant'), the study of meaning, usually applied to language. It focuses on the relationship between signs and symbols and what they stand for, what they represent. In olfaction the semantic mechanism is where an odour acquires a meaning and a label, and thus enters the semantic odour memory.

SENSITISATION REACTION: Contact sensitisation is an allergic reaction to an antigen that manifests as itching and inflammation.

SEROTONERGIC MECHANISM: acting in relation to serotonin.

SEROTONIN: 5-hydroxytriptamine – a monoamine neurotransmitter that contributes to feelings of wellbeing and happiness.

SHAMAN: a practitioner who enters an altered state of consciousness to commune with the spirit world in order to act as a diviner, healer or teacher.

SILLAGE: refers to the scented trail left in the air as its wearer passes by; likened to the 'wake' in the water left by a boat, or the vapour trail of an aeroplane. Some fragrances have this quality more than others.

SOLVENT EXTRACTION: the separation of soluble matter from a natural source of plant material, oleo-gum resin or oleoresin, using a pure, volatile solvent. At the end of the process, the solvent is recovered by vacuum distillation, leaving behind the product containing the odorous portion of the material. The product is a concrete, which can be further treated to produce an absolute or a resinoid, which in some cases may be distilled to produce a volatile oil.

SOMATIC: relating to the body.

SOMMELIER: a knowledgeable and educated wine professional.

SOPORIFIC: induces sleep.

SPADIX: a racemose inflorescence where the flowers are without stalks and borne on a fleshy axis. The spadix is found in the Arum family, where it secretes a sticky, insect-attracting substance, and is usually surrounded by a large bract or spathe. This can be highly coloured and petal-like, adapted to attract pollinating insects. An example is the *Anthurium*.

STAMEN: the male reproductive organ of a flowering plant; differentiated into a narrow stalk called the *filament*, which supports the *anther*. Yellow pollen grains (microspores) are formed in pollen-sacs in the anther.

STEAM DISTILLATION: a process of distillation in which steam, under pressure, is used to heat a charge in a still, and release and vaporise the volatile molecules. The volatile portion is then condensed back into liquid form and collected in a receiver vessel.

STIGMA AND STYLE: the *stigma* is the receptive tip of the carpel, which receives pollen at germination, and on which the pollen grain germinates. The *style* is the sterile part of the carpel between the ovary and the stigma, and it ensures that the stigma is presented in an effective place for pollination.

STYRAX (STORAX): obtained from the tree *Liquidambar orientalis*; a gum with a sweet balsamic scent that exudes from the heartwood if the bark is injured.

SUBTLE BODY: in Sufism the 'most sacred body', in Taoism the 'diamond body', and in Tibetan Buddhism the 'light' or 'rainbow body'. This is a concept that beyond the physical body, there are layers that represent subtle planes of existence. *Prana* refers to the subtle energy that moves through energy channels (*nadis*), and psychic centres (*chakras*) of the subtle body.

SYMPATHETIC MAGIC: a type of magic based on imitation or correspondence. The 'Law of Similarity' is that 'like produces like' and the 'Law of Contact' suggests that 'an effect resembles its cause'.

SYMPATHETIC AND PARASYMPATHETIC NERVOUS SYSTEMS: two of the three branches of the autonomic nervous system. The sympathetic system controls the internal organs, and the parasympathetic system controls the rest and relaxation responses.

TA'IF: a region on the Hijaz plateau in the Sarawat Mountains of Saudi Arabia, renowned for growing grapes and roses, and also for honey.

TANTRIC YOGA: a practice that aims to expand awareness in all states of consciousness and create inner peace, harmony and order, through mantras, poses, sense withdrawal, breath regulation, mental concentration and meditation. Tantra was a style of religious ritual and meditation that emerged around the fifth century CE and embraces the concept that the universe is a manifestation of divine energy.

TAXA: plural of taxon; a rank in biological classification.

TERPENOID: a term used to denote a molecule based on the isoprene unit (a five-carbon structure). A monoterpenoid has ten carbon atoms, and a sesquiterpenoid has 15.

THIRD EYE: the inner eye which allows perception beyond normal sight. It is located at the *ajna* or brow chakra (between the eyebrows).

TINCTURE: in perfumery, an alcoholic extract of aromatic material prepared by maceration. Tinctures of ambergris, castoreum, civet and musk were widely used in early perfumery.

TOP NOTE: the initial sensory impact of an aromatic material or perfume, dominated by the most volatile constituents and some of the moderately volatile constituents; has short lasting power.

TRAIT ABSORPTION: a personality trait where there is a predisposition to become deeply immersed in sensory or mystical experiences, or altered states of consciousness. A person who is open to experience, open to hypnotic suggestion, and has imagination and the ability for dissociation will have a high trait absorption score.

TRANSMIGRATION OF THE SOUL: reincarnation from human into human, or human into animal or plant life. A pure life would lead to reincarnation into a higher form in the next life.

TRANSMUTATION OF THE SOUL: in terms of reincarnation, signifies a change from a lower to a higher form, for example from animalic to angelic.

TRIGEMINAL: the trigeminal nerve is the fifth cranial nerve, with three branches (ophthalmic, maxillary and mandibular), and is the principal sensory nerve of the face. The trigeminal component of olfaction is the sensation of hot, cold, tingling or irritation; for example, the smell of menthol is perceived as 'cooling'.

TRIMURTI (HINDU): a composite image of Brahma the creator, Shiva the destroyer and Vishnu the regenerator.

TRYPTAMINES: these are biochemicals such as the monoamine alkaloids – for example, psilocybin in plants and fungi, but also in the brain, where they function as neurotransmitters. Serotonin (feelings of wellbeing) and melatonin (the sleep–wake cycle) are in the class of tryptamines.

UMBEL: a flower-head composed of a number of small flowers, all of which are borne on short stalks arising from a single point at the tip of the main stem – as in, for example, the African lily and some members of the Allium family (not to mention the family Umbelliferae).

VACUUM DISTILLATION: fractional distillation under a vacuum, which reduces the temperature required for the charge to reach boiling point; this eliminates thermal stress.

VACUUM STRIPPING: evaporation of the product of solvent extraction in a vacuum, to remove traces of solvent that remain in the product.

VAPOUR: a gas, under specific conditions where a slight increase of pressure, or decrease in temperature, will result in condensation into the liquid phase.

VETIVONE: α- and β- vetivones are chemicals belonging to the family of sesquiterpenoids. They are named after the aromatic plant in which they are important constituents – *Vetiveria zizanoides*, a grass whose tough, fibrous roots yield the essential oil of vetiver.

VOLATILE: descriptive of a substance which evaporates when exposed to air. The term also applies to the low boiling point constituents of natural aromatic materials – for example, plant volatile oils.

VOLATILITY: the rate at which a substance evaporates. The concept of volatility has led to the classification of essential oils and aromatic extracts as top, middle and base notes.

WATER DISTILLATION: a distillation process suitable for a limited range of aromatic materials, where boiling water is in direct contact with the charge in the still.

Z- PREFIX: abbreviation of the German *zusammen*, 'together', and referring to the *cis*-form of a pair of isomers.

Classification of Fragrance

Fragrance family	Typical examples, houses, launch dates and composers	Some key notes or accords that contribute to main characteristics
Floral (mostly 'feminine')		
Floral green	*Chanel No.19* (Chanel 1970, Henry Robert)	Galbanum and hyacinth, rose, orris.
	Grand Amour (Annick Goutal 1996, composer unknown)	Green notes, hyacinth, lily, honeysuckle, rose, jasmine, amber, vanilla.
	Envy (Gucci 1997, Maurice Roucel)	Green apple, hyacinth, lily of the valley, jasmine, violet, woods.
Floral fruity	*Calyx* (Prescriptives 1987, Sophia Grojsman)	Peach, apricot, guava, tagetes, lily of the valley, lily, jasmine, raspberry.
	Jaïpur (Boucheron 1994, Sophia Grojsman)	Apricot, plum, rose.
	Petite Chérie (Annick Goutal 1998, composer unknown)	Pear, peach, rose, coumarin, vanilla.
	Sira des Indes (Patou 2006, Jean-Michel Duriez)	Fruity (pear, banana), champaca, vanilla.
Floral fresh	*Diorissimo* (Dior 1956, Edmond Roudnitska)	Lily of the valley, boronia, jasmine, sandalwood, civet.
	Escada (Escada 1990, composer unknown)	Bergamot, galbanum, hyacinth, peach, jasmine, tuberose, narcissus, cedar, amber, sandalwood, vanilla.
	Parfum d'Été (Kenzo 1993, Christian Mathieu and Jean-Claude Deville)	Green note, hyacinth, lily of the valley, sandalwood, cedarwood, musk.

Floral	*Joy* (Jean Patou 1935, Henri Alméras)	Rose and jasmine, ylang, tuberose.
	Fidji (Guy Laroche 1966, Josephine Catapano)	Carnation and orris, spices, sandalwood, patchouli.
	Paris (Yves Saint Laurent 1983, Sophia Grojsman)	Violet and rose, orange blossom.
	Carnal Flower (Frédéric Malle 2005, Dominique Ropion)	Tuberose, jasmine, orange blossom.
	Iris Silver Mist (Serge Lutens, 1994, Maurice Roucel)	Orris root.
Floral aldehydic	*Chanel No. 5* (Chanel 1921, Ernest Beaux)	Aldehydes, citrus, jasmine, rose, lily of the valley, orris, ylang.
	Chamade (Guerlain 1969, Jean Paul Guerlain)	Galbanum, hyacinth, blackcurrant bud, lilac, jasmine, ylang, rose.
	Rive Gauche (Yves Saint Laurent 1971, composer unknown)	Aldehydes, rose, jasmine.
	White Linen (Lauder 1978, Sophia Grojsman)	Aldehydes, rose, lily of the valley, jasmine, ylang.
Floral sweet	*Après l'Ondée* (Guerlain 1905, Jacques Guerlain)	Violet, anise, carnation, hawthorn, ylang, orris, vanilla, benzoin, styrax, heliotrope.
	L'Heure Bleue (Guerlain 1912, Jacques Guerlain)	Neroli, clove, rose, ylang, carnation, orris, vanilla, benzoin.
	Poison (Dior 1985, Jean Guichard)	Rose, tuberose, vanilla, opopanax.

Fragrance family	Typical examples, houses, launch dates and composers	Some key notes or accords that contribute to main characteristics
Oriental Oriental ambery, has 'gourmand' vanilla characteristics while the spicy type is typified by clove, cinnamon, etc.; sometimes dry-woody.		
Oriental ambery	*Jicky* (Guerlain 1889, Aimé Guerlain)	Jasmine, patchouli, vanilla, benzoin, 'amber', tonka.
	Shalimar (Guerlain 1925, Jacques Guerlain)	Patchouli, rose, jasmine, orris, opopanax, vanilla, benzoin, tonka, balsams.
	Angel (Thierry Mugler 1992, Oliver Cresp and Yves de Chiris)	Ethylmaltol, 'caramel', 'chocolate', vanilla, honey, bergamot, patchouli.
Oriental spicy	*Opium* (Yves Saint Laurent 1977, Jean-Louise Sieuzac)	Mandarin, pimento, bay, carnation, benzoin, tolu, vanilla.
	Cinnabar (Lauder 1978, composer unknown)	Clove, cinnamon, patchouli, ylang, jasmine, orris.
Chypre 'feminine' Typically has a citrus accord over an oakmoss base, patchouli is usually present. The animalic variant has often dry-leathery characteristics.		
Chypre fruity	*Mitsouko* (Guerlain 1919, Jacques Guerlain)	Bergamot, peach, jasmine, oakmoss, benzoin.
	So Pretty (Cartier 1995, Jean Guichard)	Blackcurrant, mandarin, rose, iris.
Chypre floral animalic	*Cuir de Russie* (Chanel 1924, Ernest Beaux)	Orange blossom, orris, carnation, leather, vetiver, cade, amber, opopanax, styrax, vanilla, heliotrope.
	Miss Dior (Dior 1947, Jean Carles and Serge Heftler Louiche)	Aldehydes, galbanum, jasmine, patchouli, amber, vetiver, oakmoss.
	Mystère (Rochas 1978, Nicolas Mamounas)	Coriander, hyacinth, rose, cedar, oakmoss, and patchouli.

Chypre floral	*Knowing* (Lauder 1988, composer unknown)	Green notes, floral accord, patchouli, oakmoss, honey, musk, amber, civet.
	Aromatics Elixir (Clinique 1972, unknown)	Bergamot, rose, patchouli, vetiver, sandalwood, civet, oakmoss, cistus, musk.
Chypre fresh	*Ô* (Lancôme 1969, Robert Gonnon)	Bergamot, citrus, basil, rose, jasmine, vetiver, oakmoss.
	Diorella (Dior 1972, Edmond Roudnitska)	Citrus, basil, melon, jasmine, oakmoss, patchouli, vetiver.
	Cristalle (Chanel 1993, Jacques Polge, who reworked Henri Robert's original 1947 version)	Citrus, basil, cumin, peach, jasmine, melon, oakmoss, musk, civet, patchouli.
Chypre green	*Alliage* (Lauder 1972, composer unknown)	Green accord, galbanum, jasmine, pine needle, oakmoss.

Chypre 'masculine'

Chypre woody, leathery and citrus are often classed as 'masculine' fragrances. The woody type is often characterised by patchouli, sandalwood and vetiver. The leathery type has a dry-smoky accord, the fresh type can include green herbaceous notes, and the citrus type has an eau de cologne top note.

Chypre woody	*Vetiver* (Guerlain 1961, Jean Paul Guerlain)	Bergamot, vetiver, clary, orris, carnation, sandalwood, oakmoss, myrrh, leather, civet, tonka, amber.
Chypre leathery	*Knize Ten* (Knize 1924, Vincent Roubert and François Coty)	Citrus, geranium, cedar, leather, musk, moss, amber, castoreum, vanilla.
	Aramis (Aramis 1965, Bernard Chant)	Artemisia, aldehydes, jasmine, patchouli, leather, oakmoss.
	Yatagan (Caron 1976, Vincent Marcello)	Lavender, wormwood, artemisia, geranium, pine, patchouli, castoreum, leather.
	Derby (Guerlain 1985, Jean Paul Guerlain)	Bergamot, artemisia, pimento, rose, leather vetiver, sandalwood.
Chypre fresh	*Eau Sauvage* (Dior 1966, Edmond Roudnitska)	Bergamot, lemon, basil, jasmine, patchouli, oakmoss.

Fragrance family	Typical examples, houses, launch dates and composers	Some key notes or accords that contribute to main characteristics
Chypre 'masculine'		
Chypre citrus	*Eau d'Hermès* (Hermès 1982, Edmond Roudnitska)	Lemon, bergamot, petitgrain, rosemary, jasmine, lavender, lily of the valley, caraway, musk, moss, sandalwood, cedarwood.
Fougère Based on lavender, oakmoss and coumarin (tonka); often classed as masculine but originally intended for women.		
Fougère lavender	*Oxford and Cambridge Traditional Lavender* (Czech and Speake 1994, John Stephen)	Bergamot, rosemary, peppermint, lavender, oakmoss.
Fougère aromatic	*Paco Rabanne pour Homme* (Paco Rabanne 1973, Jean Martel)	Bergamot, lavender, rosemary, bay laurel, clary, carnation, geranium, tree moss.
	Jules (Dior 1980, composer unknown)	Artemisia, bergamot, wormwood, bay laurel, jasmine, cyclamen, leather, moss, tonka, castoreum.
Fougère fresh	*Azzaro pour Homme* (Azzaro 1978, Gérard Anthony, Martin Heiddenreich and Richard Wirtz)	Lavender, bergamot, clary, lemon, petitgrain, basil, patchouli, caraway, juniper berry, amber, oakmoss, tonka.
	Calvin (Calvin Klein 1981, composer unknown)	Lavender, anise, geranium, patchouli, moss, amber.
	Jazz (Yves Saint Laurent 1988, Jean-François Latty)	Lavender, basil, anise, geranium, fern, cedar, leather, tonka, olibanum.
Fougère woody ambery	*Fougère Royale* (Houbigant 1882, unknown)	Lavender, clary, bergamot, petitgrain, geranium, oakmoss, musk, tonka, hay, vanilla.
	Rive Gauche pour Homme (Yves Saint Laurent 2003, Jacques Cavallier)	Bergamot, anise, rosemary, lavender, geranium, clove, vetiver, guaiacwood, patchouli.

Oriental 'masculine'
Masculine variants include the spicy type which is often dry-fresh, while the ambery type is sweeter, with honey or vanilla notes.

Oriental spicy	*Héritage* (Guerlain 1992, Jean Paul Guerlain)	Bergamot, lemon, rose, bay, cinnamon, cedar, patchouli, tonka.
	Equipage (Hermès 1970, Guy Robert)	Clary, carnation, cinnamon, oakmoss, tonka.
Oriental ambery	*Habit Rouge* (Guerlain 1965, Jean Paul Guerlain)	Bergamot, lemon, pimento, carnation, patchouli, vanilla, amber.

Tabac
Tabac fragrances are characterised by a tobacco note.

'Feminine'	*Tabac Blond* (Caron 1919, Ernest Daltroff)	Rose, floral, tobacco.
	Tabac (La Via del Profumo, date unknown, Dominique Dubrana)	Tobacco leaf, vanilla, cistus, tonka.

Aquatic and marine
Cool, green, melon-like cucumber-like, watery notes.
Often characterised by 'Calone'.

Aquatic floral fresh	*Acqua di Giò* (Armani 1995, composer unknown)	Citrus, pineapple, aquatic, lily of the valley, hyacinth.
	L'Eau d'Issey (Issey Miyake 1992, Jacques Cavallier)	Aquatic note, rose water, green note, floral – lily, peony, and freesia.
	Flower (Kenzo 2000, Alberto Morilla)	Hawthorn, rose, cassie, violet top, blackcurrant bud, opopanax and musk, Hedione (green, fresh).
Aquatic citrus	*Acqua di Giò pour Homme* (Armani 1996, composer unknown)	Citrus, marine, rosemary, cedarwood, musk.
Marine	*Sel de Vetiver* (The Different Company, 2006, Céline Ellena)	Citrus, cardamom, geranium, iris, patchouli, sea salt, vetiver.
	Sandflowers (Montale, 2008? Pierre Montale)	Juniper, marine, oakmoss.

Sources

Compiled and adapted from the Haarmann and Reimer Genealogies in Glöss 1995.

Classifications suggested by Turin and Sanchez 2009.

Supplemented by the manufacturers' commercial marketing materials, accessed online.

Notes on the compilation of the table

Every effort has been made to give examples that are very typical of their types, and which are likely to remain in production for some time; they could be seen as 'reference' fragrances. Most of these are 'classic fragrances' – that is, they have already been in production for many years and have remained popular, or have gained 'cult status'. In some cases the originals have been reformulated; the dates given relate to the original release. The lists of 'ingredients' are obviously not complete – however, the notes mentioned are important in the olfactory profile of the fragrance, and are intended only to give a sense of its characteristics.

Ambergris

Ambergris is possibly one of the most interesting perfume materials – however, because it is derived from a pathological secretion of the whale, it falls outside the scope of this book. Ambergris can be found washed up on the shores of New Zealand, Australia and the Indian Ocean, and it has long held an important place in perfumery, and also as a medicine, aphrodisiac and incense. The name translates as 'grey amber', which gives a clue to its appearance. Originally it was thought to be bird excrement, or congealed gum or bitumen, or even a marine fungus. However, it is none of these; it is a pathological secretion that occurs in just 1 per cent of adult male sperm whales. The formation of ambergris can only be described as natural alchemy, where water, air and sunlight transform malodorous matter into a rare and costly perfume material.

The 50-tonne sperm whale, *Physeter macrocephalus*, feeds on squid and cuttlefish, consuming around a tonne of food a day. The indigestible parts of the squid – the beak-like mouth parts, the lenses of the eyes and an internal organ known as the 'pen' – begin to accumulate, conglomerate and irritate the whale's four stomachs. Normally, every few days this will be vomited out into the sea. However, sometimes the mass passes on from the stomach into the intestines, where it continues to irritate whilst becoming saturated with faeces, and this eventually blocks the rectum. As a result, more water will be absorbed from the intestines and eventually the mass becomes condensed and smooth, so that the faeces can pass again. The entire process can repeat several times, each time increasing the size of the obstruction. Kemp (2012) tells us that the largest piece of ambergris on record was from a whale killed in 1953, weighing almost half a tonne.

Sometimes the whale can pass the obstruction, but at other times it is fatal, causing the intestines to rupture. Either way, the blackened, sticky mass enters the ocean waters, where it can remain for decades, floating just under the surface. It is the time spent in the sea that transforms the appearance and odour of ambergris. When expelled, it looks like tar and has, unsurprisingly, a faecal smell. With time, and the influence of salt water, sunlight, waves and tides, it shrinks, becomes smoother, lighter grey in colour and more stone-like, with black flecks. The smell changes beyond recognition – it becomes complex and reminiscent of tobacco, musty and woody, like old furniture, earthy and seaweed-like. Although it looks like a stone, it will soften at 60°C, and will melt in boiling water.

According to Jouhar (1991) there are ten distinct types of ambergris. The best is pure white or silver grey from New Zealand. Other types are golden from the coast of North Africa; golden grey from the Gulf of Aden; pale yellow from Australia; dark grey or black with golden striations from the Azores; hard black from all parts of the world; dry and dark grey from the Persian Gulf; and dark reddish-brown from Madagascar.

Ambergris is one of the most valuable natural substances, costing around US$20 per gram – around half the price of gold. It is no wonder, then, that beachcombers in New Zealand walk for miles in the hope of finding this 'floating gold'. Not only is its formation a unique process, it is also a unique raw material in perfumery. Although it is derived from a mammal, it does not smell 'animalic' like other animal-derived perfume materials, such as castoreum, civet and musk. Also, because some whales eliminate ambergris naturally, it can be collected without causing any further suffering.

The original formulae of some of the classic fine fragrances, such as the floral-aldehydic *Chanel No.5* (Ernest Beaux 1921) and the warm, sweet ambery *Shalimar* (Jacques Guerlain 1925), contained the alcoholic tincture of ambergris. However, it is very rare, and very expensive. Also, in recent years, there has been a steadily increasing demand for products free of animal ingredients, and so ambergris is no longer part of mainstream/commercial perfumery. Although ambergris can be found on the beach, it was also once supplied by whalers, and this practice is not acceptable to the vast majority of people. Modern trade in ambergris is difficult to clarify, too, because of differing restrictions enforced by the various countries involved.

So in order to find something that could replace ambergris in perfumery, there have been several attempts to discover its fragrance 'markers' and synthesise substitutes. In 1820 chemists at the School of Pharmacy in Paris investigated ambergris in both its raw form and the tincture. They discovered that white crystals formed in the filtered tincture, and named this *ambrein* – however, ambrein itself is odourless. Awano *et al.* (2005) identified 31 constituents in ambergris tincture, which they classed as degradation products of ambrein, including two novel cyclic acetals. The first of these had a sweet, warm, amber-like odour, and the second had a long-lasting, gentle note of ambergris. Neither was detected in the raw ambergris, so they were presumed to be artefacts of the tincture-making process, and it was suggested that they were promising substances for future use in perfumery. According to Kemp (2012), mature ambergris contains the tobacco-like dihydro-γ-ionone, the seawater-like butanal, the mouldy, faecal α-ambrinol and ambergris oxide, which is the component with the odour most like ambergris. Synthetic substitutes include 'Ambrox' and 'Synambrane', but according to perfumers they do not smell like 'the real thing'.

A few artisan perfumers will use a tincture made from ambergris sourced from the beach. Other perfumers will use naturals such as labdanum – the oleo-resin from the flowering shrub *Cistus ladaniferus* – which has a rich, sweet, balsamic odour that is reminiscent of ambergris. Indeed, an ambergris 'base' can be constructed using labdanum, olibanum (frankincense) and vanilla.

APPENDIX C
Fragrance and the Four Elements

The western concept of the 'Four Elements' has its roots in the ancient Greek philosophies of Empedocles, Aristotle and Hippocrates. The Four Elements could be said to represent ways of feeling and behaving, consciousness and individual perceptions. Using this framework we can develop a new set of correspondences which can illustrate the potential effects of the fragrances of plant-derived aromatics on the psyche. These are presented below.

Element	Realm/Jungian concept	Potential effects	Fragrance types and characteristics
Air	Mental realm/ Thinking	To support mental activity, to stimulate creativity and generation of ideas.	Green, herbal, minty, coniferous, anise, cineolic, camphoraceous, pine-like, sharp/ citrus, fresh, penetrating, diffusive.
Fire	Spiritual realm/ Intuition	To stimulate, invigorate and uplift.	Spicy, caryophyllaceous (clove-like), floral/ fruity, peppery, pungent, rich, warm.
Earth	Physical, material realm/Sensing	To relax, comfort, ground and nurture.	Balsamic, caramel, earthy, lemony, soft, heavy, musty, rich, smooth, sweet and warm, sensual.
Water	Emotional realm/ Feeling	To anchor, reduce anxiety, promote a sense of ease and adaptability, to balance.	Citrus/sweet, rosy, floral/sweet, floral/ green, fruity/green, agrestic/hay/grass, woody/fresh, woody/soft.

Developing Sensory Appreciation of Plant Aromatics, Essential Oils, Absolutes and Fragrances

Aromatic plant materials

Sensory appreciation can begin with an exploration of the aromas of *natural plant materials*, such as fresh and dried herbs, fruits, spices, wood, conifer leaves and twigs and scented flowers. These materials are easily obtained, and provide most of the odour types and characteristics that are necessary for experiential learning. You should maintain records of all sensory impressions. Once the associations between the odour and the source have been made – that is, once the connections between sensory perception and a verbal label have been established – an olfactory memory has been created. Attempting identification is also recommended. This involves 'blind' sampling, where the scents are presented in the absence of visual identification and knowledge of the source; and this will obviously require assistance.

A systematic approach to sampling aromatic plant materials, coupled with keeping records of your sensory impressions, gives a very good base from which to explore the aromas of *essential oils and absolutes*. These are much more concentrated and intense aromas, and often do not smell like their natural counterparts until diluted. Essential oils are usually liquids, although they vary in viscosity ('thickness') from being less viscous than water (like the citrus oils), to more viscous than water (like sandalwood). Some absolutes have a liquid form, such as rose, jasmine and orange blossom. Others have a paste-like consistency, and some resinoids, such as benzoin, are hard and brittle. These can be purchased as alcohol extraits (a 10–30% concentration is ideal), or diluted in an odourless solvent such as dipropylene glycol (DPG); and these preparations are preferable for sensory exercises. The supplier should be able to provide not only botanical authentication but also safety data for all products, and this should be checked and consulted before using aromatic extracts.

Sensory exercises

It is important that sensory exercises are conducted in peace and quiet, and in an ordered and methodical manner. Everything that is required should be at hand, including the samples, blotters, notebook and pencil. Ideally, the environment should be warm, free of draughts, well ventilated, and away from other smells. It is also important to feel relaxed and comfortable before commencing. All aromatic extracts should be carefully applied to blotters ('smelling strips'), not sampled directly from the bottle. This is so that the different phases of fragrance can be appreciated, and this cannot be achieved otherwise. Always label the blotter before use, with a reference and the time; it can be folded across its length to form a 45° bend at both ends to create a 'handle' and an elevated tip for the sample, so that you can put the strip aside without the sample touching anything else. Then dip the blotter in the aromatic extract, up to 0.5cm, or dispense one drop on the tip. If an alcoholic extrait is being sampled, always wait for the alcohol to evaporate, as alcohol will temporarily 'numb' the olfactory receptors.

In active smelling, technique is important. The nose adapts to odours very quickly, so it is important to work quickly at first. First impressions should be gathered before fatigue sets in. The eyes should be closed to eliminate visual distractions, and the awareness should be directed to the odour. Sniff the sample, it is not necessary to inhale,[1] but concentrate on the impressions and record perceptions of the top notes immediately. Check this from time to time over the next five minutes, observing for changes. Then put the blotter aside, and take a short break before assessing the next sample. Return to the smelling strips at intervals (15 minutes and 45 minutes) to assess the different notes, looking for the body and dryout phases. In the case of the citrus oils, the body notes will emerge very quickly, and the dryout will be barely perceptible, even after just 30 minutes. The body notes of other oils, typically those classed as middle notes, will begin to emerge after 15–45 minutes, and their dryouts anywhere between 90 minutes and several hours. However, the dryouts of base notes, such as sandalwood and vetiver, will be present on the smelling strip for several days. So the sampling time should be managed accordingly. In each session, it is best to limit the sampling to two or three materials. It is also possible to 'fatigue' your nose to top notes just before smelling the middle notes, or to fatigue your nose to the middle notes before smelling base notes, and by doing this you can get a better clarity of each phase.

When learning about odour types and characteristics, it is suggested that the process is structured, by selecting samples that have the attributes for a particular set of odours. For example, when exploring the woody family, choose Virginian cedar as the 'reference' for wood, and let this enter your olfactory memory, complete with its characteristics. Other woods, such as sandalwood or Atlas cedarwood, can then be sampled; note their differing characteristics. Record your olfactory impressions, using the standard odour vocabulary to identify the different characteristics. Table 6.1 is a guide for this part of the process, and you can find reliable odour descriptions throughout the chapters on the aromatic plants and their extracts.

The process cannot be rushed. The aim is to determine the 'personality' of each scent – its character, duration, how it evolves over time. The goal (apart from

---

1   Prolonged inhalation of fragrances can influence the autonomic nervous system and elicit mental and emotional changes; here we are concerned with their olfactory characteristics.

pleasure) is to learn to smell with awareness, to stimulate the olfactory receptors and build an olfactory memory.

Identification and discrimination

Just as with the natural plant materials, blind sampling can be used, with assistance, to test progress with identification. If you close your eyes and a blotter is presented to you, can you describe the attributes of the odour, and perhaps name it? Again, record-keeping is important, whether of errors or successful identifications.

The 'odd man out' test (or 'triangle test') tests the ability to discriminate between odours. The simplest way of carrying this out is to have someone prepare three blotters, each labelled with a code and the numbers 1, 2 and 3. Two of the blotters should have the same sample applied, and the third should be different – but not too different. The samples could be, for example, lemon and grapefruit, or French lavender and Spanish lavender, or jasmine *sambac* and jasmine *grandiflorum*. When you are presented with the blotters, can you tell which two are the same, and which one is different? Can you describe the difference? Can you identify the samples?

Complex mixtures

Once you are further along the olfactory path, you might want to explore what happens with different combinations of oils and absolutes. You can start with simple binary combinations, prepared by putting three drops of each of two oils into a small, clean bottle. Dip the blotter, let it absorb, and notice what you perceive. It will probably be fairly easy to sense some of the characteristics of the two components. With help, this can be done 'blind'. Ask someone to prepare a combination that is unknown to you – can you discriminate, can you identify the components? Then you can begin to explore what happens with mixtures of three or more oils. In Roudnitska's words:

> When introduced into a mixture, the odour ceases to be one entity and interacts freely with other odorous bodies. Take note of everything that comes to mind, using the words which arise naturally; if they enable a thought to be more precise, if they surround the contours of the odours without ambiguity. Avoid 'almost' at any cost. Try to find the words that unequivocally define the impression so that twenty years later, if confronted with the same impression, the same words come to mind. (Roudnitska 1991, cited in Aftel 2008, pp.60–61)

In Chapter 8, when discussing the composition and olfactory profile of pennyroyal essential oil, we discovered that although its individual components make a contribution to the odour, it is their proportions and combinations that give pennyroyal its aromatic signature (Díaz-Maroto *et al.* 2007). In other words, the scent of each oil or absolute, and indeed each aromatic plant, is given by many constituents, each of which has its own characteristics, and their relative proportions will also have a major impact on the aroma. So the whole fragrance is something much, much more than the sum of the parts. When the already complex essential oils and absolutes are combined, the potential for creating new effects is vast. However, it is not only the combinations of ingredients; it is also their ratios that will determine the nature of the new aroma. In reality, the potential for creating new fragrances is infinite. Moreover, the process of this creation, which involves active olfaction and complete focus on scent, can have effects which can be compared to concentrative meditation. For an exploration of this and the composition of a natural fragrance, see Chapter 6 in Lawless (2009).

Appreciating olfactory art

> In the art of perfumes, Beauty is eternal and universal and follows the rules of Nature. (Corfan 2013)

The sensory appreciation of fragrances is also rewarding. The same learning process can be applied to commercially available and niche and artisan fragrances. Learn to recognise the fragrance families (see Appendix A), and take note of all your olfactory impressions: the characteristics of the top, heart and drydown notes, the diffusiveness, the persistence, how a fragrance evolves. Compare the scents on blotters and on skin – your own and that of others. These fragrances are created to be worn, not evaporated on blotters, and sometimes this is the only way that the true nature of a fragrance can be understood. This way, more characteristics can be identified. Which fragrances leave a trail in the air, and which ones stay close to the skin? Can you discern the structure – is it traditional, like Jean Paul Guerlain, or modern, like Sophia Grojsman or Jean-Claude Ellena? Can you discern the 'signature' of certain perfumers, like Edmond Roudnitska? If you have the opportunity, explore vintage fragrances and compare them with their modern counterparts. Compare your perceptions with the commercial descriptions and the critics. Enjoy the world of olfactory art.

References

Ackerman, D. (1990) *A Natural History of the Senses*. London: Phoenix.

Afoakawa, E.O. (2008) 'Cocoa and chocolate consumption – are there aphrodisiac and other benefits for human health?' *South African Journal of Clinical Nutrition 21*, 3, 107–113.

Aftel, M. (2008) *Essence and Alchemy: A Natural History of Perfume*. Layton, UT: Gibbs Smith.

Akhondzadeh, S., Fallah-Pour, H., Afkham, K., Jamshidi, A.-H. and Khalighi-Cigaroudi, F. (2004) 'Comparison of Crocus sativus L. and imipramine in the treatment of mild to moderate depression: a pilot double-blind randomized trial.' *BMC Complementary and Alternative Medicine 4*, 12.

Akhondzadeh, S., Tahmacebi-Pour, N., Noorbala, A.-A., Amini, H. *et al.* (2005) 'Crocus sativus L. in the treatment of light to moderate depression: a double-blind, randomized, and placebo-controlled trial.' *Phytotherapy Research 19*, 148–151.

Alaoui-Ismaïli, O., Vernet-Maury, E., Dittmar, A., Delhomme, G. and Chanel, J. (1997) 'Odor hedonics: connection with emotional response estimated by autonomic parameters.' *Chemical Senses 22*, 237–248.

Alavi, D. (2012) *Le Snob: Perfume*. London: Hardie Grant Books.

Al Bawaba (2010) 'Future of ancient trade in aromatic wood uncertain.' Available at www.albawaba.com/news/future-ancient-trade-aromatic-wood-uncertain, accessed on 14 May 2013.

Alderete, E., Erickson, P.I., Kaplan, C.P. and Pérez-Stable, E.J. (2010) 'Ceremonial tobacco use in the Andes: implications for smoking prevention among indigenous youth.' *Anthropology and Medicine 17*, 1, 27–39.

American Medical Association (1993) *Guides to the Evaluation of Permanent Impairment* (4th Edition). Chicago, IL: AMA.

Amoore, J.E. (1963) 'The stereochemical theory of olfaction.' *Nature 198*, 271–272.

Anderson, B.M., Rizzo, M., Block, R.I., Pearlson, G.D. and O'Leary, D.S. (2010) 'Sex, drugs, and cognition: effects of marijuana.' *Journal of Psychoactive Drugs 42*, 4, 413–424.

Ansari, B.A.S. (1976) 'Abu Bakr Muhammad Ibn Yahya: universal scholar and scientist.' *Islamic Studies 15*, 3, 155–166. Islamabad: Islamic Research Institute.

Antoninetti, M. (2011) 'The long journey of Italian grappa: from quintessential element to local moonshine to national sunshine.' *Journal of Cultural Geography 28*, 3, 375–398.

Arena, J.M. (1973) *Poisoning: Toxicology, Symptoms, Treatments*. Springfield IL: Charles C. Thomas.

Arroyo, S. (1975) *Astrology, Psychology and the Four Elements: An Energy Approach to Astrology and Its Use in the Counselling Arts*. Nevada: CRCS Publications.

Aschenbrenner, K., Hummel, C., Teszmer, K., Krone, F. *et al.* (2007) 'The influence of olfactory loss on dietary behaviours.' *Laryngoscope 118*, 135–144.

Attar, F. (1984) *The Conference of the Birds*, trans. A. Darbandi and D. Davies. London: Penguin.

Attar, F. (1990) *Mantegh-e-Tir (Farsi version)*. Iran: Ayandeh.

Austin, D.F. (2004) *Florida Ethnobotany*. London: CRC Press.

Awano, K., Ishizaki, S., Takazawa, O. and Kitahara, T. (2005) 'Analysis of ambergris tincture.' *Flavour and Fragrance Journal 20*, 18–21.

Ayabe-Kanamura, S., Schicker, I., Laska, M., Hudson, R. *et al.* (1998) 'Differences in perception of everyday odors: a Japanese–German cross-cultural study.' *Chemical Senses 23*, 31–38.

Baggott, M.J., Erowid, E., Erowid, F., Galloway, G.P. and Mendelson, J. (2010) 'Use patterns and self-reported effects of Salvia divinorum: an internet-based survey.' *Drug and Alcohol Dependence 111*, 250–256.

Balacs, T. (1998/1999) 'Research reports.' *International Journal of Aromatherapy 9*, 2, 86–88.

Baldovini, N., Delasalle, C. and Joulain, D. (2011) 'Phytochemistry of the heartwood from fragrant Santalum species: a review.' *Flavour and Fragrance Journal 26*, 7–26.

Ballard, C.G., O'Brien, C.T., Reichelt, K. and Perry, E.K. (2002) 'Aromatherapy as a safe and effective treatment for the management of agitation in severe dementia: the results of a double-blind, placebo-controlled trial with melissa.' *Journal of Clinical Psychiatry 63*, 555–558.

Baranauskiene, R., Venskutonis, P.R. and Demyttenaere, J.C.R. (2005) 'Sensory and instrumental evaluation of sweet marjoram (Origanum majorana L.) aroma.' *Flavour and Fragrance Journal 20*, 492–500.

Barkat, S., Le Berre, E., Coureaud, G., Sicard, G. and Thomas-Danguin, T. (2012) 'Perceptual blending in odor mixtures depends on the nature of odorants and human olfactory expertise.' *Chemical Senses 37*, 159–166.

Baron, R.A. (1983) '"Sweet smell of success?" The impact of pleasant scents on evaluations of job applicants.' *Journal of Applied Psychology 68*, 709–713.

Baron, R.A. (1988) 'Perfume as a Tactic of Impression Management in Social and Organizational Settings.' In S. Van Toller and G.H. Dodd (eds) *Perfumery: The Psychology and Biology of Fragrance.* London: Chapman and Hall.

Baron, R.A. (1997) 'The sweet smell of…helping: effects of pleasant ambient fragrances on prosocial behaviour in shopping malls.' *Personality and Social Psychology Bulletin 23*, 5, 498.

Başer, K.H.C., Demirci, B., Dekebo, A. and Dagne, E. (2003) 'Essential oils of some Boswellia spp., myrrh and opopanax.' *Flavour and Fragrance Journal 18*, 153–156.

Batchelder, T. (2004) 'The cultural pharmacology of chocolate.' Townsend Letter for Doctors and Patients, November 2004, 103–106.

Bateson, P. (1983) 'Optimal Outbreeding.' In P. Bateson (ed.) *Mate Choice.* Cambridge: Cambridge University Press.

Baumann, L.S. (2007) 'Less-known botanical cosmeceuticals.' *Dermatologic Therapy 20*, 330–342.

Baylac, S. and Racine, P. (2003) 'Inhibition of 5-lipoxygenase by essential oils and other natural fragrant extracts.' *International Journal of Aromatherapy 13*, 2/3, 138–142.

Baylac, S. and Racine, P. (2004) 'Inhibition of human leukocyte elastase by natural fragrant extracts of aromatic plants.' *International Journal of Aromatherapy 14*, 4, 179–182.

Bazzali, O., Tomi, F., Casanova, J. and Bighelli, A. (2012) 'Occurrence of C8–C10 esters in Mediterranean Myrtus communis L. leaf essential oil.' *Flavour and Fragrance Journal 27*, 335–340.

Behl, T.N.S. (2008) 'Fleeting fragrance.' Available at http://businesstoday.intoday.in/story/fleeting-fragrance/1/2521.html, accessed on 14 May 2013.

Benson, S.G. and Dundis, S.P. (2003) 'Understanding and motivating health care employees: integrating Maslow's hierarchy of needs, training and technology.' *Journal of Nursing Management 11*, 315–320.

Bischoff, K. and Guale, F. (1998) 'Australian tea tree (*Melaleuca alternifolia*) oil poisoning in three purebred cats.' *Journal of Veterinary Diagnostic Investigation 10*, 208–210.

Blacow, N.W. (1972) *Martindale: The Extra Pharmacopoeia* (26th Edition). London: Pharmaceutical Press.

Bloom, W. (2011) *The Power of Modern Spirituality.* London: Piatkus.

Bonfils, P., Faulcon, P., Tavernier, L., Bonfils, N. and Malinvaud, D. (2008) 'Home accidents associated with anosmia.' *La Presse Médicale 37*, 742–745.

Bowles, E.J. (2003) *The Chemistry of Aromatherapeutic Oils* (3rd Edition). Crow's Nest, Australia: Allen and Unwin.

Brechbill, G.O. (2007) *Classifying Aroma Chemicals.* New Jersey: Fragrance Books.

Brooks, J.E. (1952) *The Mighty Leaf: Tobacco through the Centuries.* Boston, MA: Little, Brown and Company.

Brophy, J.J. and Doran, J.C. (2004) 'Geographic variation in oil characteristics in *Melaleuca ericifolia*.' *Journal of Essential Oil Research,* January/February 2004.

Buchbauer, G. (1996) 'Methods in aromatherapy research.' *Perfumer and Flavorist 21*, 31–36.

Buchbauer, G., Dietrich, H., Karamat, E., Jirovetz, L., Jager, W. and Plank, C. (1991) 'Aromatherapy: evidence for sedative effects of the essential oil of lavender after inhalation.' *Journal of Biosciences 46*, 1067–1072.

Buchbauer, G., Jirovetz, L., Jager, W., Plank, C. and Dietrich, H. (1993) 'Fragrance compounds and essential oils with sedative effects upon inhalation.' *Journal of Pharmaceutical Sciences 82*, 6, 660–664.

Burfield, T. (2002) 'Cedarwood oils.' *The Cropwatch Series.* Available at www.cropwatch.org, accessed on 30 November 2011.

Burfield, T. (2004) 'Rosewood sustainability: critical assessment of the May and Barata paper.' *The Cropwatch Series.* Available at www.cropwatch.org/cropwatch6.htm, accessed on 30 November 2011.

Burns, L.M. and Harper, M. (2012) 'Making a connection through colour: even before a product is sampled, consumers have formed an idea about how the fragrance should smell, likely based on its colour.' *Global Cosmetic Industry*, January–February 2012, 28.

Burr, C. (2007) *The Perfect Scent*. New York, NY: Picador.

Byrne-Quinn, J. (1988) 'Perfume, People, Perceptions and Products.' In S. Van Toller and G.H. Dodd (eds) *Perfumery: The Psychology and Biology of Fragrance*. London: Chapman and Hall.

Byron, E. (2013) 'Uncork the nose's secret powers.' *The Wall Street Journal,* 12 February 2013.

Cabo, Y., Crespo, M.E., Jimenez, J., Navarro, C. *et al.* (1987) 'Sur l'huile essentielle de *Salvia lavandulaefolia vahl* subsp. *Oxydon.*' *Plantes Médicinales et Phytothérapie 21*, 2, 116–121.

Cadby, P., Ellis, G., Hall, B., Surot, C. and Vey, M. (2011) 'Identification of the causes of an allergic reaction to a fragranced consumer product.' *Fragrance and Flavour Journal 26*, 2–6.

Cahill, L., Haier, R.J., Fallon, J., Alkire, M.T. *et al.* (1996) 'Amygdala activity at encoding correlated with long-term free recall of emotional information.' *Proceedings of the National Academy of Science USA 93*, 8016–8021

Calkin, R. (1999) 'The fragrance of old roses.' *Historic Rose Journal.* Available at www.historicroses.org/index.php?id=38, accessed on 30 May 2013.

Calkin, R.R. and Jellinek, J.S. (1994) *Perfumery: Practice and Principles*. New York, NY: John Wiley and Sons.

Cappello, G., Spezzaferrp, M., Grossi, L., Manzoli, L. and Marzio, L. (2007) 'Peppermint oil (Mintoil) in the treatment of irritable bowel syndrome: a prospective double blind placebo-controlled randomized trial.' *Digestive and Liver Disease 39*, 6, 530–536.

Caseau, B. (1994) *The Use and Meaning of Fragrances in the Ancient World and Their Christianization (100–900 ad)*. Princeton University, PhD thesis.

Castel, C., Fernandez, X., Filippi, J.-J. and Brun, J.-P. (2009) 'Perfumes in Mediterranean antiquity.' *Flavour and Fragrance Journal 24*, 326–334.

Cernoch, J. and Porter, R. (1985) 'Recognition of maternal axillary odors by infants.' *Child Development 56*, 1593–1598.

Chen, D. and Haviland-Jones, J. (2000) 'Human olfactory communication of emotion.' *Perceptual and Motor Skills 91*, 3, 771.

Chishti, M. (1991) *The Traditional Healer's Handbook: A Classic Guide to the Medicine of Avicenna*. Rochester, VT: Healing Arts Press.

Chishti, M. (2003) *Medicines for the Soul: Spiritual Aromatherapy Practitioner's Handbook*. USA: The Chishti Co.

Chishti, M. (2005) *Eastern Spiritual Aromatherapy*. USA: The Chishti Co.

Chrea, C., Grandjean, D., Delplanque, S., Cayeux, I. *et al.* (2009) 'Mapping the semantic space for the subjective experience of emotional responses to odours.' *Chemical Senses 34*, 49–62.

Chu, S. (2008) 'Olfactory conditioning of positive performance in humans.' *Chemical Senses 33*, 65–71.

Chu, S. and Downes, J.J. (2000) 'Odour-evoked autobiographical memories: psychological investigations of Proustian phenomena.' *Chemical Senses 25*, 111–116.

Classen, C. (1992) 'The odor of the other – olfactory symbolism and cultural categories.' *Ethos 20*, 133–166.

Classen, C., Howes, D. and Synnott. A. (1994) *Aroma: The Cultural History of Smell*. London: Routledge.

Collins, J.J. (1968) 'A descriptive introduction to the Taos peyote ceremony.' *Ethnology 7*, 4, 427.

Corbin, A. (1996) *The Foul and the Fragrant: Odour and the Social Imagination*. London: Macmillan Publishers.

Corfan, O. (2010) 'Linden blossom CO2 extraction.' Available at www.1000fragrances.blogspot.co.uk/2010/03/linden-blossom-CO2-extract.html, accessed on 14 February 2013.

Corfan, O. (2013) '14 February 2013.' www.1000fragrances.blogspot.co.uk, accessed on 14 February 2013.

Costa, R., Dugo, P., Navarra, M., Raymo, V., Dugoa, G. and Mondello, L. (2010) 'Study on the chemical composition variability of some processed bergamot (*Citrus bergamia*) essential oils.' *Flavour and Fragrance Journal 25*, 4–12.

Cowley, J.J., Johnson, A.L. and Brooksbank, B.W.L. (1977) 'The effect of two odorous compounds on performance of an assessment-of-people test.' *Psychoneuroendocrinology 2*, 159–172.

Craffert, P.F. (2011) 'Shamanism and the shamanic complex.' *Biblical Theology Bulletin: A Journal of Bible and Theology 41*, 3, 151–161.

Criley, R.A. (2001) 'What is the true *Plumeria* fragrance?' Available at www.ctahr.hawaii.edu/tpss/digest/hd102/hd102_3.html, accessed on 15 February 2013.

Crisinel, A.-S. and Spence, C. (2012) 'A fruity note: cross-modal associations between odors and musical notes.' *Chemical Senses 37*, 151–158.

Curtis, V. and Biran, A. (2001) 'Dirt, disgust and disease.' *Perspectives in Biological Medicine 44*, 17–30.

Dalton, P. (1996) 'Cognitive aspects of perfumery.' *Perfumer and Flavorist 21*, 13–20.

Dalton, P. and Wysocki, C.J. (1996) 'The nature and duration of adaptation following long-term exposure to odors.' *Perception and Psychophysics 58*, 781–792.

Dannaway, F.R. (2010) 'Strange fires, weird smokes and psychoactive combustibles: entheogens and incense in ancient traditions.' *Journal of Psychoactive Drugs 42*, 4, 485–497.

Das Gupta, L. (2012) 'Meaning making in artistic perfumery.' Lecture by Dr Claus Noppeney at Esxence 2012. Available at www.basenotes.net/content/3-features, accessed on 26 April 2012.

Davies, S.J., Harding, L.M. and Baranowski, A.P. (2002) 'A novel treatment for postherpetic neuralgia using peppermint oil.' *Clinical Journal of Pain 18*, 3, 200–202.

Davis, F. (1979) *Yearning for Yesterday: A Sociology of Nostlagia*. New York, NY: Free Press.

Davis, P. (1991) *Subtle Aromatherapy*. Saffron Walden: C.W. Daniel Company.

Degel, J. and Köster, E.P. (1999) 'Odors: implicit memory and performance effects.' *Chemical Senses 24*, 317–325.

Dehghan, G.R., Shahverdi, A.R., Amin, G., Abdollah, M. and Shafiee, A. (2007) 'Chemical composition and antimicrobial activity of essential oil of *Ferula szovitsiana* D.C.' *Flavour and Fragrance Journal 22*, 224–227.

Deikman, A.J. (1982) *The Observing Self: Mysticism and Psychotherapy*. Boston, MA: Beacon Press.

Delort, E. and Jaquier, A. (2009) 'Novel terpenyl esters from Australian finger lime (*Citrus australasica*) peel extract.' *Flavour and Fragrance Journal 24*, 123–132.

Demattè, M.L., Sanabria, D., Sugarman, R. and Spence, C. (2006) 'Cross-modal interactions between olfaction and touch.' *Chemical Senses 31*, 291–300.

Deterre, S., Rega, B., Delarue, J., Decloux, M., Lebrun, M. and Giampaoli, P. (2011) 'Identification of key aroma compounds from bitter orange (*Citrus aurantium* L.) products: essential oil and macerate-distillate extract.' *Flavour and Fragrance Journal 27*, 77–88.

Díaz-Maroto, M.C., Castillo, N., Castro-Vázquez, L., González-Viñas, M.A. and Pérez-Coello, M.S. (2007) 'Volatile composition and olfactory profile of pennyroyal (*Mentha pulegium* L.) plants.' *Flavour and Fragrance Journal 22*, 114–118.

Diego, M.A., Jones, N.A., Field, T., Hernandez-Reif, M. *et al.* (1998) 'Aromatherapy positively affects mood, EEG patterns of alertness and math computations.' *International Journal of Neuroscience 96*, 217–224.

Dobetsberger, C. and Buchbauer, G. (2011) 'Actions of essential oils on the central nervous system: an updated review.' *Flavour and Fragrance Journal 26*, 5, 300–316.

Donna, L. (2009) 'Fragrance perception: is everything relative?' *Perfumer and Flavorist 34*, 26–35.

Donoyama, N. and Ichiman, Y. (2006) 'Which essential oil is better for hygienic massage practice?' *International Journal of Aromatherapy 16*, 3, 175–179.

Douek, E. (1988) 'Foreword – Abnormalities of Smell.' In S. Van Toller and G.H. Dodd (eds) *Perfumery: The Psychology and Biology of Fragrance*. London: Chapman and Hall.

Douglas, M. (1975) *Implicit Meanings*. London: Routledge and Kegan Paul.

Drobnick, J. (2012) 'Towards an olfactory art history: the mingled, fatal and rejuvenating perfumes of Paul Gauguin.' *Senses and Society 7*, 2, 196–208.

DuBois, T.A. (2009) *An Introduction to Shamanism*. Cambridge: Cambridge University Press.

Dugo, P., Bonaccorsi, I., Ragonese, C., Russo, M. *et al.* (2011) 'Analytical characterisation of mandarin (*Citrus deliciosa* Ten.) essential oil.' *Flavour and Fragrance Journal 26*, 34–46.

Durgnat, R. (1969) 'Symbolism and the Underground.' *The Hudson Review 22*, 3, 457.

Edwards, M. (2008) *Fragrances of the World: Parfums du Monde 2008* (24th Edition). Sydney: Fragrances of the World.

Elliot, M.S.J., Abuhamdah, S., Howes, M.-J.R., Lees, G. *et al.* (2007) 'The essential oils from *Melissa officinalis* L. and *Lavandula angustifolia* Mill. as potential treatment for agitation in people with severe dementia.' *International Journal of Essential Oil Therapeutics 1*, 4, 143–152.

Engen, T. (1988) 'The Acquisition of Odour Hedonics.' In S. Van Toller and G.H. Dodd (eds) *Perfumery: The Psychology and Biology of Fragrance*. London: Chapman and Hall.

Erligmann, A. (2001) 'Sandalwood oils.' *International Journal of Aromatherapy 11*, 4, 186–192.

Evans, S. (2002) 'The scent of a martyr. Exploring the tradition of the "aroma of sanctity" among Christian saints as an explanation of divine communication.' *Numen: International Review for the History of Religions 49*, 193–211.

Evans, W.C. (1989) *Trease and Evans' Pharmacognosy* (13th Edition). London: Ballière Tindall.

Fernandez, X., Castel, C., Lizzani-Cuvelier, L., Delbecque, C. and Venzal, S.P. (2006) 'Volatile constituents of benzoin gums: Siam and Sumatra, Part 3. Fast characterisation with an electronic nose.' *Flavour and Fragrance Journal 21*, 439–446.

Ferrence, S.C. and Bendersky, G. (2004) 'Therapy with saffron and the goddess at Thera.' *Perspectives in Biology and Medicine 47*, 2, 199–226.

Figueiredo, A.C. and Miguel, M.G. (2010) 'Aromatic plants, spices and volatiles in food and beverages.' *Flavour and Fragrance Journal 25*, 251–252.

Fischer-Rizzi, S. (1990) *Complete Aromatherapy Handbook*. New York, NY: Sterling.

Forbes, P.D. Urbach, F. and Daviesm R.E. (1977) 'Phototoxicity testing of fragrance raw materials.' *Food and Cosmetics Toxicology 15*, 1, 55–60.

Fortineau, A.-D. (2004) 'Chemistry perfumes your daily life.' *Journal of Chemical Education 81*, 1, 45–50.

Franchomme, P. and Pénoël, D. (1990) *L'aromathérapie Exactement*. Limoges: Jallois.

Franzoi, S.L. and Herzog, M.E. (1987) 'Judging physical attractiveness: what body aspects do we use?' *Personality and Social Psychology Bulletin 13*, 19–33.

Frasnelli, J., Lundström, J.N., Boyle, J.A., Katsarkas, A. and Jones-Gotman, M. (2011) 'The vomeronasal organ is not involved in the perception of endogenous odors.' *Human Brain Mapping 32*, 450–460.

Frawley, D. and Lad, V. (1986) *The Yoga of Herbs*. Twin Lakes, CO: Lotus Press.

Freyberg, R. and Ahren, M.-P. (2011) 'A preliminary trial exploring perfume preferences in adolescent girls.' *Journal of Sensory Studies 26*, 3, 237–243.

Friedlander, S. (1992) *The Whirling Dervishes*. New York, NY: State University of New York Press.

Fujii, N., Abla, D., Kudo, N., Hihara, S., Okanoya, K. and Iriki, A. (2007) 'Prefrontal activity during *koh-do* incense discrimination.' *Neuroscience Research 59*, 257–264.

Fukui, H., Toyoshima, K. and Komaki, R. (2011) 'Psychological and neuroendocrinological effects of odor of saffron (*Crocus sativus*).' *Phytomedicine 18*, 726–730.

Gali-Muhtasib, H., Hilan, H. and Khater, C. (2000) 'Traditional uses of *Salvia libanotica* (East Mediterranean sage) and the effects of its essential oils.' *Journal of Ethnopharmacology 71*, 3, 513–520.

Gattefossé, M. (1992) 'René-Maurice Gattefossé – the father of modern aromatherapy.' *International Journal of Aromatherapy 4*, 2, 18–22.

Gauguin, P. (1957) *Noa Noa: A Journal of the South Seas*, trans. O.F. Theis. New York, NY: Farrar, Straus and Giroux.

Geiger, J.L. (2005) 'The essential oil of ginger, *Zingiber officinale*, and anaesthesia.' *International Journal of Aromatherapy 15*, 1, 7–14.

Gell, A. (1977) 'Magic, Perfume, Dream…' In I. Lewis (ed.) *Symbols and Sentiments: Cross-cultural Studies in Symbolism*. London: Academic Press.

Gilbert, A. (1997) 'The evolving links between scent and odour.' *Perfumer and Flavorist 22*, 4, 53–54.

Gilbert, A. (2008) *What the Nose Knows*. New York, NY: Crown Publishers.

Gilbert, A.N., Martin, R. and Kemp, S.E. (1996) 'Cross-modal correspondence between vision and olfaction: the colour of smells.' *American Journal of Psychology 109*, 335–351.

Gilbert, N. (2013) 'Greatest Hits: Antoine Lie.' Available at www.basenotes.net/content/1543-Greatest-Hits-Antoine-Lie, accessed on 25 January 2013.

Gilman, S.L. and Xun, Z. (eds) (2004) *Smoke: A Global History of Smoking*. London: Reaktion Books.

Gimelli, S.P. (2001) *Aroma Science*. Weymouth: Micelle Press.

Glaser, G. (2002) *The Nose: A Profile of Sex, Beauty and Survival*. New York, NY: Atria Books.

Glicksohn, J. (1998) 'States of consciousness and symbolic cognition.' *The Journal of Mind and Behaviour 19*, 105–118.

Glicksohn, J. and Berkovich Ohana, A. (2011) 'From trance to transcendence: a neurocognitive approach.' *The Journal of Mind and Behavior 32*, 1, 49–62.

Glöss, W. (ed.) (1995) *Fragrance Guide: Fragrances on the International Market*. Hamburg: Verlag Glöss.

Gobel, H., Schmidt, G., Dworschak, M., Stolze, H. and Heuss, D. (1995) 'Essential plant oils and headache mechanisms.' *Phytomedicine 2*, 2, 93–102.

Goode, J.A. (2000) 'Sending out an SOS: semiochemicals in nature.' *Biologist 47*, 5, 247–250.

Goodrich, K.R. (2012) 'Floral scent in Annonaceae.' *Botanical Journal of the Linnean Society 169*, 262–279.

Goody, J. (1993) *The Culture of Flowers*. Cambridge: Cambridge University Press.

Gordon, L. (1980) *A Country Herbal*. Devon: Webb and Bower Publishers.

Gottfried, J.A. and Dolan, R.J. (2003) 'The nose smells what the eye sees: cross-modal visual facilitation of human olfactory perception.' *Neuron 39*, 375–386.

Graves, R. (1992) *The Greek Myths Combined Edition*. London: Penguin Books. (First published in 1955 in two volumes by Pelican Books.)

Gray. R. (2011) 'Why your special perfume is a very personal choice.' *The Sunday Telegraph*, 9 October.

Greenway, F.L., Frome, B.M., Engels, T.M. and McLellan, A. (2003) 'Temporary relief of postherpetic neuralgia pain with topical geranium oil.' *American Journal of Medicine 115*, 7, 586–587.

Grieve, M. (1992) *A Modern Herbal*. London: Tiger Books International. (Original work published in 1931.)

Griffiths, J.G. (1970) *Plutarch's De Iside et Osiride*. Wales: University of Wales.

Guéguen, N. (2012) 'The sweet smell of…courtship: effects of pleasant ambient fragrance on women's receptivity to a man's courtship request.' *Journal of Environmental Psychology 32*, 2, 123–125.

Gupta, C.S. (2013) 'Pandanus.' Available at www.fragantica.com/news/Pandanus-3998.html, accessed on 14 February 2013.

Hanson, J.R. (2010) 'Natural products from the hallucinogenic sage.' *Science Progress 93*, 2, 171–180.

Haque, M.H. and Haque, A.U. (1999) 'Haque Inc. European Patent no.1 059 086.' *Chemical Abstracts 134*, 25349.

Harris, B. (2006) 'Research reports.' *International Journal of Aromatherapy 16*, 1, 51–54.

Harvey, S.A. (1998) 'St Ephrem on the scent of salvation.' *Journal of Theological Studies 49*, 1. Available at http://jts.oxfordjournals.org, accessed on 30 January 2012.

Heffern, R. (2010) 'The catechism of our senses: earth and spirit.' *National Catholic Reporter 46*, 16, 19.

Helgeson, L.A. (2011) 'Fragrance in Roses.' Available at www.ars.org/?page_id=3043, accessed on 11/02/2013.

Hernandez Salazar, L.T., Laska, M. and Rodriguez Luna, E. (2003) 'Olfactory sensitivity for aliphatic esters in spider monkeys *Ateles geoffroyi*.' *Behavioural Neuroscience 117*, 1142–1149.

Herz, R.S. (2000) 'Scents of time.' *The Sciences*, July/August 2000, 34–39.

Herz, R.S. (2005) 'Odor-associative learning and emotion: effects on perception and behaviour.' *Chemical Senses 30*, 1, 1250–1251.

Herz, R.S. and Cahill, E.D. (1997) 'Differential use of sensory information in sexual behaviour as a function of gender.' *Human Nature 8*, 275–286.

Herz, R.S. and Inzlicht, M. (2002) 'Sex differences in response to physical and social factors involved in human mate selection: the importance of smell for women.' *Evolution and Human Behaviour 23*, 359–364.

Heuberger, E., Hongratanaworakit, T., Bohm, C., Weber, R. and Buchbauer, G. (2001) 'Effects of chiral fragrances on human autonomic nervous system parameters and self-evaluation.' *Chemical Senses 26*, 281–292.

Heuberger, E., Hongratanaworakit, T. and Buchbauer, G. (2006) 'East Indian sandalwood and α-santalol odor increase physiological and self-rated arousal in humans.' *Planta Medica 72*, 9, 792–800.

Hewitt, K. (2011) 'The "feeling of knowing," the psychedelic sensorium, and contemporary neuroscience: shifting contexts for noetic insight.' *Senses and Society 6*, 2, 177–202.

Hicks, A., Hicks, J. and Mole, P. (2011) *Five Element Constitutional Acupuncture* (2nd Edition). London: Elsevier.

Higuchi, T., Shoji, K., Taguchi, S. and Hatayama, T. (2005) 'Improvement of nonverbal behaviour in Japanese female perfume-wearers.' *International Journal of Psychology 40*, 2, 90–99.

Hill, J.H. (1992) 'The flower world of old Uto-Aztecan.' *Journal of Anthropological Research 48*, 2, 117–144.

Hirsch, H. (2013) 'Cosmetics and gender: perfumes in medieval legal Muslim sources.' *Household and Personal Care Today 8*, 1, 13–16.

Hirsch, A., Ye, Y., Lu, Y. and Choe, M. (2007) 'The effects of the aroma of jasmine on bowling score.' *International Journal of Essential Oil Therapeutics 1*, 79–82.

Hodgson, R.W. (1967) 'Horticultural Varieties of *Citrus*.' In W. Reuther, H.J. Webber and L.D. Batchelor (eds) *The Citrus Industry* (Revised Edition). Berkeley, CA: University of California Press.

Holland, R.W., Hendriks, M. and Aarts, H. (2005) 'Smells like clean spirit: nonconscious effects of scent on cognition and behaviour.' *Psychological Science 16*, 9, 689–693.

Hollister, L.E. (1986) 'Health aspects of cannabis.' *Pharmacological Reviews 38*, 1, 1–20.

Holmes, P. (1994) *The Energetics of Western Herbs. Volume I.* Boulder, CO: Snow Lotus Press.

Holmes, P. (1996) 'Ginger – warmth and soul strength.' *International Journal of Aromatherapy 7*, 4, 16–19.

Holmes, P. (1997) 'Patchouli – the colours within the darkness.' *International Journal of Aromatherapy 8*, 1, 18–22.

Holmes, P. (1998) 'Jasmine – queen of the night.' *International Journal of Aromatherapy 8*, 4, 8–12.

Holmes, P. (1998/1999) 'Frankincense oil – the rainbow bridge.' *International Journal of Aromatherapy 9*, 4, 156–161.

Holmes, P. (2001) *Clinical Aromatherapy.* Boulder, CO: Tigerlily Press.

Hongratanaworakit, T. (2009) 'Relaxing effects of rose on humans.' *Natural Products Communications 4*, 2, 291.

Hongratanaworakit, T. (2010) 'Stimulating effect of aromatherapy massage with jasmine oil.' *Natural Products Communications 5*, 1, 157.

Hongratanaworakit, T. and Buchbauer, G. (2004) 'Evaluation of the harmonizing effect of ylang ylang on humans after inhalation.' *Planta Medica 70*, 7, 632–636.

Hongratanaworakit, T. and Buchbauer, G. (2006) 'Relaxing effect of ylang ylang on humans after transdermal absorption.' *Phytotherapy Research 20*, 9, 758–763.

Hongratanaworakit, T. and Buchbauer, G. (2007a) 'Chemical composition and stimulating effect of *Citrus hystrix* oil on humans.' *Flavour and Fragrance Journal 22*, 5, 443–449.

Hongratanaworakit, T. and Buchbauer, G. (2007b) 'Autonomic and emotional responses after transdermal absorption of sweet orange oil in humans: placebo controlled trial.' *International Journal of Essential Oil Therapeutics 1*, 29–34.

Hongratanaworakit, T., Heuberger, E. and Buchbauer, G. (2004) 'Evaluation of the effects of East Indian sandalwood oil and α-santalol on humans after transdermal absorption.' *Planta Medica 70*, 1, 3–7.

Hosoi, J. and Tsuchiya, T. (2000) 'Regulation of cutaneous allergic reaction by odorant inhalation.' *Journal of Investigative Dermatology 114*, 541–544.

Hossain, M.M. (2011) 'Therapeutic orchids: traditional uses and recent advances – an overview.' *Fitoterapia 82*, 102–140.

Hosseinzadeh, H., Ziaee, T. and Sadeghi, A (2008) 'The effect of saffron, *Crocus sativus* stigma extract and its constituents, safranal and crocin on sexual behaviours in normal male rats.' *Phytomedicine 15*, 6–7, 491–495.

Howard Hughes Medical Institute (2004) 'Linda B. Buck, PhD.' Available at www.hhmi.org/research/nobel/buck.html, accessed on 18 July 2013.

Howell, T.H. (1987) 'Avicenna and his regimen of old age.' *Age and Ageing 16*, 1, 58–59.

Howes, D. (1998) 'Sensory healing.' *International Journal of Aromatherapy 8*, 4, 18–26.

Hudson R. (1999) 'From molecule to mind: the role of experience in shaping olfactory function.' *Journal of Comparative Physiology A*, 185, 297–304.

Hummel, T. and Nordin, S. (2011) 'SOSI White Paper: Quality of life in olfactory dysfunction.' Sense of Smell Institute. Available at www.yumpu.com/en/document/view/9622830/quality-of-life-in-olfactory-dysfunction-the-sense-of-smell-institute, accessed on 18 July 2013.

Hunt, H. (2005) 'Synesthesia, metaphor and consciousness: a cognitive developmental perspective.' *Journal of Consciousness Studies 12*, 12, 26–45.

Hunt, H.T. (2012) 'A collective unconscious reconsidered: Jung's archetypal imagination in the light of contemporary psychology and social science.' *Journal of Analytical Psychology 57*, 1, 76–98.

Huxley, A. (1954) *The Doors of Perception.* London: Chatto and Windus.

Ibn Sina, A.A. (1993) *Al-Qanun Fi'l-Tibb (The Canon of Medicine), Book I,* trans. J. Hamdard. Delhi: Jamia Hamdard.

Iijima, M., Osawa, M., Nishitani, N. and Iwata, M. (2009) 'Effects of incense on brain function: evaluation using electroencephalograms and event-related potentials.' *Neuropsychobiology 59*, 80–86.

Ilmberger, J., Heuberger, E., Mahrhofer, C., Dessovic, H., Kowarik, D. and Buchbauer, G. (2001) 'The influence of essential oils on human attention. 1: Alertness.' *Chemical Senses 26*, 239–245.

Innocenti, G., Dall'Acqua, S., Scialino, G., Banfi, E. *et al.* (2010) 'Chemical composition and biological properties of *Rhododendron anthopogon* essential oil.' *Molecules 15*, 4, 2326–2338.

International School of Aromatherapy (1993) *A Safety Guide on the Use of Essential Oils.* London: Natural by Nature Oils.

Ispahany, B. (trans.) (1956) *Islamic Medical Wisdom, the Tibb al-A'imma.* Qum, Iran

Jacob, T. (1999) 'Human Pheromones.' Available at www.cf.ac.uk/biosi/staff/jacob/teaching/sensory/pherom.html, accessed on 28 December 2012.

Jay, M. (2010) *High Society: Mind-Altering Drugs in History and Culture.* London: Thames and Hudson.

Jellinek, P. (1949) *Praktikum des Modernen Parfümeurs.* Translated as *The Practice of Modern Perfumery* (1959) (trans. A.J. Kraijkeman). London: Leonard Hill.

Jellinek, P. (1951) *Die Psychologischen Grundlagen der Parfümerie. Untersuchungen über die Wirkung von Gerüchen auf das Gefühlsleben.* Heidelberg: Hüthig.

Jellinek, J.S. (1997a) 'Psychodynamic odor effects and their mechanisms.' *Perfumer and Flavorist 22,* 29–41.

Jellinek, P. (1997b) 'The Psychological Basis of Perfumery.' In J.S. Jellinek (ed.) *The Psychological Basis of Perfumery* (4th Edition). London: Chapman and Hall.

Jennings-White, C., Dolberg, D.S. and Berliner, D.L. (1994) 'The human vomeronasal system.' *Psychoneuroendocrinology 19,* 673–686.

Jiang, H., Xiao, L. Zhao, Y., Ferguson, D. *et al.* (2006) 'A new insight into *Cannabis sativa* (Cannabaceae) utilisation from 2500-year old Yanghai Tombs, Xin jiang, China.' *Journal of Ethnopharmacology 108,* 414–422.

Johnson, M.W., MacLean, K.A., Reissig, C.J., Prisinzano, T.E. and Griffiths, R.R. (2011) 'Human psychopharmacology and dose-effects of salvinorum A, a kappa opioid agonist hallucinogen present in the plant *Salvia divinorum.*' *Drug and Alcohol Dependence 115,* 150–155.

Joichi, A., Yomogida, K., Awano, K. and Uedo, Y. (2005) 'Volatile components of tea-scented modern roses and ancient Chinese roses.' *Flavour and Fragrance Journal 20,* 152–157.

Jouhar, A.J. (ed.) (1991) *Poucher's Perfumes, Cosmetics and Soaps. Volume 1: The Raw Materials of Perfumery* (9th Edition). London: Chapman and Hall.

Joulain, D. and Tabacchi, R. (2009) 'Lichen extracts as raw materials in perfumery. Part 1: Oakmoss.' *Flavour and Fragrance Journal 24,* 49–61.

Jung, C.G. (1970) *The Structure and Dynamics of the Psyche* (Collected Works of C.G. Jung Volume 8). Princeton, NJ: Princeton University Press. (Original works first published 1913–1935.)

Kaiser, R. (2006) *Meaningful Scents around the World.* Zurich: Verlag Helvetica Chimica Acta and Wiley-VCH.

Kaiser, R. (2011) 'Perfumes preserved.' *Nature 470,* 464.

Kanafani, A. (1983) *Aesthetics and Ritual in the United Arab Emirates: The Anthropology of Foods and Personal Adornment among Arabian Women.* Beirut: American University of Beirut.

Kar, K., Puri, V.N., Patnaik, G.K., Sur, R.N. *et al.* (1975) 'Spasmolytic constituents of *Cedrus deodora* (Roxb.) Loud: pharmacological evaluation of himachol. *Journal of Pharmaceutical Science 64,* 2, 258–262.

Katzer, G. (2013) 'Southernwood.' Available at http://gernot-katzers-spice-pages.com/engl/Arte_abr.html, accessed on 18 July 2013.

Kemp, C. (2012) *Floating Gold: A Natural (and Unnatural) History of Ambergris.* Chicago, IL: University of Chicago Press.

Kemp, S.E. and Gilbert, A.N. (1997) 'Odor intensity and color lightness are correlated sensory dimensions.' *American Journal of Psychology 110,* 35–36.

Kennedy, D.O., Dodd, F.L., Robertson, B.C., Okello, E.J. *et al.* (2010) 'Monoterpenoid extract of sage (*Salvia lavandulaefolia*) with cholesterinase-inhibiting properties improves cognitive performance and mood in healthy adults.' *Journal of Psychopharmacology 25,* 1088

Khan, M., Verma, S.C., Srivastava, S.K., Shawl, A.S. *et al.* (2006) 'Essential oil composition of *Taxus wallichiana* Zucc. from the Northern Himalayan region of India.' *Flavour and Fragrance Journal 21,* 772–775.

King, J.R. (1983) 'Have the scents to relax?' *World Medicine 19,* 29–31.

King, J.R. (1988) 'Anxiety Reduction Using Fragrances.' In S. Van Toller and G.H. Dodd (eds) *Perfumery: The Psychology and Biology of Fragrance.* London: Chapman Hall.

Kirk-Smith, M. (1995) *The Physiological and Psychological Effects of Fragrances.* In ISPA Conference Proceedings. Kingston-upon-Hull: ISPA.

Kirk-Smith, M. and Booth, D.A. (1992) 'Effects of natural and synthetic odorants on mood and perception of other people.' Abstracts of Xth Congress of ECRO (European Chemoreception Research Organisation), Munich, 23–28 August, p.72.

Kirk-Smith, M.D., Van Toller, S. and Dodd, G.H. (1983) 'Unconscious odour conditioning in human subjects.' *Biological Psychology 17*, 221–231.

Klimes, I. and Lamparsky, D. (1976) 'Vanilla volatiles – a comprehensive analysis.' *International Flavours Food Additives 7*, 272–291.

Knaapila, A., Tuorila, H., Silventoinen, K., Wright, M.J. *et al.* (2008) 'Environmental effects exceed genetic effects on perceived intensity and pleasantness of several odours: a three-population twin study.' *Behavioural Genetics 38*, 484–492.

Knasko, S.C. (1989) 'Ambient odour and shopping behaviour.' *Chemical Senses 14*, 718.

Knasko, S.C. (1993) 'Performance, mood, and health during exposure to intermittent odors.' *Archives of Environmental Health 48*, 5, 305–309.

Knasko, S. (1997) 'Ambient odour – effects on human behaviour.' *International Journal of Aromatherapy 8*, 3, 28–33.

Knasko, S., Gilbert, A.N. and Sabini, J. (1990) 'Emotional state, physical well-being, and performance in the presence of feigned ambient odour.' *Journal of Applied Social Psychology 20*, 1345–1357.

Komori, T. (2009) 'Effects of lemon and valerian inhalation on autonomic nerve activity in depressed and healthy subjects.' *International Journal of Essential Oil Therapeutics 3*, 1, 3–8.

Köster, E.P., Degel, J. and Piper, D. (2002) 'Proactive and retroactive interference in implicit odor memory.' *Chemical Senses 27*, 191–206.

Kuiate, J. R., Bessière, J.M., Vilarem, G. and Amvam, Z. (2006) 'Chemical composition and antidermatophytic properties of the essential oils from leaves, flowers and fruits of *Cupressus lusitanica* Mill. from Cameroon.' *Flavour and Fragrance Journal 21*, 693–697.

Kurose, K., Okamura, D. and Yatagai, M. (2007) 'Composition of the essential oils from the leaves of nine *Pinus* species and the cones of three *Pinus* species.' *Flavour and Fragrance Journal 22*, 10–20.

Lachenmeier, D. W. (2008) 'Absinthe.' *Medizinische Monatsschrift für Pharmazeuten* 31, 101.

Lachenmeier, D.W. (2010) 'Wormwood (*Artemisia absinthium* L.) – a curious plant with both neurotoxic and neuroprotective properties?' *Journal of Ethnopharmacology 131*, 1, 224–227.

Laska, M., Bauer, V. and Hernandez Salazar, L.T. (2007) 'Self-anointing behaviour in free-ranging spider monkeys (*Ateles geoffroyi*) in Mexico.' *Primates 48*, 160–163.

Laska, M. and Ringh, A. (2010) 'How big is the gap between olfactory detection and recognition of aliphatic aldehydes?' *Attention, Perception and Psychophysics 72*, 3, 806–812.

Laska, M., Weiser, A. and Hernandez Salazar, L.T. (2005) 'Olfactory responsiveness to two odorous steroids in three species of nonhuman primates.' *Chemical Senses 30*, 505–511.

Laska, M., Weiser, A. and Hernandez Salazar, L.T. (2006) 'Sex-specific differences in olfactory sensitivity for putative human pheromones in nonhuman primates.' *Journal of Comparative Psychology 120*, 106–112.

Lawless, A. (2009) *Artisan Perfumery or Being Led by the Nose.* Stroud: Boronia Souk.

Lawless, A. (2010a) 'The Ordinary Mind, Perfume and Natural Health.' Available at www.aleclawless.blogspot.co.uk, accessed on 21 June 2012.

Lawless, A. (2010b) 'Victorian Pharmacy.' Available at www.aleclawless.blogspot.co.uk, accessed on 29 November 2012.

Lawless, A. (2011) 'Absolute Knownsense.' Available at www.aleclawless.blogspot.co.uk, accessed on 25 June 2012.

Lawless, J. (1992) *The Encyclopaedia of Essential Oils.* Dorset: Element Books.

Lawless, J. (1994) *Aromatherapy and the Mind: An Exploration into the Psychological and Emotional Effects of Essential Oils.* London: Thorsons.

Leela, N.K., Vipin, T.M., Shafeekh, K.M., Priyanka, V. and Rema, J. (2009) 'Chemical composition of essential oils from aerial parts of *Cinnamomum malabatrum* (Burman f.) Bercht and Presl.' *Flavour and Fragrance Journal 24*, 13–16.

Leffingwell, J.C. and Associates (1999–2001) 'Olfaction – a Review.' Available at www.leffingwell.com/olfaction.htm, accessed on 28 December 2011.

Le Guérer, A. (1994) *Scent: The Mysterious and Essential Powers of Smell.* London: Chatto and Windus.

Lehrner, J., Marwiski, G., Lehr, S., Johren, P. and Deecke, L. (2005) 'Ambient odours of orange and lavender reduce anxiety and improve mood in a dental office.' *Physiology and Behaviour 86*, 92–95.

Lenochová, P., Vohnoutová, P., Roberts, S.C., Oberzaucher, E., Grammer, K. and Havlíček, J. (2012) 'Psychology of fragrance use: perception of individual odor and perfume blends reveals a mechanism for idiosyncratic effects on fragrance choice.' *PLoS ONE 7*, 3, e33810, 1–10.

Li, S., Chen, L., Xu, Y., Wang, L. and Wang, L. (2012) 'Identification of floral fragrances in tree peony cultivars by gas chromatography-mass spectrometry.' *Scientia Horticulturae 142*, 158–165.

Li, W., Moallem, I., Paller, K.A. and Gottfried, J.A. (2007) 'Subliminal smells can guide social preferences.' *Psychological Science 18*, 12, 1044–1049.

Linck, V.M., da Silva, A.L., Figueiró, M., Caramão, E.B., Moreno, P.R.H. and Elisabetsky, E. (2010) 'Effects of inhaled linalool in anxiety, social interaction and aggressive behaviour in mice.' *Phytomedicine 17*, 679–683.

Lind, E.M. (1998) 'Profile of tuberose.' *Aromatherapy Quarterly 56*, 17–20.

Lindqvist, A. (2012) 'Perfume preferences and how they are related to commercial gender classifications of fragrances.' *Chemical Perception 5*, 197–204.

Lis-Balchin, M. (1995) *The Chemistry and Bioactivity of Essential Oils.* Surrey: Amberwood Publishing.

Liu, J.R., Sun, X.R., Doug, H.W., Sun, C.H. *et al.* (2008) *International Journal of Cancer 122*, 2689.

Livermore, A. and Laing, D.G. (1996) 'Influence of training and experience on the perception of multicomponent odor mixtures.' *Journal of Experimental Psychology, Human Perception and Performance 22*, 267–277.

Lombion-Pouthier, S., Vandel, P., Nezelhof, S., Haffen, E. and Millot, J.-L. (2006) 'Odor perception in patients with mood disorders.' *Journal of Affective Disorders 90*, 187–191.

Loret, V. (1949) 'La resine de terebinth (sonter) chez les anciens egyptiens.' Cairo: Recherches d'archéologie et philologic et d'histoire. Tome XIX.

Łuczaj, Ł. (2011) 'Herbal bouquets blessed on Assumption Day in South-eastern Poland: Freelisting versus photographic inventory.' Available at www.ethnobotanyjournal.org/vol9/i1547-3456-09-001.pdf, accessed on 18 July 2013.

Ludvigson, H.W. and Rottman, R. (1989) 'Effects of ambient odours of lavender and cloves on cognition, memory, affect and mood.' *Chemical Senses 14*, 4, 525–536.

Ludwig, A.M. (1967) 'The trance.' *Comprehensive Psychiatry 8*, 7–15.

McClintock, M.K., Bullivant, S., Jacob, S., Spencer, N., Zelano, B. and Ober, C. (2005) 'Human body scents: Conscious perceptions and biological effects.' *Chemical Senses 30*, (Suppl.1) i135–i137.

McMahon, C. (2011a) 'Monograph: Poplar Bud (*Populus balsamifera*).' Available at www.whitelotusblog.com/2011/07monograph-poplar-bud-populus.html, accessed on 3 December 2011.

McMahon, C. (2011b) 'Monograph: Lotus, Pink (*Nelumbo nucifera*).' Available at www.whitelotusblog.com/2011/07monograph-lotus-pink-nelumbo-nucifera.html, accessed on 3 December 2011.

McMahon, C. (2011c) 'Monograph: Frangipani (*Plumeria alba*).' Available at www.whitelotusblog.com/2011/07monograph-frangipani-plumeria-alba.html, accessed on 3 December 2011.

Malnic, B., Hirono, J., Sato, T. and Buck, L.B. (1999) 'Combinatorial receptor codes for odours.' *Cell 96*, 5, 713–723.

Manetta, C., Sales-Wuillemin, E., Gaillard, A. and Urdapilleta, I. (2011) 'Verbal representation of fragrances: Dependence of specific task.' *Journal of Applied Social Psychology 41*, 3, 658–681.

Manniche, L. (1999) *Sacred Luxuries: Fragrance, Aromatherapy and Cosmetics in Ancient Egypt.* London: Opus Publishing.

Marchais-Roubelat, A. and Roubelat F. (2011) 'The Delphi method as a ritual: inquiring the Delphic Oracle.' *Technological Forecasting and Social Change 78*, 1491–1499.

Marcotullio, M.C., Santi, C., Mwankie, G.N.O.M. and Curini, M. (2009) 'Chemical composition of the essential oil of *Commiphora erythraea*.' *Natural Products Communications 4*, 12, 1751–1754.

Margetts, E.L. (1967) 'Miraa and myrrh in East Africa: clinical notes about *Catha edulis*.' *Economic Botany 21*, 4, 358–362.

Maric, Y. and Jacquot, M. (2012) 'Contribution to understanding odour–colour associations.' *Food Quality and Preference*, 11 May 2012.

Martí, D., Pérez-Gracia, M.T., Blanquer, A., Villagrasa, V., Sanahuja1, M.A. and Moreno, L. (2007) '*Thymus piperella* (L.) essential oil: an alternative in the treatment of diarrhoea.' *Flavour and Fragrance Journal 22*, 201–205.

Martinetz, D., Lohs, K. and Janzen, J. (1989) *Weihrauch und Myrrhe*. Stuttgart: WVG.

Martins, Y., Preti, G., Crabtree, C.R., Runyan, T., Vainius, A.A. and Wysocki, C.J. (2005) 'Preference for human body odours is influenced by gender and sexual orientation.' *Psychological Science 16*, 694–701.

Maruyama, N., Ishibashi, H., Hu, W., Morofuji, S. and Yamaguchi, H. (2006) 'Suppression of carrageenan and collagen induced inflammation in mice by geranium oil.' *Mediators of Inflammation 3*, 1–7.

Masayoshi, M. (ed.) (2010) *Citrus Essential Oils: Flavour and Fragrance*. Hoboken, NJ: John Wiley and Sons.

Masters, R. and Houston, J. (1966) *The Varieties of Psychedelic Experience*. New York, NY: Dell Publishing.

Matsubara, E., Fukagawa, M., Okamoto, T., Ohnuki, K., Shimizu, K. and Kondo, R. (2011) 'The essential oil of *Abies sibirica* (Pinaceae) reduces arousal levels after visual display terminal work.' *Flavour and Fragrance Journal 26*, 204–210.

Maury, M. (1989) *Marguerite Maury's Guide to Aromatherapy – The Secret of Life and Youth: A Modern Alchemy*. Saffron Walden: C.W. Daniel Co. (Original work published in English in 1961.)

Mediavilla, V. and Steinemann, J. (date unknown) 'Essential oil of *Cannabis sativa* L. strains.' Available at www.internationalhempassociation.org.jiha/jiha4208html, accessed on 29 November 2011.

Melnyk, J.P. and Marcone, M.F. (2011) 'Aphrodisiacs from plant and animal sources: a review of current literature.' *Food Research International 44*, 840–850.

Menezes Júnior, A. and Moreira-Almeida, A. (2009) 'Differential diagnosis between spiritual experiences and mental disorders of religious content.' *Revista de Psiquiatra Clínica 36*, 2, 69–76.

Mensing, J. and Beck, C. (1988) 'The Psychology of Fragrance Selection.' In S. Van Toller and G.H. Dodd (eds) *Perfumery: The Psychology and Biology of Fragrance*. London: Chapman Hall.

Meredith, M. (2001) 'Human Vomeronasal Organ function: a critical review of best and worst cases.' *Chemical Senses 26*, 433–445.

Mertens, M., Buettner, A. and Kirchoff, E. (2009) 'The volatile constituents of frankincense – a review.' *Flavour and Fragrance Journal 24*, 279–300.

Michael, A. (2013) 'Cannabis essential oil.' Available at www.hermitageoils.com/cannabis-essential-oil, accessed on 3 February 2013.

Milinski, M. and Wedekind, C. (2001) 'Evidence for MHC-correlated perfume preferences in humans.' *Behavioural Ecology 12*, 2, 140–149.

Miller, A.G. and Morris, M. (1988) *Plants of Dhofar: The Southern Region of Oman. Traditional, Economic and Medicinal Uses*. Muscat, Oman: Office of the Advisor for Conservation of the Environment, Diwan of the Royal Court, Sultanate of Oman.

Miller, G. (2004) 'Axel and Buck 2004 Nobel Prize.' *Science 306*, 5694, 207.

Mills, S. and Bone, K. (2000) *Principles and Practice of Phytotherapy: Modern Herbal Medicine*. Edinburgh: Churchill Livingstone.

Mirahmadi, S.N. and Mirahmadi, H. (2005) *The Healing Power of Sufi Meditation*. Fenton, MI: Naqshbandi Haqqani Sufi Order of America.

Mitchell, D., Khan, B. and Knasko, S.C. (1995) 'There's something in the air: effects of congruent or incongruent ambient odour on consumer decision making.' *Journal of Consumer Research*, September 1995.

Moeran, B. (2007) 'Marketing scents and the anthropology of smell.' *Social Anthropology 15*, 2, 153–168.

Moeran, B. (2009) 'Making scents of smell: manufacturing and consuming incense in Japan.' *Human Organisation 68*, 4, 439–264.

Monti-Bloch, L and Grosser, B.I. (1991) 'Effect of putative pheromones on the electrical activity of the human vomeronasal organ and olfactory epithelium.' *Journal of Steroid Biochemical and Molecular Biology 39* (4B), 573–582.

Morie, J.F. (2008) 'Ontological implications of being in immersive virtual environments.' *Engineering Reality of Virtual Reality*, 2008, 6804.

Morikawa H. *et al.* (1995) *Eucalyptus Absorbs Nitrogen Dioxide*. Hiroshima, Japan: Faculty of Science, Hiroshima University.

Morita, K. (1992) *The Book of Incense: Enjoying the Traditional Art of Japanese Scents*. Tokyo: Kodansha International.

Morita, E., Fukuda, S., Nagano, J., Hamajima, N. *et al.* (2007) 'Psychological effects of forest environments on healthy adults: Shinrin-yoku (forest air bathing, walking) as a possible method of stress reduction.' *Public Health 121*, 54–63.

Morrant, J.C.A. (1993) 'The wing of madness: the illness of Vincent van Gogh.' *Canadian Journal of Psychiatry 38*, 480–484.

Morris, B. (1998) 'The powers of nature.' *Anthropology and Medicine 5*, 1, 81–101.

Morris, E.T. (1984) *Fragrance: The Story of Perfume from Cleopatra to Chanel.* New York, NY: Scribner.

Morris, N., Birtwistle, S. and Toms, M. (1995) 'Anxiety reduction.' *International Journal of Aromatherapy 7*, 2, 33–39.

Moss, M., Cook, J., Wesnes, K. and Duckett, P. (2003) 'Aromas of rosemary and lavender essential oils differentially affect cognition and mood in healthy adults.' *International Journal of Neuroscience 113*, 15–38.

Moss, M., Hewitt, S. and Moss, L. (2008) 'Modulation of cognitive performance and mood by aromas of peppermint and ylang ylang.' *International Journal of Neuroscience 118*, 59–77.

Moss, M., Howarth, R., Wilkinson, L. and Wesnes, K. (2006) 'Expectancy and the aroma of Roman chamomile influence mood and cognition in healthy volunteers.' *International Journal of Aromatherapy 16*, 2, 63–73.

Moussaieff, A., Rimmerman, N., Bregman, T., Straiker, A. *et al.* (2008) 'Incensole acetate, an incense component, elicits psychoactivity by activating TRPV3 channels in the brain.' *Journal of the Federation of American Societies for Experimental Biology 2*, 8, 3024–3034.

Müller, M. and Buchbauer, G. (2011) 'Essential oil components as pheromones: a review.' *Flavour and Fragrance Journal 26*, 357–377.

Naef, R. (2011) 'The volatile and semi-volatile constituents of agarwood, the infected heartwood of *Aquilaria* species: a review.' *Flavour and Fragrance Journal 26*, 73–89.

Natural History Museum (date unknown) 'Citrus: Seeds of Trade.' Available at www.nhm.ac.uk/nature-online/life/plants-fungi/seeds-of-trade, accessed on 20 February 2013.

Needham, J. (1974) *Science and Civilization in China. Vol. 5, Parts 1 and 2.* Cambridge: Cambridge University Press.

Nagai, H., Nakagawa, M., Nakamura, M., Fujii, W., Inui, T. and Asakura, Y. (1991) 'Effects of odours on humans. (II) Reducing effects of mental stress and fatigue.' *Chemical Senses 16*, 198.

O'Brien, D (1969) *Empedocles' Cosmic Cycle: A Reconstruction from the Fragments and Secondary Sources* (Cambridge Classical Studies). Cambridge: Cambridge University Press.

Ohloff, G. (1994) *Scent and Fragrances: The Fascination of Odors and Their Chemical Perspectives.* Berlin and New York, NY: Springer.

Okugawa, H., Ueda, R., Matsumoto, K., Kawanishi, K. and Kato, K. (2000) 'Effects of sesquiterpenoids from "Oriental incenses" on acetic acid-induced writhing and D2 and 5-HT2A receptors in rat brain.' *Phytomedicine 7*, 417–422.

Olsson, S., Barnard, J. and Turri, L (2006) 'Olfaction and identification of unrelated individuals: examination of the mysteries of human odor recognition.' *Journal of Chemical Ecology 32*, 1635–1645.

Omato, A., Yomogida, K., Nakamura, S., Hashimoto, S., Arai, T. and Furukawa K. (1991) 'Volatile components of *Plumeria* flowers. Part I. *Plumeria rubra* forma *acutifolia* (Poir.) Woodson cv. Common Yellow.' *Flavour and Fragrance Journal 6*, 277–279.

Omato, A., Nakamura, S., Hashimoto, S. and Furukawa K. (1992) 'Volatile components of *Plumeria* flowers. Part II. *Plumeria rubra* L.cv Irma Bryan.' *Flavour and Fragrance Journal 7*, 33–35.

Omori, H., Nakahara, K. and Umano, K. (2011) 'Characterisation of aroma compounds in the peel extract of Jabara (*Citrus jabara* Hort. ex Tanaka).' *Flavour and Fragrance Journal 26*, 396–402.

Ostad, S.N. *et al.* (2001) 'The effect of fennel essential oil on uterine contraction as a model for dysmenorrhoea, pharmacology and toxicity.' *Journal of Ethnopharmacology 76*, 299–304.

Paolini, J., Desjobert, J.M., Costa, J., Bernadidni, A.F. *et al.* (2006) 'Composition of essential oils of *Helichrysum italicum* (Roth) G. Don fil subsp. *italicum* from Tuscan archipelago islands.' *Flavour and Fragrance Journal 21*, 805–808.

Patil, J.R., Jaiprakasha, G.K., Murthy, K.N.C., Tichy, S.E., Chetti, M.B. and Patil, B.S. (2009) 'Apoptosis-mediated proliferation inhibition of human colon cancer cells by volatile principles of *Citrus aurantifolia*.' *Food Chemistry 114*, 1351–1358.

Patnaik, G.K. *et al.* (1977) 'Spasmolytic activity of sesquiterpenes from *Cedrus deodora*.' *Indian Drug Manufacturing Association Bulletin (VII)*, 18, 238–242.

Patra, M., Shahi, S.K., Midgley, G. and Dikshit, A. (2002) 'Utilisation of sweet fennel oil as natural antifungal against nail-infective fungi.' *Flavour and Fragrance Journal 17*, 91–94.

Pekala, R.J., Wenger, C.F. and Levine, R.L. (1985) 'Individual differences in phenomenological experience: states of consciousness as a function of absorption.' *Journal of Personality and Social Psychology 48*, 125–132.

Pennacchio, M., Jefferson, L. and Havens, K. (2010) *Uses and Abuses of Plant-Derived Smoke: Its Ethnobotany as Hallucinogen, Perfume, Incense, and Medicine.* New York, NY: Oxford University Press.

Perry, N.S.L., Bollen, C., Perry, E.K. and Ballard, C. (2003) '*Salvia* for dementia therapy: review of pharmacological activity and pilot tolerability clinical trial.' *Pharmacology, Biochemistry and Behaviour 75*, 651–659.

Piesse, C.H. (1891) *Piesse's Art of Perfumery* (5th Edition). London: Piesse and Lubin.

Porcherot, C., Delplanque, S., Raviot-Derrien, S., Le Calvé, B. *et al.* (2010) 'How do you feel when you smell this? Optimization of a verbal measurement of odor-elicited emotions.' *Food Quality and Preference 21*, 938–947.

Porter, R., Balogh, R.D., Cernoch, J. and Franchi, C. (1986) 'Recognition of kin through characteristic body odours.' *Chemical Senses 11*, 389–395.

Potterton, D. (ed.) (1983) *Culpeper's Colour Herbal.* London: W. Foulsham and Company.

de Pradier, E. (2006) 'A trial of a mixture of three essential oils in the treatment of postoperative nausea and vomiting.' *International Journal of Aromatherapy 16*, 1, 15–20.

Prashar, A., Locke, I.C. and Evans, C.S. (2004) 'Cytotoxicity of lavender oil and its major components to human skin cells.' *Skin Proliferation 37*, 221–229.

Prehn-Kristensen, A., Wiesner, C., Bergmann, T.O., Wolff, S. *et al.* (2009) 'Induction of empathy by the smell of anxiety.' *PloS ONE 4*, 6, e5987.

Price, S. and Price, L. (2007) *Aromatherapy for Health Professionals* (3rd Edition). Edinburgh: Churchill Livingstone.

Prisinzano, T.E. (2005) 'Psychopharmacology of the hallucinogenic sage *Salvia divinorum.*' *Life Sciences 78*, 5, 527–531.

Rabin, M.D. and Cain, W.S. (1986) 'Determinants of measured olfactory sensitivity.' *Perception and Psychophysics 39*, 281–286.

Radin, D. (2006) *Entangled Minds: Extrasensory Experiences in a Quantum Reality.* New York, NY: Paraview Pocket Books.

Rapaport, D. (1951) 'Toward a Theory of Thinking.' In D. Rapaport (ed.) *Organization and Pathology of Thought.* New York, NY: Columbia University Press.

Rapaport, D. (1967) 'States of consciousness: A psychopathological and psychodynamic view.' In M.M. Gill (ed.) *The Collected Papers of David Rapaport.* New York, NY: Basic Books.

Reither, C., Doenlen, R., Pacheco-Lopez, G., Neimi, M. *et al.* (2008) 'Behavioural conditioning of immune functions: how the central nervous system controls peripheral immune responses by evoking associative learning processes.' *Reviews in the Neurosciences 19*, 1–17.

Roberts, S.C., Little, A.C., Lyndon, A., Roberts, J. *et al.* (2009) 'Manipulation of body odour alters men's self-confidence and judgements of their visual attractiveness by women.' *International Journal of Cosmetic Science 31*, 47–54.

Robbins, G. and Broughan, C. (2007) 'The effects of manipulating participant expectations of an essential oil on memory through verbal suggestion.' *International Journal of Essential Oil Therapeutics 1*, 2, 56–60.

Roth, B.L., Baner, K., Westkaemper, R., Siebert, D. *et al.* (2002) 'Salvinorin A, a potent naturally occurring non-nitrogenous κ-opioid receptor agonist.' *Proceedings of the National Academy of Sciences 99*, 11934–11939.

Rotton, J. (1983) 'Affective and cognitive consequences of malodourous pollution.' *Basic and Applied Social Psychology 4*, 171–191.

Rotton, J., Barry, T., Frey, J. and Soler, E. (1978) 'Air pollution and interpersonal attraction.' *Journal of Applied Social Psychology 8*, 57–71.

Roudnitska, E. (1991) 'The Art of Perfumery.' In P.M. Müller and D. Lamparsky (eds) *Perfumes: Art, Science and Technology.* London: Elsevier.

Rout, P.K., Naik, S.N. and Rao, Y.R. (2006) 'Composition of the concrete, absolute, headspace and essential oil of the flowers of *Michelia champaca* Linn.' *Flavour and Fragrance Journal 21*, 906–911.

Roux, G. (1976) *Delphes: son oracle et ses dieux.* Paris: Les Belles Lettres.

Sacks, O. (1985) *The Man who Mistook his Wife for a Hat.* London: Picador.

Safarinejad, M.R., Shafiei, N. and Safarinejad, S. (2010) 'An open label, randomised, fixed-dose, crossover study comparing efficacy and safety of sildenafil citrate and saffron (*Crocus sativus* Linn.) for treating erectile dysfunction in men naïve to treatment.' *International Journal of Impotence Research 22*, 4, 240–250.

Saiyudthong, S., Ausavarungnirun, R., Jiwajinda, S. and Turakitwanakan, W. (2009) 'Effects of aromatherapy massage with lime essential oil on stress.' *International Journal of Essential Oil Therapeutics 3*, 2, 76–80.

Salonia, A., Fabbri, F., Zanni, G., Scavini, M. *et al.* (2006) 'Chocolate and women's sexual health: an intriguing correlation.' *The Journal of Sexual Medicine 3*, 3, 476–482.

Saniotis, A. (2010) 'Evolutionary and anthropological approaches towards understanding human need for psychotropic and mood altering substances.' *Journal of Psychoactive Drugs 42*, 4, 477–484.

Santana, A., Ohashi, S., de Rosa, L. and Green, C.L. (1997) 'Brazilian rosewood oil.' *International Journal of Aromatherapy 8*, 3, 16–20.

Santos, D.V., Reiter, E.R., DiNardo, L.J. and Costanzon, R.M. (2004) 'Hazardous effects associated with impaired olfactory function.' *Archive Otolaryngol Head Neck Surgery 130*, 317–319.

Satou, T., Kasuya, H., Takahashi, M., Murakami, S. *et al.* (2011a) 'Relationship between duration of exposure and anxiolytic□like effects of essential oil from *Alpinia zerumbet.*' *Flavour and Fragrance Journal 26*, 180–185.

Satou, T., Matsuura, M., Takahashi, M., Umezu, T. *et al.* (2011b) 'Anxiolytic-like effect of essential oil extracted from *Abies sachalinensis.*' *Flavour and Fragrance Journal 26*, 416–420.

Saucier, C. (2010) 'The sweet sound of sanctity: sensing St Lambert.' *Senses and Society 6*, 1, 10–27.

Sayyah, M., Soroukhani, G., Peirovi, A. and Kamalinejad, A. (2003) 'Analgesic and anti-inflammatory activity of the leaf oil of Lauris nobilis Linn.' *Phytotherapy Research 17*, 7, 733–736.

Schaal, B., Marlier, L. and Soussignan, R. (1998) 'Olfactory function in the human foetus: evidence from selective neonatal responsiveness to the odour of amniotic fluid.' *Behavioural Neuroscience 112*, 1438–1449.

Schier, V. (2010) 'Probing the mystery of the use of saffron in medieval nunneries.' *Senses and Society 5*, 1, 57–72.

Schifferstein, H.N.J. and Tanudjaja, I. (2004) 'Visualising fragrances through colours: the mediating role of emotions.' *Perception 33*, 1249–1266.

Schifferstein, H.N.J., Talke, K.S.S. and Oudshoorn, D.-J. (2011) 'Can ambient scent enhance the nightlife experience?' *Chemosensory Perception 4*, 55–64.

Schiffman, S.S., Sately-Miller, E.A., Suggs, M.S. and Graham, B.G. (1995a) 'The effect of pleasant odours and hormone status on mood of women at midlife.' *Brain Research Bulletin 36*, 1, 19–29.

Schiffman, S.S., Suggs, M.S. and Sately-Miller, E.A. (1995b) 'Effect of pleasant odours on mood of males at midlife: comparison of African-American and European-American men.' *Brain Research Bulletin 36*, 1, 31–37.

Schilling, B., Kaiser, R., Natsch, A. and Gautschi, M. (2010) 'Investigation of odours in the fragrance industry.' *Chemoecology 20*, 135–147.

Schinde, U.A., Kulkarni, K.R., Phadke, A.S., Nair, A.M. *et al.* (1999a) 'Mast cell stabilising and lipoxygenase inhibitory activity of *Cedrus deodora* (Roxb.) Loud. wood oil.' *Indian Journal of Experimental Biology 37*, 3, 258–261.

Schinde, U.A., Phadke, A.S., Nair, A.M., Mungantiwar, A.A., Dikshit, V.J. and Saraf, M.N. (1999b) 'Studies on the anti-inflammatory and analgesic activity of *Cedrus deodora* (Roxb.) Loud. wood oil.' *Journal of Ethnopharmacology 65*, 1, 21–27.

Schleidt, M., Hold, B. and Attili, G. (1981) 'A cross-cultural study on the attitude towards personal odours.' *Journal of Chemical Ecology 7*, 19–31.

Schleidt, M. and Genzel, C. (1990) 'The significance of mother's perfume for infants in the first weeks of their life.' *Ethology and Sociobiology 11*, 145–154

Schmidt, G., Romero, A.L., Sartoretto, J.L., Caparroz-Assef, S.M., Bersani-Amado, C.A. and Cuman, R.K. (2009) 'Immunomodulatory activity of *Zingiber officinale* Roscoe, *Salvia officinalis* L. and *Syzygium aromaticum* L. essential oils: evidence for humor- and cell-mediated responses.' *Journal of Pharmacy and Pharmacology 61*, 7, 961–967.

Schnaubelt, K. (1995) *Advanced Aromatherapy: The Science of Essential Oil Therapy.* Rochester, VT: Healing Arts Press.

Schnaubelt, K. (1999) *Medical Aromatherapy: Healing with Essential Oils.* Berkeley, CA: Frog Books.

Semb, G. (1968) 'The detectability of the odor of butanol.' *Perception and Psychophysics 4*, 335–340.

Seo, H.-S., Arshamian, A., Schemmer, K., Scheer, I. *et al.* (2010) 'Cross-modal integration between odours and abstract symbols.' *Neuroscience Letters 478*, 175–178.

Seo, H.-S. and Hummel, T. (2011) 'Auditory–olfactory integration: congruent or pleasant sounds amplify odor pleasantness.' *Chemical Senses 36*, 301–309.

Seo, H.-S., Guarneros, M., Hudson, R., Distel, H. *et al.* (2011) 'Attitudes toward olfaction: a cross-regional study.' *Chemical Senses 36*, 177–187.

Seol, G.H., Shim, H.S., Kim, P.-J., Li, K.H. *et al.* (2010) 'Antidepressant-like activity of *Salvia sclarea* is explained by modulation of dopamine activities in rats.' *Journal of Ethnopharmacology 130*, 1, 187–190.

Serpico, M. and White, R. (2000) 'The botanical identity and transport of incense during the Egyptian New Kingdom.' *Antiquity 74*, 884–897.

Seth, G., Kokate, C.K. and Varma, K.C. (1976) 'Effect of essential oil of *Cymbopogon citratus* Stapf. on the central nervous system.' *Indian Journal of Experimental Biology 14*, 3, 370–371.

Shamsa, A., Hosseinzadeh, H., Molaei, M., Shakeri, M.T. and Rajabi, O. (2009) 'Evaluation of *Crocus sativa* L. (saffron) on male erectile dysfunction: a pilot study.' *Phytomedicine 16*, 8, 690–693.

Sharer, R.J. (1994) *The Ancient Maya* (5th Edition). Palo Alto, CA: Stanford University Press.

Shawe, K. (1996) 'Essential oils and their biological roles.' *Aromatherapy Quarterly 50*, 3, 23–27.

Shen, J., Niijima, A., Tanida, M., Horri, Y., Maeda, K. and Nagai, K. (2005a) 'Olfactory stimulation with scent of lavender affects autonomic nerves, lipolysis and appetite in rats.' *Neuroscience Letters 383*, 188–193.

Shen, J., Niijima, A., Tanida, M., Horii, Y., Maeda, K. and Nagai, K. (2005b) 'Olfactory stimulation with scent of grapefruit oil affects autonomic nerves, lipolysis and appetite in rats.' *Neuroscience Letters 380*, 289–294.

Siegel, R.K., Collings, P.R. and Diaz, J.L. (1977) 'On the use of *Tagetes lucida* and *Nicotiana rustica* as a Huichol smoking mixture: the Aztec "Yahutli" with suggestive hallucinogenic effects.' *Economic Botany 31*, 1, 16–23.

Silva, I., Rocha, S.M. and Coimbra, M.A. (2010) 'Quantification and potential aroma contribution of β-ionone in marine salt.' *Flavour and Fragrance Journal 25*, 93–97.

Soeda, S. *et al.* (2001) 'Crocin suppresses tumor necrosis factor-α-induced cell death of neuronally differentiated PC-12 cells.' *Life Science 69*, 2887–2898.

Soković, M.D., Brkiç, D.D., Džamiç, A.M. Ristiçd, M.S. and Marinc, P.D. (2009) 'Chemical composition and antifungal activity of *Salvia desoleana* Atzei and Picci essential oil and its major components.' *Flavour and Fragrance Journal 24*, 83–87.

Sorensen, J.M. (2000) '*Melissa officinalis.*' *International Journal of Aromatherapy 10*, 1/2, 7–15.

Soulier, J.-M. (1995) 'The *Thymus* genus.' *Aromatherapy Records 1*, 38–56.

Spence, C. (2008) 'Multisensory Perception.' In H. Blumenthal (2008) *The Fat Duck Cookbook*. London: Bloomsbury.

Spinney, L. (2011) 'You smell flowers, I smell stale urine.' *Scientific American 304*, 2, 5.

Stamelman, R. (2006) *Perfume – Joy, Obsession, Scandal, Sin: A Cultural History of Fragrance from 1750 to the Present*. New York, NY: Rizzoli.

Stansfield, W.D. (2012) 'Science and the senses: perceptions and deceptions.' *The American Biology Teacher 74*, 145–150.

Steele, J.J. (1994) 'Foreword.' In J. Lawless (1994) *Aromatherapy and the Mind: An Exploration into the Psychological and Emotional Effects of Essential Oils*. London: Thorsons.

Stella, L., Vitelli, M.R., Palazzo, E., Olivia, P. *et al.* (2010) '*Datura stramonium* intake: a report of three cases.' *Journal of Psychoactive Drugs 42*, 4, 507–512.

Stewart, S. (2007) *Cosmetics and Perfumes in the Roman World*. Stroud: Tempus Publishing.

Stevenson, R.J. (2010) 'An initial evaluation of the functions of human olfaction.' *Chemical Senses 35*, 3–20.

Stevenson, R.J., Oaten, M., Case, T.I., Repacholi, B.M. and Wagland, P. (2010) 'Children's response to adult disgust elicitors: development and acquisition.' *Developmental Psychology 46*, 1, 165–177.

Stoddart, D.M. (1988) 'Human Odour Culture: A Zoological Perspective.' In S. Van Toller and G.H. Dodd (eds) *Perfumery: The Psychology and Biology of Fragrance*. London: Chapman Hall.

Sullivan, R.J. and Hagen, E.H. (2002) 'Psychotropic substance-seeking: evolutionary pathology and adaptation.' *Addiction 97*, 389–400.

Svoboda, K.P. and Greenaway, R.I. (2003) 'Lemon-scented plants.' *International Journal of Aromatherapy 13*, 1, 23–32.

Svoboda, R.E. (1984) *Prakruti: Your Ayurvedic Constitution.* Albuquerque, NM: Geocom.

Svoboda, R.E. (2003) *Ayurveda: Life, Health and Longevity.* Albuquerque, NM: Ayurvedic Press.

Tajajuddin, A.S., Latif, A. and Qasmi, I.A. (2003) 'Aphrodisiac activity of 50% ethanolic extracts of *Myristica fragrans* Houtt. (nutmeg) and *Syzgium aromaticum* (L) Merr. and Perry (clove) in male mice: a comparative study.' *BMC Complementary and Alternative Medicine 3*, 6.

Tajajuddin, A.S., Latif, A., Qasmi, I.A. and Amin, K.M.Y. (2005) 'An experimental study of the sexual function improving effect of *Myristica fragrans* Houtt. (nutmeg).' *BMC Complementary and Alternative Medicine 5*, 16.

Takakai, I., Bersani-Amado, L.E., Vendruscolo, A., Sartoretto, S.M. *et al.* (2008) 'Anti-inflammatory and antinociceptive effects of *Rosmarinus officinalis* L. essential oil in experimental animal models.' *Journal of Medicinal Food 11*, 4, 741–746.

Tayoub, G., Schwob, I., Bessière, J.M., Rabier, J. *et al.* (2006) 'Essential oil composition of leaf, flower and stem of Styrax (*Styrax officinalis* L.) from south-eastern France.' *Flavour and Fragrance Journal 21*, 809–812.

Teerling, A., Nixdorf, R.R. and Koster, E.P. (1992) 'The effect of ambient odours on shopping behaviour.' Abstracts of Xth Congress of ECRO (European Chemoreception Research Organisation), Munich, 23–28 August.

Tester-Dalderup, C.B.M. (1980) 'Drugs Used in Bronchial Asthma and Cough.' In M.N.G. Dukes (ed.) *Meyler's Side Effects of Drugs* (9th Edition). Amsterdam: Excerpta Medica.

Thompson, C.W. (2011) 'Linking landscape and health: the recurring theme.' *Landscape and Urban Planning 99*, 187–195.

Thompson, R.C. (1908) 'Assyrian prescriptions for diseases of the head.' *American Journal of Semitic Languages 24*, 323–353.

Thompson, R.C. (1924) *The Assyrian Herbal.* London: Lusac.

Tilley, C. (2006) 'The sensory dimensions of gardening.' *Senses and Society 1*, 3, 311–330.

Tisserand, R. (1985) *The Art of Aromatherapy.* Saffron Walden: C.W. Daniel Company. (First published in 1977.)

Tisserand, R. (1988) 'Essential Oils as Therapeutic Agents.' In S. Van Toller and G.H. Dodd (eds) *Perfumery: The Psychology and Biology of Fragrance.* London: Chapman Hall.

Tisserand, R. and Balacs, T. (1995) *Essential Oil Safety: A Guide for Health Care Professionals.* London: Churchill Livingstone.

Tohar, N., Mohd, M.A., Jantan, I. and Awang, K. (2006) 'A comparative study of the essential oils of the genus *Plumeria* Linn. from Malaysia.' *Flavour and Fragrance Journal 21*, 859–863.

Tonutti, I. and Liddle, P. (2010) 'Aromatic plants in alcoholic beverages: a review.' *Flavour and Fragrance Journal 25*, 341–350.

Torii, S. (1997) 'Odour mechanisms: the psychological benefits of odours.' *International Journal of Aromatherapy 8*, 3 34–39.

Torii, S. and Fukada, H. (1985) 'Effects of odours on the contingent negative variation (CNV).' *Proceedings of the 19th Japanese Symposium on Taste and Smell*, 65–68.

Torii, S., Fukada, H., Kanemoto, H., Miyanchi, R., Hamauzu, Y. and Kawasaki, M. (1988) 'Contingent Negative Variation and the Psychological Effects of Odour.' In S. Van Toller and G.H. Dodd (eds) *Perfumery: The Psychology and Biology of Fragrance.* London: Chapman Hall.

Tsachaki, M., Arnaoutopoulou, A.P., Margomenou, L., Roubedakis, S.C. and Zabetakis, L. (2010) 'Development of a suitable lexicon for sensory studies of the anise-flavoured spirits ouzo and tsipouro.' *Flavour and Fragrance Journal 25*, 468–474.

Tsunetsugu, Y., Park, B.-J. and Miyazaki, Y. (2010) 'Trends in research related to "Shinrin-yoku" (taking in the forest atmosphere or forest bathing) in Japan.' *Environmental Health Preventative Medicine 15*, 27–37.

Tubaro, A., Giangaspero, A., Sosa, S., Negri, R. *et al.* (2010) 'Comparative topical anti-inflammatory activity of cannabinoids and cannabivarins.' *Fitoterapia 81*, 816–819.

Turin, L. (1996) 'A spectroscopic mechanism for primary olfactory reception.' *Chemical Senses 21*, 773–791.

Turin, L. (2006) *The Secret of Scent.* London: Faber and Faber.

Turin, L. and Sanchez, T. (2009) *Perfumes: The A–Z Guide.* London: Profile Books.

Turner, R. (1993) 'Absinthe – the green fairy.' *International Journal of Aromatherapy 5*, 2, 24–26.

Turner, V. (1969) *The Ritual Process*. London: Routledge and Kegan Paul.

Tzvi, N. (2011) 'Peddling scents: merchandise and meaning in 2 Corinthians 2:14–17.' *Journal of Biblical Literature 130*, 3, 543–547.

Ubukata, Y., Hanafusa, M., Hayashi, S., Hashimoto, S., Honda, K. and Kujo, M. (2002) 'Essential oil constituents of the Ukon-no-Tachibana (*Citrus tachibana*) in Heian-Jingu shrine.' In *International Symposium on the Chemistry of Essential Oils, Terpenes and Aromatics, Tokushima, Japan 1*, 3, 8–9.

US Department of Health and Human Services (USDHHS) (2007) *Drug Abuse Warning Network, 2005: National Estimates of Drug-Related Emergency Department Visits.* Rockville, MD: USDHHS.

Valder, C., Neugbauer, M., Meier, M. and Kohlenberg, B. (2003) 'Western Australian sandalwood oil – new constituents of Santalum spicatum (R.Br.) A. DC. (Santalaceae).' *Journal of Essential Oil Research*, May/June.

Valentin, D., Dacremont, C. and Cayeux, I. (2011) 'Does short-term odour memory increase with expertise? An experimental study with perfumers, flavourists, trained panellists and novices.' *Flavour and Fragrance Journal 26*, 408–415.

Valnet, J. (1982) *The Practice of Aromatherapy*. Saffron Walden: C.W. Daniel Company. (Originally published in 1980 in French as *Aromathérapie* by Libraire Maloine, Paris.)

Van Toller, S. (1999) 'Assessing the impact of anosmia: review of questionnaires' findings.' *Chemical Senses 24*, 705–712.

Veluthoor, S., Kelsey, R.G., González-Hernández, M.P., Panella, N., Dolan, M. and Karchesy, J. (2011) 'Composition of the heartwood essential oil of incense cedar (*Calocedrus decurrens* Torr.).' *Holzforschung 65*, 333–336.

Videault, S. (2002) '*Kyphi*.' Available at www.mail-archive.com/eristocracy@merrymeet.com/msg00132, accessed on 4 April 2013.

Viroxis (1999) 'Viroxis secures sandalwood supply agreement with TFS Corporation.' Available at www.viroxis.com/oct09.pdf.

Voinchet, V. and Giraud-Robert, A.-M. (2007) 'Utilisation de l'huile essentielle d'hélichryse italienne et de l'huile végétale de rose musquée après intervention de chirurgie plastique réparatrice et esthétique.' *Phytothérapie 2*, 67–72.

Vosnaki, E. (2011) 'Chanel Gardenia vintage vs. modern Les Exclusifs Gardenia: Fragrance review and history.' Available at www.perfumeshrine.blogspot.co.uk, accessed on 6 February 2013.

Waghchaure, C.K., Tetlai, P., Gunale, V.R., Antia, N.H. and Birdi, T.J. (2006) 'Sacred groves of Parinche Valley of Pune District of Maharashtra, India and their importance.' *Anthropology and Medicine 13*, 1, 55–76.

Wajs, A., Bonikowski, R. and Kalemba, D. (2008) 'Composition of essential oil from seeds of *Nigella sativa* L. cultivated in Poland.' *Flavour and Fragrance Journal 23*, 126–132.

Warren, C. and Warrenburg, S. (1993) 'Mood benefits of fragrance.' *International Journal of Aromatherapy 5*, 2, 12–16.

Warrenburg, S. (1995) 'Effects of fragrance on emotions: moods and physiology.' *Chemical Senses 30* (Supplement 1), i248–i249.

Waskul, D.D, Vannini, P. and Wilson, J. (2009) 'The aroma of recollection: olfaction, nostalgia, and the shaping of the sensuous self.' *Senses and Society 4*, 1, 5–22.

Wasson, G.R. (1963) *Soma, the Divine Mushroom of Immortality*. Ethnomycological Studies I. New York, NY: Harcourt, Brace and World.

Watt, M. and Sellar, W. (1996) *Frankincense and Myrrh*. Saffron Walden: C.W. Daniel Company.

Weber, S.T. and Heuberger, E. (2008) 'The impact of natural odours on affective states in humans.' *Chemical Senses 33*, 441–447.

Wedekind, C., Seebeck, T., Bettens, F. and Paepke, A.J. (1995) 'MHC-dependent mate preferences in humans.' *Proceedings of the Royal Society of London, Series B. Biological Sciences 260*, 245–249.

Weisfeld, G., Czilli, T., Phillips, K., Gall, J. and Lichtman, C. (2003) 'Possible olfaction-based mechanisms in human kin recognition and interbreeding avoidance.' *Journal of Experimental Child Psychology 85*, 279–295.

Weiss, E.A. (1997) *Essential Oil Crops*. Wallingford: CAB International.

Wesson, D.W. and Wilson, D.A. (2010) 'Smelling sounds: olfactory–auditory sensory convergence in the olfactory tubercle.' *Journal of Neuroscience 30*, 3013–3021.

Weyerstahl, P., Marschall, H., Weirauch, M., Thefeld, K. and Surburg, H. (1998) 'Constituents of commercial labdanum oil.' *Flavour and Fragrance Journal 13*, 295–318.

Williams, D.G. (1995a) *Historical Development of Perfumery. Part 5 Diploma Perfumery Correspondence Course.* London: Perfumery Education Centre.

Williams, D.G. (1995b) *Odours: Their Description and Classification. Part 1 Diploma Perfumery Correspondence Course.* London: Perfumery Education Centre.

Williams, D.G. (1995c) *Aromatic Materials from Natural Sources. Part 2 Diploma Perfumery Correspondence Course.* London: Perfumery Education Centre.

Williams, D.G. (1995d) *Aromatic Chemicals. Part 3 Diploma Perfumery Correspondence Course.* London: Perfumery Education Centre.

Williams, D.G. (1996) *The Chemistry of Essential Oils.* Dorset: Micelle Press.

Williams, D.G. (2000) *Lecture Notes on Essential Oils.* Peterborough: Eve Taylor.

Wilson, E.O. (1984) *Biophilia.* Cambridge, MA: Harvard University Press.

Witzel, M. (2011) 'Shamanism in northern and southern Eurasia: their distinctive methods of change of consciousness.' *Social Science Information 50*, 1, 39–61.

Wolinski, S. (1991) *Trances People Live: Healing Approaches in Quantum Psychology.* Las Vegas, NV: Bramble Books.

Wrzesniewski, A., McCauley, C. and Rozin, P. (1999) 'Odor and effect: individual differences in the impact of odor on liking for places, things and people.' *Chemical Senses 24*, 713–721.

Wysocki, C.J., Louie, J., Leyden, J.J., Blank, D. *et al.* (2008) 'Cross-adaptation of a model human stress-related odour with fragrance chemicals and ethyl esters of axillary odorants: gender-specific effects.' *Flavour and Fragrance Journal 24*, 209–218.

Zaidia, S.M.A., Pathan, S.A., Singh, S., Jamil, S.S., Ahmad, F.J. and Khar, R.K. (2009) 'Chemical composition, neurotoxicity and anticonvulsant profile of *Lavandula stoechas* L. essential oil.' *The International Journal of Essential Oil Therapeutics 3*, 4, 136–141.

Zarzo, M. and Stanton, D.T. (2009) 'Understanding the underlying dimensions in perfumers' odor perception space as a basis for developing meaningful odor maps.' *Attention, Perception and Psychophysics 71*, 225–247.

Zavazava, N., Westphal, E. and Muller-Ruchholtz, W. (1990) 'Characterisation of soluble HLA molecules in sweat and quantitative HLA differences in serum of healthy individuals.' *Journal of Immunogenetics 17*, 387–394.

Zhang, X.L., Liu, Y.Y., Wei, J.H., Yun Yang, Y. *et al.* (2012) 'Production of high-quality agarwood in *Aquilaria sinensis* trees via whole-tree agarwood-induction technology.' *Chinese Chemical Letters 23*, 727–730.

Further Reading

Publications

Afnan, S.M. (1958) *Avicenna: His Life and Works*. London: G. Allen and Unwin.

As-Suyuti, J.A. (1994) *As-Suyuti's Medicine of the Prophet*. London: Ta-Ha Publishers.

Glicksohn, J. and Berkovich Ohana, A. (2011) 'From trance to transcendence: a neurocognitive approach.' *The Journal of Mind and Behavior 32*, 1, 49–62.

Hewitt, K. (2011) 'The "feeling of knowing," the psychedelic sensorium, and contemporary neuroscience: shifting contexts for noetic insight.' *Senses and Society 6*, 2, 177–202.

Jay, M. (2010) *High Society: Mind-Altering Drugs in History and Culture*. London: Thames and Hudson.

Kabbani, M.H. (2005) *The Sufi Science of Self-Realization*. Fenton, MI: Islamic Supreme Council of America.

Khan, M.S. (1986) *Islamic Medicine*. London: Routledge and Kegan Paul.

Lawless, J. (1994) *Aromatherapy and the Mind: An Exploration into the Psychological and Emotional Effects of Essential Oils*. London: Thorsons.

Lawless, A. (2009) *Artisan Perfumery: Or Being Led by the Nose*. Stroud: Boronia Souk.

Morris, E.T. (1984) *Fragrance: The Story of Perfume from Cleopatra to Chanel*. New York, NY: Scribner.

Nasr, S.H. (1993) *An Introduction to Islamic Cosmological Doctrines*. New York, NY: State University of New York Press.

Stamelman, R. (2006) *Perfume – Joy, Obsession, Scandal, Sin: A Cultural History of Fragrance from 1750 to Present*. New York, NY: Rizzoli.

Aromachemicals

Brechbill, G.O. (2007) *Classifying Aroma Chemicals*. Tenafly, NJ: Fragrance Books. (Available online as a pdf at www.perfumerbook.com/Classifying%20Aroma%20Chemicals.pdf.)

Turin, L. (2006) *The Secret of Scent: Adventures in Perfume and the Science of Smell*. London: Faber and Faber.

Recommended websites
Fragrance

1000 Fragrances – Octavian Sever
www.1000fragrances.blogspot.co.uk

Basenotes
www.basenotes.net

Grain de Musc
http://graindemusc.blogspot.co.uk

Perfume Shrine
www.perfumeshrine.blogspot.co.uk

Fragrance safety

International Fragrance Association
www.ifraorg.org

Research Institute for Fragrance Materials
www.rifm.org

Fragrance Index

Subject Index

Author Index